Critical Care Paramedic

Workbook

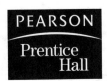

BRADY

Critical Care Paramedic

Workbook

Scott R. Snyder, BS, NREMT-P

BRYAN E. BLEDSOE, DO, FACEP, EMT-P
Adjunct Associate Professor of Emergency Medicine
The George Washington University Medical Center
Washington, DC
and
Emergency Physician
Midlothian, Texas

RANDALL W. BENNER, MEd, MICP, NREMT-P
Director, Emergency Medical Technology Program
Instructor, Department of Health Professions
Youngstown State University
Youngstown, Ohio

PEARSON
Prentice
Hall

Upper Saddle River, New Jersey 07458

Publisher: Julie Levin Alexander
Publisher's Assistant: Regina Bruno
Executive Editor: Marlene McHugh Pratt
Senior Managing Editor for Development:
  Lois Berlowitz
Project Development: TripleSSS Press Media
  Development
Assistant Editor: Matthew Sirinides
Director of Marketing: Karen Allman
Executive Marketing Manager: Katrin Beacom
Marketing Coordinator: Michael Sirinides
Managing Editor for Production: Patrick Walsh
Production Liaison: Faye Gemmellaro
Production Editor: Heather Willison, Carlisle
  Publishing Services
Manufacturing Manager: Ilene Sanford
Manufacturing Buyer: Pat Brown
Senior Design Coordinator: Christopher Weigand
Cover Designer: Michael Ginsberg
Cover Photo: Mark Ide
Composition: Carlisle Publishing Services
Printing and Binding: Bind Rite Graphics
Cover Printer: Phoenix Color

NOTICE ON CARE PROCEDURES

It is the intent of the authors and publisher that this workbook be used as part of a formal EMT-Paramedic program taught by qualified instructors and supervised by a licensed physician. The procedures described in this workbook are based upon consultation with EMT and medical authorities. The authors and publisher have taken care to make certain that these procedures reflect currently accepted clinical practice; however, they cannot be considered absolute recommendations.

The material in this workbook contains the most current information available at the time of publication. However, federal, state, and local guidelines concerning clinical practices, including, without limitation, those governing infection control and universal precautions, change rapidly. The reader should note, therefore, that the new regulations may require changes in some procedures.

It is the responsibility of the reader to familiarize himself or herself with the policies and procedures set by federal, state, and local agencies as well as the institution or agency where the reader is employed. The authors and the publisher of this workbook disclaim any liability, loss, or risk resulting directly or indirectly from the suggested procedures and theory, from any undetected errors, or from the reader's misunderstanding of the text. It is the reader's responsibility to stay informed of any new changes or recommendations made by any federal, state, and local agency as well as by his or her employing institution or agency.

NOTICE ON CPR AND ECC

The national standards for Cardiopulmonary Resuscitation (CPR) and Emergency Cardiovascular Care (ECC) are reviewed and revised on a regular basis and may change slightly after this manual is printed. It is important that you know the most current procedures for CPR and ECC, both for the classroom and your patients. The most current information may be obtained from the appropriate credentialing agency.

Pearson Education Ltd.
Pearson Education Singapore, Pte. Ltd.
Pearson Education Canada, Ltd.
Pearson Education—Japan
Pearson Education Australia Pty., Limited

Pearson Education North Asia Ltd.
Pearson Educación de Mexico, S.A. de C.V.
Pearson Education Malaysia, Pte. Ltd.
Pearson Education, Upper Saddle River, New Jersey

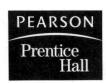

10 9 8 7 6 5 4 3 2 1
ISBN: 0-13-225892-7

CONTENTS

Critical Care Paramedic Workbook

INTRODUCTION
The Self-Instructional Workbook
Critical Care Paramedic

Welcome to the self-instructional workbook for *Critical Care Paramedic*. This workbook is designed to be used either in conjunction with your instructor or as a self-study guide you use on your own.

This workbook features many different ways to help you learn the material necessary to become a critical care paramedic and includes the following:

Features

Review of Chapter Objectives
Each chapter of *Critical Care Paramedic Workbook* begins with objectives that identify the important information and principles addressed in the chapter reading. To help you identify and learn this material, each workbook chapter reviews the important content elements addressed by these objectives as presented in the text.

Case Study Review
Each chapter of *Critical Care Paramedic Workbook* includes a case study that introduces and highlights important principles presented in the chapter. The workbook reviews these case studies and points out much of the essential information and many of the applied principles they describe.

Content Review
Each chapter of *Critical Care Paramedic Workbook* presents an extensive narrative explanation of the principles of critical care paramedic practice. The workbook chapter (or chapter section) contains multiple choice questions to test your reading comprehension of the textbook material and to give you experience for taking typical emergency medical service examinations.

Emergency Drug Cards
At the end of the workbook are emergency drug cards, which are designed to help you practice your knowledge of individual drugs. The cards contain the name, class, actions, indications, contraindications, side effects, dosage, and special considerations for each drug.

Acknowledgments

Reviewers
The following reviewers provided many excellent suggestions for improving this workbook. Their assistance is greatly appreciated.

Vicki Bacidore, RN, MS
Loyola Emergency Medical Services
Loyola University Medical Center
Maywood, Illinois

Steve Maffin, EMT-P
Training Coordinator
Lancaster Fire Department
Lancaster, Ohio

Scott F. McConnell, CCEMT-P, NREMT-P, MICP, FPC
AHA Training Center Coordinator
Capital Health System
Emergency Services Training Center
Trenton, New Jersey

HOW TO USE
The Self-Instructional Workbook
Critical Care Paramedic

The self-instructional workbook accompanying *Critical Care Paramedic* may be used as directed by your instructor or independently by you during your course of instruction. The following recommendations listed below are intended to guide you in using the workbook independently.

- Examine your course schedule and identify the appropriate text chapter or other assigned reading.

- Read the assigned chapter in *Critical Care Paramedic* carefully. Do this in a relaxed environment, free from distractions, and give yourself adequate time to read and digest the material. The information presented in *Critical Care Paramedic* is often technically complex and demanding, but it is very important that you fully comprehend it. Be sure that you read the chapter carefully enough to understand and remember what you have read.

- Carefully read the Review of Chapter Objectives at the beginning of each workbook chapter (or section). This material includes both the objectives listed in *Critical Care Paramedic* and narrative descriptions of their content. If you do not understand or remember what is discussed from your reading, refer to the referenced pages and reread them carefully. If you still do not feel comfortable with your understanding of any objective, consider asking your instructor about it.

- Reread the case study in *Critical Care Paramedic*, and then read the Case Study Review in the workbook. Note the important points regarding assessment and care that the Case Study Review highlights, and be sure that you understand and agree with the analysis of the call. If you have any questions or concerns, ask your instructor for clarification.

- Do the Content Review questions at the end of each workbook chapter (or section), answering each question carefully. Do this in a quiet environment, free from distractions, and allow yourself adequate time to complete the exercise. Correct your self-evaluation by reviewing the answers at the back of the workbook, and determine the percentage you have answered correctly (the number you got right divided by the total number of questions). If you have answered most of the questions correctly (85 to 90 percent), review those that you missed by rereading the material on the pages listed in the Answer Key and be sure you understand which answer is correct and why. If you have more than a few questions wrong (less than 85 percent correct), look for incorrect answers that are grouped together. This suggests that you did not understand a particular topic in the reading. Reread the text dealing with that topic carefully, and then retest yourself on the questions you answered incorrectly. If your incorrect answers are spread throughout the chapter content, reread the chapter and retake the Content Review to ensure that you understand the material. If you don't understand why your answer to any question is incorrect after reviewing the text, consult your instructor.

During your completion of the workbook exercises, if you have any questions that either the textbook or workbook doesn't answer, write them down and ask your instructor about them. Paramedic critical care is a complex and complicated subject, and answers are not always black-and-white. It is also common for different EMS systems to use differing methods of care. The questions you bring up in class, and your instructor's answers to them, will help you expand and complete your knowledge of paramedic critical care.

Introduction to Critical Care Transport

Review of Chapter Objectives

Upon completion of this chapter, the student should be able to:

1. **Define and give examples of behavior that characterizes the health care professional.**   **p. 3**

   A health care professional is a member of the health care continuum who is not only an expert in her chosen field, but engages in behavior that reflects her dedication, respect, and loyalty to both the profession and the patients she cares for. There are many behaviors and attitudes that characterize the health care professional, and they do not come easy. Learning to adopt these attitudes and making these behaviors a habit takes hard work, effort, and perhaps, most of all, persistence. Calvin Coolidge said, "Nothing in this world can take the place of persistence. Talent will not; nothing is more common than unsuccessful people with talent. Genius will not; unrewarded genius is almost a proverb. Education will not; the world is full of educated derelicts. Persistence and determination alone are omnipotent." President Coolidge realized that natural talent, brains, and letters after your name do not necessarily make you successful or, for that matter, a professional. There is something more that is required, something that separates the professional health care provider from the unprofessional. He called that something persistence and determination; today, we tend to refer to that something as effort and attitude.

   We all recognize a professional attitude when we see it. Professionals set high goals for themselves, their crew, their organization, and their profession, and then strive to achieve those goals. They earn the respect and confidence of their colleagues by the things they do everyday, whether they are being watched or not. Professionals place the patient first, not their egos. Professionals take continuing and refresher training seriously, and practice their skills to the point of mastery and beyond. They check their equipment, recognize the importance of response times, and are willing to critically review their performance and recognize mistakes. After recognizing a mistake, a professional acknowledges it, learns from it, and tries to never repeat it. Effort is required along with this attitude because the health care professional is presented every day with the opportunity to relax that attitude. Maybe you're having a bad week and don't feel like being nice, maybe you would rather go play softball with your friends rather than attend a training session, or maybe you are working with an unprofessional, senior partner who is intimidating you to engage in unprofessional behavior. The opportunities to adopt, and the number of excuses for, an unprofessional attitude are myriad, every day. This is why it takes effort to make these professional behaviors a habit.

   Maintaining professionalism requires effort and attitude. But the result of that effort and attitude—the admiration and respect of one's peers—is the highest compliment a person can receive. True professionals establish excellence as their goal and never allow themselves to become satisfied with their performance. Professionalism is an attitude, not a matter of pay. It cannot be bought, rented, bestowed, or faked. Although a young industry, EMS has achieved recognition as a bona fide allied health care profession. Gaining professional stature is the result of many hard-working, caring individuals who have refused to compromise their standards, and it is up to you, as a critical care paramedic candidate, to carry the torch that was lit by those before you.

2. Provide a brief overview of the history of critical care transport.   p. 4

The specialization of hospitals in the 1980s resulted in the need to transport patients from unspecialized to specialized facilities. Some patients who required transport were in an ICU setting, receiving complicated care that made transfer by the standard ambulance crew impossible. As such, a nurse from either the receiving or transporting hospital would accompany the patient during transport. This model presented a number of difficulties, including increased out-of-service time for the ambulance, and the problems associated with the nurse operating in an unfamiliar out-of-hospital environment. These difficulties notwithstanding, it was the nursing shortage of the late 1980s and early 1990s that strained this transport model the greatest. As a result of the shortage, fewer nurses were available to accompany patients on interfacility transports.

Both air and surface transport agencies were then forced to staff their transport units with nurses to ensure that the continuation of the same level of care was provided during the interfacility transport. The role of the critical care paramedic (CCP) became more defined during this period, especially in aeromedicine. As aeromedical transport matured, service providers began staffing ground transport units with crew configurations that included CCPs. As demand for ground critical care transport (CCT) increased, it became obvious that there was a need for paramedics who had critical care training to handle the vast majority of these ground transports. CCP training programs were developed by several ground and aeromedical operations to meet local demand. As the demand for CCPs grew, there was a push to develop and standardize the CCP educational curriculum. Educators in Maryland, Iowa, and Texas were the vanguard of the initial CCP curriculum development. These programs operated independently, and no single accrediting body oversaw the process. This independent trend continues today, with numerous, if not countless, CCP education programs offered throughout the United States, all without standardization.

Presently, CCT transport units are seemingly ubiquitous, and CCT is a frequently utilized, cost-effective method of transporting critically ill or injured patients between medical facilities.

3. Define the role of the critical care paramedic.   p. 8

The role of the critical care paramedic varies significantly between agencies. They may be assigned to dedicated ground critical care transport units, standard EMS units that are summoned when needed for CCT, or dedicated air (fixed wing and/or rotor) critical care transport units. Some hospitals operate CCT services as part of their emergency department (ED) or intensive care unit (ICU), with the CCP working in the ED or ICU, when not on a CCT.

The composition of the critical care (CC) team is driven by the specific needs of the patient and system. Dual RN, dual CCP, and RN/CCP are common crew configurations in the United States. In order to meet an increasing demand for service, some critical care paramedics have elected to specialize in specific areas of critical care transport such as neonatal or pediatric transport. Such units, by necessity, are typically found in the larger cities and are usually operated by a children's hospital.

No standardized or universally accepted method of certification exists for the CCP, though the Board for Critical Care Transport Paramedic Certification (BCCTPC), an affiliate of the International Association of Flight Paramedics (IAFP), offers a Certified Flight Paramedic (FP-C) certification.

Like the paramedic, the CCP must function under the authority of a licensed physician. Care is guided by medical protocols and standing orders that provide guidelines and direction for care of individual patients. CCP protocols are customized for the specific patient population being cared for, and the skill set practiced by the CCP is usually more advanced than that of a normal paramedic. A much more expansive formulary places additional responsibility on the CCP, who must be intimately familiar with all the medications available for his use.

4. **List the duties of the critical care paramedic in preparation for handling critical care transport patients.** p. 8

Duties of the critical care paramedic performed in preparation for handling CCT patients include:
a. Skills maintenance
b. Pre-shift equipment check

5. **List the duties of the critical care paramedic during a critical care transport.** p. 9

Duties of the CCP during transport may include:
a. Positive interaction with the transporting facility
b. Full and complete patient assessment
c. Establishing contact with medical control and delivering patient report
d. Rendering of patient care in accordance with medical control or standing orders
e. Performance of patient care skills which may include:
  1. Rapid sequence induction/intubation (RSI)
  2. Central venous line placement
  3. Arterial line placement
  4. Pericardiocentesis
  5. Intraosseous needle placement
  6. Arterial blood gas interpretation
  7. Interpretation of common laboratory studies
  8. Continuous waveform capnography
  9. Management of complicated pharmacologic infusions
  10. Mechanical ventilation including PEEP (positive end-expiratory pressure)
  11. Thoracic needle and tube decompression
  12. Escharotomy
  13. Intra-aortic balloon pump management
  14. Management of invasive hemodynamic monitors
  15. Surgical cricothyrotomy
f. Packaging of patient for transport
g. Continuing of care during transport
h. Effective patient transfer at receiving facility
i. Delivery of patient report and paperwork to receiving care team

6. **List the duties of the critical care paramedic after a critical care transport.** p. 11

Duties of the CCP after completion of a critical care transport may include:
a. Timely return of transport unit to service
b. Critical evaluation of care rendered

7. **Define and give examples of professional ethics.** p. 12

Ethics are the standards of conduct, often self-imposed, that govern a group of professionals. An example of the application of professional ethics within the CCT profession is the providing of emotional care and support to patients and their family members. While the holding of a hand or the offering of some words of comfort is not required by law, we recognize that both are important aspects of patient care, and frequently employ them in practice.

8. **List the post-graduation responsibilities of the critical care paramedic.** p. 12

a. Stay abreast of current developments
b. Maintain continuing education

9. **State the benefits and responsibilities of continuing education for the critical care paramedic.** p. 13

As a critical care paramedic, you are responsible for keeping pace of changes in the dynamic field of critical care medicine. Benefits of continuing education include skills maintenance, clinical adeptness, and patient care that are up-to-date with current trends and standards. Journals, trade shows, hospital workshops/courses, grand rounds, CD or web-based programs, textbooks, and skills workshops are some of the methods that can be employed to meet continuing education requirements.

10. List some national organizations for critical care paramedics. p. 13

    a. National Association of Critical Care Paramedics (NACCP)
    b. International Flight Paramedics Association (IFPA)
    c. National Association of EMS Physicians (NAEMSP)
    d. National Association of Emergency Medical Technicians (NAEMT)

11. Describe the major benefits of subscribing to professional journals. p. 13

Your CCP education is not finished with the completion of a CCP course; rather, it has only just begun. Critical Care Medicine (CCM) and CCT are highly technical and ever-evolving fields, and it is essential that the CCP stay abreast of developments in CCM and CCT to provide the best patient care possible. This can be accomplished through the following:

    a. Self-study
    b. Textbooks, periodicals, trade journals
    c. Continuing medical education (CME)
    d. Refresher courses
    e. Online and computer-based education
    f. Attending professional conferences, trade shows
    g. Attending "Grand Rounds" at local medical school
    h. Rotations through ED, ICU, OR

Case Study

The pager vibrates against your side alerting you to the call, but fortunately does not disturb anyone else in the lecture hall. Since you sat in the back, near the door, anticipating just such a contingency, you're able to leave without any significant commotion. A quick phone call to the dispatcher informs you that you are needed for a transfer from a small rural hospital about 70 miles from the tertiary hospital at which your program is based. The request is for the transport of a male patient who has suffered an acute myocardial infarction. Although the transferring hospital is served by a paramedic level service, it has become the rule for the area hospitals to request your service for any transfer that involves a critically ill patient. It seems that with the increase in specialization of some hospitals and the decrease in services at others, the demand for interfacility transfers increases year after year. It has also become evident that the complexity of the medical problems of the patients being transferred has increased dramatically. In fact, you now regularly perform skills and care for patients that you would not have imagined when you first became a paramedic.

While waiting for the elevator, you are struck by the irony that the lecture you just left at the medical college was on advances in the primary surgical management of acute myocardial infarctions. You wonder if it is going to be "one of those days." While riding the elevator to the roof-based helipad, you reflect on how fortunate you are to have the medical college available to your program for continuing medical education. At a recent national EMS conference, a colleague who works at a program from a rural area was discussing the difficulty in obtaining quality CME and keeping current on medical advancements. She subscribes to all available professional journals and attends as many conferences as possible, expending a great deal of effort and expense to remain up to date. As a dedicated professional you know that you would also do whatever it took to stay current, but are glad for the incredible CME opportunities that are present in your workplace.

Arriving on the roof of the parking garage, you move the gear-laden stretcher from the storage room to the back of the helicopter where the flight nurse assists you in its loading. At the beginning of your shift, you had performed a meticulous inventory check to ensure the availability of all necessary equipment and supplies. That effort now pays off as the helicopter is airborne within 10 minutes of the request.

En route to the sending facility, you discuss the case with Paul, the flight nurse on your shift. At this particular service, all transfers are performed with a paramedic and a nurse, unlike the last critical care transport service you worked for where the team makeup varied significantly depending on the patient's needs. Your role and responsibilities varied greatly with each individual team makeup. For this transfer, you and Paul agree that he will assume the lead role as care provider and you will assist him with the technical aspects of care. Often, based on the patient's needs, this role is reversed and Paul assists you in the lead role.

The transfer was performed without incident. After the equipment is restocked, you head for the Emergency Department to see what interesting cases have come in while you were gone. As you are nearing the triage desk, the pager begins to vibrate again, making you do an about-face and head for the elevator. It is apparently going to be "one of those days."

DISCUSSION QUESTIONS

1. What developments have contributed to the increased use of critical care transport services?
2. What types of behaviors exemplify the health care professional?
3. Give some examples of the role of the critical care paramedic before, during, and after a critical care transport.

Content Review

MULTIPLE CHOICE

_____ 1. Which of the following is not a behavior that characterizes the health care professional?
  A. Providing emotional support to a patient
  B. Making an effort to attend a Critical Care Transport conference
  C. Refusing to accept a transport because you have had issues with the receiving physician in the past
  D. Refusing to allow a family member to accompany the patient during transport because you believe there would be a safety risk in doing so

_____ 2. Which of the following events led to the development of the Geneva treaty, which established rules related to the care of injured soldiers on the field of battle?
  A. The Geneva Convention of 1864
  B. The Civil War in 1865
  C. The Napoleonic Wars in the 1790s
  D. The formation of the American Red Cross in 1865

_____ 3. The well-known nurse who founded the American Red Cross and traveled the battlefield with army ambulances during the Civil War was:
  A. Rosa Parks.   C. Dorothea Dix.
  B. Wendy Stock.   D. Clara Barton.

_____ 4. Motorized ambulances were first used in 1899 by:
  A. Michael Reese Hospital in Chicago.
  B. Saint Vincent's Hospital in New York.
  C. Bellevue Hospital in New York.
  D. Commercial Hospital in Cincinnati.

_____ 5. _____ introduced advanced life support to the prehospital setting in Belfast, Northern Ireland, in the late 1950s.
  A. Dr. Eugene Nagel
  B. Dr. J. F. Pantridge
  C. Dr. Michael Reese
  D. Dr. R. Adams Crowley

_____ 6. The development of which document was meant to be a guide map for EMS into the 21st century?
   A. The White Paper
   B. Accidental Death and Disability: The Neglected Disease of Modern Society
   C. Consolidated Omnibus Budget Reconciliation Act
   D. EMS Agenda for the Future

_____ 7. Helicopters were first used for transport during:
   A. the Prussian siege of Paris.
   B. World War II.
   C. the Korean War.
   D. the Vietnam War.

_____ 8. In 1969, the first aircraft used for ambulance work began flying for:
   A. the Maryland State Police.
   B. Saint Anthony's Hospital in Denver, CO.
   C. REACH Air Ambulance in Santa Rosa, CA.
   D. Samaritan Air Evac in Phoenix, AZ.

_____ 9. In 1972, _____ began the first helicopter service dedicated exclusively to patient care.
   A. the Maryland State Police
   B. Saint Anthony's Hospital in Denver, CO
   C. REACH Air Ambulance in Santa Rosa, CA
   D. Samaritan Air Evac in Phoenix, AZ

_____ 10. Dr. W. E. Dandy is credited with establishing the first Intensive Care Unit (ICU) in the United States, a _____ at the _____.
   A. Neurosurgical ICU, Sarah Morris Hospital in Chicago, IL
   B. Premature Infant ICU, Sarah Morris Hospital in Chicago, IL
   C. Neurosurgical ICU, Crowley Shock Trauma Center in Baltimore, MD
   D. Neurosurgical ICU, the Johns Hopkins Hospital in Baltimore, MD

_____ 11. Mechanical ventilation became widely available in the United States and Europe in the 1950s due in large part to the:
   A. polio epidemic of 1947–1948.
   B. influenza epidemic of 1945–1946.
   C. Second World War in the early 1940s.
   D. Korean War in the 1950s.

_____ 12. By 1958, approximately what percentage of community hospitals in the United States with more than 300 beds had an ICU?
   A. 15 percent
   B. 20 percent
   C. 25 percent
   D. 30 percent

_____ 13. Which of the following is not a goal of the American Association of Critical-Care Nurses (AACN) CCRN Certification Program?
   A. To train the critical care nurse to work in the prehospital environment
   B. To establish the body of knowledge necessary for CCRN certification
   C. To test, through written examination, the common body of knowledge needed to function effectively within the critical care setting
   D. To assist and promote continued professional development of critical care nurses

_____ 14. Composition of the critical care team is best determined by the:
   A. cost and availability of staffing.
   B. opinion of the program Medical Director.
   C. geographical location of transporting and receiving facilities.
   D. specific needs of the patient and the system.

©2007 Pearson Education, Inc.
Critical Care Paramedic

_____ 15. _____ describes the conduct or qualities that characterize a practitioner in a particular field or occupation.
   A. Ethics
   B. Morals
   C. Professionalism
   D. Attitude

_____ 16. _____ are the standards that govern the conduct of members of a particular group.
   A. Ethics
   B. Morals
   C. Professionalism
   D. Attitude

_____ 17. Which of the following is a true statement regarding professional attitude?
   A. Professionals set high standards for themselves, their crew, their agency, and their system.
   B. Professionals require little continuing training because they already possess a solid knowledge base.
   C. Professionals do not need skill refreshing, as they have proven their mastery of their required skill set.
   D. Professionals demand, and receive, higher compensation for their work.

_____ 18. One of the best ways to ensure that you will never perform an unethical act as a critical care paramedic is to:
   A. always do for the patient what you would want done for yourself.
   B. always place the patient's welfare above everything but your own safety.
   C. consult with a police officer or lawyer, if possible, whenever an ethical dilemma presents itself.
   D. honor the wishes of family members if the patient is unable to make decisions for himself.

2 Critical Care Ground Transport

Review of Chapter Objectives

Upon completion of this chapter, the student should be able to:

1. **Discuss the history of critical care ground transport.**   p. 18

   Critical care ground transport has its roots in the Korean and Vietnam Wars, where the advantages of rapid air transport of wounded soldiers to definitive medical care was first introduced. The first helicopter program dedicated exclusively to patient care was started in 1972 at Saint Anthony's Hospital in Denver, Colorado, and additional programs soon followed, based primarily out of major hospitals in urban areas. The initial purpose of these programs was to respond to on-scene emergencies and rural hospitals, transporting patients to the helicopter programs home facility.

   Aeromedical critical care programs also evolved, with many services opting to staff ground units separate from the air component of the program. Advantages to having a separate ground component include the ability to transport patients in bad weather, the lower cost of operating a ground transport unit, faster transport times in some situations, and a less inherent risk in ground transport. Air medical services that do not have a ground component will frequently contract with an established EMS ground service to provide an ambulance, driver, and assistant to the aeromedical crew, who utilize their own equipment.

2. **Contrast the benefits and limitations of various ambulance types including ground ambulances, rotor-wing aircraft, and fixed-wing aircraft.**   p. 19

   Advantages of ground transport compared to air transport include faster departure times, a larger patient compartment, lower transport costs, a relative immunity to changing weather conditions, and increased safety. Ground transport can often be faster than air when factors such as short travel distances, aircraft warm-up and shutdown times, and the time required for nonflight activities are considered. Other advantages of ground transport include the absence of severe environmental stressors inherent in air transport, such as decreased oxygen levels, acceleration/deceleration forces, gas volume changes with altitude, cabin pressurization, humidity, noise, and vibration.

   Advantages of air transport compared to ground transport include faster travel times and shorter prehospital times over large distances.

3. **Discuss the role of funding as it pertains to critical care transport.**   p. 19

   Fees collected for service from patients and third-party payers provide much of the revenue for the majority of transport program operations. Systems may also receive financial support through government-based tax revenue, while funds generated from hospitalization after transport can also contribute to transport program reimbursement. Medicare reimbursements are an important part of the transport program revenue stream, and new fee schedules that recognize the role of the critical care ambulance may allow for greater reimbursement than for regular ALS level ambulances. Specifically, the new fee schedules recognize the higher educational level of the critical care transport team, and the subsequent higher level of care it can provide.

4. **Discuss the advantages and disadvantages of various critical care crew configurations. p. 20**

Influences on the staffing configurations of CCT ambulances can vary widely between agencies or geographical areas, and can be influenced by legislative initiative, the local medical community, and a patient's individual needs.

Members of the CCT can include, but are not limited to, EMTs, paramedics, critical care paramedics, registered nurses, nurse practitioners, respiratory therapists, physician assistants, and physician residents. Regardless of the staffing configurations on a critical care transport unit, the local medical community must be comfortable with, and trust, the education, critical thinking skills, and care provided by the transport team.

EMTs are often assigned to critical care ground transport teams in the role of vehicle operator, or to assist with basic patient care. Paramedics, already accustomed to a relatively autonomous clinical environment, can typically be expected to perform well in the critical care environment after completion of critical care transport training. The critical care paramedic skill set includes, but is not limited to, advanced airway management techniques, chest tube monitoring, thoracic escharotomy, surgical cricothyroidotomy, transvenous pacing, central venous catheter maintenance/interpretation, use of intra-aortic balloon pumps, blood and blood by-product administration and monitoring, electrolyte interpretation, arterial blood gas measurement, basic radiography interpretation, ventilator management, 12-lead ECG interpretation, pulse oximetry and capnogram interpretation, use of intracranial pressure monitoring lines, venous cutdown, use of infusion pumps, and advanced pharmacologic interventions.

5. **Detail the equipment typically used in modern critical care transport.**   **p. 21**

Generally speaking, the critical care ground transport ambulance will have all of the equipment found in a paramedic-level ambulance, such as intubation equipment, medications, and ECG monitors. Specialized equipment may include medication pumps, automatic ventilators, automatic blood pressure monitors, central venous and arterial catheter hemodynamic monitors, and intra-aortic balloon pumps.

Case Study

You are called to transport a patient from a Critical Access hospital that has eight inpatient beds and no ICU. As Sharon, your EMT driver, slides the transmission selector to neutral and pulls the air brake on, you slide down out of the passenger seat and walk to the side door of the big Type I ambulance. Your partner Bill, who is also a critical care paramedic, has already loaded the necessary equipment on the stretcher. Your patient is a 65-year-old woman in diabetic ketoacidosis who is intubated and on an insulin drip. She needs to be transported for ICU admission to the regional medical center, about 50 miles away. Although the medical center has an air medical program, experience has taught the sending hospital that due to logistical issues (neither the sending nor receiving hospitals have on-site helipads), the actual prehospital time difference is negligible, and, therefore, they rarely use the helicopter service.

You mentally double check the gear Bill has selected for this transport. The transport ventilator, 3 channel IV pump, critical care monitor, equipment stand, and oxygen/assessment bag are securely strapped to the cot. As your team moves the stretcher toward the three-bed emergency department, you reflect on how much your service has changed over the past 10 years. Initially, your agency primarily provided 911-type service. If called to transfer a critical care patient, they would send two EMTs in a regular Type II ambulance to take the patient, the nurse, and the hospital equipment to the receiving facility. Now, primarily as a result of increased government funding, your service has highly trained critical care paramedics with specialized equipment and vehicles to perform these transports. When necessary, your agency even has the ability to call in critical care nurses and/or a respiratory therapist to assist you.

The transport goes very well, and after turning your care over to the patient's nurse, you complete the paperwork and return to the ambulance bay. Sharon and Bill already have the rig back in service when you get there. The possibility of a long mid-morning break comes to mind. As Sharon calls your unit back in service, you realize that a break is not in your immediate future as she begins to write down the details of the next transfer request.

DISCUSSION QUESTIONS

1. What are some of the advantages and disadvantages of ground ambulances for critical care transports?
2. What are some of the advantages and disadvantages of various critical care crew configurations?
3. What types of equipment are considered standard on a critical care unit?

Content Review

MULTIPLE CHOICE

_____ 1. Which organization developed the first helicopter program dedicated exclusively to patient care in 1972?
   A. Saint Anthony's Hospital in Denver, CO
   B. Bellevue Hospital in New York City, NY
   C. Saint Vincent's Hospital in New York City, NY
   D. Maryland State Police in Baltimore, MD

_____ 2. Advantages of critical care ground transport over air transport include all of the following except:
   A. the ability to transport patients in bad weather.
   B. shorter transport times over long distances.
   C. absence of severe environmental stressors in ground transport.
   D. less inherent risk in ground transport.

_____ 3. Which of the following practitioners is the least likely to be a member of a critical care transport team?
   A. physician assistant   C. attending physician
   B. resident physician   D. basic EMT

_____ 4. Which of the following skills can be expected to be part of the skill set of the critical care paramedic?
   A. intra-aortic balloon pump insertion
   B. arterial cannulation
   C. cesarean section
   D. intracranial pressure monitoring

_____ 5. EMTs are often assigned to critical care transport ground teams, and their duties typically include:
   A. vehicle operation and assistance with basic patient care.
   B. patient care decision making.
   C. the provision of advanced life support.
   D. completion of the patient care report.

6. Which of the following is not a piece of specialized equipment typically found on a critical care transport ambulance?
   A. medication pump
   B. automatic ventilator
   C. portable radiograph
   D. automatic blood pressure monitor

7. Factors that can contribute to faster travel times by ground ambulance over air ambulance include all of the following except:
   A. aircraft start-up and shutdown times.
   B. short travel distances.
   C. nonflight activities.
   D. lower operation costs.

8. Which of the following statements regarding funding for critical care transport services is true?
   A. Critical care transport services are disqualified from receiving funding from government-based tax revenue.
   B. Funds generated from hospitalization after transport can contribute to transport program reimbursement.
   C. Medicare allows for a higher level of reimbursement for transports that meet specialty care transport guidelines.
   D. Fees collected for service from patients and third-party payers provide little of the revenue for the majority of transport program operations.

9. Which of the following statements regarding specialty care transport (SCT) is true?
   A. SCT is necessary when patient care requires the services of more than one health professional.
   B. SCT is necessary when a patient's ongoing care may require future attention from a specialty service.
   C. SCT is defined as the hospital-to-hospital transport of a critically injured or ill patient by a ground ambulance at a level of service beyond the scope of normal EMT-Paramedic training.
   D. The presence of a registered nurse is required on all transports designated as an STC by Medicare.

10. Which of the following transports would most likely meet Medicare's requirement for specialty care transport?
   A. a stable 33-year-old female complaining of a headache requiring BLS transport from an ED to a local medical center for an MRI
   B. a stable 13-year-old male with a suspected fractured ulna after a 5-foot fall from a tree, requiring transport from his home to a local ED
   C. a 22-year-old male asthmatic, unresponsive to inhaled beta-agonists, requiring transport from a rural community health clinic to a tertiary care facility
   D. a 1-day-old female, born 38 days premature, with difficulty breathing, requiring transport from a community OB unit to an NICU at a regional tertiary care facility

Critical Care Aerial Transport

Review of Chapter Objectives

Upon completion of this chapter, the student should be able to:

1. Identify the administrative structure and functions of the administrative team.   **p. 27**

All air medical organizations have an administrative team that directs the daily operations of the transport program. Administrative structure varies greatly between organizations, with some utilizing large administrative teams consisting of multiple, base site managers, outreach teams, and clinical coordinators, while some organizations utilize a more utilitarian approach. There is no right or wrong administrative approach, and each organization's administration is tailored to meet the demands of that organization's specific situation. Two basic components shared by all administrative teams are the program director and the medical director. The program director coordinates both the daily operations and the long-term goals and issues of the flight program, such as organization strategy and growth. Specific responsibilities of the program director include the creation of administrative policy, the ensuring of continuous quality improvement, the maintenance of fleet aircraft, maintenance of the communications center, preparation and planning of the operating budget, determination of direct marketing and growth strategies, and acting as the public figurehead of the organization. Very often, some of these responsibilities are delegated to a Director of Operations and/or a Director of Communications.

Responsibilities of the medical director include the creation of medical protocols, the ensuring of adequate training for new flight crew members, the provision of continuing medical education, periodic competency testing, and the provision of online medical direction.

Both the program director and the medical director commonly have input on the crew configurations of the critical care transport team. Crew configuration is usually determined by mission and patient need, and most programs opt for a dual provider crew made up of one RN and an RN or paramedic partner.

2. Discuss the importance of a comprehensive communication center.   **p. 29**

The communication center is often referred to as the heart of the air medical transport organization, and its responsibilities include the receiving of incoming requests for transport, and the gathering of required information such as coordinates, ground contact frequencies, destinations, and patient information. In addition, in-flight and follow-up duties, including following the flight of the aircraft, communications with security at the receiving hospital, and callbacks to the requesting agency are included in the scope of the communications center's responsibility.

3. Discuss the indications and benefits of fixed-wing transport. p. 29

In the United States, indications for fixed-wing transport (i.e., a plane) include transport distances of greater than 100 nautical miles, and the presence of weather that prohibits the use of rotor-winged (i.e., a helicopter) aircraft. Benefits of fixed-winged aircraft include the provision of a highly trained medical crew and their specialized equipment, the ability to fly in bad weather, increased transport range, and increased cost effectiveness.

While the planning of a fixed-wing transport within the country of origin is similar to that of a rotor-wing transport, international transports require a substantial amount of additional planning. Additional considerations include the arranging of safe passage into foreign airspace, assuring efficient and safe refueling and ground transport, and the assuring of air medical crew safety in foreign, and potentially unfriendly, countries.

4. Describe the indications and benefits of rotor-wing transport. p. 30

Aeromedical transports utilizing rotor-winged aircraft represent the majority of air medical transports in the United States; in other countries, rotor-winged aircraft are used to a lesser degree. Rotor-winged aircraft are generally used for transports located within a 100-nautical mile radius of their base. Large-frame, rotor-winged aircraft are desirable for servicing remote geographical areas far from tertiary care facilities, as they can cruise at high rates of speed and can carry large fuel loads, which allow for rapid transport times and fewer refueling delays. In addition, large airframes can perform rescue work, can better accommodate multiple-patient loads, and also have the benefit of more workspace for the air medical crew. Disadvantages of large-frame aircraft include the need for a large, sturdy landing site, and higher operating expenses including original cost, maintenance, and fuel, when compared to small-frame aircraft.

Small airframes are justified in situations where the transport service operates relatively close to tertiary care facilities or has several additional medical helicopters available for multiple-patient missions, and have the benefit of being less expensive to operate. While some small air-frame aircraft are capable of dual-patient loads, the additional loss of already limited cabin space can make such transports challenging for the air medical crew. Even with a single patient, small-frame rotor-winged aircraft have limited workspace, and air medical crew size is often limited to two providers. In many small airframes, some area of the patient may be out of reach during transport, and the aircraft may have weight restrictions that limit the combined crew and patient load.

Benefits of rotor-winged aircraft include the provision of highly trained medical crew and their specialized equipment, decreased response times over long distances compared to ground units, decreased out-of-hospital transport time compared to ground transport (in most cases), the ability to land in remote locations, and the ability to perform rescue work.

5. Describe the indications for calling for air medical transport. p. 40

Indications for air medical transport include medical emergencies, trauma emergencies, and missions involving search and rescue where the utilization of a rotor-winged aircraft may prove beneficial. While exact launch criteria involving clinical status, mechanism of injury, and transport time of air versus ground transport often varies by region, the following list of questions prepared by the National Association of EMS Physicians' Air Medical Task Force can help shape the ultimate decision to utilize air medical transport:
1. Does the patient's clinical condition require minimization of time spent out of the hospital environment during the transport?
2. Does the patient require specific or time-sensitive evaluation or treatment that is not available at the referring facility?
3. Is the patient located in an area that is inaccessible to ground transport?
4. What are the current and predicted weather situations along the transport route?
5. Is the weight of the patient (plus the weight of required equipment and transport personnel) within allowable ranges for air transport?
6. For interhospital transport, is there a helipad or airport near the referring hospital?
7. Does the patient require critical care life support (e.g., monitoring personnel, specific medications, specific equipment) during transport that is not available with ground transport options?

©2007 Pearson Education, Inc.
Critical Care Paramedic

8. Would use of local ground transport leave the local area without adequate emergency medical services coverage?
9. If local ground transport is not an option, can the needs of the patient (and the system) be met by an available regional ground critical care transport service (i.e., specialized surface transport systems operated by hospitals and/or air medical programs)?

In cases of trauma, indications for helicopter transport are similar to the indications for trauma center care, and include both mechanism of injury and clinical criteria. Keep in mind, however, that recent studies have indicated that mechanism of injury criteria are poor predictors of which patients will benefit from helicopter transport to a trauma center. Overall, limited research is available that specifically supports when, or when not, to utilize critical care transport services, both in the trauma and nontrauma scenario. Until more concrete data is available to help in decision making, logistical considerations, clinical judgment, and medical oversight should all influence the decision to utilize aeromedical and critical care transport services.

The National Association of EMS Physicians (NAEMSP), Air Medical Physician Association (AMPA), and Association of Air Medical Services (AAMS) have collaborated to produce the most comprehensive guidelines, to date, for the dispatch of air medical critical care transport teams in cases of trauma, interfacility, and nontrauma transports. For scene calls with trauma, the NAEMSP recommends the following criteria:

1. General trauma and mechanism of injury considerations
   a. Trauma Score < 12
   b. Unstable vital signs (e.g., hypotension or tachypnea)
   c. Significant trauma in patients < 12 years old, > 55 years old, or pregnant patients
   d. Multisystem injuries (e.g., long-bone fractures in different extremities; injury to more than two body regions)
   e. Ejection from vehicle
   f. Pedestrian or cyclist struck by motor vehicle
   g. Death in same passenger compartment as patient
   h. Ground provider perception of significant damage to patient's passenger compartment
   i. Penetrating trauma to the abdomen, pelvis, chest, neck, or head
   j. Crush injury to the abdomen, chest, or head
   k. Fall from significant height
2. Neurologic considerations
   a. Glasgow Coma Scale score < 10
   b. Deteriorating mental status
   c. Skull fracture
   d. Neurologic presentation suggestive of spinal cord injury
3. Thoracic considerations
   a. Major chest wall injury (e.g., flail chest)
   b. Pneumothorax/hemothorax
   c. Suspected cardiac injury
4. Abdominal/pelvic considerations
   a. Significant abdominal pain after blunt trauma
   b. Presence of a "seatbelt" sign or other abdominal wall contusion
   c. Obvious rib fracture below the nipple line
   d. Major pelvic fracture (e.g., unstable pelvic ring disruption, open pelvic fracture, or pelvic fracture with hypotension)
5. Orthopedic/extremity considerations
   a. Partial or total amputation of a limb (exclusive of digits)
   b. Finger/thumb amputation when emergent surgical evaluation (or replantation) is indicated and rapid surface transport is not available
   c. Fracture or dislocation with vascular compromise
   d. Extremity ischemia
   e. Open long-bone fractures
   f. Two or more long-bone fractures

6. Major burns
    a. > 20 percent body surface area
    b. Involvement of face, head, hands, feet, or genitalia
    c. Inhalational injury
    d. Electrical or chemical burns
    e. Burns with associated injuries
7. Patients with near-drowning injuries

For interfacility transfers, the NAEMSP recommends the following criteria for air medical critical care transport:
1. Trauma: Injured patients constitute the diagnostic group for which there is best evidence to support outcome improvements from air transport.
    a. Depending on local hospital capabilities and regional practices, any diagnostic consideration (suspected, or confirmed as with referring hospital radiography) listed previously under "scene" guidelines may be sufficient indication for air transport from a community hospital to a regional trauma center.
    b. Additionally, air transport may be appropriate when initial evaluation at the community hospital reveals injuries or potential injuries requiring further evaluation and management beyond the capabilities of the referring hospital.
2. Cardiac: Patients with certain cardiac conditions may be candidates for air transport.
    a. Acute coronary syndromes with time-critical need for urgent interventional therapy (e.g., cardiac catheterization, intra-aortic balloon pump placement, emergent cardiac surgery) unavailable at the referring center
    b. Cardiogenic shock (especially in presence of, or need for, ventricular assist devices or intra-aortic balloon pumps)
    c. Cardiac tamponade with impending hemodynamic compromise
    d. Mechanical cardiac disease (e.g., acute cardiac rupture, decompensating valvular heart disease)
3. Critically ill, medical, or surgical patients: Examples of conditions where air transport may be appropriate include:
    a. Pretransport cardiac/respiratory arrest.
    b. Requirement for continuous intravenous vasoactive medications or mechanical ventricular assist to maintain stable cardiac output.
    c. Risk for airway deterioration (e.g., angioedema, epiglottitis).
    d. Acute pulmonary failure and/or requirement for sophisticated, pulmonary, intensive care during transport.
    e. Severe poisoning or overdose requiring specialized toxicology services.
    f. Urgent need for hyperbaric oxygen therapy (e.g., vascular gas embolism, necrotizing infectious process, carbon monoxide toxicity).
    g. Requirement for emergent dialysis.
    h. Gastrointestinal hemorrhages with hemodynamic compromise.
    i. Surgical emergencies, such as fasciitis, aortic dissection or aneurysm, or extremity ischemia.
    j. Pediatric patients for whom referring facilities cannot provide required evaluation and/or therapy.
4. Obstetric: Examples of conditions where air transport may be appropriate include:
    a. Reasonable expectation that delivery of infant(s) may require obstetric or neonatal care beyond the capabilities of the referring hospital.
    b. Active premature labor when estimated gestational age is < 34 weeks or estimated fetal weight is < 2,000 grams.
    c. Severe pre-eclampsia or eclampsia (pregnancy-induced hypertension).
    d. Third-trimester hemorrhage.
    e. Fetal hydrops.
    f. Maternal medical conditions (e.g., heart disease, drug overdose, metabolic disturbances) that may cause premature birth.
    g. Severe, predicted, fetal heart disease.
    h. Acute abdominal emergencies (i.e., likely to require surgery) when estimated gestational age is < 34 weeks or estimated fetal weight is < 2,000 grams.

5. Neurological: Examples of conditions where air transport may be appropriate include:
   a. Central nervous system hemorrhage.
   b. Spinal cord compression by mass lesion.
   c. Evolving ischemic stroke (i.e., potential candidate for lytic therapy).
   d. Status epilepticus.
6. Neonatal: Examples of instances where air medical dispatch may be appropriate include:
   a. Gestational age < 30 weeks, body weight < 2,000 grams, or complicated neonatal course (e.g., perinatal cardiac/respiratory arrest, hemodynamic instability, sepsis, meningitis, metabolic derangement, temperature instability).
   b. Requirement for supplemental oxygen exceeding 60 percent, continuous positive airway pressure (CPAP), or mechanical ventilation.
   c. Extrapulmonary air leak, interstitial emphysema, or pneumothorax.
   d. Medical emergencies, such as seizure activity, congestive heart failure, or disseminated intravascular coagulation.
   e. Surgical emergencies, such as diaphragmatic hernia, necrotizing enterocolitis, abdominal wall defects, intussusception, suspected volvulus, or congenital heart defects.
7. Other: Air medical dispatch may also be appropriate in miscellaneous situations.
   a. Transplant
      1. Patient has met criteria for brain death, and air transport is necessary for organ salvage.
      2. Organ and/or organ recipient requires air transport to the transplant center in order to maintain viability of time-critical transplant.
   b. Search-and-rescue operations are generally outside the purview of air medical transport services, but, in some instances, helicopter EMS may participate in such operations.
   c. Patients known to be in cardiac arrest are rarely candidates for air medical transport.

6. Indicate general considerations that go into planning and implementing a critical care flight mission. p. 40

Once the decision to initiate critical care transport has been made, the following guidelines should be utilized:
1. Patients requiring critical interventions should be provided those interventions in the most expeditious manner possible.
2. Patients who are stable should be transported in a manner that best addresses the needs of the patient and the system.
3. Patients with critical injuries or illnesses resulting in unstable vital signs require transport to a center capable of providing definitive care by the fastest available modality, and with a transport team that has the appropriate level of care capabilities.
4. Patients with critical injuries or illnesses should be transported by a team that can provide intratransport critical care services.
5. Patients who require high-level care during transport, but do not have time-critical illness or injury, may be candidates for ground critical care transport (i.e., by a specialized ground critical care transport vehicle with level of care exceeding that of local EMS) if such service is available and logistically feasible.

7. Discuss the advantages and disadvantages of air medical transport. p. 45

Advantages of air medical transport over regular ALS ground transport include decreased out-of-hospital times, access to remote locations, access to specialty teams, and access to highly trained, medical personnel with specialized skills. Disadvantages of air medical transport include limitations on the number of patients that can be transported, patient and crew size, and available workspace. In addition, bad weather and the need for frequent maintenance can limit the availability of air medical ambulances compared to ground ambulances, and air medical transport is more expensive.

Specific advantages of rotor-winged transport include decreased response time under distances of 100 nautical miles compared to both fixed-wing aircraft and ground units, a decreased prehospital transport time, and the availability of highly trained medical crews and specialized equipment. Disadvantages include the inability to fly in bad weather conditions, and a relatively limited availability of rotor-wing ambulances compared to ground ambulances.

Specific advantages of fixed-wing aircraft include decreased response times to patients when transport distances exceed 100 nautical miles compared to both rotor-wing aircraft and ground ambulances, decreased prehospital transport times, the availability of highly trained medical crews and their specialized equipment, and less susceptibility to bad weather than rotor-wing aircraft. Disadvantages include the need for an airport, extra transport legs between airports and health care facilities, greater susceptibility to weather than ground transport, and the fact that fixed-wing transport is a less desirable transport mode for critically ill or injured patients.

8. Identify proper packaging of the air medical patient. p. 46

Preparation for transport in the air medical environment often varies slightly from the preparation of the ground transport patient. As the treatment of critical patients often requires the use of much equipment, the setup and placing of equipment should be done in an organized fashion so that it can be easily accessed when needed. This includes not only properly securing equipment in an accessible location, but also securing wires and hoses, such as by coiling unneeded length and securing with tape to prevent them from becoming entangled, being pinched, or accidentally cut with sheers. Consider labeling coiled IV tubing to better identify its role; this can easily be accomplished by simply writing on the tape used to secure the coiled tubing. When not in use, medical equipment may be stowed in compartments accessible only from outside the aircraft, making it challenging, and unadvisable, to access such equipment if needed while caring for a patient. In such instances, it is necessary to land the aircraft to retrieve needed equipment, increasing risk and lengthening transport time. As such, consideration much be taken prior to takeoff as to which equipment may be needed during patient transport, and said equipment brought into, and secured properly within, the cabin.

Often, patients must be placed on a stretcher or litter specific for the aircraft being used, requiring transfer between the sending agencies stretcher and that of the flight crew. A foil or some other impermeable layer is often used to "wrap up" the patient, protecting her from the environment, as well as helping to prevent contamination of the aircraft and equipment with blood or other body fluids. Every effort should be made to protect the patient from wind, rain, and extremes of temperature.

Conscious patients are sometimes offered the use of a headset, allowing for improved communication between him and the air medical crew. Headsets also have the benefit of protecting the patient's hearing, and earplugs should be provided if a headset is not available.

Case Study

As the ambulance rolls out onto the tarmac, you radio Emily, the pilot, to let her know about the arrival of your patient. She tells you that she is going to get an updated weather report, advise the communications center, and return to help with loading as soon as possible.

Your patient, an 80-year-old man who suffered a stroke while on vacation here in Arizona, is being transferred home for long-term care. The long-term care facility where your patient will be placed is just south of Albany, NY, approximately 2,100 miles away. Although your patient is stable, his CVA left him with left hemiplegia and he is ventilator-dependent, making a commercial flight impossible. After introductions are made, and a thorough patient assessment is performed in the ambulance, the patient is packaged for transport. The ventilator circuit and monitor leads are attached, and excess tubing and wires are coiled and taped to keep them from tangling. The patient has a slight build and is easily moved into the fuselage of the aircraft. With a recheck of the patient to confirm that all is in order, and a "thumbs up" to the pilot, the aircraft begins to taxi toward the runway.

The transport is without incident, and in four and one-half hours, the aircraft begins its long descent into Albany. Your communications center has already arranged ground transport in Albany, and, as your plane taxis to the parking area, you are pleased to see the ambulance on the tarmac. After introductions are made and a patient care report is given, the loading process is reversed to move the patient from the aircraft into the ambulance. After saying good-bye to your patient and watching the ambulance pull away, Emily advises you that the communications center has given you a transfer for tomorrow from New York City to Paris.

DISCUSSION QUESTIONS

1. What are some indications for the use of air medical transport?
2. What are the benefits of rotor-wing and fixed-wing transport?
3. What factors should be considered in the proper packaging of a patient for air transport?

Content Review

MULTIPLE CHOICE

_____ 1. Which of the following is not considered a normal responsibility of a critical care transport program's program coordinator?
   A. the creation of administrative policy
   B. the provision of online medical direction
   C. determination of marketing and growth strategies
   D. acting as the public figurehead of the organization

_____ 2. Responsibilities of a critical care transport program's medical director might include all of the following except:
   A. the ensuring of adequate training for new flight crewmembers.
   B. periodic competency testing.
   C. the creation of medical protocols.
   D. the coordination of daily operations and long-term program goals.

_____ 3. Crew configuration of a critical care air ambulance is usually determined by:
   A. mission and patient need.
   B. economic status of the transport program.
   C. health care provider unions.
   D. local and institution politics.

_____ 4. Responsibilities of the communications center typically include all of the following except:
   A. callbacks and follow-up with the requesting agency.
   B. the gathering of required mission information.
   C. following of the flight during the mission.
   D. providing a verbal patient report to receiving facility.

_____ 5. Which of the following statements regarding fixed-wing air medical transport is true?
   A. Indications for fixed-wing transport include travel distances of less than 100 nautical miles.
   B. Fixed-wing aircraft are as limited by weather conditions as are rotor-winged aircraft.
   C. International transports require a substantial amount of additional planning, as compared to transports within the United States.
   D. Aeromedical transports using fixed-wing aircraft represent the majority of air medical transports in the United States every year.

_____ 6. Which of the following statements regarding rotor-wing air medical transport is true?
   A. Small airframes are typically used when travel distances are large, and when limited air medical resources are available.
   B. Use of rotor-winged aircraft rather than fixed-wing aircraft usually results in a shorter prehospital time when travel distances are less than 100 nautical miles.
   C. Most small-frame rotor aircraft are capable of carrying dual-patient loads while still allowing adequate cabin space for the air medical crew.
   D. Compared to small-frame rotor aircraft, large-frame rotor aircraft offer the advantage of faster cruising speed and better fuel economy.

_____ 7. Packaging considerations for the air ambulance patient include all of the following except:
   A. coiling and securing all unneeded lengths of tubing and wires.
   B. securing the patient to a litter or stretcher that is compatible to the aircraft securing system.
   C. ensuring that all equipment is placed on the floor to prevent it from falling on the patient during transport.
   D. protecting the patient from wind, rain, and temperature extremes.

_____ 8. Advantages of fixed-wing aircraft over rotor-winged aircraft include:
   A. decreased response times to patients when transport distances exceed 100 nautical miles.
   B. decreased response times when transport distances are less than 100 nautical miles.
   C. the ability to perform rescue work.
   D. the provision of a highly trained medical crew and specialized equipment.

_____ 9. Advantages of rotor-winged aircraft over fixed-wing aircraft include:
   A. the ability to travel at high cruising speeds.
   B. the ability to land in remote locations without a runway.
   C. greater workspace and patient accessibility.
   D. the need for a smaller air medical crew.

_____ 10. Proper packaging of a patient prior to air medical transport includes all of the following except:
   A. placing all medical equipment located in outside compartments into the cabin prior to takeoff.
   B. securing all equipment in an accessible location.
   C. protecting the patient from the elements.
   D. providing the patient with a headset.

Altitude Physiology

Review of Chapter Objectives

Upon completion of this chapter, the student should be able to:

1. Detail the various atmospheric levels and the characteristics of each.   **p. 50**

The atmosphere can be thought of as an ocean of gases composed primarily of nitrogen, oxygen, argon, and trace gases. The atmosphere exists as four distinct, readily identifiable layers known as the troposphere, stratosphere, mesosphere, and thermosphere. The troposphere is located from the Earth's surface to a height of about 5–9 miles, and is the level in which air medical transports, and all weather, occur. The stratosphere extends from the troposphere to a height of about 31 miles, where transition to the mesosphere occurs. The outermost atmospheric layer, the thermosphere, begins at the outer border of the mesosphere, located about 53 miles above the Earth's surface, and extends to a height of about 372 miles.

2. Detail the three physiologically important atmospheric zones.   **p. 51**

The Earth's atmosphere can be divided into three atmospheric zones, the boundaries of which are based on physiologic research into the human body's response to altitude. These three atmospheric zones are the physiological zone, the physiologically deficient zone, and the space-equivalent zone.

The physiological zone extends from sea level to a height of about 10,000 feet. Adequate oxygen for human survival without protective equipment exists in this zone, and the human body is well adapted to exist here. Rapid ascent or descent between altitudes within the physiologic zone can produce ear or sinus trapped-gas problems and other minor issues.

The physiologically deficient zone extends from an altitude of 10,000 feet to about 50,000 feet. At these altitudes, decreased barometric pressure and oxygen can cause hypoxia in unprotected individuals, and issues occurring secondary to trapped and evolved gases are common. Fixed-wing aeromedical aircraft, which commonly fly at 5,000–15,000 feet, often operate within this zone, and jet aircraft may cruise at altitudes as high as 35,000 feet. Internal cabins in fixed-wing aircraft are pressurized and provide a higher oxygen content to prevent hypoxia. Supplemental oxygen is required if a loss of cabin pressure occurs within this atmospheric zone.

The space-equivalent zone can be thought of as outer space, in which there is no protection from the uninhabitable environment other than sealed cabins and pressure suits. Unprotected humans can expect such pleasantries as hypoxia, radiation effects, and ebullism should they be exposed to the space-equivalent environment. Ebullism, the boiling of body fluids, occurs at an altitude of about 63,500 feet (Armstrong's line), and results from the lowering of total barometric pressure to less than the vapor pressure of water.

3. **Define and describe the significance of the following gas laws:**

Dalton's law p. 53

Definition: The total pressure of a gas mixture in a container equals the sum of the partial pressures of the individual gases.

Equation: $P_t = P_1 + P_2 + P_3 + \ldots$

Where: P_t = total pressure of the gas mixture

P_1, P_2, P_3, and so on = the partial pressures of the gases in the mixture

Partial pressure = pressure of a single gas in a mixture as if that gas alone occupied the container.

Significance: Dalton's law says that gases in a mixture will act independent of one another, as long as the temperature is not too cold or the gas is not compressed (we're talking *really* cold and *really* compressed). For our purposes, gases will behave according to Dalton's law on the Earth's surface, and in flight. Gases will act independently of one another in a mixture because there is, on an atomic level, an enormous amount of space between gas molecules rendering them, in effect, by themselves. Now, cool or compress a gas, and the individual gas molecules come closer together and interact, and Dalton's law does not hold. Recognizing that gases in a mixture act independently from one another allows us to consider their contributions to the overall pressure of the mixture independently, a term called partial pressure. The partial pressure of a gas is determined by the equation $P_A = X_A \times P$, where P_A = the pressure of gas A, X_A = the mole fraction of gas A (its weight), and P = the total pressure of the gas mixture. The partial pressure of oxygen, and any other gas, can be determined by the partial pressure equation: $PO_2 = 0.21 \times 760$ mmHg = 159.6 mmHg at sea level.

Boyle's law p. 53

Definition: At constant temperature, the volume of a gas is inversely related to its pressure.

Equation: $P_1 V_1 = P_2 V_2$

Where: P = the pressure of gas in a container

V = the volume of gas in a container

Significance: Simply stated, Boyle's law says that in a closed container, as pressure increases, volume decreases, and as pressure decreases, volume increases. At 18,000 feet, gas in a closed container will attempt to expand to twice its normal volume at sea level. In air medical transport, the closed containers we are concerned with include endotracheal tube cuffs, and the bowel and lungs in the patient. As air pressure decreases with altitude, trapped gases will expand, possibly resulting in equipment failure or tissue injury. The reverse is true as an aircraft descends but pressurized aircraft cabins minimize these effects. Specific problems that can occur during flight that are directly related to Boyle's law include pain from trapped gas expansion, changes in respiratory rate and depth, and a rise in endotracheal tube cuff pressure, leading to pressure necrosis of the tracheal mucosa.

Charles' law p. 55

Definition: The volume of a fixed amount and pressure of gas is directly proportional to it's temperature.

Equation: $\dfrac{V_1}{T_1} = \dfrac{V_2}{T_2}$

Where: V = the volume of gas

T = the temperature of gas in K

Significance: Charles' law can be used to predict the volume of gas at any given temperature. Simply stated, gas expands when heated and volume increases, and gas contracts when cooled and volume decreases. Although a patient can experience temperature decreases at altitude, the resultant contraction of trapped gases in no way compensates for the expansion of trapped gases secondary to the decrease in pressure.

Gay-Lussac's law   p. 56

Definition: For a fixed amount of gas at a fixed volume, pressure is proportional to temperature.

Equation: $\dfrac{P_1}{T_1} = \dfrac{P_2}{T_2}$

> Where: P = pressure
> T = temperature

Significance: Gay-Lussac's law once again illustrates how a trapped gas (fixed volume) will react to changes in the surrounding environment; specifically, in this case, how the pressure changes with the temperature. The pressure of trapped gas increases as the gas warms, and decreases as the gas cools. A clinical application of Gay-Lussac's law can be appreciated by noting how the pressure in a gas cylinder (i.e., oxygen, nitrous oxide) decreases with the temperature. In theory and practice, gas reserves in an unprotected cylinder will be lower than expected at altitude, or even at sea level on a cold day.

Henry's law   p. 57

Definition: The amount of gas that will dissolve into a solution is directly proportional to the partial pressure of the gas above the solution.

Equation: Concentration of gas in a solution = partial pressure of gas × solubility coefficient

Significance: When gas is in contact with the surface of a liquid, the amount of gas that will go into the liquid (into solution) is proportional to the partial pressure of the gas; the greater the partial pressure of a gas (the more of it), the greater the amount of that gas that will dissolve into the liquid. Because of differences in chemical and physical properties, different gases dissolve into liquids at different rates, or with varying "ease," which is why a gas' solubility coefficient is considered in the equation. Thus, for a known partial pressure of a gas, Henry's law can be used to predict the amount of gas that will go into a solution. A clinical application of Henry's law can be appreciated by considering that at altitude, where there is a lower partial pressure of oxygen as compared to at sea level, less oxygen is available to dissolve into blood plasma, and arterial oxygen content (the amount of gas in the liquid) decreases.

Graham's law   p. 57

Definition: The relative rates at which two gases, under identical conditions of temperature and pressure, will diffuse varies inversely to the square roots of their respective molecular masses.

Equation: $\sqrt{\dfrac{M_1}{M_2}} = \dfrac{V_2}{V_1}$

Significance: Graham's law is fairly intuitive in that it says a smaller gas molecule will dissolve faster than a larger one. It is used to determine the diffusion rates of gases. Graham's law explains why carbon dioxide, with a 22 × greater solubility in plasma than oxygen, is not present in amounts 22 × greater than oxygen. With a larger mass, carbon dioxide's diffusion rate is slower than that of oxygen.

Fick's law   p. 58

Definition: The net diffusion rate of a gas across a fluid membrane is: (1) proportional to the difference in partial pressure, (2) proportional to the area of the membrane, and (3) inversely proportional to the thickness of the membrane.

Equation: none

Significance: When combined with Graham's law, Fick's law can be used to determine the exchange rates of gases across membranes, such as the alveolar-capillary membrane.

Avogadro's law   p. 58

Definition: At a fixed temperature and pressure, an equal number of molecules of gas occupy the same volume.

Equation: $n_1 \times V_1 = n_2 \times V_2$

> Where: n = number of moles of gas
> V = volume

Significance: The equation for Avogadro's law states that the volume of a gas increases as the number of molecules of gas increases. This makes intuitive sense, as one would expect the volume of anything to increase as you add more "stuff" to it. An exception occurs if a container's volume remains fixed; in such a case, adding more gas increases pressure, as volume cannot increase to compensate for the increased number of gas molecules.

Ideal gas law   p. 59

Definition: The ideal gas law is an equation derived from the relationship of Boyle's, Charles', and Avogadro's laws, and relates the temperature, pressure, and volume of a gas.

Equation: $PV = nRT$

> Where: P = pressure in atmosphere
> V = volume
> n = number of moles of gas present
> R = proportionality constant
> T = temperature in K

Significance: Ideal gases are ones that obey Charles' and Boyle's laws exactly. Many common or real gases, such as oxygen and carbon dioxide, behave enough like ideal gases at ambient temperature and pressure to use the ideal gas equation to calculate values such as pressure, volume, temperature, and number of moles of gas. Real gases do deviate from ideal gases at low temperatures and high pressures, but again, differences from ideal gases are negligible, even at altitudes normally experienced during flight.

4. Discuss the stresses of altitude and flight including:

Hypoxia   p. 60
Hypoxia is one of the most frequently encountered problems in aviation medicine, and is defined as an inadequate supply of oxygen for normal cellular function. Hypoxemia, an end result of hypoxia, is a deficiency of oxygen in the blood. Types of hypoxia include hypoxic hypoxia, anemic hypoxia, stagnant hypoxia, and histotoxic hypoxia.

Barometric pressure   p. 62
Changes in barometric pressure that accompany flight have direct implications for flight medicine, and are predictable in accordance to Boyle's law. The lower barometric pressure experienced high altitude causes trapped air to expand. Specifically, problems such as changing pressure in PASG, variations in respiratory rate and depth, changes in intravenous flow rates, pain from trapped gas expansion (in viscera or sinuses), and changes in endotracheal tube cuff pressure occur with variations in barometric pressure. Generally, these issues are mostly a concern with fixed-wing flight, as these aircraft cruise at high altitudes; rotor-wing aircraft cruise at lower altitudes. Fixed-wing aircraft pressurize the internal cabin pressure to the equivalent of 5,000 to 8,000 feet to avoid such issues.

Fatigue   p. 63
Factors that contribute to fatigue in the patient and air medical crew include the general health of the individual, smoking history, alcohol use, aircraft vibration and noise, temperature changes, disturbances in circadian rhythms, diet, dehydration, hypoxia, gravitational forces, barometric changes, and emotional stress. Fatigue can be minimized with adequate rest, hydration, and diet, and by eliminating unhealthy habits such as smoking and alcohol use.

Thermal   p. 63
Temperature decreases with altitude, and can cause stress on the body. Specifically, hypothermia (and hyperthermia) increases oxygen demand. As a result, hypoxia is worsened with decreases in temperature. In addition, variations in ambient atmospheric temperature can create turbulence, which can create psychological stress as well as fatigue, disorientation, and motion sickness.

Dehydration   p. 63
At altitude, air is drier as well as colder, and can worsen existing dehydration. Fluid replacement should be considered early, and humidified oxygen utilized to minimize drying of the respiratory mucosal membranes.

Humidity is the concentration of water vapor in the atmosphere. The amount of water vapor in the atmosphere at any given time is usually less than the amount required to saturate the air, and cooler air holds less water than does warm air.

The relative humidity is the percent of saturation humidity, or how much water vapor the air is holding compared to how much it could hold at a certain temperature. It is determined by dividing the actual vapor density of air by the saturation vapor density and multiplying by 100 percent. The relative humidity can change if available water vapor or temperature changes.

The dew point is the temperature at which relative humidity reaches 100 percent. At the dew point temperature, atmospheric air will be holding all of the water vapor it can, and is said to be saturated. We recognize when the dew point has been reached when it rains, or when water droplets, or dew, start to form inside whatever closed environment we are in, such as an aircraft cabin.

Noise   p. 64
Noise created from the engines, propellers, and rotors of aircraft pose a significant hazard for air medical crews. Long-term hearing loss is a real risk, and efforts should be made to protect both the crew and patient from noise exposure by utilizing helmets, headsets, or earplugs. In addition, noise can interfere with procedures such as lung auscultation and blood pressure determination.

Vibration   p. 64
Vibration in an aircraft can occur in all three axes (X, Y, and Z) and is transferred to the occupants of the vehicle. Energy that is absorbed from vibration is broken down into heat, which increases metabolic rate and results in peripheral vasoconstriction, redistribution of blood, and overriding of the body's cooling mechanisms.

Gravitational forces   p. 64
Gravitational forces, or G-forces, are force changes that occur with acceleration. Luckily, the G-forces created by the majority of aircraft used for aeromedical purposes are not significant. G-forces measure the rate of change in velocity of an object, or its acceleration, and are described by Newton's three laws of motion.

1. First Law: A body in motion (or at rest) tends to remain in motion (or at rest) unless it is acted upon by an outside force.
2. Second Law: The relationship between an object's mass (m) and its acceleration (a) and the applied force (F) is $F = ma$.
3. Third Law: For every action, there is an equal and opposite reaction.

The three types of accelerative forces that can develop in flight occur in specific circumstances. Linear acceleration results from a change in speed without a change in direction, as when an aircraft takes off or changes its forward air speed. Radial, or centripetal, acceleration occurs when the aircraft changes direction without changing speed, as when it banks or turns. Angular acceleration occurs when the aircraft changes both speed and direction, a situation that occurs when an aircraft enters a spin.

G-forces, and the direction at which the body receives them, can be considered utilizing the XYZ axis. Positive G ($+Gz$) forces occur when a seated body accelerates upwards, in a head-first direction. Inertial forces act in the opposite direction, toward the feet. As a result, the body is forced down into the seat. Negative G ($-Gz$) forces occur when a seated body is accelerated downward, in a feet-first direction. Inertial forces act in the opposite direction, toward the feet, lifting the body from the seat. Forward transverse G ($+Gx$) forces occur when a seated body is accelerated forward, with the resultant forces acting across the body in an anterior to posterior direction. Backward transverse ($-Gx$) forces occur when a seated body decelerates, with the resultant forces acting across the body in a posterior to anterior direction. Right- or left-lateral G ($+/-Gy$) forces occur when the accelerative force acts across a lateral, or shoulder-to-shoulder, direction.

Several factors determine the effect that G-forces will have on the human body. These factors include intensity, duration, rate of onset, body area affected, and impact direction. Generally speaking, the greater the intensity, duration, rate of onset, and body surface area affected, the greater the physiologic effects of G-forces are. In addition, the human body has less tolerance for Gz forces than for Gx forces.

Third spacing   p. 66

Third spacing of fluids, the movement of fluid from the intravascular space to the interstitial space, occurs secondary to increased intravascular pressure and increased cell membrane permeability, and can be aggravated by stressors typical of flight, such as temperature changes, vibration, and G-forces. Third spacing occurs more frequently during long-distance, high-altitude flights.

Spatial disorientation   p. 67

Spatial disorientation is the inability to determine one's position, attitude, and motion relative to the surface of the Earth or fixed objects on the ground. Disorientation occurs when a person's visual, vestibular, and proprioceptive systems provide the brain with erroneous information with regard to orientation. All air crew members are at risk, regardless of flight experience, and when it affects pilots, the results can be catastrophic. When a pilot experiences spatial disorientation, he may rely on the false information that his senses provide him rather than on the accurate information provided by instruments, thereby resulting in a crash.

There are three types of spatial disorientation. Type I (unrecognized) occurs when a crew member does not recognize that he is experiencing spatial disorientation. His misperceptions are wrongfully corroborated by his other senses. Type II (recognized) spatial disorientation occurs when the pilot recognizes that a problem exists, but does not recognize it as spatial disorientation; the pilot may believe that a control is malfunctioning. In type III (incapacitating) spatial disorientation, the crew member is overwhelmed by the inability to orient himself and is subsequently unable to perform his duties. Methods of preventing spatial disorientation include flying only when visual reference points are available, trusting your instruments, and avoiding fatigue, hypoglycemia, hypoxia, and anxiety. In addition, utilizing scanning techniques, and not staring at lights, helps to prevent spatial disorientation. Providing a tactile reference during flight may assist in preventing spatial disorientation in patients.

Flicker vertigo   p. 67

Vertigo is a disturbance of inner ear equilibrium characterized by a sensation of spinning; it is often described as a feeling that you or the environment is moving when no movement is occurring. The three sensory systems important in maintaining equilibrium and balance are the visual, vestibular, and proprioceptive systems. An excess of stimulation from either of the systems that cannot be compensated for by the others can result in vertigo. In the absence of visual stimuli (reference point), the vestibular and proprioceptive systems are unreliable in flight, explaining why flying over water, or any other situation where there is no fixed ground reference point, is so dangerous.

Pathological vertigo occurs secondary to abnormal sensory signals from peripheral sensors or abnormal signal processing by the central nervous system. Physiological vertigo occurs secondary to overstimulation of one of the three sensory systems. An example of physiological vertigo is flicker vertigo.

Flicker vertigo is created by light sources that emit flickering light at rates of 4–20 cycles per second. Sources of such light include sunlight interrupted by propellers of rotors, flashing aircraft anticollision lights, rotating beacons or strobes, fluorescent lights, and television screens. Preventative measures include avoiding looking at flashing lights, and the use of sunglasses or caps.

5. List the four types of hypoxia.   p. 60

The four types of hypoxia include hypoxic hypoxia, anemic hypoxia, stagnant hypoxia, and histotoxic hypoxia. Hypoxic hypoxia occurs secondary to inadequate atmospheric oxygen or inadequate gas exchange at the alveolar-capillary membrane. Altitude hypoxia, the most common cause of hypoxia in aviation, occurs secondary to the decreased partial pressure of atmospheric oxygen at altitude. Anemic hypoxia results from a reduced oxygen-carrying capacity of hemoglobin in the blood, and can occur in conditions such as anemia, blood loss, carbon monoxide poisoning, or toxic methemoglobinemia. Stagnant hypoxia occurs when cardiac output fails to meet the body's metabolic demand, resulting in shock. Histotoxic hypoxia occurs when tissues are unable to utilize available oxygen secondary to poisoning of the cellular machinery that utilizes oxygen for energy. In other words, there is no oxygen deficiency at the cellular level, but rather an inability to utilize the available oxygen at the cellular level. A common poison that can result in histotoxic hypoxia is cyanide.

©2007 Pearson Education, Inc.
Critical Care Paramedic

6. Detail the signs and symptoms of hypoxia.   p. 61

The subjective and objective symptoms of hypoxia tend to worsen as altitude is gained. Objective symptoms at 10,000 feet include hyperventilation and impaired performance. At 18,000 feet, cyanosis, confusion, poor judgment, and muscular uncoordination are common. At altitudes greater than 20,000 feet, jerking of the upper limbs, seizures, and rapid unconsciousness are seen. Subjective symptoms at 5,000 feet include blurred vision and/or tunnel vision. Air hunger, apprehension, fatigue, headache, nausea, dizziness, and hot and cold flashes are common at altitudes of 10,000 feet, and numbness, tingling, euphoria, and belligerence are often seen at altitudes of about 15,000 feet.

Stages of hypoxia include the indifferent stage, compensatory stage, disturbance stage, and the critical stage. The indifferent stage is typified by subtle changes that are not easily observable. Heart and respiratory rate increase slightly, and night vision decreases by up to 28 percent. During the compensatory stage, the heart and respiratory rate continue to increase to compensate for the decreased FiO_2, and night vision is further decreased by up to 50 percent. During the disturbance stage, the body's normal physiological compensatory responses are inadequate and hypoxia is evident, both to the subject affected and to bystanders. The subject may experience air hunger, headache, decreased level of consciousness, euphoria, amnesia, belligerence, and nausea and vomiting (usually seen in children). Additional objective findings include impairment to the senses, mental processes, psychomotor functions, and changes in personality traits. In the critical stage of acute hypoxia, near complete mental and physical incapacitation results in loss of consciousness, seizures, respiratory failure, and death.

7. Describe the effective performance time.   p. 62

Effective performance time is the amount of time a person can perform flight duties in an environment with inadequate oxygen levels.

8. Describe the time of useful consciousness.   p. 62

The time of useful consciousness is measured from the time of exposure to an oxygen-deficient environment until useful consciousness is lost.

9. Discuss the pathophysiology and treatment of high-altitude pulmonary edema.   p. 68

High-altitude pulmonary edema (HAPE) is best described as pulmonary edema following ascent to altitude. It is a common condition encountered in mountaineering, but not in aviation, as cabins of high-flying aircraft are pressurized to lower altitude equivalents. HAPE is associated with a rapid ascent to altitudes greater than 8,000 feet, and lack of acclimatization increases the risk. It usually occurs after 48–96 hours at altitude, and is the most common cause of death from high-altitude illness.

Current theory suggests that increases in altitude result in an increased intracapillary pressure, promoting the leakage of plasma and protein across the capillary membrane and into the alveoli and interstitial space. Following descent, pulmonary artery pressure decreases, edema is corrected, and the basement membrane repairs itself. Descent to a lower altitude results in immediate improvement in the clinical condition.

Signs and symptoms of HAPE include crackles in at least one lung field, orthopnea, the production of pink, frothy sputum, a high-altitude cough, fever, cyanosis, tachycardia, and tachypnea. Treatment priorities include the application of airway control, supplemental oxygen, and immediate descent. Breathing assistance in the form of BVM ventilations, CPAP, or BiPAP may be necessary, and morphine and nifedipine can be considered in the treatment of HAPE.

10. Describe problems associated with altitude with which the critical care paramedic must be familiar.   p. 68

In addition to HAPE, HACE, and decompression, all previously described, the critical care paramedic should be familiar with other problems that may occur and may have a direct impact on the well-being of the patient and crew.

Decompression sickness is a condition characterized by a variety of symptoms that occurs from exposure to abruptly lower barometric pressure resulting in the dissolution of gas into the bloodstream. The same principles that apply to decompression sickness in divers apply to humans at altitude; compressed gas (in a pressurized cabin) is breathed, gas is absorbed into the bloodstream, and rapid decompression (think of a diver ascending too quickly) leads to the dissolution of gas (primarily nitrogen) in the bloodstream and the formation of gas bubbles.

It is uncommon for decompression sickness to occur below altitudes of 18,000 feet, and the incidence of decompression sickness is small below altitudes of 25,000–30,000 feet. The risk of decompression sickness following rapid decompression is only slightly greater than after a slow decompression, and is greater as the duration of exposure is lengthened.

Hypothermia secondary to exposure to cold, high-altitude atmosphere can vary in extent and severity depending on duration of exposure, severity of exposure, and the effectiveness of protective clothing worn by the individual.

Trapped gas emergencies can occur in the middle ear, sinuses, and teeth. During both ascent and descent, the middle ear may be unable to equalize with the ambient air pressure. A common cause is occlusion of the eustachian tube as a result of anatomical variation or swelling from infection or trauma. Symptoms include pain or pressure in the middle ear, muffled hearing, dizziness, and tinnitus. Middle ear pressure can be equalized with various maneuvers such as swallowing, yawning, tensing of the throat muscles, the Valsava maneuver, or chewing gum.

As with the middle ear, and for the same reasons, the sinuses may be unable to equalize with the ambient air pressure. In 70 percent of cases, the frontal sinuses are involved, with the maxillary sinuses being the next most frequently involved. Pain with descent occurs in 90 percent of cases, but can occur on ascent as well. With maxillary sinus involvement, pain can radiate to the teeth of the upper jaw and is often mistaken for a toothache. Unlike middle ear pressure, there are no maneuvers to alleviate sinus pressure.

The onset of barodentalgia varies between individuals, but usually develops between 5,000–15,000 feet and may or may not increase in severity as altitude increases. Pain is usually relieved upon descent, which can help distinguish it from maxillary sinus pain. The mechanism of barodentalgia is not fully understood, but it is associated with preexisting dental pathology such as carious teeth and those with fillings or pulpitis; healthy teeth do not seem to be affected.

11. Discuss the pathophysiology and treatment of high-altitude cerebral edema. p. 69

High-altitude cerebral edema (HACE) is cerebral edema following ascent to altitude, and is largely considered to be the end stage of acute mountain sickness (AMS). At altitudes greater than 5,280 feet, AMS affects every individual to some degree, with severity varying between individuals.

Current theory suggests that hypoxia-induced changes in the blood-brain barrier and increased cerebral blood flow lead to vasogenic edema and increased intracranial pressure. Signs and symptoms of HACE include headache, insomnia, anorexia, nausea, dizziness, weakness, altered mental status, and a decreasing level of consciousness.

Treatment priorities include airway and breathing control, supplemental oxygen administration, and rapid descent from altitude. In addition, steroids such as dexamethasone may decrease fluid loss from the cerebral microvasculature. Antiemetics such as prochloperazine (Compazine) and promethazine (Phenergan) can be used to alleviate nausea. Prophylactic treatment with acetazolamide (Diamox) is suggested for those individuals who will ascend to 10,000 feet. Acetazolamide increases the renal excretion of bicarbonate, producing a mild acidosis that can counter the respiratory alkalosis that occurs secondary to hyperventilation at altitude. The resultant mild acidosis may also act as a respiratory stimulant, decreasing the nocturnal periodic breathing that is typical at altitude.

12. Understand the consequences should there be a rapid decompression of the aircraft cabin at altitude. p. 69

Decompression is the loss of cabin pressure in an aircraft that is at altitude, and can be categorized as slow or rapid. Slow decompression occurs when a cabin seal develops a leak, and the insidious effects of slowly developing hypoxia are a significant danger. Rapid decompression, which can occur with the perforation of the aircraft wall or loss of a canopy or hatch, is significantly more destructive and considered more dangerous.

The principal factors that determine the rate and time of decompression include the size of the opening, the volume of the cabin, and the pressure ratio and differential between the cabin and atmospheric environments.

Physical characteristics of rapid decompression include noise, fogging, temperature changes, and flying debris. Some degree of noise will accompany decompression, with larger violations in the pressure seal resulting in louder noise production. Fogging can result during a rapid decompression as air pressure and temperature in the cabin are reduced. As the dew point is met, the cabin air's capacity to hold water vapor diminishes, and water vapor precipitates as fog and may freeze if the ambient temperature is cold enough. The rapid displacement of large volumes of air can result in unsecured items taking flight, and being extracted through the opening in the cabin wall.

Physiological effects of rapid decompression include hypoxia and pulmonary, ear and sinus, and gastrointestinal issues created by expanding gas. Hypoxia is the most significant issue following cabin decompression, and the use of supplemental oxygen during decompression can assist in the prevention, or at least attenuation, of hypoxia. The lungs are extremely vulnerable during decompression, with expansion injury likely if expanding air cannot escape through an open airway, as in cases of mechanical ventilation or breath holding. Pain production and injury to the middle ear and paranasal sinuses may occur during rapid decompression, and injury to the gastrointestinal tract is possible as well. In addition, abdominal distension secondary to trapped gas expansion can impede diaphragm movement and can result in respiratory impairment, and increased vagal stimulation secondary to increased intraabdominal pressure may result in cardiovascular depression.

13. **Discuss preventative measures the critical care paramedic can employ in order to reduce the effects of stressors that may occur during flight.** p. 73

Practices that can be utilized to minimize stress include the avoidance of smoking, gas-producing foods and liquids, chewing gum on ascent, and flying with a "head cold," congestion, or ear infection. In addition, being well rested, and remaining in your seat, properly restrained (to reduce vibration), can help reduce stress. Finally, in the unlikely event of an emergency, the air medical crew member should consider the time of useful consciousness and act accordingly.

Case Study

As the aircraft levels out of a turn, you unbuckle your seat belt and shimmy closer to your patient so that you can reassess him. The pilot informs you that your altitude is now 28,000 feet and the estimated arrival time to Chicago is a little under five hours.

Your patient is a 35-year-old male who was on holiday in the United Kingdom when he was involved in a serious motor vehicle crash. He is being transferred to a facility closer to home in the United States. The patient sustained multiple injuries in the accident including a lacerated liver, a right hemopneumothorax, and a subdural hematoma. It has been five days since the accident and he is relatively stable. His pneumothorax was nearly resolved on x-ray, but the chest tube has been left in place as a precaution against possible redevelopment. Although the additional tubes complicate the packaging of the patient, you are happy to know that, with the pressure changes en route and even the rare possibility of decompression at altitude, you will not have to worry about the development of a tension pneumothorax.

During your check of the airway, you palpate the pilot balloon of the endotracheal tube to ensure that the lower atmospheric pressure at altitude does not significantly increase the pressure within the cuff. During report, you were told that the patient received a blood transfusion two days ago, and that this morning's lab report showed a hemoglobin value of 11 g/dL and a hematocrit of 34 percent. Although essentially normal, these values are still low enough to raise concern for the possibility of anemic hypoxia. The patient's ventilator had been set at 40 percent FiO_2 at the sending ICU, but you increase the FiO_2 to 60 percent for the transfer to help prevent hypoxia from both anemia and the decreased partial pressure of oxygen at altitude. You pay close attention to the cardiac, SpO_2, and $ETCO_2$ monitors during the flight, realizing that the noise and vibration in the cabin make physical examinations more difficult. The cabin remains a little chilly, so you make sure the edges of the blankets are tucked in after your assessment. The patient had been specifically loaded head first into the aircraft in semi-Fowler's position to help reduce cerebral edema from any G-forces produced by the aircraft movement.

With checks every 10 minutes while en route, the trip is completed without incident and your patient is delivered to the awaiting ground critical care transport team without change. As the ambulance pulls away, your pilot helps you load the equipment back in the aircraft, before you head to the lounge. It's time for a nice long meal break and a good night's sleep.

DISCUSSION QUESTIONS

1. In brief, what is the practical significance of gas physics and physiology as it relates to "stressors of altitude"?
2. Describe some methods to combat "stressors of altitude."
3. What are some "stressors of flight"?
4. Describe some methods to combat "stressors of flight."

Content Review

MULTIPLE CHOICE

_____ 1. The _____ is located between 53 and 372 miles high.
A. troposphere
B. stratosphere
C. mesosphere
D. thermosphere

_____ 2. Weather, as well as all air medical flights, occurs in the:
A. troposphere.
B. stratosphere.
C. mesosphere.
D. thermosphere.

_____ 3. The atmosphere is composed primarily of:
A. nitrogen, oxygen, carbon monoxide, and trace gases.
B. nitrogen, oxygen, argon, and trace gases.
C. oxygen, nitrogen, carbon dioxide, and xenon.
D. oxygen and carbon dioxide.

_____ 4. The three zones of the atmosphere, from the surface of the Earth outward, are the:
A. physiologically deficient zone, physiological zone, and outer space.
B. physiological zone, physiologically deficient zone, and outer space.
C. physiological zone, physiologically deficient zone, and the space-equivalent zone.
D. near-Earth zone, physiologically deficient zone, and space-equivalent zone.

_____ 5. The human body is well adapted to survive in the:
A. space-equivalent zone.
B. physiologically deficient zone.
C. near-Earth zone.
D. physiological zone.

_____ 6. The physiologically deficient zone extends from about:
A. 5,000–10,000 feet.
B. 10,000–15,000 feet.
C. 10,000–50,000 feet.
D. 15,000–25,000 feet.

_____ 7. Rotor-wing aircraft typically operate in the:
A. space-equivalent zone.
B. physiologically deficient zone.
C. near-Earth zone.
D. physiological zone.

_____ 8. 1 atm is equal to:
A. 760 mmHg.
B. 1.01325 Bar.
C. 29.92 inches Hg.
D. all of the above.

_____ 9. The four gases that impact aviation medicine are:
   A. water vapor, carbon monoxide, oxygen, and nitrogen.
   B. oxygen, carbon dioxide, nitrogen, and water vapor.
   C. oxygen, carbon dioxide, nitrogen, and trace gases.
   D. oxygen, carbon monoxide, nitrogen, and trace gases.

_____ 10. Which gas law states that the total pressure in a container is the sum of the partial pressures of all the gases in the container?
   A. Dalton's law   C. Henry's law
   B. Boyle's law   D. Gay-Lussac's law

_____ 11. Which gas law states that the volume of a gas is inversely proportional to its pressure, assuming that temperature remains constant?
   A. Graham's law   C. Henry's law
   B. Boyle's law   D. Gay-Lussac's law

_____ 12. Which gas law states that the volume of a quantity of gas, held at constant pressure, varies directly with the temperature of the gas?
   A. Graham's law   C. Charles' law
   B. Boyle's law   D. Fick's law

_____ 13. Which gas law states that the amount of pressure of a fixed amount of gas, at a fixed volume, is proportional to the temperature?
   A. Graham's law   C. Henry's law
   B. Avogadro's law   D. Gay-Lussac's law

_____ 14. Which gas law states that at equilibrium, the amount of gas dissolved in a given volume of liquid is directly proportional to the partial pressure of that gas in the gas phase above the liquid surface?
   A. ideal gas law   C. Henry's law
   B. Avogadro's law   D. Gay-Lussac's law

_____ 15. Which gas law states that the rate at which a gas diffuses is inversely proportional to the square root of its density?
   A. ideal gas law   C. Graham's law
   B. Avogadro's law   D. Gay-Lussac's law

_____ 16. Which gas law states that equal volumes of all gases under identical conditions of pressure and temperature contain the same number of molecules?
   A. Avogadro's law   C. Graham's law
   B. ideal gas law   D. Fick's law

_____ 17. Which gas law states that the net diffusion of a gas across a fluid membrane is proportional to the difference in partial pressure across the membrane, proportional to the area of the membrane, and inversely proportional to the thickness of the membrane?
   A. ideal gas law   C. Henry's law
   B. Avogadro's law   D. Gay-Lussac's law

_____ 18. Which type of gas obeys Boyle's law, Charles' law, and Avogadro's law exactly?
   A. an ideal gas   C. carbon dioxide
   B. oxygen   D. a stable gas

_____ 19. Your patient, a 32-year-old male with a pneumothorax, is intubated prior to rotor-wing air transport. As the aircraft ascends to its cruising altitude of 3,800 feet, you would expect that, to some degree, the endotracheal tube cuff volume would:
   A. decrease in accordance with Henry's law.
   B. increase in accordance with Boyle's law.
   C. increase in accordance with Dalton's law.
   D. decrease in accordance with Boyle's law.

_____ 20. During your routine pre-shift equipment check in your heated hanger, you note that your portable oxygen cylinder has 1,500 lbs of pressure. The oxygen cylinder is placed in an unheated, outside storage compartment, and the aircraft is placed outside in 42°F weather. Later that day, you arrive on a scene call and note that the oxygen cylinder is cold to the touch. Assuming that the oxygen has not been used and there are no leaks, you would expect the pressure in the cylinder to:
A. be the same as during checkout.
B. have decreased in accordance with Charles' law.
C. have decreased in accordance with Gay-Lussac's law.
D. have increased in accordance with Charles' law.

_____ 21. A nonrebreather mask with an oxygen flow rate of 15 lpm is placed on a patient who is breathing normally at 16 times a minute. You would expect arterial oxygen concentration to:
A. decrease in accordance with Gay-Lussac's law.
B. increase in accordance with Gay-Lussac's law.
C. increase in accordance with Henry's law.
D. increase in accordance with Avogadro's law.

_____ 22. In emphysema, alveolar tissue is destroyed and replaced with scar tissue, resulting in decreased alveolar surface area and a thickened and scarred capillary-alveolar membrane. With regard to oxygen diffusion across the remaining alveolar membrane, you could expect:
A. decreased diffusion in accordance with Fick's law.
B. decreased diffusion in accordance with Avogadro's law.
C. diffusion to remain the same in accordance with the ideal gas law.
D. increased diffusion in accordance with Gay-Lussac's law.

_____ 23. Stressors of altitude include all of the following except:
A. fatigue.
B. vibration.
C. hypoxia.
D. dehydration.

_____ 24. Stressors of flight include all of the following except:
A. gravitational forces.
B. spatial disorientation.
C. thermal changes.
D. flicker vertigo.

_____ 25. Your patient has experienced a chemical inhalation that has burned and disrupted his alveolar-capillary membrane, resulting in poor gas exchange and a PaO_2 of 62 mmHg. Which of the following categories of hypoxia does this situation represent?
A. anemic hypoxia
B. hypoxic hypoxia
C. stagnant hypoxia
D. histotoxic hypoxia

_____ 26. Your patient has suffered a massive AMI resulting in cardiogenic shock and a PaO_2 of 68 mmHg. Which of the following categories of hypoxia does this situation represent?
A. anemic hypoxia
B. hypoxic hypoxia
C. stagnant hypoxia
D. histotoxic hypoxia

_____ 27. Your patient has ingested a poison that disrupts the mitochondrial utilization of oxygen, resulting in a PaO_2 of 59 mmHg. Which of the following categories of hypoxia does this situation represent?
A. anemic hypoxia
B. hypoxic hypoxia
C. stagnant hypoxia
D. histotoxic hypoxia

_____ 28. A pediatric patient presents with a PaO_2 of 61 mmHg secondary to an autoimmune hemolysis triggered by an infection. Which of the following categories of hypoxia does this situation represent?
A. anemic hypoxia
B. hypoxic hypoxia
C. stagnant hypoxia
D. histotoxic hypoxia

_____ 29. A fixed-wing aircraft develops a slow pressure leak while at altitude, resulting in a decrease in available atmospheric oxygen. One of the air medical crew members notes that she can't catch her breath, is tachycardic, tachypnic, and has a headache. Based on her symptoms, she is most likely in which stage of hypoxia?
- A. indifferent stage
- B. compensatory stage
- C. disturbance stage
- D. critical stage

_____ 30. The term _____ is used to describe the time period from the point of exposure to an oxygen-deficient environment until useful consciousness is lost.
- A. time of useful consciousness
- B. effective performance time
- C. time of useful performance
- D. effective consciousness time

_____ 31. Factors that contribute to patient and air medical crew fatigue include all of the following except:
- A. alcohol use.
- B. temperature changes.
- C. aircraft vibration and noise.
- D. dew point changes.

_____ 32. Which of the following statements regarding humidity and dew point is true?
- A. The relative humidity is the percent of saturation humidity compared to the amount of water vapor in the air.
- B. The relative humidity of air does not change unless the dew point and air temperature are equal.
- C. When the air temperature and dew point temperature are equal, water precipitates.
- D. Relative humidity is the temperature at which the dew point reaches 100 percent.

_____ 33. Air at altitude:
- A. is colder and dryer.
- B. can worsen existing dehydration.
- C. can necessitate the need for usual fluid replacement earlier.
- D. all of the above.

_____ 34. Identify the type of force appreciated during takeoff or changes in forward airspeed.
- A. linear acceleration
- B. radial acceleration
- C. angular acceleration
- D. centripetal force

_____ 35. The effects of accelerative forces experienced during flight are dependent on several factors including:
- A. altitude.
- B. atmospheric pressure.
- C. barometric pressure.
- D. rate of onset.

_____ 36. Which of the following statements regarding the third spacing of fluids is true?
- A. Third spacing occurs more frequently with long-distance, high-altitude flights.
- B. Third spacing occurs secondary to increased intravascular pressure and decreased cell membrane permeability.
- C. The prophylactic use of diuretics is recommended to prevent third spacing during flight.
- D. Special disorientation can aggravate third spacing of fluids.

_____ 37. An air medical pilot is experiencing an overwhelming sensation of movement and cannot orient himself with visual cues or aircraft instruments. Which category of spatial disorientation is he experiencing?
- A. Type IV (unrecognized)
- B. Type II (recognized)
- C. Type III (incapacitating)
- D. Type IV (debilitating)

_____ 38. All of the following are methods to prevent spatial disorientation except:
- A. flying only when visual reference points are available.
- B. chewing gum during flight.
- C. utilizing effective scanning techniques.
- D. never staring at lights.

_____ 39. Vertigo can best be described as:
   A. a disturbance of inner ear equilibrium characterized by a sensation of spinning.
   B. the inability to determine one's position, attitude, and motion relative to the surface of the Earth or fixed objects.
   C. the effects of accelerative forces including dizziness, nausea, and vomiting.
   D. cerebellar disturbances resulting in a sensation of spinning.

_____ 40. You are cruising back to your base at an altitude of 1,800 feet above sea level. While staring at the helicopter's anticollision lights, you develop a sensation that the aircraft is moving around you. You are most likely suffering from:
   A. air sickness.   C. flicker vertigo.
   B. vertigo.   D. altitude sickness.

_____ 41. High-altitude pulmonary edema (HAPE) can best be described as:
   A. pulmonary edema secondary to cardiac complications of altitude.
   B. pulmonary edema following ascent to altitude.
   C. a frequent hazard of aviation medicine.
   D. the movement of fluid across the alveolar-capillary membrane.

_____ 42. Which of the following statements regarding the pathophysiology of high-altitude pulmonary edema (HAPE) is false?
   A. Intracapillary pressure increases with altitude.
   B. Increases in intracapillary pressure disrupt the capillary basement membrane.
   C. Decreased arterial oxygen partial pressure results in increased capillary-alveolar membrane permeability.
   D. Plasma and proteins leak across the capillary-alveolar membrane into the alveoli and interstitial space.

_____ 43. The treatment of high-altitude pulmonary edema (HAPE) may include all of the following except:
   A. supplemental oxygen administration.   C. morphine administration.
   B. immediate descent.   D. diuretic administration.

_____ 44. High-altitude cerebral edema (HACE) can best be described as:
   A. cerebral edema following ascent to altitude.
   B. altered mental status and loss of consciousness following ascent to altitude.
   C. increased intracranial pressure following ascent to altitude.
   D. the end stage of severe mountain sickness (SMS).

_____ 45. Which of the following statements regarding the pathophysiology of high-altitude cerebral edema (HACE) is false?
   A. Hypoxia induces changes in blood-brain barrier permeability.
   B. Increased cerebral blood flow leads to increased intracranial pressure.
   C. Cerebral endothelium permeability occurs secondary to hypoxia.
   D. Protein leakage into cerebral tissue results in increased osmotic flow and increased intracranial pressure.

_____ 46. Signs and symptoms of high-altitude cerebral edema (HACE) include:
   A. headache, dizziness, altered mental status, and decreased level of conscious.
   B. difficulty breathing, tachycardia, and tachypnea.
   C. dizziness, weakness, seizures, and respiratory arrest.
   D. altered mental status, decreased level of consciousness, coma, and seizures.

_____ 47. Treatment for high-altitude cerebral edema (HACE) includes all of the following except:
   A. prophylactic use of acetazolamide.
   B. administration of prochlorperazine or promethazine.
   C. administration of osmotic diuretics such as bumex.
   D. rapid descent from altitude.

©2007 Pearson Education, Inc.
Critical Care Paramedic

_____ **48.** A loss of cabin pressure at altitude secondary to a perforation of the cabin wall that results in unsecured items becoming airborne is termed a:
A. rapid decompression.
B. destructive decompression.
C. slow decompression.
D. violation decompression.

_____ **49.** Factors that control the rate of decompression include all of the following except the:
A. size of the opening.
B. pressure ratio between the cabin and atmosphere.
C. temperature of the atmosphere.
D. volume of the cabin.

_____ **50.** Which of the following is not a physical characteristic of rapid decompression?
A. fogging
B. noise
C. temperature change
D. increased barometric pressure

_____ **51.** Which of the following statements regarding trapped gas emergencies is true?
A. During ascent, gas trapped in body cavities compresses.
B. Ear pain can occur when the middle ear is unable to equalize with the eustachian tube.
C. Pain from trapped gas in the sinuses occurs only on ascent.
D. Carious teeth and pulpitis are thought to contribute to barodentalgia.

_____ **52.** Which of the following is not a recommended way of reducing stress in the aeromedical workplace?
A. using decongestants such as diphenhydramine
B. avoiding gas-producing foods and liquids
C. avoiding flying with "head colds," congestion, or ear infections
D. remaining in one's seat, properly restrained

_____ **53.** Your patient is a 43-year-old male CAO in severe respiratory distress, being transported from a ski resort located at 10,300 feet. Ski patrol reports the patient flew into town this morning from sea level and immediately went skiing, reaching altitudes as high as 14,000 feet on the mountain. The patient describes an acute onset of shortness of breath that became worse over 2 hours. He has no PMH, takes no medications, and has no allergies. Vital signs: HR = 140 and regular, RR = 22 and labored, BP = 138/80, SpO_2 = 83 percent on room air, temperature = 100.6°F tympanic. Physical exam reveals crackles and wheezing to the lower and mid lobes bilaterally. Based on the clinical findings, which of the following would be the best treatment for this patient?
A. intubation, supplemental oxygen, cardiac monitoring, IV access, morphine IV, nifedipine IV, and immediate descent
B. oxygen via nonrebreather mask 15 lpm, cardiac monitoring, IV access, and immediate descent
C. RSI, intubation, positive pressure ventilation with supplemental oxygen, morphine IV, and immediate descent
D. oxygen via nasal cannula 4 lpm, cardiac monitoring, IV access, and immediate descent

_____ **54.** Your patient is a 33-year-old male ice climber who presents unconscious at a campground at 11,000 feet. His climbing partners describe a 2-day history of headache and dizziness that progressed to odd behavior, altered mental status, and eventual unconsciousness. Vital signs: HR = 92 regular, R = 10 shallow, BP = 142/96, SpO_2 = 92 percent. You note that the patient is unresponsive to painful stimuli. Based on the clinical findings, which of the following would be the best treatment for this patient?
A. oxygen via nonrebreather mask 15 lpm, IV access, cardiac monitoring, and prochlorperazine IV
B. oxygen via nonrebreather mask 15 lpm, IV access, cardiac monitoring, prochlorperazine IV, acetazolamode IV, and rapid descent
C. intubation, positive pressure ventilation with supplemental oxygen, IV access, cardiac monitoring, acetazolamode IV, and rapid descent
D. intubation, positive pressure ventilation with supplemental oxygen, IV access, cardiac monitoring, and acetazolamode IV

5 Flight Safety and Survival

Review of Chapter Objectives

Upon completion of this chapter, the student should be able to:

1. Name and discuss several facets of rotor-wing (and fixed-wing) transportation imperative to the safe completion of each mission. p. 80

Air medical transport is a unique work environment with numerous inherent dangers. The flight crew is responsible for patient and crew safety, and safe operations require effective leadership, team member coordination, and assertiveness. Aeromedicine is not inherently dangerous, but it can be unforgiving; lack of operation and safety knowledge can contribute to risk, and lax attitudes can contribute to failure. Having a "safety conscious" attitude is a must in this industry.

Flight safety can be defined as those plans that are incorporated into daily flight operations that serve to eliminate or reduce risk so that each mission can be undertaken without incident. The goals of flight safety are to assess risk, prioritize identified risks, minimize risk with the implementation of safety plans, and to establish a monitoring system to determine the risk reduction program effectiveness.

Flight safety awareness programs are usually facilitated by a safety committee, commonly made up of representatives from management, flight crew members (pilots and medical crew), and maintenance and communications personnel. Responsibilities of the safety committee include the maintaining of an open forum to identify risk, the integration of identified risks into risk reduction programs, and the establishment of a review process to keep risk appreciation current.

The National Transportation Safety Board (NTSB) is an independent federal agency charged by Congress to investigate every civil aviation accident in the United States. NTSB studies and recommendations are often utilized by program safety committees and incorporated into daily safety practice. For example, in the late 1980s, the NTSB made recommendations to the Federal Aviation Administration (FAA), Association of Air Medical Services (AAMS), and the National Aeronautics and Space Administration (NASA) after an investigation into medical flight accidents. Recommendations included improved, poor-weather, piloting education; prioritizing incoming calls; aircraft interior enhancements to improve crew safety; and ongoing research into the risks and hazards associated with flight programs.

Safety consciousness is an important component of a flight safety program, and is defined as the ability of flight crew members to actively look for risks. The degree of safety consciousness can vary between individuals, with some individuals willing to take "acceptable risks." It is generally accepted that an individual's "acceptable risk" should not be greater than that of other crew members. If one crew member feels that a mission carries too much risk, the mission is cancelled, as the perception of risk affects job performance, increasing the incidence of errors.

It is the responsibility of the aeromedical crew to ensure that every mission meets established safety needs, and the following list offers examples of components of aeromedical transport that crew members need to be constantly attentive to.
1. Following all program preflight guidelines
2. Ensuring that the aircraft is ready to take off
3. Noting any irregularities to the takeoff or landing locations
4. Preparing all on-board equipment for flight
5. Use of safety devices (helmets, clothing, restraint systems)
6. Proper securing of patient within aircraft
7. Utilizing proper communication channels
8. Adequate use of interior lighting during night missions
9. Isolation of the pilot and aircraft controls from the patient compartment
10. Maintaining good personal, physical, and mental health

2. Briefly describe the following helicopter components:

Airframe (p. 82): The main structure of the aircraft to which all other components are attached.

Fuselage (p. 83): The external body of the aircraft that surrounds the airframe and components.

Tail boom (p. 83): The tail boom extends aft of the airframe and serves as both attachment points for horizontal and vertical stabilizers, and as a housing for the tail rotor.

Tail rotor system (p. 83): The small, vertical rotor at the distal end of the tail boom. The tail rotor compensates for torque created by the turning of the main rotor system.

Main rotor system (p. 83): The large, horizontal blades located above the fuselage that produce aircraft lift and thrust.

Engines (p. 83): The engines supply power to both rotor systems. They are attached to the airframe (frequently located above the patient compartment), and are protected externally by cowls and coverings.

Transmission (p. 84): Connected to both the engine and the rotor systems, the transmission converts power from the engines into rotational power that is transferred to the main and tail rotors via drive shafts.

Landing gear (p. 84): Landing gear can come in the form of skids, floats, wheels, or retractable gear.

Horizontal and vertical stabilizers (p. 84): Attached to the tail boom, they provide stabilization to the aircraft while airborne. The size and physical appearance of stabilizers differ between aircraft models.

3. Briefly describe the following helicopter flight controls:

Collective pitch control (p. 85): Large, round level located at the pilot's side. The collective controls altitude by changing the pitch angle of the rotor blades; the sharper the pitch angle, the more air is directed downward, causing the aircraft to rise.

Cyclic pitch control (p. 86): The "stick" located between the pilot's legs. The cyclic controls aircraft direction and airspeed; moving the cyclic forward tilts the rotor system forward and results in air being directing downward and aft, thus moving the aircraft forward and up.

Throttle (p. 86): The "twisting" handle on the collective pitch control lever, the throttle controls the RPM of the rotor system and provides the thrust necessary for flight. It is analogous to the gas pedal in a car.

Foot pedals (p. 86): Located at the pilot's feet, the foot pedals control the pitch angle of the tail rotor blades which prevents the aircraft from spinning uncontrollably, and also allows for the turning of the aircraft.

4. Describe the importance of the pilot safety brief.   **p. 88**

The pilot safety brief is conducted prior to the start of each mission, and helps to maintain a safe environment by promoting communication between crew members, reinforcing the need for effective communication between pilots and medical crews. Issues discussed can include the current or forecasted weather conditions, aircraft weights and balances, fuel capacity, and operational issues.

5. List and describe the common hazards of operating around a helicopter.   p. 89

Main rotor system: Helicopter main rotor systems usually consist of two to five blades turning at speeds of 290 to 400 rpm, reaching speeds of up to 500 mph at the blade tips. Wind gusts may lower the blade tips to within 4 feet of the ground while the blades are turning at low rpm. All personal gear and equipment should be adequately secured and protected from rotor wash to prevent airborne objects from causing injury or being pulled into the rotor system.

Tail rotor: Compared to the main rotor system, the tail rotor system is much lower to the ground, increasing the possibility for serious injury or death. As it spins at greater than 2,000 rpm, it is virtually impossible to visualize.

Rotor wash: Rotor wash produced while the rotor systems are spinning can propel objects at high rates of speed. During warm up and cool down, wind speeds of 25 mph are typical, and wind speeds in excess of 50–150 mph are possible during operational power.

Landing zone issues: Landing zone hazards include utility poles, trees, fences, and power wires, and should be identified to the pilot to ensure safe operations. All crew members should be observant for obstacles during landing, takeoff, and while on scene.

Approaching/departing the aircraft: Approaching and departing the aircraft, even for crew members, is done at the pilot's discretion. Operating around a "hot" aircraft should be done within direct visual contact with the pilot, which is best achieved by positioning oneself at the 10 or 2 o'clock position with regard to the nose of the aircraft. The pilot will indicate when it is safe to operate around the aircraft, usually with a "thumbs up" signal.

Air traffic: All crew members should share the responsibility of identifying other aircraft in your aircraft's airspace, utilizing the clock code to relay location information to the pilot.

6. Explain the importance of perimeter guards at landing zones.   p. 90

Perimeter guards are essential to safe flight operations at an incident scene landing zone. The perimeter guard should position himself not less than 50 feet from the nose of the aircraft, remaining in visual contact with the pilot at all times. All movement to and from the aircraft should occur via the perimeter guard. The guard, who has no direct involvement in patient care, extrication, or rescue, is focused on the job at hand, in order to protect persons around the aircraft. In addition, a tail guard should be utilized whenever personnel will be around the rear of the aircraft (as when loading a patient), to prevent individuals from walking into the tail rotor.

7. Understand the importance of proper rest and nutrition for the flight paramedic.   p. 90

The aeromedical environment is both physically and mentally demanding, and requires physical stamina and emotional stability; adequate rest and nutritional habits are necessary to meet these demands. Crew members should be well rested prior to their shift, ideally having 8–10 hours of uninterrupted sleep. Rest periods during shifts are recommended, if possible, during periods of low call volume.

As the stressors of flight combined with poor nutritional intake can affect performance, flight crew personnel must maintain adequate intake throughout their duty period. Due to the possibility of significant time periods between meals, flight crew members should consider ingesting several, small, high-energy meals throughout their shift.

8. Describe the various types of personal protection equipment, and understand the importance of their use.   p. 91

Personal protective equipment available to flight crew members includes helmets, fire-resistant clothing, protective footwear, hearing protection, and eye protection. Helmets are typically constructed of a graphite or Spectra composite shell and provide protection to the wearer's head, eyes, and ears, both on scene and in the aircraft. Helmet use is not an industry standard, and their utilization is up to the individual and/or his flight program.

Fire-resistant clothing protects crew members from burns in cases of post-accident fire. The clothing can withstand high temperature for about 20 seconds, hopefully allowing the wearer to remove herself from the environment. Typically, a one-piece "coverall" type of style is utilized, with a Kevlar or Nomex fiber uniform worn over cotton, silk, or wool undergarments. Gloves, constructed of Nomex or leather, provide protection to the hands.

Protective footwear is especially important on scene calls. Characteristics of a good boot include leather construction; thick, oil resistant soles; steel toes; support above the ankle; and vents to prevent moisture buildup.

Hearing protection is beneficial in reducing long-term hearing loss. Types of hearing protection include headphones, helmets, earplugs, and earmuffs. Eye protection reduces the risk of eye injury on scene, and can also decrease exposure risk during transports.

9. **List and describe the responsibilities (duties) of each air medical crew member:**

Preflight duties (p. 92): Preflight procedures are tasks completed prior to a mission that ensure safety. A preflight "walk around" can ensure that the ground around the aircraft is free of debris that may be blown or picked up by the rotor systems, and any aircraft issues that may compromise safety are identified. A popular mantra is "cords, covers, and cowlings." All electrical cords should be removed from their attachment points on the aircraft and properly secured, and all rotor tie-down straps should be removed and properly stored. All vent, window, and fuel covers should be removed and properly stored. All engine casing cowlings should be secured, and all locking mechanisms engaged. All equipment should be secured inside the cabin, and each individual should be properly restrained in his seat. The internal communication systems should be activated, and "sterile cockpit" rules respected. No nonessential communications should take place during liftoff, taxiing, and landing.

In-flight duties (p. 94): In-flight duties are those procedures performed while the aircraft is en route to its destination to ensure the highest degree of safety. All crew members should be restrained at all times, though brief periods of unrestrained activity are acceptable if patient care demands it. All crew members should remain on the internal communications system, and all equipment should be secured unless its use demands otherwise. Whenever possible, all crew members should actively scan for the presence of hazards such as other aircraft, buildings, wires, and towers. Hazards are identified to the pilot utilizing the clock method.

Post-flight duties (p. 95): Post-flight duties are procedures performed during the landing and exiting of the aircraft. A "fly around" is performed above the landing zone to identify potential hazards, and all crew members not involved in other tasks should assist. During a "hot unload," the patient is removed from the aircraft while the engines are running. Predetermination of responsibilities during patient removal is essential to protect the crew, patient, and any receiving staff assisting the crew. The air crew should be cognizant of all bystanders and care providers approaching the aircraft, and should provide direction to ensure safety. All individuals operating about the aircraft should be cognizant of the location of exhaust vents and tail rotor. All individuals should exit from under the main rotor system at the front of the aircraft, keeping their heads low, as the rotor blades can "flap" with wind gusts. If the helicopter is sitting on uneven ground, all exiting from under the main rotor system should take place on the downhill side.

10. **Understand and be able to utilize the clock code in relation to describing objects' position to the aircraft.**   p. 94

The clock-code system assumes that the nose of the aircraft is pointing at the 12 o'clock position, rendering 3 o'clock off to the right side, 9 o'clock to the left, and 6 o'clock to the rear. In addition, the term "low" is used to identify objects below the level of the aircraft, and "high" used for those objects above.

11. Discuss the additional duties of the medical flight crew in instances of in-flight or post-accident emergencies.   pp. 97, 98

In-flight emergency responsibilities are not left up to chance. Air medical programs will generally assign specific responsibilities to specific crew members. During an in-flight emergency, crew members should first, and foremost, follow any directions issued by the pilot. In addition, crew members should confirm that an emergency exists, and relay as much information as possible to the communications center, including current coordinates and a brief description of the emergency. To help prevent a post-emergency fire, the power inverter should be disabled and the main oxygen supply shut off. The patient should be prepared for an emergency landing by ensuring that he is in a supine position, and that all belts and straps are secure. Crew members other than the pilot should prepare for the emergency landing by tightening all safety straps and harnesses and assuming a survival position.

Post-accident duties should be performed immediately following an unplanned landing by those crew members not incapacitated by the event, regardless of impact severity. All crew members should meet with other surviving crew members at a predetermined location. Attempted rescue of other surviving crew members trapped in the wreckage should be undertaken with scene safety in mind. Survivors should be assessed for injuries, and attempts at stabilization made. Supplies should be salvaged from the wreckage, and the emergency locator transmitter (ELT) located and its activation assured. Unless the unplanned landing took place in a populated area, all survivors should remain with the aircraft.

12. Describe the "rule of threes" as it pertains to survival situations.   p. 99

The "rule of threes" states that a person can survive 3 minutes without oxygen, 3 hours in extreme weather without shelter, 3 days without water, and 3 weeks without food. In survival situations, this mantra will help prioritize the surviving air crews' actions.

13. Be able to discuss common strategies to provide shelter, food, and water in a survival situation.   p. 100

Obtaining or creating shelter is the first component of a survival situation. Shelter provides protection, aids in heat preservation, and provides a psychological boost. The aircraft fuselage should be used, if possible, or a shelter constructed if the fuselage is uninhabitable. If forced to construct a shelter, one should build, in order, a roof, floor, windward wall, and remaining walls. In addition to providing heat and being a strong psychological boost, a fire provides a method for drying wet clothes, and providing light and signal smoke.

Hydration is imperative in survival situations, and a water source should be sought early in the event. If water is unavailable, consider recovering IV and irrigation supplies from the aircraft wreckage, and consider collecting condensation or melting snow.

Food procurement is the last priority in a survival situation, as one's body fat, carbohydrate, and protein stores will be an adequate energy supply for days. Rationing of available food to keep all crew members healthy is advisable, and care should be taken if edible food sources from the surrounding environment will be ingested, as gastrointestinal illness can lead to dehydration and death.

Case Study

The aircraft heat has been on since takeoff and you still feel a chill up your spine. It's mid-January and the temperature has not reached above 10°F in four days. Looking forward and down through the chin bubble of the Bell 407, you see nothing but the stark, white ground. Since the severe winter weather of the past two days blanketed the area, even the evergreen color of the hemlock forest below is muted white.

You are responding to the scene of a teenager whose snowmobile fell through the ice approximately two hours ago. The GPS gives an ETA of six minutes to the scene and both you and the pilot are straining your eyes to locate the landing zone (LZ). Looking over the landscape, you can't help but wonder how long it would take your aircraft to be found if it was forced down in these woods. It has been at least 30 minutes since you have seen a building or even a road. What if another storm was to move into the area and no one could fly?

During the pilot's safety brief this morning, equipment weight concerns were discussed, and, even though this particular aircraft has such a limited useful payload, you feel glad that part of it is absorbed by the cold weather survival gear. You think using the "rule of threes," that in this weather you might make it three hours without survival gear before exposure set in. That thought quickly fades from your mind as you and the pilot both see the LZ. "There it is," the pilot announces over the intercom, "red lights 10 o'clock low." The pilot banks the aircraft to the left and begins a high, clockwise, reconnaissance orbit of the LZ. No hazards are noted, and, after conferring with the LZ coordinator, the pilot announces that you are turning for final approach to landing. After landing and confirming with the pilot that it is OK to exit the aircraft, you place the clear visor of your helmet down, secure the side door, and move directly to the 10 o'clock position to make eye contact with the pilot. He gives you the "OK" sign with finger and thumb indicating it is safe to move out under the rotors to the awaiting ambulance.

After assessing the patient, you determine that he will need his airway secured. You advise the pilot of that fact and of the patient's approximate weight by portable radio. After intubating and securely packaging the patient, you let the pilot know that you are ready to load. After gently sliding a tapered spine board under the patient, you enlist the help of three other rescue personnel on scene to carry the patient to the aircraft. Returning to the 12 o'clock position, you note that the pilot has locked open the side door of the aircraft and motions to you that it is OK to approach. As you load the patient into the port side of the helicopter, the pilot stands aft of the door to act as a guard and prevent any personnel from approaching the tail boom area, a procedure used even though the tail rotor is not in motion at this time. After the patient and equipment are well secured, you survey the area visible to you outside the aircraft and announce over the intercom, "All set back here. You are clear left, right, and above."

The flight and patient transfer at the trauma center are without incident. While finishing the run report in the ED, it occurs to you that you have finally stopped feeling chilled, and you ask Karen, the ED receptionist, "How many months until spring?"

DISCUSSION QUESTIONS

1. What is flight safety?
2. What procedures can help a program ensure flight safety?
3. What are some common survival strategies to provide shelter, fire, and water in a survival situation?

Content Review

MULTIPLE CHOICE

_____ 1. Flight safety can best be defined as:
   A. eliminating all risks involved with flight operations.
   B. plans that are incorporated into daily flight operations that help to reduce or eliminate risk.
   C. a course offered by the NTSB, required for all air medical crew members.
   D. tracking the progress of all flights to ensure that safety standards are adhered to.

_____ 2. Air medical flight program safety committees are usually made up of representatives from:
   A. management, maintenance, communications, and flight crews.
   B. board members, management, medical personnel, and pilots.
   C. NTSB, flight crews, management, and communications.
   D. local EMS services, management, flight crews, and communications.

©2007 Pearson Education, Inc.
Critical Care Paramedic

_____ 3. An air medical crew consisting of a pilot, nurse, and paramedic are dispatched to a rural hospital for a transfer to their tertiary care facility. The pilot reports that the radar shows heavy rain and lightning storms along the route of travel. Based on the weather report, the paramedic states that he is uncomfortable proceeding with the mission. According to the theory of safety consciousness, which of the following scenarios is most likely to occur?
   A. The pilot and nurse will pressure the paramedic into proceeding with the mission.
   B. The paramedic should be disciplined for not wanting to proceed with the mission.
   C. The mission will be refused, and possibly attempted if, and when, the weather improves.
   D. The pilot and nurse should proceed without the paramedic.

_____ 4. The _____ of a helicopter extends aft of the airframe and serves both as attachment points for horizontal and vertical stabilizers and as a housing for the tail rotor.
   A. tail rotor   C. tail boom
   B. transmission   D. fuselage

_____ 5. The _____ of a helicopter is connected to both the engine and the rotor systems and converts power from the engines into rotational power that is transferred to the main and tail rotors via drive shafts.
   A. engines   C. tail rotor system
   B. main rotor system   D. transmission

_____ 6. The _____ is located between the pilot's legs, and controls aircraft direction and airspeed.
   A. cyclic pitch control   C. collective pitch control
   B. throttle   D. foot pedal

_____ 7. Which of the following statements regarding the pilot safety brief is false?
   A. The pilot safety brief is conducted prior to the start of every mission.
   B. The pilot safety brief helps maintain a safe environment by encouraging communication between crew members.
   C. Issues discussed in the pilot's safety brief can include weather reports, weight limits and balances, and fuel capacity.
   D. The pilot safety brief is targeted at newer, less experienced members of the flight team.

_____ 8. Common hazards associated with operating around a running helicopter that is on the ground in a landing zone include the:
   A. tail rotor, main rotor system, hypoxia, and rotor wash.
   B. rotor wash, main rotor system, and tail rotor.
   C. air traffic, rotor wash, main rotor system, and tail rotor.
   D. cabin decompression, rotor wash, main rotor system, and tail rotor.

_____ 9. Which of the following best describes who is responsible for identifying other aircraft in your helicopter's airspace?
   A. all crew members, all of the time
   B. all crew members not involved in patient care at the time
   C. the pilot only
   D. air medical crew only

_____ 10. Which statement regarding the role of the perimeter guard is true?
   A. The perimeter guard should not have any additional responsibilities at the scene.
   B. The perimeter guard should be located within 50 feet of the nose of the aircraft, in visual contact with the pilot.
   C. The perimeter guard controls movement to and from the front and rear of the aircraft.
   D. The perimeter guard is responsible for relaying all radio communications between the helicopter and the ground crew.

_____ 11. Which of the following statements regarding rest and nutrition for the flight crew member is true?
  A. Flight crew members should "load up" with large meals prior to their shift, in anticipation of inadequate time available for meals.
  B. Air crew members should get eight to ten hours of total sleep in the 24 hours preceding a shift.
  C. Flight crew members should attempt to eat several small, high-energy meals throughout their shift.
  D. Rest periods during periods of low call volume are not recommended.

_____ 12. Personal protection equipment for air crew members might include all of the following except:
  A. protective footwear.   C. helmets.
  B. fire-resistant clothing.   D. ballistic vests.

_____ 13. All of the following are examples of procedures performed during a preflight check except:
  A. clearing ground debris around the aircraft.
  B. scanning for obstructions such as wires, towers, or buildings.
  C. securing all equipment within the aircraft cabin.
  D. activating internal communication systems.

_____ 14. While in flight, you note the presence of another helicopter directly off the right side of your aircraft and below your horizontal plane. Which of the following best illustrates the proper way of describing the other helicopter's position to your aircraft's pilot?
  A. three o'clock low   C. twelve o'clock high
  B. nine o'clock low   D. on the right

_____ 15. Which of the following is not a post-accident duty for air crew members?
  A. meeting with other survivors at a predetermined location
  B. locating the ELT and assuring that it is activated
  C. for accident sites located in unpopulated areas, forming search parties to locate help
  D. salvaging usable supplies from the wreckage

_____ 16. The "rule of threes" states that a person can survive:
  A. three seconds without oxygen, three minutes in extreme weather, three days without water, and three weeks without food.
  B. three minutes in extreme weather, three days without water, and three weeks without food.
  C. three minutes with an occluded airway, three hours submerged in cold water, three days without food, and three weeks without water.
  D. three minutes without oxygen, three hours in extreme weather without shelter, three days without water, and three weeks without food.

_____ 17. You, your pilot, and your nurse partner have survived, uninjured, a crash landing of your helicopter into a remote, mountainous area. It is January, snow is falling, and the temperature is 24°F. After self-extrication, assessment for injuries, and securing the ELT and assuring that it is transmitting, the three of you discuss what your first actions should be. Which of the following would be the best action to undertake first?
  A. creating/finding shelter
  B. salvaging water from the wreckage
  C. rationing available food
  D. hiking toward a town you know is about 10 miles away

Patient Assessment and Preparation for Transport

Review of Chapter Objectives

Upon completion of this chapter, the student should be able to:

1. **Understand the differences between the prehospital assessment and the critical care provider assessment.** p. 106

   In the prehospital environment, paramedics are accustomed to formulating a management plan based primarily on their clinical assessment findings. In the critical care environment, the paramedic will often utilize a working diagnosis that has been formulated by a team of medical professionals, including physicians, nurses, respiratory therapists, and others.

2. **Identify the steps necessary to obtain comprehensive objective and subjective assessment data through history taking, physical examination techniques, and review of pre-existing medical documentation.** p. 107

   Patient assessment is the one skill that is performed on every patient. As in the prehospital environment, a patient assessment is performed prior to treatment, is an ongoing process, and should be used in concert with acquired diagnostic and laboratory data to form a working diagnosis to determine management strategy. While having a structured assessment technique is important to ensure consistency, situations may present themselves that demand a more dynamic assessment strategy. A structured assessment will usually consist of taking a history, performing a physical examination, and reviewing pre-existing medical documentation. In addition, much information can be obtained from dispatch information, and, while not a formal part of the physical assessment, such information should be included in your assessment, when appropriate.

   Pre-arrival information gathered by the communications/dispatch center is often provided by the transferring care facility or on-scene personnel, and may allow the transport crew to begin forming a differential diagnosis and preparing anticipated equipment or personnel. Pre-arrival information may include a chief complaint or reason for transport, history of present illness (HPI) or nature of illness (NOI), interventions performed and any responses, current status of the patient, and any expected interventions that may be necessary during transport.

   Obtaining a patient history includes understanding the past medical history (PMH) and HPI or NOI. Obtaining a complete HPI/NOI is necessary to effectively plan interventions and anticipate complications, and is especially important in the critical care environment because of the higher acuity and higher level of care required for these patients. Often, the transporting facility will have PMH and HPI/NOI information readily available. However, it is common for transporting facilities not to have such information available if the patient has been in their care for a short period of time, and on-scene calls are notorious for their lack of available information. In such cases, utilizing the SAMPLE and OPQRST methods of information procurement will prove useful and sufficient, as in the prehospital environment. Important PMH information, as in the prehospital environment, includes the identification of chronic illnesses, prescribed medications and compliance, and known allergies. In addition, appreciation of the MOI during a scene size-up may aid in understanding the HPI. Scene size-up is not limited to the out-of-hospital environment. Interfacility missions commonly include hospital personnel from numerous departments who may not be familiar with critical care transport or flight medicine. Just as you would quickly evaluate a first responder's familiarity with your roles and responsibilities, the critical care transport paramedic needs to evaluate a transporting facility's personnel and aid those who need direction as to how to properly and constructively contribute to the transport effort. The steps necessary to "control a scene" are the same in the interfacility realm as they are on scene; take BSI precautions, determine MOI/NOI, determine if additional resources are needed (or if there are too many), access the necessity for cervical spine protection, and determine the number of patients.

The completion of a physical exam in the critical care transport environment is similar to that performed in the prehospital environment and follows the initial assessment/detailed assessment format that is ubiquitous in emergency care. The goal of the initial assessment (or primary exam) is to find and correct any potentially life-threatening situations, such as airway compromise, breathing inadequacy, or gross hemorrhaging; in other words, taking care of the ABCs. To be specific, a general impression is determined, a mental status assessment performed, and then an assessment made of airway, breathing, and circulation. The initial assessment is sometimes referred to as the rapid physical exam, in which a head-to-toe exam is performed, rapidly, with the intention of identifying and correcting potentially life-threatening injuries.

After potential life-threats have been corrected, a detailed physical exam should be performed. The goals of the detailed exam are to identify non-life-threatening injuries and to assess the adequacy of interventions performed during the initial/rapid assessment. A methodical, systematic method of performing a detailed assessment is desirable, as it ensures consistency and completeness. The detailed physical exam is a bit more involved at the critical care level compared to the prehospital, requiring a bit of a more detailed overview than was provided for the initial exam. As with a prehospital detailed (or secondary) exam, the exam performed by the critical care paramedic will follow a head-to-toe approach, but will involve a more thorough and involved assessment, sometimes utilizing tools not available to the prehospital paramedic.

A detailed assessment of the head starts with reassuring airway patency. The pupils should be examined, and the inner eye examined with an ophthalmoscope. Mucous membranes and conjuntiva should be assessed, as should the structural integrity of the skin and skeletal components. The ears and nasal cavity can be examined with an otoscope as needed.

Assessment of the neck includes an inspection of the trachea and jugular veins, and palpation of the cervical spine and soft tissue for crepitus or subcutaneous emphysema. Auscultation can be performed for the presence of carotid bruits, and a review of imaging studies (CT or X-ray) performed to identify bone or soft-tissue injury or foreign bodies.

Inspection, palpation, and percussion of the anterior, posterior, and lateral chest walls should be performed to identify any obvious trauma, and auscultation of lung and heart sounds performed. In addition, chest tubes, central venous catheters, and needle decompression sites should be identified and inspected. A review of imaging studies (CT, X-ray, ultrasound) should be performed, as well, to identify traumatic or medical insult.

The abdomen should receive a normal assessment that includes inspection, auscultation, palpation, and percussion for injury or pathology. In addition, identification and evaluation of interventions performed and indwelling devices inserted is required. Abdominal and intestinal drainage devices, NG/OG tubes, and transabdominal feeding tubes are examples of some of the devices commonly encountered in critical care transport. Imaging studies, such as ultrasound or CT scans, should be evaluated when available.

As with the abdomen, the pelvis/genitourinary exam should include the normal inspection, auscultation, palpation, and percussion for injury or pathology. Identification and evaluation of procedures, such as insertion of urinary catheters (superpubic, Foley, or Texas catheters), fixation devices, and rectal tubes should also be done. Also, imaging studies such as X-rays, CT scans, or cystography should be included in your assessment.

In addition to the normal inspection of the extremities and determination of sensory, circulatory, and motor function, X-rays are helpful in identifying injury.

A review of pre-existing medical documentation includes considering all previous assessments performed prior to your arrival, and assessing diagnostic studies performed. Diagnostic study results that may be useful in clinical decision making include laboratory tests, ECGs, pulmonary function tests, echocardiography, ultrasound, and CT and MRI imaging.

3. Explain how to categorize a patient's physiologic status as either a high or low priority. p. 110

Categorizing a patient's physiologic status requires consideration of clinical assessment findings, diagnostic study findings, and experience. Specific information to be considered includes the patient's current mental status and trends in GCS scoring. Respiratory rate and breathing adequacy, and information garnered from studies such as peak flow, capnography, and pulse oxymetry can be useful. If a patient is being mechanically ventilated, ventilator compliancy should also be considered. The cardiovascular and peripheral perfusion assessment can produce information, such as heart rate and rhythm, capillary refill, skin characteristics, and hemodynamic pressures. Laboratory and blood chemistry findings, as well as imaging study findings, are also valuable tools to help in categorizing a patient's physiologic status.

4. Be able to incorporate all assessment and pertinent diagnostic findings into a working field impression or diagnosis for management. p. 118

It is typical for a critical care transport team to share the patient care workload, with one individual interacting with the transporting agency (receiving a patient report, reviewing diagnostic and laboratory test results, reviewing paperwork), while the other performs the patient assessment. At some point, all transport team members and at least one caregiver from the transporting facility should get together and integrate all the information that has been acquired to that point. There must be agreement as to the MOI/NOI, HPI, interventions that have been rendered, patient response to interventions, current clinical status, interventions needed now, and consideration of anticipated interventions that may be required while in transport.

5. Become familiar with procedures to minimize complications of critical care transports. p. 120

For interfacility transports, several important documents need to be prepared prior to departing from the transporting facility. These documents are outlined in EMTALA/COBRA legislation and typically include paperwork that contains the following:
1. Physician certification that the risks of transport do not outweigh the anticipated benefits
2. Written request by the patient for transport, free of duress
3. Documented, advanced acceptance of the patient by the receiving facility
4. Signed consent for transport
5. Medical orders for the transporting team
6. Copies of medical records, tests, and studies, unless transport delays will jeopardize patient outcome

Proper preparation for transport can significantly reduce complications common to critical care transport. If the patient is intubated, breath sounds should be auscultated before, and after, packaging or moving the patient to confirm tube placement. In addition, a cervical collar should be placed prior to transport to limit head and cervical mobility, both causes of tube displacement. All IV lines should be identified, separated, and labeled to promote rapid identification, and all medications should be transferred to IV pumps. All cables, such as ECG or defibrillation cables, should be labeled and isolated to prevent tangling. In addition, a quick "policing" of the work area should be performed to ensure that no equipment is left on scene or at the transporting facility.

Case Study

"Your patient is in the ER and will be going to the ICU at University," crackles the speaker as the dispatcher finishes giving the transfer details. "Okay, we're en route," you respond into the mike. While on the way, you remember how, when you first became a paramedic, your mind used to race with all the "what ifs" about the scene and the patient's condition. Now, with several years of experience and a lot more confidence, your mind no longer races around. However, you still find it useful to start integrating the available dispatch information about the transfer to help form a plan of action.

The patient is an 8-year-old boy who accidentally hanged himself while playing in a tree. He was taken by local EMS to a small, rural ED approximately 60 miles from University Hospital. The patient is intubated and remains unresponsive. This particular ED has a reputation with your service's critical care transport teams for presenting "train wrecks" to crews for transfer. With this in mind, you discuss with your crew the equipment you will most likely need, and contingency plans in case the patient worsens during transfer. After conferring with Jan, your CCRN partner on this crew, it is decided that she will be the lead provider on this transfer.

Upon arrival at the sending facility, Jan seeks out the physician in charge while you and Bill, the EMT/Driver on the crew, collect the necessary equipment on the stretcher. As you and Bill approach the patient's room, Jan returns and gives you a report on what she learned from the physician. The patient was swinging in a tree from a chain dog leash when it got caught around his neck and strangled him. His older sister quickly removed the chain but he was apneic and pulseless on EMS arrival. BLS recovered a pulse and respirations en route to the hospital, but the patient has remained unresponsive.

While Jan reviews the transfer paperwork, including the ED chart with labs and X-rays and the COBRA/EMTALA forms, you begin your assessment. During your initial assessment, it is immediately obvious that the patient is critically ill and high priority. He is unresponsive with a GCS of 1-1T-2 for a total of 4T. He is intubated and on a ventilator. A quick glance at the monitors indicates that his SpO_2 and vital signs are within normal limits. Continuing with your detailed physical exam you find: HEENT—face and scalp without evidence of soft-tissue trauma, and pupils are of equal size without hyphema, but slightly dilated and poorly reactive to light. Ears and nose are without discharge or hemotympanum, mouth without evidence of soft-tissue trauma, and 6.0 mm cuffed endotracheal tube is well secured, measuring 18 cm at lip line. You also observe the following:

- Cervical collar in place, anterior neck with ecchymosis and edema but no subcutaneous emphysema noted
- Cross table c-spine film without obvious fractures; a CT scan was not performed
- Chest—no evidence of soft-tissue trauma; chest X-ray shows the tip of the endotracheal tube to be 3 cm above the carina, but is otherwise unremarkable
- Abdomen—soft, without evidence of soft-tissue trauma
- Pelvis—stable, without evidence of soft-tissue trauma, 12 French Foley catheter in place draining clear, yellow urine with 300 ml out since it was placed
- Extremities—strong peripheral pulses in all extremities without evidence of trauma

You report your findings to Jan. She has reviewed the labs and advises you that the patient initially had a respiratory acidosis, but that the most recent blood gas shows that this has resolved. She was told that CT scans were not performed because the scanner is down. She learned that the patient was bolused with mannitol approximately 15 minutes ago, and is actually going to the ED at University Hospital, not the ICU. After log rolling the patient to a spine board and fully immobilizing him, you adjust the ventilatory rate of your transport ventilator to keep the $ETCO_2$ at approximately 28 mmHg. The patient is quickly moved to the ambulance and transport is begun. Although serial assessments show no significant improvement in the patient's status en route, he at least arrives at University Hospital ED without any further deterioration. While moving the patient over to the ED stretcher, a full report is given and patient care is turned over to the staff there.

DISCUSSION QUESTIONS

1. What are some differences between the prehospital assessment and the critical care transport team assessment?

©2007 Pearson Education, Inc.
Critical Care Paramedic

2. What steps should be performed to assure that all necessary patient assessment data is gathered before transport is begun?

3. What are some procedures to minimize complications of critical care transports?

Content Review

MULTIPLE CHOICE

_____ 1. Information that may be gathered from pre-arrival information that may assist in developing an initial assessment and management plan includes all of the following except:
   A. reason for transport.
   B. interventions performed.
   C. response to interventions performed.
   D. patient insurance information.

_____ 2. Which of the following is not an acceptable reason for activation of a critical care team for interfacility transport?
   A. The patient will benefit from the rapid transport provided by an aircraft.
   B. An unstable, uninsured patient at a private community hospital requires transport to a local university hospital that usually provides care to uninsured individuals.
   C. The patient and his family request transfer to a different facility.
   D. A small, rural hospital does not have the resources to care for the patient.

_____ 3. Your critical care team is dispatched to a rural ED to transfer an unconscious and intubated male with a head injury secondary to a high-speed MVA rollover. The scene size-up for this interfacility transfer is most likely to include:
   A. BSI precautions, determining the NOI, considering the need for additional resources, and determining the number of patients.
   B. BSI precautions, identifying the officer in charge, and considering the need for additional resources.
   C. determining the NOI, considering the need for additional resources, determining the need for cervical spine precautions, and assuring that the scene is clear of gas, oil, or other combustibles.
   D. BSI precautions, identifying the officer in charge, considering the MOI, and assuring that the vehicle is properly stabilized.

_____ 4. EMTALA/COBRA legislation assures that all of the following information is obtained prior to transport except:
   A. signed patient consent for transport.
   B. proof of medical insurance.
   C. medical orders for the transporting team.
   D. copies of available medical records and lab and imaging results.

_____ 5. Patient packaging prior to transport that might help prevent in-flight difficulties includes:
   A. identifying, separating, and labeling IV lines.
   B. backboarding every patient to facilitate transfer between the hospital and transport stretchers.
   C. resting all equipment within reach and clearly visible on the patient's legs.
   D. monitoring pulse oxymetry before, and after, moving intubated patients to ensure that the endotracheal tube has not become dislodged.

_____ 6. The goal of the initial assessment and rapid physical exam is to:
   A. identify and address all injuries the patient has sustained.
   B. identify and correct potential life-threatening injuries only.
   C. secure a patent airway and assess breathing.
   D. identify any lost vital body functions.

_____ 7. The goal of the detailed physical exam is to:
   A. reassess any corrective procedures performed in the initial assessment.
   B. perform a head-to-toe exam.
   C. identify non-life-threatening problems and reassess the adequacy of interventions performed in the initial exam.
   D. assess those areas and systems not assessed in the initial assessment.

_____ 8. During the performance of a detailed physical exam of the head, a critical care paramedic may assess:
   A. the retina with an otoscope.
   B. the tympanic membrane with an ophthalmoscope.
   C. a previously inserted NG or OG tube for proper placement and patency.
   D. the presence of adventitious lung sounds.

_____ 9. Assessment of the chest should include inspecting for:
   A. thoracostomy tubes.   C. J-tubes.
   B. T-tubes.   D. urinary catheters.

_____ 10. Which of the following best represents the progression of initial airway maintenance?
   A. Manual airway technique, suctioning, BLS airway adjunct, endotracheal intubation, and transtracheal airway.
   B. Suctioning, manual airway technique, endotracheal intubation, and transtracheal airway.
   C. Suctioning, BLS airway adjunct, endotracheal intubation, and transtracheal airway.
   D. Manual airway technique, suctioning, CombiTube, BLS airway adjunct, endotracheal intubation, and transtracheal airway.

_____ 11. Components of circulatory and cardiac system assessment during the initial assessment may include all of the following except:
   A. determining heart rate and rhythm.
   B. reviewing IV access and fluids and medications administered.
   C. assessing skin temperature, color, and condition.
   D. blood and laboratory tests.

_____ 12. You and your partner are dispatched to a local ED to transport a 33-year-old male patient who has had an AMI and requires balloon angioplasty at a local university hospital. Upon arrival, your partner goes to receive the patient report from the transferring physician, and you go to the "critical care" room to meet and assess the patient. You find nine persons in the room with the patient, and are finding it difficult to get to the patient's side to perform an assessment. At this point, the best course of action would be to:
   A. announce that you are part of the transport team and demand to be let near the patient.
   B. find the charge nurse and ask him to help clear the room of all nonessential personnel.
   C. attempt to obtain patient information from a nurse.
   D. sit back and wait for the room to clear out while trying to stay out of the way.

_____ 13. Topics discussed with patient family members prior to transport commonly include:
   A. detailing the events that will take place during transport.
   B. the name, location, and phone number of, and directions to, the receiving facility.
   C. a brief helicopter safety orientation.
   D. detailing the events that have taken place up to that point.

_____ 14. You have determined that your unconscious patient does not have an adequate airway. Which of the following best describes what your next actions should be?
   A. Open the airway manually, suction, insert a BLS airway adjunct, and assess breathing.
   B. Open the airway manually, insert a BLS airway adjunct, intubate, and assess breathing.
   C. Suction the airway, intubate, and then assess breathing.
   D. Determine if the patient is a candidate for RSI.

©2007 Pearson Education, Inc.
Critical Care Paramedic

Airway Management and Ventilation

Review of Chapter Objectives

Upon completion of this chapter, the student should be able to:

1. **Discuss the importance of airway management and ventilation in modern critical care transport.**   **p. 127**

   Airway management is an important skill, and one that the critical care paramedic (CCP) is likely to utilize frequently. More directly, as a CCP, you are likely to be called upon to manage both routine and difficult airways much more often than you ever would in the prehospital environment. As such, it is imperative that the CCP possess excellent airway management skills and master the procedures employed to manage difficult airways. In addition to the more frequent need for airway management, the CCP will often perform mechanical ventilation for longer periods of time as compared to their noncritical care colleagues, further stressing the need for airway mastery.

2. **Discuss the advantages and disadvantages of the following specialized laryngoscope blades.**

   Grandview™   **p. 129**

   The Grandview™ blade's unique design has an 80 percent wider blade surface area and a more anatomically appropriate curve, and is more effective in displacing the tongue and allowing for an improved view of the glottic structures. In addition, the blade design reduces the need to reposition the blade in the oropharynx. Its proprietary lamp provides more light than standard bulbs, and it fits all standard laryngoscope handles. It is available in adult and pediatric sizes.

   Viewmax™   **p. 129**

   The Viewmax™ blade is used in a similar fashion to a traditional curved blade, and contains a patented lens system housed in a viewing tube that runs the length of the blade. The lens system refracts the image 20° from the horizontal, allowing for better visualization of anterior anatomy through the eyepiece. The Viewmax™ blade fits Greenspec fiber-optic laryngoscope handles, and is available in both adult and pediatric sizes.

3. **Detail the use of the gum elastic bougie in advanced airway management.**   **p. 129**

   The gum elastic bougie (oddly named, as it is neither made of gum or elastic!), a.k.a. the Eschmann tracheal tube introducer, is a straight, semi-rigid stylet used to facilitate the passage of an endotracheal tube into the trachea. It is 60–70 cm in length, and has a tip bent at 30° at about 3.5 cm from distal end. The gum elastic bougie is used with endotracheal tubes sized 6.0 or greater, and aids in directing the tube tip under the epiglottis and into the trachea. Its use is indicated for all Cormack-Lehane grade 3 or higher views of the epiglottis.

The procedure for use is as follows:

1. Under direct laryngoscopy, the tip of the bougie is oriented anteriorly at the midline and inserted under the epiglottis into the trachea.
2. If the bougie is placed into the trachea, the operator should be able to feel tracheal rings as the distal tip is "bounced" over the trachea.
3. Continue inserting the bougie into the trachea until resistance is felt.
   a. Resistance felt when tip reaches carina
   b. Typically between 25–40 cm
4. If no "bumps" are felt from the tracheal rings and/or if the bougie meets no resistance, remove the bougie, reventilate if necessary, and reattempt insertion.
5. If the bougie has been properly inserted in the trachea, maintain laryngoscope and bougie in place while an assistant threads an endotracheal tube over the bougie and into the larynx.
6. If endotracheal tube impinges on the posterior cartilages or tracheal ring, rotate the tube counterclockwise, while advancing slowly.
7. Once the endotracheal tube is in place, hold it firmly at the lip, remove the bougie, inflate the distal cuff, and confirm tube placement.

4. Describe the use of the following blind nasotracheal intubation adjunct devices.

Burden nasoscope   **p. 131**

The Burden nasoscope is a disposable, single-use device used to facilitate blind nasotracheal intubation. It is a stethoscope with an in-line diaphragm that connects the proximal end of an endotracheal tube via a 15-mm connector. The user confirms tracheal placement of the endotracheal tube by auscultating breath sounds through the earpieces, as with a normal stethoscope.

Beck airway airflow monitor (BAAM)   **p. 132**

The Beck airway airflow monitor (BAAM) is another disposable device used to facilitate blind nasotracheal intubation. The BAAM connects to the proximal end of an endotracheal tube via a 15-mm connector, and produces an audible whistling sound as air moves through the endotracheal tube with inspiration and exhalation. The whistling becomes louder as the distal end of the tube is directed closer to the glottic opening; tracheal placement dramatically increases the intensity of the whistling. Conversely, loss of whistling indicates esophageal placement of the endotracheal tube.

5. Describe the application of the BURP maneuver and the advantage it may offer.   p. 133

The BURP maneuver—Backward, Upward, Rightward Pressure—consists of direct manipulation of the larynx under direct laryngoscopy by the intubator and is used to improve visualization of the larynx. Utilization of the BURP maneuver can improve a Cormack-Lehane grade 2 or 3 view of the glottis by at least one grade.

    The procedure is as follows:

1. The laryngoscope is held in the left hand and inserted into the airway while sweeping the tongue to the left and lifting the jaw, as normal.
2. If the glottis structures are not visible, the right hand is used to reach around the patient and grasp the thyroid cartilage between the thumb and forefinger.
3. The thyroid cartilage is manipulated as needed to achieve an optimal view of the glottis.
4. When the laryngoscopist has an optimal view of the glottic structures, the assistant holds the larynx in position, freeing the laryngoscopist's right hand for intubation.
5. While still under direct laryngoscopy, the trachea is intubated.

6. Detail the indications, contraindications, and technique for the following intubation techniques:

Digital intubation   **p. 133**

Indications:

1. Laryngoscopy equipment is unavailable or not working.
2. Visualization of glottic structures is impossible because of:
   a. trauma.
   b. blood or vomit in the airway.

3. Potential cervical spine injury
4. Instances where poor lighting, patient positioning, and other situations make laryngoscopy impossible
    a. Prehospital environment
5. Rescue airways are unavailable or have failed.

Contraindications:

1. Conscious patient
2. Presence of gag reflex

Procedure:

1. If cervical spine injury is suspected, provide immobilization from superior position.
2. Insert stylet into endotracheal tube and form a "J" shape.
3. Place a bite block between the patient's molars to protect the intubator's fingers.
4. If the intubator is right handed, he should kneel at the patient's left shoulder, facing caudad.
5. Insert the left middle and index fingers into the patient's mouth.
6. "Walk" the fingers and hand down midline into the hypopharynx.
7. Palpate the arytenoid cartilage posterior and epiglottis anterior, to the glottis, and lift the glottis with the middle finger.
8. Insert the endotracheal tube into the patient's mouth, anterior to your fingers.
9. Advance the tube with your right hand, using the left index finger to keep the tube pressed against the middle finger as a guide.
10. Use the middle and index fingers to direct the tube into the glottic opening and through cords and into the trachea.
11. Hold the tube firmly in place, carefully remove the left hand from the patient's mouth without displacing the tube, inflate the distal cuff, and confirm tube placement.

Sky hook technique   p. 135
Indications:

1. Intubator cannot get into normal, superior position for intubation
    a. Patient trapped in sitting position in vehicle
    b. Patient sitting upright in chair, on stretcher
2. Direct visualization of the glottis is difficult.

Contraindications:

1. None specified

Procedure:

1. Perform cervical spine stabilization if needed.
2. The intubator stands behind the patient or at his side, situation permitting, with prepared endotracheal tube in hand.
3. The assistant moves in front of the patient, situation permitting, and inserts a laryngoscope (Macintosh #3 or #4 blade) into the patient's mouth, and lifts, or "hooks" the patient's tongue and jaw at 90° to the patient's vertical axis. This had the same effect as a jaw-thrust/chin-lift maneuver.
4. The intubator looks into the patient's airway, visualizes the glottic opening, and inserts the endotracheal tube.

Lighted stylet   p. 137
Indications:

1. Visualization is difficult under direct laryngoscopy.
2. Limited cervical mobility, need for cervical stabilization

Contraindications:

1. Although there aren't specific contraindications, bright ambient light, dark skin pigmentation, and excessive adipose tissue may decrease transillumination.

Procedure:

1. Prepare the endotracheal tube on the stylet per the manufacturer's instructions.
2. With the patient supine and the head in neutral position, kneel at the patient's side, facing cephalad.
3. Ensure that the patient's neck is exposed.
4. Turn on the lighted stylet.
5. With the nondominant hand, grasp and lift the patient's jaw and tongue.
6. Keeping the stylet/tube midline, insert it into the patient's mouth and advance to the hypopharynx.
7. Continue to advance the stylet/tube, "hooking" under the epiglottis and into the trachea.
8. Observe the well-defined circumferential transillumination of the patient's anterior neck.
9. Advance and secure the endotracheal tube.
10. Confirm proper endotracheal tube placement.

Retrograde Intubation   p. 140

Indications:

1. Direct orotracheal intubation is impossible.

Contraindications:

1. Inability to identify laryngeal landmarks
2. Presence of a cervical mass
3. Inability of the patient to open his mouth

Procedure:

1. Position the patient with his head extended and his anterior neck readily accessible and fully exposed.
2. Prepare the anterior neck with povidone/iodine or a similar antiseptic solution.
3. Identify the cricothyroid cartilage.
4. Using a large-bore needle attached to a syringe containing 1–2 cc of normal saline, advance the needle cephalad into the tracheal lumen.
5. Confirm tracheal placement of the needle tip by aspirating air and observing bubbles in the syringe.
6. While firmly securing the needle in place, remove the syringe from the needle hub.
7. Insert the guidewire into the trachea through the needle and advance the wire into the pharynx.
8. Under direct laryngoscopy, the assistant should identify the guidewire in the pharynx and grasp it with forceps, pulling the wire through while taking care not to pull the distal end of wire through the needle. The distal end of the wire can be secured with a hemostat clamp to prevent it from retreating through the needle.
9. Slide the guide catheter over the proximal end (in assistant's hand) of guidewire, into airway, advancing until resistance is felt.
10. Advance the endotracheal tube over the guide catheter into the airway until resistance is met.
11. While holding the endotracheal tube firmly, remove the clamp on the guidewire at the needle and pull the guidewire and guide catheter out through the patient's mouth.
12. Advance the endotracheal tube to the proper depth in the trachea.
13. Secure the endotracheal tube and confirm proper placement.

7. **List the four phases of rapid-sequence intubation (RSI) pharmacology.**   p. 142

The four phases of RSI pharmacology are: induction, premedication, neuromuscular blockade, and maintenance therapy.

8. **List the indications for RSI.**   p. 142

Indications for RSI include:

1. Impending respiratory failure secondary to pulmonary disease, such as COPD, asthma, CHF, or pneumonia.
2. Acute airway disorder that threatens airway patency, such as airway burns, laryngeal or upper airway trauma, and epiglottitis.

©2007 Pearson Education, Inc.
Critical Care Paramedic

3. Altered mental status with significant risk of vomiting and aspiration. Examples include: a GCS < 8, alcohol or drug intoxication, and status epilepticus.

9. Detail the role of analgesics and hypnotics in RSI.   p. 142

Analgesics and hypnotics are used as induction agents in RSI, and are intended to provide sedation prior to paralysis. It is important to remember that paralytic agents do not affect the patient's mental status, and that the use of a paralytic agent alone may result in a patient who is paralyzed but fully conscious, coherent, and able to feel pain and understand what is going on around him. The use of an induction agent will render the patient unable to appreciate, respond to, or recall the procedure.

10. Review and detail the following induction agents:

Thiopental Sodium (Pentothal)   p. 143
- Short-acting barbiturate
  - CNS depressant
- Onset of action: 10 to 20 seconds
- Duration of effect: 5 to 10 minutes
- Dose: 2 to 5 mg/kg IV
- Significant hemodynamic effects
  - Worsens hypotension
  - Decreases ICP
- Ideal for head-injured patients

Methohexital (Brevital)   p. 143
- Barbiturate similar to thiopental.
- Onset of action: < 1 minute
- Duration of effect: 5–7 minutes
- Dose: 1 to 2 mg/kg IV

Etomidate (Amidate)   p. 143
- Short-acting, nonbarbiturate hypnotic agent
- Attractive safety profile
- Onset of action: 10 to 20 seconds
- Duration of effect: 3 to 5 minutes
- Dose: 0.2 to 0.3 mg/kg IV over 15 to 30 seconds

Propofol (Diprivan)   p. 143
- Highly lipid soluble, easily crosses blood-brain barrier
- Onset of action: 10 to 20 seconds
- Duration of effect: 10 to 15 minutes
- Dose: 1 to 3 mg/kg IV
- Causes apnea early in RSI attempt

Fentanyl (Sublimaze)   p. 143
- Short-acting opiate
  - Chemically unrelated to morphine
- Widely used in anesthesia
- Onset of action: immediate
- Duration of effect: 30 to 60 minutes
- Dose: 2 to 10 mcg/kg IV

Morphine   p. 143
- Less effective than fentanyl
- Hemodynamic properties make it unattractive
- Onset of action: 3 to 5 minutes
- Duration of effect: 2 to 7 hours
- Dose: 0.1 to 0.2 mg/kg IV

Ketamine   p. 144
- Dissociative drug
  - Used in pediatric anesthesia and veterinary medicine
- Patient appears awake, is deeply anesthetized
- Causes catecholamine release
  - Increases sympathetic nervous system tone
  - Increases HR, CO, BP
  - May increase ICP
- Onset of action: 45 to 60 seconds
- Duration of effect: 10 to 20 minutes
- Dose: 1 to 4 mg/kg IV

Midazolam (Versed)   p. 144
- Popular induction agent for prehospital RSI
- Potent amnesic effects
- 2–4 times more potent than diazepam
- Onset of action: 1 to 2 minutes
- Duration of effect: 30 to 60 minutes
- Dose: 0.1 to 0.3 mg/kg IV
  - May be administered IM

Diazepam (Valium)   p. 144
- Features similar to midazolam
- Not water soluble, less potent
- Greater potential for hypotension
- Onset of action: 2 to 4 minutes
- Duration of effect: 30 to 90 minutes
- Dose: 0.25 to 0.4 mg/kg IV

Lorazepam (Ativan)   p. 144
- Long-acting benzodiazepine
- Useful for long-term sedation after intubation
- Onset of action: 1 to 5 minutes
- Duration of effect: 1 to 2 hours
- Dose: 50 mcg/kg IV

11. **Discuss the importance of premedication in high-risk patients undergoing RSI.**   p. 145

A patient's condition may demand the use of some medications prior to the administration of a neuromuscular blocking agent. Premedications serve to blunt the adverse side effects associated with both neuromuscular blocking agents, and laryngoscopy and intubation. Specific premedication agents, and their profiles, include:

Lidocaine
- Thought to prevent rise in ICP
  - Patients with possible head injury
  - Patients with CNS pathology
- Suppresses cough reflex and increases in airway resistance
- Dysrhythmia control
- Dose: 1.0–1.5 mg/kg IVP 2 to 3 minutes prior to intubation

Atropine
- Used in adults exhibiting, or at high risk for developing, bradycardia
- Reduces succinylcholine and laryngoscope-induced bradycardia in children
- Indicated in all patients < 3 years of age
- Dose
  - Adult: 0.5 mg IVP
  - Peds: 0.01 mg/kg IVP

Defasciculating Agents

- Defasciculating dose of neuromuscular blocking agent can attenuate fasciculations seen with succinylcholine use.
- All of the neuromuscular agents can be administered at defasciculating dose prior to administration of succinylcholine.
- Agents:
  - Vecuronium
  - Pancuronium
  - Rocuronium
  - Succinylcholine

12. Detail the pharmacokinetics, including onset of action and duration of effect for the following nondepolarizing blockers:

Pancuronium (Pavulon) p. 146

- Nondepolarizing agent
- Does not cause fasciculations
- Advantage of rapid onset offset by long duration of action
  - Can be a disadvantage in instances of failed intubation
- Onset of action: 3 to 5 minutes
- Duration of effect: 60 minutes
- Dose: 0.1–0.2 mg/kg

Vecuronium (Norcuron) p. 146

- Nondepolarizing agent
- Does not cause fasciculations
  - Commonly used as a defasciculating agent prior to administration of succinylcholine
  - 0.01 mg/kg IV
- Generally considered a second-line paralytic if succinylcholine contraindicated
- Onset of action: 2 to 3 minutes
- Duration of effect: 45 minutes
- Dose:
  - Priming dose 0.01 mg/kg
  - Effective dose 0.1–0.2 mg/kg

Atracurium (Tracrium) p. 146

- Nondepolarizing agent
- Does not cause fasciculations
- Useful in patients with liver and kidney disease
  - Not excreted via renal, hepatic mechanisms
- Onset of action: 30 to 60 minutes
- Duration of effect: 20 to 30 minutes
- Dose: 0.5 mg/kg IV

Rocuronium (Zemuron) p. 146

- Nondepolarizing agent
  - Does not cause fasciculations
- Short onset of action makes it a good choice for patients with contraindications to succinylcholine
- Onset of action: 30 to 60 seconds
- Duration of effect: 30 to 60 minutes
- Dose: 0.6 mg/kg IV, adults and children

13. Contrast the pharmacology of depolarizing and nondepolarizing neuromuscular blocking agents. p. 146

In order to understand the pharmacological differences between the neuromuscular blocking agents (NMBAs), it is necessary to understand the anatomy and physiology of the neuromuscular junction. Under normal conditions, acetylcholine (ACh) is produced by the nerve and stored in vesicles located in the synaptic knob. Nerve stimulation results in movement of the vesicles to the presynaptic membrane, where they fuse with the membrane and release their ACh into the neuromuscular junction (synaptic cleft). ACh diffuses across the neuromuscular junction and binds to ACh receptors on the postsynaptic membrane, promoting muscle fiber depolarization that propagates into a muscular contraction. The effects of ACh are temporary, as the postsynaptic membrane and neuromuscular junction contain the enzyme acetylcholinesterase (AChE, or cholinesterase), which hydrolizes ACh into acetate and choline. Choline is actively absorbed by the synaptic knob and is used to synthesize additional ACh, while acetate diffuses into surrounding cells and tissues, where it is metabolized.

NMBAs are either agonists to ACh (depolarizers of the motor end plate) or antagonists to ACh (nondepolarizers of the motor end plate). Depolarizing agents, succinylcholine being by far the most popular, act by binding tightly to, and depolarizing, ACh receptors. After the initial depolarization, the depolarizing agent continues to occupy the ACh receptor, preventing repolarization and another depolarization. This is why the administration of a depolarizing agent is typified by a period of fasciculations (initial depolarization) followed by paralysis (continued occupation of the ACh receptor). In addition, succinylcholine is not hydrolyzed by AChE, but by pseudocholinesterase, an enzyme synthesized by the liver and present in plasma, not at the neuromuscular junction, which contributes to its long duration of action. There is no reversal agent for succinylcholine.

Nondepolarizing agents, in contrast, cause paralysis by tightly binding to the ACh receptor, preventing ACh from binding, which of course is required for motor end plate depolarization and muscular contraction. Since the binding of a nondepolarizing agent does not result in depolarization, fasciculations are not a result of their administration. As nondepolarizing agents are competitive inhibitors of ACh, any increase in the amount of ACh in the neuromuscular junction will decrease their effectiveness. As such, agents that inhibit the action of cholinesterase in the synaptic cleft, such as neostigmine or pyridostigmine, will act as reversal agents for nondepolarizing NMBAs.

14. Discuss the lack of effect of neuromuscular blocking agents on mental status and pain sensation. p. 148

Neuromuscular blocking agents (NMBAs) act on postsynaptic cholinergic nicotinic receptors in the neuromuscular junction located at the motor end plate. NMBAs have no sedation effect on the CNS, have no effect on pain receptors in the brain (such as opiate receptors), and have no effect on peripheral sensory nerves. As such, while a patient may be paralyzed after the administration of a NMBA, they are still conscious, cognizant, and able to feel pain, hence the need for the administration of a rapid-acting induction agent prior to the administration of NMBAs and any intubation attempt.

15. Describe the need for a reversal agent for neuromuscular blockade and detail medications used. p. 149

Reversal agents for neuromuscular blocking agents (NMBAs) are limited to nondepolarizing agents only; no reversal agents exist for depolarizing NMBAs. Specifically, acetylcholinesterase (AChE) inhibitors prevent AChE from breaking down ACh in the neuromuscular junction, thereby prolonging the effect of ACh, and allowing it to better compete with the nondepolarizing agent that has been administered, thus, increasing ACh receptor stimulation and muscle depolarization. Specific medications and their doses include:

- Neostigmine: 0.05 mg/kg not to exceed 5 mg slow IVP
- Pyridostigmine: 0.2 mg/kg slow IVP
- Edrophonium: 0.5 mg/kg slow IVP

16. Discuss the need for a rescue airway anytime RSI is considered. p. 151

Simply put, if you are going to perform an RSI, you had better have a rescue airway available. Administration of a neuromuscular blocking agent results in paralysis of all skeletal muscles, including those responsible for respiration. In the event of a failed intubation, manually opening the airway and providing ventilation may prove difficult or impossible. In such cases, the use of a rescue airway is necessary to assure proper ventilation and oxygenation to avoid hypoxia and death.

17. Discuss the indications, contraindications, insertion, and removal of the following rescue airways:

Endotracheal CombiTube (ETC) p. 151
Indications:

- Failed intubation: "can't intubate, can't ventilate" situation
- Patient unconscious, absent gag reflexes
- Upper gastrointestinal or GI bleeding that threatens airway

Contraindications:

- Responsive patients with gag reflex intact
- Patients with known esophageal disease
- Caustic ingestions
- FBAO or obstruction secondary to pathology
- Patient < 4 feet or > 7 feet tall

Insertion:

1. Lubricate the distal end of the CombiTube with a water-soluble lubricant.
2. Perform jaw thrust on patient, keeping head in neutral position.
3. Insert the distal end of the CombiTube through the mouth into the posterior hypopharynx and advance until the patient's teeth lie between the two heavy black vertical lines on the tube.
4. Inflate the large, proximal pharyngeal cuff (blue pilot balloon) with 85 or 100 mL of air utilizing the syringe provided. The pilot balloon will have the appropriate air volume clearly printed on it, as well as a "No. 1" indicating that it is to be inflated first, for example, "No. 1—85 mL" or "No. 1—100 mL."
5. Do not hold the device as you inflate the pharyngeal cuff. The CombiTube may rise out of the patient's mouth slightly as the cuff is inflated.
6. Inflate the distal cuff with 12 or 15 mL of air, depending on the size device use. The pilot balloon will be white, and have "No. 2—12 mL" or "No. 2—15 mL" clearly printed on it.
7. Attach a BVM to the proximal end of the CombiTube and attempt to ventilate, and then confirm breath sounds.

Removal:

1. Deflate the distal and pharyngeal cuffs by attaching a syringe to their pilot balloons.
2. Pull the CombiTube out of the airway in an anatomically correct fashion.

Pharyngotracheal Lumen (PtL) Airway p. 153
Indications:

- Failed intubation: "can't intubate, can't ventilate" situation
- Patient unconscious, absent gag reflexes
- Upper gastrointestinal or GI bleeding that threatens airway

Contraindications:

- Responsive patients with gag reflex intact
- Patients with known esophageal disease
- Caustic ingestions
- Pediatric patients

Insertion:

1. Place the patient in the supine position.
2. Hyperextend the patient's head if no cervical spine injury is suspected.
3. Lubricate the tip of PtL with a water-soluble lubricant.
4. Perform a jaw lift.

5. With the other hand, hold the PtL airway so that its curve matches the anatomical curve of the pharynx.
6. Insert the tip into the patient's mouth and advance carefully behind the tongue until the PtL teeth strap touches the patient's teeth. Secure the restraining strap around the patient's head.
   a. Modest resistance may be encountered. Do not force the PtL into the airway. If the tube does not advance, withdraw and start again, redirecting the PtL tip.
7. When the PtL has been inserted, inflate both cuffs with a bag-valve mask (BVM) into the No. 1 inflation valve.
8. Attempt to ventilate the patient's lungs through the No. 2 tube (short, green tube).
   a. Immediately ventilate tube No. 2 (short, green tube).
   b. Observe chest rise on ventilation.
   c. Auscultate for bilateral breath sounds.
   d. Auscultate the abdomen for absence of gurgling.
9. If the chest rises and falls as expected, breath sounds are heard, and no gurgling is noted in the epigastric area, the long tube and cuff are located in the esophagus. Continue to ventilate the patient.
10. If the chest does not rise and/or lung sounds are not auscultated, remove the stylet from tube No. 3 (long, clear tube) and ventilate through that tube.
    a. Observe chest rise on ventilation.
    b. Auscultate for bilateral breath sounds.
    c. Auscultate the epigastric area for gurgling. If the chest rises, breath sounds are obvious, and no gurgling is noted in the epigastric area, the trachea has been intubated. Continue to ventilate the patient through tube No. 3.

Removal:

1. Disconnect the BVM from the device.
2. Deflate the pharyngeal and distall cuffs via the No.1 valve.
3. Perform a jaw lift.
4. Pull the device out, following the anatomical curve of the patient's airway.

Laryngeal Mask Airway (LMA) p. 155
Indications:

- Failed intubation: "can't intubate, can't ventilate" situation
- Patient unconscious, absent gag reflexes

Contraindications:

- Presence of a gag reflex

Insertion:

1. Completely deflate the cuff by aspirating the pilot balloon.
2. Lubricate both sides of the LMA with a water-soluble lubricant.
3. Perform a head-tilt/chin-lift maneuver.
4. Insert the LMA into the oropharynx with the laryngeal surface directed caudally, pressing the device onto the hard palate and advancing it over the back of the tongue, using your fingers to "push" the cuff as far down into the airway as your index finger will allow. Use your other hand to grasp the proximal end of the LMA and push the device into its final seated position.
5. Inflate the collar with the appropriate amount of air (varies with size of the device) or until there is no leak with BVM ventilations.
6. Attach a BVM to the proximal end of the LMA and attempt to ventilate and confirm lung sounds.

Removal:

1. Deflate cuff by aspirating with syringe.
2. Remove LMA by pulling on distal end, following the curve of the airway.

©2007 Pearson Education, Inc.
Critical Care Paramedic

Indications:

Same as LMA

Contraindications:

Same as LMA

Insertion:

1. Same as LMA
2. ETT passed through device lumen into trachea

Removal:

1. If endotracheal tube has not been inserted, the device is removed in the same fashion as the LMA.
2. If endotracheal tube has been inserted through device lumen into trachea:
   a. Inflate the endotracheal tube cuff and confirm tube placement.
   b. Deflate the intubating laryngeal mask airway's cuff.
   c. Remove the 15-mm adapter from the proximal end of the endotracheal tube.
   d. Carefully remove the device from the airway and off the proximal end of the endotracheal tube.
   e. Reattach the 15-mm adapter to the end of the endotracheal tube and continue ventilation.
   f. Secure the endotracheal tube.

18. Compare and contrast the use of needle cricothyrotomy and frank surgical airways in critical care transport.   p. 160

Surgical airways should be utilized only after failed orotracheal intubation. The indication for the need to perform a surgical airway is the inability to ventilate or intubate a patient by oral or nasal routes. Contraindications to performing surgical airways in the field include the ability to ventilate or intubate by oral or nasal routes, inability to identify anatomical landmarks, and the presence of any morphology or pathology that will prevent a successful procedure.

Needle cricothyrotomy should be viewed as an airway that is a temporizing measure only; it is used as a "bridge" until a surgical cricothyrotomy or some other definitive airway can be secured. The procedure utilizes a transtracheal (via the cricothyroid membrane), large-bore (14 gauge or higher) needle. Compared to a surgical cricothyrotomy, it is easier to initiate and has fewer complications. The use of a transtracheal jet insufflator is helpful in achieving the tidal volumes necessary for adequate ventilation of the lungs, as a BVM is generally regarded as inadequate for providing anything even approaching normal ventilation. Potential complications of needle cricothyrotomy include barotraumas, hemorrhaging, subcutaneous emphysema, and hypoventilation secondary to a misplaced catheter (not in trachea), insufficient equipment (BVM), or the incorrect use of a jet insufflator.

Open cricothyrotomy involves opening an airway at the cricothyroid membrane and placing an endotracheal or tracheostomy tube into the trachea. While cricothyrotomy does have its advantages—it can be performed rapidly, and does not manipulate the cervical spine—there is enormous potential for complication, including, misplacement of the endotracheal tube into a false passage, laryngeal or thyroid trauma with resultant hemorrhage, laryngeal nerve and vocal cord damage, and subcutaneous emphysema.

19. Describe the process of identifying the possible difficult airway.   p. 167

There are some common factors among difficult airways, including, historical factors, anatomical factors, and issues with intubation technique. Historical factors that can alert the intubator that an airway may be difficult include a documented history of difficult airway management, and a history of patient difficulty with anesthesia; both of these factors illustrate the importance of obtaining a thorough patient history, and the need for the paramedic to inquire as to these specifics, if intubation is anticipated.

Upper airway anatomy differs greatly among individuals, and several factors are associated with difficult airway, none of which is a reliable indicator by itself. Specific factors associated with the difficult airway are a short or thick neck, and a restricted range of motion, as is present with the need for cervical spine stabilization or in instances of cervical spine pathology that limit extension and flexion. In addition, the presence of malocclusion or an overbite can hinder laryngoscopy, as can a short mandible or a mouth opening less than 3 cm (3 finger breadths) wide. Obesity and anatomical distortion secondary to trauma or pathology complicate laryngoscopy, and every paramedic with any intubation experience is familiar with the difficulties involved with visualizing an anterior larynx. An anterior larynx will manifest morphologically as a short thyromental distance, and a thyromental distance less than 3 cm is considered problematic.

Numerous assessment systems based on visible anatomy have been developed to aid the intubator in identifying those airways that have potential for difficulty, with the Mallampati, Cormack and Lehane, and POGO grading systems perhaps the most widely known and used. The Mallampati classification system is an assessment based on the visual assessment of oropharyngeal anatomy, which is scored on a scale of 1 to 4; the higher the score, the more difficult the intubation. To perform the exam, a patient must be sitting up with his mouth open as wide as possible, and protrude his tongue to the best of his ability, allowing the visible oropharyngeal anatomy to be assessed. The four classes in the Mallampati classification system are as follows:

- Class 1: Uvula and tonsils completely visible
- Class 2: Upper half of uvula, tonsils visible
- Class 3: Hard and soft palate visible
- Class 4: Only hard palate visible

Obviously, asking a patient who is in respiratory extremis to sit up, open his mouth, and stick out his tongue is a bit unrealistic, and is the limiting factor for this grading system's use in the emergency environment. It can be argued that if your patient can sit up and follow your directions to open his mouth as wide as possible and stick out his tongue long enough for you to visualize his oropharyngeal anatomy, he probably does not need intubation! The Mallampati classification does have a place in elective surgery, for instance, where it would be used to identify those potentially difficult airways prior to sedation and neuromuscular blockade. Anesthesiologists preparing for surgery frequently utilize this system.

The Cormack and Lehane grading system is used to assess glottic anatomy under direct laryngoscopy, and is as follows:

- Grade 1: Entire glottic opening and vocal cords visualized
- Grade 2: Epiglottis partially obstructs view, posterior glottic opening and posterior vocal cords visualized
- Grade 3: Epiglottis fully obstructs view of larynx, no vocal cords or posterior cartilage visualized
- Grade 4: Inability to visualize the epiglottis

The Percentage Of Glottic Opening (POGO) scale grades the percentage of glottic opening visible to the laryngoscopist and ranges from 0 (no glottis visualized = bad!) to 100 percent (the entire glottis is visible = good!).

Poor technique can make even the most assessable airway difficult, and can render a difficult airway impossible, leading to the development of inadequate ventilation, hypoxia, and death. While the critical care paramedic cannot control a patient's history or anatomy, he can control his technique. As such, frequent practice, both laboratory and clinical, a command of your equipment, and continuing education are important contributors to airway success.

20. Discuss management of the difficult airway.   p. 167

It has been estimated that 1 out of every 10 airways can be classified as "difficult," and that endotracheal intubation may be impossible in 1 out of every 100 patients utilizing conventional methods, such as laryngoscopy. The ramifications of encountering a difficult airway range from anxiety on the part of the care provider, to hypoxia and death for the patient. As such, it is important for the critical care paramedic to become adept at assessing airways and predicting which of those may prove to be difficult or near impossible to manage.

There are numerous terms used to describe the difficult airway; difficult airway refers to those situations where a conventionally trained paramedic experiences difficulty with BVM ventilation and/or endotracheal intubation. The term "difficult mask ventilation" refers to one of two situations:

- An unassisted paramedic is unable to maintain an SpO_2 > 90 percent using 100 percent oxygen and BVM ventilation on a patient whose SpO_2 was > 90 percent prior to ventilation.

©2007 Pearson Education, Inc.
Critical Care Paramedic

- An unassisted paramedic is unable to reverse or prevent signs of inadequate ventilation during BVM ventilation.

"Difficult laryngoscopy" is a term used to describe the inability to visualize the vocal cords under direct laryngoscopy, and a "difficult intubation" is one that requires more than three attempts at laryngoscopy, or greater than 10 minutes to perform.

21. Discuss the role of noninvasive monitors in airway management and ventilation.   **p. 171**

The most common methods of noninvasive respiratory monitoring in the prehospital environment are pulse oximetry and end-tidal carbon dioxide ($ETCO_2$). Pulse oximetry (SpO_2) measures hemoglobin saturation in the peripheral tissues, and can be an indication of developing hypoxia. Commonly accepted ranges and their representation of hypoxia are:

- Normal values 95 to 99 percent
- Mild hypoxia: 91 to 94 percent
- Moderate hypoxia: 86 to 90 percent
- Severe hypoxia: < 85 percent

The relationship between SpO_2 and PaO_2 is complex, but, generally speaking, the greater the PaO_2, the greater the SpO_2. Pulse oximetry is noninvasive, rapidly applied, is easy to operate, accurate, and offers continuous monitoring of peripheral oxygen delivery. False readings can result from a misplaced sensor, carbon monoxide poisoning, high-intensity lighting, or hemoglobin abnormalities.

    $ETCO_2$ monitoring can be accomplished by one of many modalities. Capnometry refers to the numerical measurement of the partial pressure of exhaled CO_2, usually in torr or mmHg. Capnography is the graphic recording or displaying of exhaled CO_2 values. A "real time" display of an $ETCO_2$ graph is called a capnogram. By measuring $ETCO_2$, we are indirectly measuring $PaCO_2$, the partial pressure of CO_2 in arterial blood, as the values are very close ($ETCO_2$ values are 1 to 2 mmHg less than $PaCO_2$). Causes of decreased $ETCO_2$ include hyperventilation, shock, cardiac arrest, pulmonary embolism, bronchospasm, and incomplete airway obstruction. Causes of increased $ETCO_2$ include hypoventilation, respiratory depression, and hyperthermia.

    Quantitative $ETCO_2$ devices, such as the capnogram, determine how much CO_2 is present. Qualitative $ETCO_2$ devices, such as colorimetric devices, detect only the presence of CO_2, not how much is present. Colorimetric devices detect exhaled CO_2 with litmus paper; H^+ ions in CO_2 cause the litmus paper to change color with each breath. Colorimetric devices are not useful in detecting the presence of hyper- or hypocarbia since they are not quantitative devices. Colorimetric devices are disposable and meant to be placed between the vent circuit (or BVM) and the endotracheal tube.

22. Describe the various phases of the capnogram and the clinical significance of each.   **p. 174**

The capnogram, a real-time waveform readout of $ETCO_2$, has 4 phases with which the critical care paramedic should be familiar. Phase 1, the respiratory baseline, corresponds with the late inspiratory/early expiratory part of the respiratory cycle, and appears as a flat line on the capnogram. It can be thought of as being analogous to the isoelectric line in an ECG, in that no CO_2 is being detected, so the readout returns to baseline. Phase II, the respiratory upstroke, represents the mixture of dead space and alveolar gases present in an exhalation. Phase III, the respiratory plateau, represents the end of exhalation, and, therefore, air from ventilated alveoli, the deepest parts of the respiratory tree. There is a nearly constant CO_2 level in Phase III, as there is very little mixing with dead space air here. As a result, CO_2 is at its highest point. Phase IV represents the inspiratory phase, and appears as a sudden downstroke back to the baseline. As inspired air will have very little CO_2 as compared to exhaled air, this is expected.

    Clinical applications of $ETCO_2$ monitoring include confirming endotracheal tube placement in patients with pulmonary perfusion, continuous monitoring of endotracheal tube placement, trend-monitoring in nonintubated patients, and evaluating the effectiveness of CPR.

23. Detail the types of mechanical ventilators used in critical care and critical care transport. p. 176

There are two types of mechanical ventilators: negative pressure ventilators and positive pressure ventilators. Negative pressure ventilators, such as the iron lung, are much too cumbersome to be utilized in the transport environment. They surround the patient's body and create a negative pressure between the patient and the inner ventilator wall that results in outward movement of the chest wall and an increase in intrathoracic volume. As intrathoracic volume increases, intrathoracic pressure decreases, and atmospheric air rushes into the lungs, much like normal respiration; in normal respiration, respiratory muscles are used to move the chest wall outward, creating an area of low pressure in the thoracic cavity, allowing air to rush into the lungs.

Positive pressure ventilators are the most frequently encountered ventilators in critical care transport, as well as in medicine. They require a closed circuit between the lungs and the ventilator (most often provided by an endotracheal tube and vent circuit tubing) to create a closed system. Positive air pressure can then be provided from the ventilator, forcing air into the lungs. Exhalation occurs passively after the positive pressure stops.

Common types of positive pressure ventilators include control, support, cycling, and triggering. Control determines how much flow the ventilator delivers, and there are three methods of control.

- Volume control: Volume is set and pressures are variable.
- Pressure control: Pressure is set and volume is variable.
- Dual control: Volume is set and limits are placed on pressure.

Support determines when the tidal volume will be delivered.

- Control mode: Ventilator delivers preset tidal volume regardless of patient effort.
- Support mode: Ventilator detects inspiratory effort by patient and supplies an assist pressure during inspiration.

Cycling determines how the ventilator switches from inspiration to expiration.

- Timed cycled: Ventilator will deliver inspiration of predetermined length of time.
- Flow cycled: Ventilator switches when predetermined pressure levels are reached.
- Volume cycled: Ventilator switches when predetermined tidal volume is reached.

Triggering determines what stimulus will trigger the ventilator to cycle to inspiration.

- Time triggered: Ventilator is set for number of breaths per minute.
- Pressure triggered: Ventilator senses patient's inspiratory effort by a decrease of pressure within the circuit, and triggers ventilation.
- Flow triggered: Ventilator senses variations in gas flow through ventilator circuit with patient's inspiratory effort, and triggers ventilation.

24. List and describe common ventilator controls. p. 177

Several parameter controls are common to most ventilators, and required parameters vary depending on patient need. Common controls include:

Mode:

The mode is the parameter by which the ventilator determines when to initiate the respiration, although the mode can vary with the patient. SIMV and Assist/Control modes are adequate starting points for most patients.

- Assist/control
  - Provides full tidal volume (TV) at preset rate.
  - Patient initiates own breath, vent assists with full TV.
  - Provides near-complete rest to ventilatory muscles.
  - Can be used in patients who are conscious, sedated, or paralyzed.
  - Can result in hyperventilation, breath stacking.
- Synchronized intermittent mandatory ventilation (SIMV)
  - Vent delivers preset TV at preset rate.

- If patient initiates own breath, vent will not provide preset breath.
- Vent does not support breath with full TV.
- Often used to "wean" patients off ventilator.
- Respiratory fatigue/failure can develop if the rate is set too slow.
- Pressure support
  - Prevent assists spontaneous breath to predetermined peak pressure.
  - Avoids asynchrony between patient and ventilator.
  - Cannot be used in patients who are comatose, heavily sedated, or paralyzed.
  - Respiratory fatigue/failure can occur if pressure support is set too low.
- Pressure control
  - Pressure and respiratory rate predetermined.
  - Ventilation delivered until predetermined pressure reached.
  - Can result in limited tidal volume.
  - Can result in low, minute ventilation.
- Positive end-expiratory pressure
  - Application of 2.5 to 10 cm/H_2O of pressure to end of expiration.
  - Prevents atelectasis.
  - Can result in:
    - Barotrauma.
    - Air trapping.
    - Increased intrathoracic pressure.
  - Airway pressure release ventilation (APRV).
    - Low level of continuous positive airway pressure (CPAP) with alternating high levels of CPAP.
      - Allows for higher tidal volume.

Sensitivity (when in assist mode), is the amount of inspiratory effort required to initiate an assisted breath.

- Common setting = −1 to −2 cm/H_2O

Minute ventilation (V_{Min}):

- V_{Min} (mL/min) = V_T (mL) × Respiratory Rate (minute)
- Normally 6 to 10 lpm in adults

Tidal volume (V_T):

- Volume of each breath
- V_T (mL) = V_A + V_D
  - V_A = alveolar air
  - V_D = dead air space
- Commonly between 5 to 15 ml/kg of ideal body weight

Respiratory rate:

- 8 to 12 breaths per minute
- 20 breaths per minute = hyperventilation

Inspiration/expiration (I/E) ratio:

- Normal setting 1:2.
- 1:4, 1:5 is commonly used in cases of restrictive airway disease to prevent air stacking.

Flow rate:

- 40 to 80 lpm commonly used.
- Patients with obstructive lung disease often require higher flow rates.

Inspired oxygen concentration (FiO_2):

- Initially set at 1.0 (100 percent)
  - Titrated down based on blood gas values
- With known blood gas values, one can predict the needed FiO_2 settings
  - $PaO_2 = FiO_2 \times (P_B - P_{H_2O}) - PaCO_2/R$

- P_B = Barometric pressure (approximately 760 mmHg at sea level)
- P_{H_2O} = Water vapor pressure (47 mmHg when air is fully saturated at 37°C)
- R = Respiratory quotient (the ration of CO_2 production to O_2 consumption—usually assumed to be 0.8)

Sigh:

- Sighing is a normal respiratory function.
- Helps prevent atelectasis.
- 1.5 to 2.0 times the normal tidal volume, 10 to 15 times per hour.

Heat/humidification:

- 37°C
- 100% humidity

Flow rate:

- Set for 60 lpm

25. Set up and select the initial ventilator settings for a simulated patient.   p. 178

Using the mechanical ventilation parameters discussed in the text, the critical care paramedic should be able to set up and select the following:

- Mode
- FiO_2
- Tidal volume (TV)
- Rate
- Inspiration/expiration ratio (I/E)
- Sigh rate
- Flow rate

26. Discuss the importance of proper documentation in critical care airway management.   p. 182

Proper documentation, not only of airway issues, but of all patient care, is important for many reasons. It must serve as an accurate record of the events that took place for other health care providers, it can be used for QA/QI purposes, and it can protect the health care provider against legal claims. Although it may not seem that way while you are writing a report at 3 A.M. "over-documentation" is more desirable than "under-documentation."

27. Detail the various methods of documenting proper endotracheal tube placement.   p. 182

- Visualization of endotracheal tube through the vocal cords
- Use of an esophageal detection device
- Use of $ETCO_2$ detection device
  - Capnometry
  - Capnography
  - Colorimetric device
- Auscultation of lung sounds
- Gastric sounds absent
- Visible chest rise and fall
- Condensation in the endotracheal tube
- Lack of gastric contents in the endotracheal tube

Case Study

The rotors are still slowly turning when the pilot gives you a "thumbs up" as a signal to head out under the main rotor to the edge of the helipad. One of the rig's medics meets you and your partner, Kate, at the edge of the pad and escorts you to sickbay. On the way down the ladder, he fills you in on the patient's condition. A 34-year-old male was working in the boiler room on a tender ship at the base of the rig when a steam line broke and severely burned his face and chest.

On arrival at sickbay, you see the patient sitting upright on the exam table with labored and stridorous respirations. The patient's face and upper chest are erythematous and edematous with large bulla present. He is alert, but is nonverbal, and in severe respiratory distress. He is receiving high-flow, high-concentration oxygen by mask and 2 large-bore IVs have been established. At this time, his SpO_2 is 88 percent with audible stridor and diminished breath sounds throughout.

With obvious concern for pending airway obstruction, you decide to secure the airway with immediate rapid sequence intubation. Because of the potential difficulty with this intubation, you and your partner decide that you will attempt the procedure as you are the most experienced with intubations. Kate draws up the medications and tells the patient to breathe as deeply as possible for the next few minutes. In the meantime, you prepare your equipment. Although you would normally use an 8.5 mm ETT for this intubation, you select an 8.0 mm tube, the tip of which you lubricate heavily in anticipation of laryngeal edema. Selecting a Viewmax™ blade to assist with visualization, you test the light and lay it to one side. You also test the CombiTube® and lay it out on the table next to the patient. If endotracheal intubation is not possible, you may be forced to use the CombiTube® to ventilate the patient. Using a sharp-tipped marker, you carefully locate and mark the patient's cricothyroid membrane in case a surgical airway becomes necessary.

Kate advises you that she has the medications drawn up and is ready to start. You lay the patient back and carefully place his head and neck in the "sniffing" position and tell your partner to give the medications. Etomidate is given for sedation, followed by succinylcholine for paralysis. Fasciculations are observed and the patient's respiratory effort ceases. After 30 seconds, you check the jaw for relaxation and find it completely lax. You tell your partner to give cricoid pressure as you open the mouth and advance the laryngoscope blade. Although the airway anatomy is distorted, you are able to make out the bottom of the glottic opening and the arytenoid cartilages. Asking Kate to give you some "BURP" brings the cords into view. Although there is clearly laryngeal edema, the tip of the tube is advanced relatively easily into the trachea. Keeping one hand on the endotracheal tube, you inflate the cuff and remove the stylet with the other, letting out a big sigh of relief in the process. Kate attaches a BVM to the tube and gives several deep, slow ventilations while you auscultate breath sounds. After hearing good breath sounds over the right and left chest and none over the epigastrium, you attach the $ETCO_2$ monitor. The monitor shows a slight increase in the slope of the plateau, but a relatively steady CO_2 concentration of 38 mmHg. The tube is secured with a plastic tube-holding device and the SpO_2 quickly increases to 94 percent. The BVM is removed and the ETT is attached to the circuit of the automatic transport ventilator for the duration of the transfer. As the patient is packaged for transport, Kate administers vecuronium and midazolam to maintain paralysis and sedation during the flight.

En route to the burn center, as the ocean falls away beneath the helicopter, you reflect on how close a call the intubation was, and how it could have been a very difficult intubation. If things had gone badly, you would've been prepared since you regularly practice your difficult airway skills.

DISCUSSION QUESTIONS

1. What are the options available for the placement of endotracheal tubes in the critical care transport setting?
2. What is the procedure for rapid sequence intubation?
3. What rescue devices or procedures are available for failed intubations in the critical care transport setting?
4. What role do noninvasive monitors play in airway management and ventilation?

Content Review

MULTIPLE CHOICE

_____ 1. All of the following are reasons that illustrate the importance of airway management in modern critical care transport except:
  A. as a critical care paramedic, you will utilize your airway skills more frequently than in the prehospital environment.
  B. airway management and mechanical ventilation is often performed for long periods of time in the critical care environment.
  C. you will tend to be presented with more difficult airways in the critical care environment.
  D. as a critical care paramedic, you will often be working alone, without a partner to assist in airway management.

_____ 2. Which of the following laryngoscope blades has a 80 percent wider surface area than traditional blades, allowing for better control of the tongue during laryngoscopy?
  A. Viewmax™   C. MacIntosh
  B. Grandview™   D. Miller

_____ 3. This semi-rigid stylet is used to facilitate the passage of an endotracheal tube into the trachea.
  A. Eschmann stylet   C. Viewmax™ blade
  B. Grandview™ blade   D. BURP maneuver

_____ 4. Which of the following devices would be the best choice to utilize to aid an intubation in which you are not able to visualize any glottic anatomy because of an extremely anterior glottis?
  A. gum elastic bougie   C. BURP maneuver
  B. Viewmax™ laryngoscope blade D. scalpel

_____ 5. Which of the following devices is not designed to facilitate nasal intubation?
  A. Beck airway airflow monitor (BAAM)   C. gum elastic bougie
  B. Burden nasoscope   D. lighted stylet

_____ 6. Which of the following statements regarding the BURP maneuver is true?
  A. The intubator uses her left hand to perform the BURP maneuver.
  B. BURP is an acronym that stands for Backward Under Respiratory Pressure.
  C. The BURP maneuver is manual manipulation of the hypopharynx to achieve a better view of glottic anatomy during laryngoscopy.
  D. Utilization of the BURP maneuver can improve a Cormack-Lehane grade 2 or 3 view of the glottis by at least one grade.

_____ 7. You are attempting to intubate a patient in cardiac arrest but are having trouble passing the endotracheal tube because you can only visualize about 50 percent of the glottic opening. Which of the following would be the least effective in assisting your intubation attempt?
  A. using a Beck airway airflow monitor (BAAM)
  B. utilizing the BURP maneuver
  C. performing a digital intubation
  D. utilizing an Eshmann stylet

©2007 Pearson Education, Inc.
Critical Care Paramedic

_____ 8. You are presented with a 32-year-old male supine on the ground, unconscious and apnic, who has a closed head injury, soft-tissue abrasions, and swelling over his larynx after being ejected from a vehicle during an MVA rollover. He accepts an OPA and is ventilated with a BVM, but starts to regurgitate vomit into his airway. The patient is suctioned, and your two attempts at endotracheal intubation are unsuccessful due to blood, vomit, and distortion of the airway anatomy from trauma. Of the following, which is the best choice to manage this patient's airway?
A. Continue to provide BVM ventilations with 100 percent oxygen while utilizing an OPA.
B. Attempt a digital intubation.
C. Perform RSI.
D. Perform a surgical cricothyrotomy.

_____ 9. Which procedure involves inserting a guidewire through the cricothyroid membrane and into the oropharynx to serve as a guide for the endotracheal tube placement into the trachea?
A. RSI
B. use of a lighted stylet
C. needle cricothyrotomy
D. retrograde intubation

_____ 10. The four phases of RSI pharmacology, in order, are:
A. induction, premedication, neuromuscular blockade, and maintenance therapy.
B. sedation, induction, neuromuscular blockade, and intubation.
C. premedication, neuromuscular blockade, intubation, and maintenance therapy.
D. sedation, neuromuscular blockade, intubation, and reassessment.

_____ 11. All of the following situations would indicate the need for RSI except:
A. an unconscious and head-injured 42-year-old female with a RR = 10 and vomit in her airway, who gags when rigid suction catheter or OPA is inserted.
B. a 24-year-old male with facial burns and stridorous respirations at 30/min after being trapped in a burning building.
C. an 18-year-old asthmatic who is unconscious in respiratory arrest.
D. a 60-year-old female with pneumonia, RR = 10 and shallow, SpO_2 = 80 percent, and altered mental status.

_____ 12. The primary reason for the use of analgesics and hypnotics in RSI is to:
A. reduce the risk of increased intracranial pressure.
B. provide sedation prior to paralysis.
C. prevent tachycardia.
D. prevent the development of fasciculations.

_____ 13. Your patient is a 42-year-old male who is unconscious with multisystem trauma after a fall off a cliff. His vital signs are: HR = 126, RR = 10 and shallow, BP = 82/52, SpO_2 = 89 percent with BVM ventilations. A medic alert bracelet says that he has end-stage renal disease and receives dialysis 2 times a week. You determine the need for RSI. Which of the following medications and doses is the most appropriate for this patient?
A. Thiopental sodium 2 to 5 mg/kg IV
B. Fentanyl 2 to 10 mcg/kg IV
C. Morphine 0.1 to 0.2 mg/kg IV
D. Diazepam 0.25 to 0.4 mg/kg IV

_____ 14. You are preparing to perform RSI on a 17-year-old male in respiratory failure secondary to status asthmaticus using succinylcholine as your neuromuscular blocking agent. His vital signs are: HR = 132, RR = 12 and labored, BP = 126/90, SpO_2 = 90 percent on 100 percent oxygen via NRM 15 lpm. Which of the following would be a proper premedication to administer to this patient?
A. Atropine
B. Lidocaine
C. Ketamine
D. Vecuronium

_____ 15. Premedications are medications used to:
A. provide sedation and analgesia prior to RSI.
B. induce paralysis prior to intubation.
C. blunt or attenuate various side effects of neuromuscular blocking agents.
D. prevent dysrhythmia during RSI.

_____ 16. Medications administered to induce muscle relaxation to facilitate endotracheal intubation are:
A. neuromuscular blocking agents.
B. premedications.
C. induction agents.
D. sedative/hypnotic agents.

_____ 17. Depolarizing blocking agents act by:
A. acting as an antagonist to ACh.
B. tightly binding to and depolarizing the ACh receptor, then continuing to occupy the receptor, preventing another depolarization.
C. causing fasciculations, thereby preventing ACh from binding to its receptors.
D. binding with pseudocholinesterase in the neuromuscular junction.

_____ 18. Administration of which of the following agents can result in fasciculations?
A. depolarizing agent
B. nondepolarizing agent
C. Vecuronium
D. Curcre

_____ 19. Which of the following statements regarding reversal agents for nondepolarizing neuromuscular blocking agents is false?
A. Neostigmine and pyridostigmine are examples of reversal agents for nondepolarizing neuromuscular blocking agents.
B. Reversal agents for nondepolarizing neuromuscular blocking agents act by inhibiting the action of cholinesterase in the synaptic cleft.
C. Reversal agents for nondepolarizing neuromuscular blocking agents increase the amount of ACh in the neuromuscular junction.
D. Reversal agents for nondepolarizing neuromuscular blocking agents decrease the amount of pseudocholinesterase in the neuromuscular junction.

_____ 20. The adult dose of succinylcholine used in RSI is:
A. 0.15 mg/kg.
B. 1.5 mg/kg.
C. 15 mg/kg.
D. 1.5 mcg/kg.

_____ 21. All of the following are considered rescue airways except:
A. endotracheal CombiTube (ETC).
B. pharyngotracheal lumen airway (PtL).
C. BVM ventilations with an OPA.
D. laryngeal mask airway (LMA).

_____ 22. The endotracheal CombiTube should not be used in a patient:
A. who is unconscious.
B. who gags when an OPA is inserted.
C. with upper gastrointestinal bleeding.
D. with a respiratory rate of 12.

_____ 23. An advantage of the pharyngotracheal lumen airway (PtL) is that:
A. it can function in either the tracheal or esophageal position.
B. endotracheal intubation can easily be performed with the PtL in place.
C. it can be used in conscious patients with a gag reflex.
D. it completely isolates the trachea and protects from aspiration.

_____ 24. All of the following are disadvantages of the laryngeal mask airway (LMA) except:
A. it cannot be used in a patient with a gag reflex.
B. it does not isolate the trachea.
C. it is designed to be inserted blindly, without the use of a laryngoscope.
D. it does not protect the airway from regurgitation and aspiration.

_____ 25. Which rescue airway device, while in place and aiding airway management, can facilitate the placement of an endotracheal tube?
   A. Eschmann stylet
   B. esophageal CombiTube (ECT)
   C. laryngeal mask airway (LMA)
   D. intubating laryngeal mask airway (LMA Fastrach®)

_____ 26. Contraindications to surgical airway include all of the following except:
   A. the inability to identify anatomical landmarks.
   B. the presence of any morphology or pathology that will prevent successful completion of the procedure.
   C. the ability to ventilate or intubate by nasal or oral routes.
   D. a documented history of hemophilia.

_____ 27. All of the following are possible complications of needle cricothyrotomy except:
   A. barotrauma.   C. reversal of hypoxia.
   B. hemorrhaging.   D. subcutaneous emphysema.

_____ 28. When performing an open cricothyrotomy, the initial incision that is made through the skin lying over the cricothyroid membrane should be:
   A. a 1- to 2-cm horizontal incision.
   B. a 1- to 2-cm vertical incision.
   C. as wide a vertical incision as necessary to pass the endotracheal tube.
   D. as narrow a horizontal incision as necessary to pass the endotracheal tube.

_____ 29. When performing an open cricothyrotomy, the second incision that is made through the cricothyroid membrane should be:
   A. a 1-cm horizontal incision.
   B. a 1-cm vertical incision.
   C. as wide a vertical incision as necessary to pass the endotracheal tube.
   D. as narrow a horizontal incision as necessary to pass the endotracheal tube.

_____ 30. Which of the following anatomical factors is associated with difficult airway?
   A. a long mandible
   B. a mouth opening greater than 3 cm (3 fingers breadths) wide
   C. presence of malocclusion or overbite
   D. posterior larynx

_____ 31. According to the Cormack and Lehane classification system, a view of the glottis in which only the epiglottis can be visualized would be considered a:
   A. Grade I view.   C. Grade III view.
   B. Grade II view.   D. Grade IV view.

_____ 32. According to the Mallampati classification system, what class of airway is typified by a view of the upper half of the uvula and tonsils?
   A. Class I   C. Class III
   B. Class II   D. Class IV

_____ 33. The term "difficult mask ventilation" is used to describe a situation in which:
   A. an unassisted paramedic is able to maintain an SpO_2 > 90 percent using only 100 percent oxygen and BVM ventilation on patient whose SpO_2 was > 90 percent prior to ventilation.
   B. an unassisted paramedic is able to reverse or prevent signs of inadequate ventilation only during BVM ventilation.
   C. both A and B.
   D. neither A nor B.

_____ 34. The term "difficult laryngoscopy" is used to describe:
   A. the inability to visualize the vocal cords under direct laryngoscopy.
   B. the inability to pass an endotracheal tube under direct laryngoscopy.
   C. an intubation that requires three or more attempts at laryngoscopy.
   D. an intubation that requires more than 10 minutes to perform.

_____ 35. The term "difficult intubation" is used to describe:
  A. an intubation that requires the use of 2 or more laryngoscopists.
  B. the inability to pass an endotracheal tube under direct laryngoscopy.
  C. intubations that require more than 3 attempts at laryngoscopy or greater than 10 minutes to perform.
  D. intubations that must be attempted in adverse conditions, such as inclement weather, poor lighting, or a lack of experienced personnel.

_____ 36. The presence of moderate hypoxia is suggested by an SpO_2 of:
  A. 95 percent.   C. 90 percent.
  B. 91 percent.   D. 84 percent.

_____ 37. Which of the following statements regarding the relationship between SpO_2 and PaO_2 is true?
  A. The greater the SpO_2, the less the PaO_2.
  B. The greater the SpO_2, the greater the PaO_2.
  C. There is no relationship between SpO_2 and PaO_2.
  D. The greater the SpO_2, the less the PaO_2 in cases of hypoxia.

_____ 38. Which method of expired CO_2 measurement presents values via a visual representation of the expired CO_2 waveform?
  A. capnogram   C. capnography
  B. capnograph   D. capnometry

_____ 39. Which method of expired CO_2 measurement presents values via a numeric display?
  A. capnogram   C. capnography
  B. capnograph   D. capnometry

_____ 40. Which of the following statements regarding end-tidal carbon dioxide ($ETCO_2$) monitoring is true?
  A. $ETCO_2$ monitoring is a minimally invasive method of measuring the levels of CO_2 in exhaled breath.
  B. When pulmonary perfusion decreases, $ETCO_2$ levels reflect ventilation efficiency, not pulmonary blood flow and cardiac output.
  C. $ETCO_2$ monitoring can provide information regarding systemic metabolism, circulation, and ventilation status.
  D. $ETCO_2$ is not as effective as pulse oximetry in verifying endotracheal tube placement in a patient with a pulse.

_____ 41. Which phase of the capnogram represents the expiration of mixed dead-space and alveolar gases?
  A. Phase I   C. Phase III
  B. Phase II   D. Phase IV

_____ 42. Which phase of the capnogram represents the inspiratory phase of the respiratory cycle?
  A. Phase I   C. Phase III
  B. Phase II   D. Phase IV

_____ 43. Which phase of the capnogram represents the early part of expiration?
  A. Phase I   C. Phase III
  B. Phase II   D. Phase IV

_____ 44. Which phase of the respiratory cycle represents the expiration of mostly alveolar gases?
  A. Phase I   C. Phase III
  B. Phase II   D. Phase IV

_____ 45. The type of ventilator utilized by the vast majority of critical care transport services is a:
  A. negative pressure ventilator.   C. volume control ventilator.
  B. positive pressure ventilator.   D. pressure ventilator.

©2007 Pearson Education, Inc.
Critical Care Paramedic

_____ 46. The stimulus that causes a ventilator to cycle to inspiration is called:
A. cycling.   C. triggering.
B. support.   D. control.

_____ 47. _____ determines how much flow a ventilator will deliver.
A. Cycling   C. Triggering
B. Support   D. Control

_____ 48. _____ determines how a ventilator switches from inspiration to expiration.
A. Cycling   C. Triggering
B. Support   D. Control

_____ 49. When _____, a ventilator is set to cycle to expiration once a set tidal volume has been delivered.
A. flow cycled   C. rate cycled
B. time cycled   D. volume cycled

_____ 50. When a ventilator is dual controlled:
A. the volume is set and the pressures are variable.
B. the volume is set and limits are placed on the pressures.
C. the pressures are set and the volume is variable.
D. both the pressure and volume are set.

_____ 51. If a ventilator is set to sense the patient's respiratory effort by detecting a decrease in circuit baseline pressure it is:
A. time triggered.   C. pressure triggered.
B. flow triggered.   D. circuit triggered.

_____ 52. In _____, a ventilator is set to deliver the preset tidal volume at a preset number of times per minute, regardless of patient effort.
A. assist/control mode   C. support mode
B. trigger mode   D. timed mode

_____ 53. In _____, a ventilator delivers a fixed tidal volume at a preset rate, and the patient can take unassisted breaths on his own, without tidal volume support.
A. assist/control mode   C. pressure support mode
B. SIMV   D. set mode

_____ 54. _____ is a mode in which a patient triggers the ventilator at a preset pressure during inspiration.
A. Pressure control   C. Assist/control
B. SIMV   D. Pressure support

_____ 55. Common settings for the sensitivity control with a patient in assist mode are:
A. 1 cm/H_2O.   C. 1 to 2 cm/H_2O.
B. −1 to −2 cm/H_2O.   D. 1:2.

_____ 56. Respiratory rate on a ventilated patient is normally set at:
A. 12 to 20/minute.   C. 8 to 12/minute.
B. 6 to 12/minute.   D. 10 to 20/minute.

_____ 57. How can minute ventilation be determined, and what is a normal value for a patient who is being mechanically ventilated?
A. Multiply the tidal volume by the respiratory rate; 6 to 10 lpm
B. Divide the tidal volume by the respiratory rate; 6 to 10 lpm
C. Multiply the respiratory rate by the tidal volume; 4 to 8 lpm.
D. Divide the respiratory rate by the tidal volume; 4 to 8 lpm

_____ 58. Which of the following I/E ratios would be best for a patient with hypercarbia secondary to an exacerbation of COPD?
A. 1:1   C. 3:1
B. 1:2   D. 1:4

_____ **59.** An inspiratory flow rate of _____ is a commonly used starting point when setting mechanical ventilator parameters.
   A. 10 to 15 lpm
   B. 15 to 25 lpm
   C. 25 to 50 lpm
   D. 40 to 80 lpm

_____ **60.** Mechanical ventilators can be set to sigh at _____ times the normal tidal volume about _____ times per hour.
   A. 5, 2
   B. 1.5 to 2, 10 to 15
   C. 1 to 2, 10 to 15
   D. 1.5 to 2, 12 to 20

©2007 Pearson Education, Inc.
Critical Care Paramedic

The Shock Patient: Assessment and Management

Review of Chapter Objectives

Upon completion of this chapter, the student should be able to:

1. Define shock.   p. 188

Shock is local or systemic hypoperfusion resulting in an inability to meet the cellular demands of tissues, organs, or organ systems, resulting in anaerobic cellular metabolism. Resulting in anaerobic cellular metabolism.

2. Describe what happens in the cell during a shock state.   p. 188

Peripheral tissues cannot store oxygen, and so rely on constant perfusion to deliver oxygen and remove metabolic waste. Oxygen uptake (a.k.a. VO_2 or oxygen consumption) is the amount of oxygen taken up and consumed by the mitochondria in the body. The metabolic requirement for oxygen (MRO_2) is the rate at which oxygen is utilized in the mitochondria to convert glucose into adenosine triphosphate (ATP) and water, both of which are products of the tricarboxylic acid (TCA) or Krebs cycle. For normal, or aerobic, metabolism to occur, VO_2 must match, or be greater than, MRO_2. Aerobic respiration results in the complete and efficient oxidation of 1 molecule of glucose, producing 36 moles of ATP and water.

If VO_2 falls below MRO_2 (supply falls below demand), oxygen uptake in the mitochondria fails to meet the metabolic demand for oxygen, and anaerobic metabolism occurs. Anaerobic metabolism results in the inefficient and incomplete breakdown of glucose into 2 molecules of ATP and pyruvic acid, which is then converted to lactic acid. So, anaerobic metabolism results not only in less energy production, but a state of acidosis. As cells are starved of energy they die, leading to tissue death, organ death, and, eventually, multi-organ and organism death.

Shock also affects the sodium/potassium (Na^+/K^+) pump. The lack of ATP production in anaerobic metabolism results in failure of the Na^+/K^+ pump, allowing Na^+ to move into the intracellular environment. An osmotic gradient is created, and water shifts along this gradient into the cell, resulting in swelling and cell lysis that can lead to clinically significant organ damage.

Dystoxia exists when ATP production is limited by the supply of oxygen, and shock is said to exist when dystoxia causes a measurable change in organ function. Under normal conditions, oxygen delivery will never be a limiting factor for cellular metabolism, as the cardiovascular system is more than adequate to supply peripheral tissues with blood. In a healthy individual, VO_2 max (the maximum amount of oxygen you can possibly metabolize at once) will be exceeded long before oxygen supply becomes a limiting factor. For example, when you become winded while running and need to slow down and rest, you have exceeded your VO_2 max, and demand for ATP has exceeded your ability to produce it (even though your cardiovascular system was capable of delivering the raw material, oxygen, to make it!) in the mitochondria.

VO_2, the amount of oxygen uptake in the mitochondria, is a function of three things:

- Cardiac output (CO)
- Available hemoglobin (Hb)
- The difference in oxygen saturation between arterial and venous blood ($SaO_2 - SvO_2$)

and is represented by the equation $VO_2 = $ Cardiac Output (CO) $\times 13.4 \times$ Hb $\times (SaO_2 - SvO_2)$. Normal $VO_2 = 100$ to 160 mL/min/m^2.
Shock can develop as a result of three situations:

1. Inadequate CO: Poor CO leads to reduced perfusion of peripheral tissues which leads to reduced oxygen supply, VO_2 falls below MRO_2, and shock develops.
2. Inadequate Hb concentration or oxygen-carrying capacity: Decreased oxygen-carrying capacity leads to decreased oxygen supply to cells, VO_2 falls below MRO_2, and shock develops.
3. Inadequate arterial oxygen saturation: Perfusion to tissues is adequate, flow-wise, but a decreased arterial oxygen saturation results in decreased oxygen supply, VO_2 falls below MRO_2, and shock develops.

3. **Identify vital organs versus nonvital organs.**   p. 192

Nonvital organs:

- Gastrointestinal tract
- Skeletal muscle
- Immune system
- Skin
- Liver
- Kidneys
- Lungs

Vital organs:

- Heart
- Brain

4. **Discuss and describe neurohumoral transmitters involved in shock.**   p. 193

The overall effects of neurohumoral transmitter release during the development of shock are increased cardiac output, vasoconstriction, electrolyte and water retention, and the increased use of alternative fuel sources. Specifically:

- Norepinephrine
  - Vasoconstriction
  - Increases cardiac contractility
- Epinephrine
  - Increases HR
  - Increases myocardial contractility
- Angiotensin II
  - Vasoconstriction
  - Promotes secretion of antidiuretic hormone
  - Increases plasma volume
- Antidiuretic hormone
  - Increases water retention in kidney
  - Increases plasma volume
- Aldosterone
  - Promotes Na$^+$ and water retention in kidneys
  - Increases plasma volume
- Cortisol
  - Suppresses immune and inflammatory response
  - Promotes protein catabolism
  - Increases blood glucose levels

©2007 Pearson Education, Inc.
Critical Care Paramedic

5. Identify the stages of shock. p. 193

The stages of shock are compensated shock, progressive shock, and decompensated shock. Compensated shock occurs when the body is able to detect the decrease in CO with feedback from chemo- and baroreceptors. Compensation for developing hemodynamic instability occurs by the release of epinephrine and norepinepherine, leading to the activation of compensatory mechanisms including increased peripheral vasoconstriction, heart rate, and myocardial contractility. Blood pressure is maintained, but compensated shock will progress to progressive shock if the insult is not recognized and corrected.

In progressive shock, developing anaerobic metabolism results in the development of hypoxia. In addition to further increases in peripheral vasoconstriction, heart rate, and myocardial contractility, water retention in the kidney is encouraged via the release of angiotensin II, antidiuretic hormone, and aldosterone.

Decompensated shock can develop suddenly, or over days, and is characterized by cellular, tissue, and, finally, organ death. Prognosis is poor, and death is certain.

6. Describe general treatment modalities involved with shock including hemodynamic monitoring. pp. 197–199

The management for shock is the same as for any critically ill patient, with the ABCDE methods utilized for prioritizing the management of life threats. Specific management for shock (i.e., antibiotic administration for septic shock) can take place after management of potential life threats, though the management of potential life-threats may help manage shock as well (fluid replacement for gross hemorrhage).

Airway management and ventilation is key, and aggressive management should be started early, with endotracheal intubation performed when necessary. Fluid resuscitation requires IV access, and 2 large-bore IV lines should be initiated if peripheral IV access is to be utilized. Central venous cannulation can be performed if peripheral IV access cannot be obtained, if the administration of large volumes of IV fluid is anticipated, or if hemodynamic monitoring is required. In cases of hypovolemic shock, the goal of fluid resuscitation is to achieve no more than 75 percent of the pre-injury blood pressure. This practice, termed "permissive hypotension," prevents the excessive bleeding and loss of coagulation factors typical with the overadministration of fluids. Crystalloid boluses of 200 ml should be administered and repeated as needed.

Hemoglobin-based oxygen-carrying solutions (HBOCs) represent a major development in emergency and critical care medicine. HBOCs contain polymerized hemoglobin that has been removed from human and bovine red blood cells, and they differ from traditional IV volume expanders in that they can transport oxygen. They are compatible with all blood types, and do not require typing, testing, or cross matching. Specific types of HBOCs include Polyheme and Hemopure.

Other volume expanders include hypertonic saline, colloids, and blood and blood products. While hypertonic saline showed some initial potential in the treatment of shock, recent evidence suggests it is no more effective than standard isotonic crystalloids. Colloids are popular outside the United States, especially in Australia, but are no more or less effective than crystalloids. Typed and cross-matched blood products are preferred for volume replacement, though O-negative can be used if time for typing and cross matching does not exist.

Pharmacologic agents used for hemodynamically significant shock unresponsive to fluid therapy include dopamine, dobutamine, epinephrine, and norepinephrine.

Hemodynamic monitoring initially takes place with uninvasive means with heart rate and rhythm determination and blood pressure. Invasive monitoring can include any of the following (normal values are provided for reference):

- Urine output: 0.5–1.0 mL/hr
- Left ventricular pressures
  - Systolic: 100–130 mmHg
  - End diastolic: 4–12 mmHg
- Left atrial (pulmonary artery wedge) pressures
  - Mean: 4–12 mmHg
  - A wave: 4–15 mmHg
  - V wave: 4–15 mmHg

- Pulmonary artery pressures:
  - Systolic: 15–30 mmHg
  - End diastolic: 6–12 mmHg
  - Mean: 9–18 mmHg
- Right ventricular pressures:
  - Systolic: 25–30 mmHg
  - End diastolic: 0–8 mmHg
- Right atrial pressures
  - Mean: 0–8 mmHg
  - A wave: 2–10 mmHg
  - V wave: 2–10 mmHg
- Cardiac output: 4–8 liters/minute
- Stroke volume: 60–130 mL
- Central venous pressure: 8–12 dynes/second
- Systemic vascular resistance (SVR): 800–1200 dynes/second
- Arterial blood gas:
  - pH: 7.35–7.45
  - PaO_2: 80–100 mmHg
  - Oxygen saturation 96–98 percent
  - $PaCO_2$: 35–45 mmHg
  - HCO_3^-: 21–28 mEq/L
  - Base/excess: ± 3 mEq/L
- Additional assessment and management may include the following standard tests:
  - Complete blood cell count and differential
  - Platelet count
  - Complete serum chemistry profile (includes electrolytes)
  - Prothrombin and activated partial thromboplastin times (PT and PTT).
  - Serum lactate
  - Urinalysis
  - Serum amylase
  - Arterial blood gases
  - 12-lead ECG
  - Pregnancy test for all females of childbearing age
  - Blood, sputum, and urine gram stains and cultures
  - Imaging tests
    - CT
    - Ultrasound
    - X-rays
    - Echocardiogram
  - Drug toxicity screening if indicated

7. Discuss the four classifications and subclassifications of shock.   pp. 200–202

Classifications of shock

- Hypovolemic
- Obstructive
- Distributive
  - Septic shock
  - Anaphylactic shock
  - Neurogenic shock
- Cardiogenic

Hypovolemic shock occurs secondary to a decrease in circulating blood volume. Etiologies include hemorrhage (trauma, GI bleeding), dehydration, and fluid shifts secondary to sepsis or burns. Signs and symptoms include altered mental status, diaphoresis, tachycardia, tachypnea, pallor, mottling, thirst, collapsed veins, increased skin turgor, decreased urine output, oliguria, concentrated urine, and hypotension. Hemodynamic monitoring will reveal decreased cardiac output (CO) and central venous pressure (CVP), and increased systemic vascular resistance (SVR) and pulmonary artery occlusion pressure (PAOP). Management of hypovolemic shock centers around volume resuscitation with crystalloids or colloids. Vasopressor agents are utilized only after adequate volume resuscitation has been attempted.

Obstructive shock occurs secondary to the impedance of normal blood flow. Etiologies include cardiac tamponade, tension pneumothorax, pericarditis, compression of the great vessels, pulmonary embolism, and aortic dissection. Signs and symptoms mirror those of hypovolemic shock and can also include those specific to the etiology. Hemodynamic monitoring will reveal a decreased CO, and increased CVP, PAOP, and SVR. Management is specific to the etiology.

Distributive shock is characterized by a decrease in vascular resistance or increased venous capacity secondary to vascular dysfunction. Hemodynamic monitoring parameters typically include an increased CO, CVP, and PAOP, and a decreased SVR. Subclassifications of distributive shock include septic, anaphylactic, and neurogenic shock. Septic shock occurs secondary to systemic infection; predisposing factors include immuno-insufficiency and nosocomial infection. Release of endotoxins by the infecting organism results in vasodilation and increased cell membrane permeability, with the end result being the third spacing of fluids and a relative intravascular hypovolemia. Signs and symptoms include fever, chills, diaphoresis, petechial rash, and pulmonary edema. Management includes identification and eradication of the source of infection, volume replacement, and vasopressors.

Anaphylactic shock is the result of an exaggerated, systemic response to an allergen, leading to profound vasodilation, third spacing of fluid, and bronchospasm. Etiologies include food and drug allergies, administration of blood products, and envenomation. Signs and symptoms, which can evolve over minutes or days, include dyspnea, bronchospasm, dysphagia, rashes, and flushing. In addition to the ABCs, management priorities include epinephrine and antihistamine administration.

Neurogenic shock results from the disruption of the sympathetic nervous system secondary to spinal cord injury, and can also occur secondary to severe head injury or migration of spinal anesthesia. A reduction in peripheral vascular resistance causes widespread vasodilation below the level of spinal cord insult; if the level of the insult is lower than T6, bradycardia develops secondary to unopposed vagal tone and a lack of compensatory tachycardia. Signs and symptoms of neurogenic shock include bradycardia, hypotension, and warm, flushed skin. Management includes volume and vasopressor administration.

Cardiogenic shock results from the heart's inability to maintain sufficient cardiac output, and is often the result of myocardial ischemia, dysrhythmia, or ventricular insufficiency; left ventricular failure will result in pulmonary hypertension and edema. Signs and symptoms vary widely with etiology, and hemodynamic monitoring typically reveals a decreased CO, and increased SVR, CVP, and PAOP. The treatment goal is to restore cardiac output with volume replacement, vasopressors, IABP placement, ventricular assist devices, pacemaker, or CABG.

Case Study

Your patient is a 74-year-old female who needs to be transferred from a two-bed rural ED to an acute care hospital approximately 40 miles away. She is being sent for a surgical consult to rule out a small bowel obstruction. The attending PA tells you that the patient presented via EMS with a 48-hour history of abdominal pain. She began vomiting feculent material shortly after the pain started. Initially, the pain was crampy in nature and intermittent, but now is constant and worsens with any movement. She has multiple air-fluid levels on the upright X-ray and the complete blood count shows an elevated white count with a "left shift." The patient's abdomen is distended with tenderness throughout and voluntary guarding is present. A nasogastric tube was placed which helped to relieve her vomiting.

The patient presents curled up in a fetal position, lying on her right side. She is guarding her belly with her hands and is in obvious pain. The patient is responsive to voice, but is moaning in pain and slow to answer questions. The NG tube is connected to low intermittent suction and is draining bilious fluid. She has cool, pale skin and a weak, radial pulse. Breath sounds are clear to auscultation bilaterally.

Her ECG shows a sinus tachycardia at 118 bpm and her blood pressure is 98/60 mmHg. The SpO$_2$ monitor shows a saturation of 95 percent on room air. With some difficulty, the patient is moved to the stretcher and packaged for transport.

Approximately 10 minutes into the transport, the patient becomes anxious, and reassessment of her vital signs shows a heart rate of 130 bpm, still in sinus tachycardia, respiratory rate of 22 breaths per minute, and blood pressure of 88/62 mmHg. The SpO$_2$ monitor is now only intermittently registering a reading of 93 percent and has a poor waveform. Adjusting the SpO$_2$ probe, you notice that her hands are cold and dusky. Opening up the IV fluid, you give the patient a 250 mL bolus of normal saline and place her on high-flow high-concentration oxygen by nonrebreather mask. After the normal saline bolus, the patient remains unchanged. After assessing the patient's lung sounds for wheezes or crackles, you listen to her heart sounds for murmurs or extra sounds. Finding none of these signs that might indicate early heart failure, you decide to give the patient another IV fluid bolus. Assuring that the patient is covered with blankets to conserve heat, you again open the IV to give another 250 cc bolus of normal saline. The patient becomes slightly less anxious, and reassessment of her vital signs shows sinus tachycardia at a rate of 122, respiratory rate of 18 breaths per minute, and blood pressure of 96/64 mmHg. The SpO$_2$ monitor still shows a poor waveform, but registers a reading of 95 percent. Advising your driver via the intercom that the patient's condition is beginning to decline, he advises you that your ETA to the receiving hospital is still 25 minutes. After updating your medical control base station, reassessment of the patient's vital signs shows a heart rate of 138, still sinus tachycardia, but now with occasional premature ventricular complexes, respiratory rate of 24 breaths per minute, and blood pressure of 70/52 mmHg. The patient's radial pulse is no longer palpable, and the SpO$_2$ monitor no longer provides a reliable waveform. Upon reassessment of breath sounds, you find some dependent crackles and expiratory wheezes bilaterally. There is now an S$_3$ sound when you auscultate the heart. Concerned that you will worsen the patient's heart failure with any further IV fluids, you decide to initiate a vasopressor infusion. After starting a dopamine infusion at 5 micrograms per kilogram per minute, you reassess your patient's vital signs. Her vital signs show a heart rate of 128, sinus tachycardia with PVCs, respirations of 20 breaths per minute, and blood pressure of 98/64 mmHg. The patient's radial pulse is now palpable, but the SpO$_2$ monitor is still not providing a reliable waveform.

With 10 minutes left of your transport, your patient's vital signs remain stable and you update medical control of her condition. On arrival to the facility, she still has stable vital signs, and after moving the patient to the ED stretcher, you update the nurses and the surgical resident on the patient's condition and treatment during the transport.

DISCUSSION QUESTIONS

1. What is shock?
2. What are the four classifications and subclassifications of shock?
3. What are the stages of shock?
4. What are some general treatment modalities for shock in the critical care transport environment?

Content Review

MULTIPLE CHOICE

_____ 1. Shock can best be defined as:
  A. inadequate cellular perfusion of peripheral tissues, organs, and organ systems leading to anaerobic respiration if left untreated.
  B. a state of local or systemic hypoperfusion resulting in an inability to meet the cellular demands of tissues, organs, or organ systems.
  C. a state of hypoperfusion leading to anaerobic respiration and inadequate cellular demand.
  D. the inability of peripheral tissues to store oxygen in times of increased oxygen demand.

_____ 2. For normal, or aerobic, metabolism to occur:
   A. VO_2 max must match or be greater than MRO_2.
   B. VO_2 must match or be less than MRO_2.
   C. VO_2 must match or be greater than MRO_2.
   D. VO_2 must match or be greater than MRO_2 max.

_____ 3. Which of the following statements regarding cellular respiration is true?
   A. Anaerobic metabolism occurs when VO_2 falls below MRO_2.
   B. Oxygen uptake (VO_2) is the maximum amount of oxygen that can be consumed by the mitochondria.
   C. Aerobic respiration results in the oxidation of 1 molecule of glucose, producing 36 moles of ATP and water.
   D. The metabolic requirement for oxygen (MRO_2) is the rate at which oxygen is utilized in the mitochondria to convert ATP and water into glucose.

_____ 4. What is dystoxia?
   A. A condition that exists when ATP production is limited by the supply of oxygen.
   B. A condition that causes a measurable change in organ function.
   C. The incomplete oxidation of glucose resulting in 2 moles of ATP and pyruvic acid.
   D. The conversion of pyruvic acid to lactic acid.

_____ 5. Lactic acid can be best described as:
   A. a toxic, metabolic by-product of anaerobic metabolism.
   B. a normal by-product of aerobic metabolism.
   C. a toxic, metabolic by-product of aerobic metabolism.
   D. a normal, immediate product of the incomplete oxidation of glucose.

_____ 6. VO_2 is a function of:
   A. anaerobic metabolism.
   B. peripheral perfusion, the number of red blood cells, and SpO_2.
   C. heart rate, hematocrit, and PaO_2.
   D. cardiac output, available hemoglobin, and the difference in oxygen saturation between arterial and venous blood.

_____ 7. The amount of oxygen transported per gram of hemoglobin is:
   A. 1.34 g.   C. 134 g.
   B. 13.4 g.   D. 0.134 g.

_____ 8. Which of the following is not a precipitator of shock?
   A. Inadequate cardiac output
   B. Increased arterial carbon dioxide saturation
   C. Inadequate oxygen-carrying capacity
   D. Inadequate arterial oxygen saturation

_____ 9. All of the following are considered nonvital organs except the:
   A. liver.   C. kidneys.
   B. lungs.   D. heart.

_____ 10. Which of the following neurohumoral transmitters, when released, does not result in the retention of water in the kidney?
   A. aldosterone
   B. angiotensin II
   C. antidiuretic hormone
   D. cortisol

_____ 11. This stage of shock is characterized by the release of epinephrine and norepinephrine resulting in the activation of compensatory mechanisms and the delaying of hypoxia.
   A. compensated shock   C. progressive shock
   B. compensatory shock   D. decompensated shock

_____ 12. Which of the following is not an indication for central venous cannulation during the treatment of shock?
   A. Peripheral IV access cannot be obtained.
   B. Vasopressor administration is required.
   C. The administration of large volumes of IV fluid is anticipated.
   D. Hemodynamic monitoring is required.

_____ 13. Permissive hypotension is the practice of:
   A. withholding vasopressor administration until after resuscitation with colloids has been attempted.
   B. administering a vasoactive medication to promote hypotension in a patient with shock.
   C. achieving no more than 75 percent of pre-injury blood pressure in a hypovolemic and hypotensive patient.
   D. achieving a blood pressure of no greater than 60 mmHg systolic during the treatment of hypotension.

_____ 14. Which of the following is not an advantage of hemoglobin-based oxygen-carrying solutions (HBOCs)?
   A. HBOCs are compatible with all blood types.
   B. HBOCs can carry oxygen.
   C. HBOCs have relatively long shelf lives (over 1 year).
   D. Cross matching and blood typing prior to HBOC administration can be performed rapidly.

_____ 15. In patients requiring volume replacement, which blood type can be used without typing and cross matching?
   A. O-positive   C. O-negative
   B. B-positive   D. A-negative

_____ 16. Your rotor-wing transport team is transporting a sedated, paralyzed, and intubated 22-year-old male with a gunshot wound to the right anterior chest who is hemodynamically stable. During transport, the vent pressure alarm activates, and over the next 30 seconds, you note that SpO_2 has decreased, BP has fallen, the patient is tachycardiac, and pronounced JVD has developed. Your partner removes the patient from the vent circuit, begins BVM ventilations, and reports that there is significant resistance to bagging. Based on the clinical information, which of the following is the most likely cause of this patient's developing shock?
   A. tension pneumothorax   C. pulmonary embolism
   B. massive hemothorax   D. cardiac tamponade

Questions 17 and 18 refer to the information provided in Question 16.

_____ 17. Based on the limited clinical information provided, what class of shock is most likely present?
   A. hypovolemic shock   C. distributive shock
   B. obstructive shock   D. cardiogenic shock

_____ 18. Based on the limited clinical information provided, which of the following would be the most appropriate immediate treatment?
   A. needle decompression of the right thoracic cavity
   B. administration of a 250 mL fluid challenge
   C. administration of 250 mL of O-negative whole blood
   D. initiation of a dopamine drip at 5–15 mcg/kg/min IV

_____ 19. What hemodynamic findings would you expect with regard to CO, SVR, CVP, and PAOP in a patient with distributive shock?
   A. CO increased, SVR increased, CVP decreased, PAOP increased
   B. CO decreased, SVR increased, CVP decreased, PAOP decreased
   C. CO increased, SVR decreased, CVP increased, PAOP decreased
   D. CO increased, SVR decreased, CVP increased, PAOP increased

_____ 20. You are presented with a 62-year-old female in moderate distress. The sending facility reports that the patient has had a 2-week history of dark, tarry stools and numerous episodes of dizziness and near-syncope with exertion for the past two days. She has a PMH significant for Type I diabetes and hypertension, for which she takes insulin and a calcium channel blocker daily. Physical exam reveals HR = 118, RR = 20 and regular, BP = 76/42, SpO_2 = 95 percent on 2 lpm via nasal cannula. A finger stick reveals a blood glucose of 98 mg/dL, and you note that her lung sounds are clear, heart sounds are normal, and her skin is cool and pale. Based on the clinical findings, what class of shock is most likely present?

A. hypovolemic shock
B. obstructive shock
C. distributive shock
D. cardiogenic shock

_____ 21. What hemodynamic findings would you expect with regard to CO, SVR, CVP, and PAOP in the patient presented in question 20?

A. CO increased, SVR increased, CVP increased, PAOP decreased
B. CO decreased, SVR increased, CVP increased, PAOP decreased
C. CO decreased, SVR increased, CVP decreased, PAOP decreased
D. CO increased, SVR decreased, CVP decreased, PAOP increased

9 Cardiac and Hemodynamic Monitoring

Review of Chapter Objectives

Upon completion of this chapter, the student should be able to:

1. Define hemodynamic monitoring. p. 206

Hemodynamic monitoring is the monitoring of various patient hemodynamic parameters in order to identify and interpret changes and trends in patient hemodynamic status and evaluate the effectiveness of treatment. Parameters monitored include, but are not limited to, electrocardiogram (ECG), arterial blood pressure (ABP), central venous pressure (CVP), cardiac output (CO), pulmonary capillary wedge pressure (PCWP), stroke volume (SV), and oxygen delivery (DO_2).

2. Define the physiological difference between noninvasive versus invasive pressure monitoring. p. 209

Noninvasive, or indirect, pressure monitoring with a sphygmomanometer is adequate for most patient care situations. While the procedure for obtaining a noninvasive arterial blood pressure is relatively simple, there are multiple sources of error, including using an inappropriate cuff size, user error, and environmental distractions. Critical care medicine often requires a more accurate blood pressure determination than is possible with noninvasive methods.

Invasive, or direct, pressure monitoring is, as the name implies, an invasive procedure requiring sophisticated equipment. In the procedure, an arterial catheter is placed into an artery, usually the femoral or radial, and filled with heparinized saline. The catheter serves as a fluid column between the blood and a transducer, able to transmit the pressure changes that occur with the pulse. The transducer receives the pressure changes from the pulse and produces a weak, electrical signal, usually strengthened with an amplifier, and sends it to an oscilloscope or graph, where the signal will be displayed for interpretation. Electronic monitors are the most often utilized, and show numerical values for systolic, diastolic, and mean arterial pressures (MAP). Frequent calibration and maintenance of equipment is required, as is the leveling and zeroing of the transducer.

The arterial waveform displayed has a characteristic morphology. An initial rapid upstroke represents the rapid ejection of blood from the left ventricle into the aorta, and follows the QRS complex on the ECG. The value measured at the peak of this upstroke is the systolic blood pressure. The dicrotic notch appears on the subsequent downstroke of the arterial waveform, and represents the slight backflow of blood in the aorta after closure of the aortic valve (in other words, the end of ventricular systole). This event corresponds with the end of ventricular repolarization, and with the T wave on an ECG. The downstroke continues after the dicrotic notch, and its value at the lowest point, the trough, is equal to the diastolic blood pressure.

The MAP is an important parameter in critical care medicine, and represents the true "driving" pressure for peripheral blood flow. MAP should be considered superior to systolic pressure for aiding in the determination of hemodynamic stability. An electronic determination of the MAP via an arterial catheter is preferred, but MAP can also be determined with the formula:

$$MAP = \frac{[(2 \times P_{\text{diastolic}}) + P_{\text{systolic}}]}{3}$$

Note that diastole counts twice as much as systole, as diastole represents two-thirds of the cardiac cycle.

3. Identify common sites for arterial line insertion (p. 211), central line insertion (p. 217), and pulmonary artery catheter insertion. (p. 222)

The most common sites for arterial catheter insertion are the radial, brachial, and femoral arteries. In addition, the brachial, axillary, or dorsalis pedis arteries may be utilized. In neonates, the umbilica or temporal arteries may be used.

Central venous lines are commonly inserted in the internal jugular, subclavian, or femoral vein. If cannulation of the deep veins proves difficult, the antecubital vein may be utilized.

Pulmonary artery catheters are inserted in the internal jugular or subclavian vein.

4. List four complications of pulmonary artery catheter insertion. p. 228

Complications of pulmonary artery catheter insertion include:

1. Pneumothorax
2. Ventricular dysrhythmia
3. Infection
4. Pulmonary artery rupture

5. Identify the waveforms of: RA, RV, PA, and PAWP. p. 224

The right arterial (RA) waveform consists of the following:

- A wave
  - First positive deflection
  - Rise in pressure due to atrial contraction
  - Follows P wave of ECG
- X descent
  - Downslope following A wave
  - Fall in pressure due to relaxation of atria
- C wave
  - Small positive deflection on downslope of A wave (X descent)
  - Bulging up of tricuspid valve early in ventricular systole
- V wave
  - First positive deflection following C wave
  - Caused by atrial filling
- Y descent
  - Follows V wave
  - Fall in pressure due to opening of tricuspid valve and ventricular filling

The right ventricular (RV) waveform morphology is as follows:

- Early, steep upstroke
  - Rapid, passive ventricular filling
- Middle, gradual upstroke
  - Slower filling period
- Late, steep upstroke
  - Ventricular filling during atrial systole and ventricular systole

Pulmonary artery (PA) waveform morphology:

- Similar to arterial pressure monitoring
- Initial upstroke
  - Blood entering the pulmonary artery during right ventricular systole
- Downstroke
  - End of right ventricular systole
- Dicrotic notch
  - Closure of pulmonic valve
- Continued downstroke
  - Pressure falls as blood moves forward in pulmonary circulation
- Nadir
  - Lowest point
  - Late right ventricular diastole
  - Pressure termed "end diastolic PA pressure"

Pulmonary artery wedge pressure (PAWP) waveform:

- A wave
  - Left atrial contraction
- V wave
  - Bulging of mitral valve into left atrium during left ventricular contraction
- C wave

6. Define normal values of: CVP, RVP, PAP, PAWP, CO/CI, MAP, SVI, SVRI, and PVRI.   **p. 230**

- CVP
  - 0–6 mmHg (5–8 mm/H_2O)
- RVP
  - Right-ventricular end-diastolic pressure: 0–8 mmHg
    - Equal to right atrial pressure when tricuspid valve is open
  - Right-ventricular systolic pressure: 15–30 mmHg
- PAP
  - 15–30 mmHg
- PAWP
  - 8–12 mmHg
- CO
  - 4–8 L/min
- CI
  - 2.5–4.0 L/minute/m^2
- MAP
  - 65–100 mmHg
- SVI
  - SVI = Cardiac Index/Heart Rate
- SVRI
  - (Mean Arterial Pressure − Right Atrial Pressure) × 80/Cardiac Index
- PVRI
  - PVRI = (PAP − PCWP) × 80/Cardiac Index

7. Identify the hemodynamic parameter that best reflects the pressure in the left ventricle.   **p. 231**

The PCWP, which best reflects the pressure in the left ventricule, is equal to the left atrial pressure that is equal to the left ventricular end-diastolic pressure. To appreciate why this is so, think of the PA catheter as a pressure sensor that can feel the pressure changes in the column of fluid (blood) contained in the pulmonary artery (where the catheter balloon is "wedged"; remember, this is a *wedge* pressure!), pulmonary capillaries, pulmonary vein, right atrium, and right ventricle. During diastole (when the mitral valve is open) the pressure sensor, wedged in the right pulmonary artery, has a clear "feel" all the way to the left ventricle. This is even easier to consider when you remember that when you feel a radial pulse, you are feeling the systolic pressure changes in the left ventricle through a column of fluid in the arterial system.

8. **Identify the hemodynamic parameter that best reflects right ventricular preload.**   **p. 231**

The CVP, which best reflects right ventricular preload, is equal to right atrial pressure, which is equal to right ventricular end-diastolic pressure when the tricuspid valve is open. The term "ventricular end-diastolic pressure" is analogous with preload.

9. **Identify from which port of a pulmonary artery catheter a mixed venous blood sample is drawn.**   **p. 234**

The distal port of a PA catheter is utilized to obtain a mixed venous blood sample.

10. **Discuss how the PA waveform changes when the pulmonary artery catheter floats from the right ventricle into the pulmonary artery.**   **p. 226**

While the right ventricular pressure (RVP) waveform and pulmonary artery pressure (PAP) waveform are very similar, there are slight differences that can, and should, be appreciated. The RVP waveform morphology is characterized by an early, rapid filling wave followed by a slow filling wave, and ends with a rapid upstroke caused by rapid ventricular filling, and systole.

The PAP waveform is similar to the arterial pressure waveform. It is characterized by a rapid upstroke followed by a slightly longer downstroke interrupted by a dicrotic notch, produced when the pulmonic valve closes.

11. **Describe how an intra-aortic balloon pump (IABP) cannula is inserted.**   **pp. 240–241**

The intra-aortic balloon pump (IABP) consists of a 30-cm polyurethane balloon attached to, and tightly wrapped around, the end of a large-bore catheter. The catheter is inserted into the femoral artery at the groin and advanced cephalad into the aorta until the distal catheter tip lies just distal to the origin of the left subclavian artery. Once in place, the balloon is unwrapped from the catheter to allow inflation.

12. **Describe how an IABP operates.**   **p. 241**

Once unwrapped from the distal catheter tip, the balloon is rapidly inflated with 35 to 40 ml of helium at the beginning of each ventricular diastole, when the aortic valve closes. The balloon is rapidly deflated at the beginning of each ventricular systole just before the aortic valve opens. Inflation of the balloon increases peak diastolic pressure, thereby increasing mean arterial pressure (MAP), and thereby, increasing blood flow to the periphery. In addition, as coronary blood flow takes place during diastole, it follows that balloon inflation and subsequent increase of peak diastolic pressure result in an increase in coronary blood flow.

An easy way of visualizing why the use of IABP will increase peripheral and coronary perfusion is to consider that the balloon, when inflated, is going to take up space in the aorta. As the balloon occupies space in the aorta, it is going to push blood away from it in the aorta; some of that blood is pushed forward in the aorta (increasing peripheral perfusion), and some of that blood will be pushed backward in the aorta, increasing coronary artery perfusion, as well as cerebral and upper body peripheral perfusion (via the brachiocephalic, left common carotid, and left subclavian arteries).

13. **Identify complications of IABP devices.**   **p. 242**

Complications of IABP devices include:

- Ruptured balloon
- Distal leg ischemia on side of insertion
- Infection of insertion site
- Catheter tip migration
  - Superior migration
  - Inferior migration

14. Describe the use of a ventricular assist device (VAD). pp. 242–243

A ventricular assist device (VAD) is a pump used to increase cardiac output (CO) in patients refractory to IABP therapy, and is commonly used in post-cardiac bypass surgery. Pumps can be placed in either or both ventricles and require an external power source. The use of a VAD is a short-term treatment, used as a bridge treatment until cardiac transplant can be performed.

Case Study

Your ground transport unit has been called to transport an 82-year-old male from a community ICU to the tertiary care center where your program is based. Your patient is post–op, day one from a ruptured appendix. Because of his atypical presentation, the appendicitis was missed on initial evaluation, and, by the time it was diagnosed, he was critically ill. He is being transferred for admission to the surgical ICU for further management of his septic shock caused by peritonitis from his ruptured appendix. He is intubated and has a propofol drip for sedation. Both the propofol and the crystalloid IV fluids are being administered through a triple lumen catheter in the right internal jugular vein. He also has an arterial line in his right radial artery. During your assessment, you note that the access insertion site dressings and the abdominal wound dressings are without evidence of hemorrhage. His skin is warm and dry, and he has a tympanic temperature of 39°C. Assessment of distal circulation in the right hand shows it is intact. Breath sounds are clear and heart sounds are without murmurs or extra sounds. This morning's chest X-ray shows that the tip of the central venous catheter is located in the superior vena cava and that there is no evidence of a pneumothorax. Observing the monitors, you see that the ECG shows sinus tachycardia at 122 beats per minute. The arterial line waveform is normal with a clear dicrotic notch, and shows a blood pressure of 88/52 mmHg with a mean arterial pressure (MAP) of 64 mmHg. The central venous line waveform is also normal and shows a central venous pressure (CVP) of 3 mmHg.

After packaging and transferring the patient to the ambulance stretcher, you secure the arterial and central venous transducers to the stretcher IV pole, leveling them with the patient's phlebostatic axis. After you are confident that they are level, you zero both lines and check that the waveforms appear normal. During the transfer, you administer a fluid bolus with good improvement in the MAP and CVP, as well as a decrease in heart rate to 110 beats per minute. With each reassessment en route, you assess and document the hemodynamic parameters, assure the waveforms appear normal, and evaluate the access site dressings for hemorrhage. The patient remains stable and arrives at the SICU without change.

DISCUSSION QUESTIONS

1. What are some benefits of invasive hemodynamic monitoring?
2. What is the method of leveling and zeroing an invasive monitor transducer?
3. What are common complications of invasive hemodynamic monitoring?

Content Review

MULTIPLE CHOICE

_____ 1. Which of the following statements regarding hemodynamic pressure monitoring is false?
    A. Parameters monitored include electrocardiogram, systemic vascular resistance, central venous pressure, and cardiac output.
    B. Hemodynamic pressure monitoring can help evaluate the effectiveness of treatments.
    C. Hemodynamic pressure monitoring can help identify trends in patient status.
    D. The majority of hemodynamic pressure monitoring does not require the use of invasive monitoring equipment.

©2007 Pearson Education, Inc.
Critical Care Paramedic   CHAPTER 9   *Cardiac and Hemodynamic Monitoring*   **89**

_____ 2. Which of the following is the correct equation for determining the mean arterial pressure
211   (MAP)?
    A. $MAP = P_{systolic} + 1/3\,(P_{systolic} + P_{diastolic})$
    B. $MAP = P_{diastolic} + 1/3\,(P_{systolic} + P_{diastolic})$
    C. $MAP = P_{diastolic} + 1/3\,(P_{systolic} - P_{diastolic})$
    D. $MAP = P_{systolic} + 1/3\,(P_{systolic} - P_{diastolic})$

_____ 3. Of the following, which is the most common site of insertion for an arterial catheter?
211   A. femoral artery   C. brachial artery
    B. radial artery   D. carotid artery

_____ 4. Of the following, which is the most common site of insertion for a central venous
216   catheter?
    A. antecubital vein   C. pulmonary vein
    B. external jugular vein   D. subclavian vein

_____ 5. Of the following, which is the most common site of insertion for a pulmonary
224   catheter?
    A. internal jugular vein   C. femoral artery
    B. pulmonary artery   D. external jugular vein

_____ 6. Complications associated with pulmonary artery catheter insertion include all of the
228   following except:
    A. pneumothorax.   C. cardiac tamponade.
    B. ventricular dysrhythmia.   D. pulmonary artery rupture.

_____ 7. Which of the following pressure waveforms has a dicrotic notch?
226   A. pulmonary artery wedge pressure   C. right ventricular pressure
    B. pulmonary artery pressure   D. right atrial pressure

_____ 8. Which of the following normal hemodynamic value ranges is incorrect?
226   A. CVP = 0–6 mmHg   C. MAP = 60–100 mmHg
    B. PAP = 8–12 mmHg   D. CO = 4–8 L/min

_____ 9. Which of the following hemodynamic values would be considered within its
215   normal range?
    A. Right ventricular end-diastolic pressure = 12 mmHg
    B. Right-ventricular systolic pressure = 5 mmHg
    C. CI = 6 L/minute/m^2
    D. MAP = 60 mmHg

_____ 10. The pulmonary capillary wedge pressure is:
231   A. determined with a central venous catheter.
    B. equal to right ventricular end-systolic pressure.
    C. less than left atrial end-diastolic pressure.
    D. equal to left ventricular end-diastolic pressure.

_____ 11. A central venous catheter can be used to determine:
215   A. MAP.   C. arterial blood gases.
    B. right ventricular preload.   D. cardiac output.

_____ 12. Which port of which hemodynamic catheter is used to obtain a mixed venous
    blood sample?
    A. proximal port of a central venous catheter
    B. yellow port of a Swan-Ganz catheter
    C. center port of a triple lumen central venous catheter
    D. distal port of a pulmonary artery catheter

©2007 Pearson Education, Inc.
Critical Care Paramedic

_____ 13. The dicrotic notch on a pulmonary artery pressure waveform is caused by the:
  A. closing of the aortic valve.
  C. closing of the pulmonic valve.
  B. end of right ventricular systole.
  D. opening of the bicuspid valve.

_____ 14. Which of the following statements regarding the IABP catheter is true?
  A. The catheter is inserted into the femoral artery.
  B. A 20-cm polyurethane balloon is attached to the distal catheter.
  C. The catheter tip is placed just distal to the origin of the brachiocephalic artery.
  D. The catheter balloon must be unwrapped from around the catheter prior to insertion.

_____ 15. Which of the following statements regarding IABP operation is true?
  A. The catheter balloon is rapidly inflated with 35 to 40 ml of helium at the beginning of each ventricular diastole.
  B. The catheter balloon is rapidly deflated at the beginning of each ventricular systole.
  C. Balloon inflation increases peak diastolic pressure, thereby increasing central venous pressure (CVP), and thereby increasing blood flow to the periphery.
  D. Coronary artery perfusion is increased during IABP operation.

_____ 16. Which of the following is NOT a complication of IABP use?
  A. Ruptured balloon
  B. Decreased peak diastolic pressure
  C. Distal leg ischemia on side of insertion
  D. Catheter tip migration

_____ 17. The main hemodynamic benefit of a ventricular assist device (VAD) is that it:
  A. increases cardiac output.
  B. increases systemic vascular resistance.
  C. decreases afterload.
  D. decreases ventricular end-diastolic pressure.

_____ 18. The phlebostatic axis is the approximate level of the:
  A. left ventricle.
  C. right ventricle.
  B. right atrium.
  D. left atrium.

_____ 19. The phlebostatic axis is located at the:
  A. fifth intercostal space, midaxillary line.
  B. fourth intercostal space, midclavicular line.
  C. fifth intercostal space, midclavicular line.
  D. fourth intercostal space, midaxillary line.

_____ 20. If the transducer of a PA catheter is zeroed at a level above the phlebostatic axis the monitor will:
  A. read an accurate pressure measurement.
  B. read an inaccurately low pressure.
  C. read an inaccurately high pressure.
  D. sound an alarm.

_____ 21. Prior to transport, you zero the transducer of a central venous catheter with the patient lying supine, and tape it to the stretcher at the level of his phlebostatic axis. During transport, the patient states he is uncomfortable lying supine and would like to sit upright. You note that his CVP = 4 mmHg, then raise the back of the stretcher upright to 80°. Which of the following CVPs might you expect to see, assuming that no hemodynamic changes have taken place?
  A. CVP = 0 mmHg
  C. CVP = 4 mmHg
  B. CVP = 2 mmHg
  D. CVP = 6 mmHg

MATCHING

Questions 22–26 refer to the following CVP waveform.

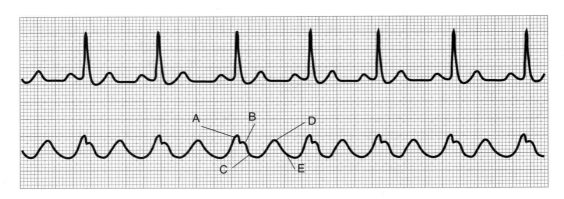

Identify the following parts of the CVP waveform:

_____ 22. Y descent

_____ 23. C wave

_____ 24. A wave

_____ 25. X descent

_____ 26. V wave

Questions 27–31 refer to the following right arterial pressure waveform.

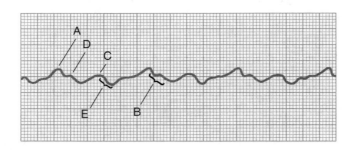

Identify the following parts of the right arterial pressure waveform:

_____ 27. Y descent

_____ 28. V wave

_____ 29. A wave

_____ 30. X descent

_____ 31. C wave

ECG Monitoring and Critical Care

Review of Chapter Objectives

Upon completion of this chapter, the student should be able to:

1. Describe how to attach ECG leads to display MCL-1 and MCL-6.   **p. 248**

MCL-1 procedure:

1. Place the RA (white) lead on the right, upper arm and the LA (black) lead on the left, upper arm.
2. Place the LL (red) lead on the fourth intercostal space, right side of sternum.
3. Place your monitor in lead III and monitor.
4. If 12-lead ECG is available, monitor lead V1 on the 12-lead.

MCL-6 procedure:

1. Leave cardiac monitor in lead III.
2. Move LL to the fifth intercostal, left midaxillary.
3. If 12-lead ECG is available, monitor lead V6 on the 12-lead.

2. Describe the management priorities of those patients at risk for complete heart block.   **p. 250**

The first priority is identifying those patients at risk for complete heart block, then shifting management priorities to prevent further ischemia and the development of heart block. Patients at risk for complete heart block include those with two separate blocks from any of the following categories:

1. Sinoatrial (SA) blocks
   a. Sinus arrest
   b. Sinus pause
   c. Sinus block
2. Atrioventricular blocks
   a. 1°HB, 2°HB TI, 2°HB TII
3. Interventricular (IV) blocks

Management priorities for these patients include increasing PaO_2, reducing cardiac workload, increasing coronary artery perfusion, and decreasing pain and anxiety. In addition, preparation for external cardiac pacing should be undertaken, with pacing pads placed on the patient prior to the initiation of transport.

3. Describe simple criteria for determining left versus right bundle branch block.   p. 257

While monitoring in MCL-1, a RSR complex greater than 120 ms wide is diagnostic for right bundle branch block (RBBB), and a QRS complex greater than 120 ms wide is diagnostic for left bundle branch block (LBBB).

In addition to the previous method, the "turn signal method" can be utilized to differentiate between LBBB and RBBB. MCL-1 or any of the precordial leads can be utilized to determine the presence of LBBB or RBBB in rhythms with a QRS > 20 ms.

Technique:

1. View the QRS of V1 (or MCL-1). It lies immediately over the right ventricle and provides the best view of the superior aspect of the interventricular septum.
2. Identify the J point of the QRS.
3. Draw a horizontal line from the J point to an intersecting line of the QRS, or to the beginning of the QRS. This will produce a triangle pointing either up or down.
   a. If the triangle points up, it indicates a right bundle branch block.
      Remember: If you push up on the vehicle's turn signal, the signal lights indicate a right turn.
   b. If the triangle points down, it indicates a left bundle branch block.
      Remember: If you pull down on the vehicle's turn signal, the signal lights indicate a left turn.

4. Using a simple chart, determine the presence of fascicular block.   p. 253

There are two ways to use the chart: If cardiac monitor does not provide axis angle:

1. Assess leads I, II, and III on ECG.
2. Determine if QRS complex is deflected more positively or negatively in each lead.
3. Compare the findings to the Rapid Axis and Hemiblock Chart.
   a. Identify the axis and hemiblock.

If axis angle is provided by cardiac monitor:

1. Compare monitor readout to Rapid Axis and Hemiblock Chart to identify axis deviation.

5. Describe the clinical significance of hemiblock.   p. 252

The clinical significance of hemiblock is:

- The mortality rate for patients having an AMI with a hemiblock is four times greater than those without a hemiblock.
- Hemiblock is a risk factor for complete heart block, since the patient is considered high risk if another block is present with hemiblock.
- In a setting of an AMI, hemiblock can indicate proximal artery occlusion.

6. Using leads MCL-1 and MCL-6, differentiate wide-complex tachycardia as either ventricular tachycardia or bundle branch block.   p. 257

The "quick VT reference" utilizing MCL-1 and MCL-6 says that VT is probably present if there is mostly positive deflection in MCL-1 (V1) and there is mostly negative deflection in MCL-6 (V6).

7. Describe criteria for Wolff-Parkinson-White syndrome.   p. 258

Criteria for Wolff-Parkinson-White syndrome includes the presence of a delta wave and a PR interval < 120 ms. The anterior and lateral ECG leads (V4-V6, I, aVL) are useful for detecting delta waves.

©2007 Pearson Education, Inc.
Critical Care Paramedic

8. Describe the assessment, management, and ECG findings of hyperkalemia and other electrolyte abnormalities.   p. 261

Hyperkalemia develops at serum levels above 5 mEq/L. Common causes of hyperkalemia include kidney failure (most common cause), acidosis, and medication or supplement overdose. Clinical and ECG manifestations are level-dependant. Expected ECG manifestations with mild hyperkalemia (< 6.5 mEq/L) include:

- Tall, tented, peaked T waves with a narrow base (QTc is still normal).
- Normal P waves

Moderate hyperkalemia (< 8 mEq/L) is characterized by:

- A wide QRS
- Broad S wave in V leads
- Left-axis deviation
- ST segment contiguous with the peaked T wave
- Flattened and diminished P wave

Severe hyperkalemia (> 8 mEq/L) is characterized by:

- Sine waves
- A lack of P waves

The management of hyperkalemia centers around three goals:

1. Stabilize the myocardial membrane.
2. Promote an intracellular shift of potassium.
3. Promote potassium excretion.

Stabilization of the myocardial membrane is achieved with the administration of calcium. An intracellular shift of potassium is promoted with the administration of insulin and glucose, bicarbonate, and beta blockers. Kayexalate (an ion-binding resin), or diuretics can be administered to aid in the excretion of potassium, and dialysis is necessary for those patients unable to produce urine because of renal failure.

9. Describe the clinical significance of prolonged QT syndrome.   p. 264

A prolonged QT interval is associated with an increased risk of syncope and sudden death from torsades de pointes. Clinical conditions that may lead to torsades include the initiation, use, or overdose of QT-prolonging drugs, myocardial ischemia or infarction, electrolyte disorders, acute bradycardia, and acute neurological events.

10. Describe the diagnosis of and clinical implications of a right ventricular infarction.   p. 266

Right ventricular infarction (RVI) is of particular concern for the critical care paramedic because of the threat of hemodynamic instability, specifically hypotension. The key to properly treating RVI is to first recognize that it is present: The critical care paramedic should develop an assessment routine that addresses the possibility. Clinical signs associated with RVI include JVD, clear lung sounds, and hypotension. The presence of ST segment changes in the inferior leads (II, III, and aVF) should alert the clinician to the possibility of RVI and prompt the immediate obtaining of a 15-lead ECG via the application of right-sided chest leads, which can effectively identify right ventricular infarction.

RVI decreases left ventricular preload; simply put, the injured right ventricle does not pump an adequate volume of blood forward to the left ventricle, resulting in decreased left ventricular preload and decreased cardiac output. The body's normal compensatory mechanisms, tachycardia and peripheral vasoconstriction, are employed to increase right ventricular preload to make up for its lack of pumping power, in accordance with the Starling mechanism (increased preload + increased myocardial stretch = increased stroke volume), and blood pressure is hopefully maintained. Now, we say that patients with RVI are "preload dependent," that is, they are dependent on an increased right ventricular preload (courtesy of compensatory tachycardia and peripheral vasoconstriction) to maintain an adequate right ventricular stroke volume to supply enough blood to the left ventricle to create a cardiac output sufficient to maintain an appropriate blood pressure. These patients are walking a hemodynamic tightrope, and any further insult may be the little nudge that results in hemodynamic compromise and hypotension. As these patients are preload dependent, part of the normal treatment of AMI, the administration of nitrates, can result in a precipitous fall in blood pressure secondary to vasodilation. As such, the administration of a small fluid bolus, 250 mL, prior to, or concurrent with, the administration of nitrates may be warranted in anticipation of a fall in blood pressure. It is not uncommon for patients to require the administration of up to a liter of fluid volume with nitrate administration. Often, patients will present with RVI and hypotension, as compensatory mechanisms were unsuccessful in maintaining blood pressure. In such cases, aggressive fluid volume administration is required to restore an adequate blood pressure prior to the administration of nitrates.

In summary, it is important to anticipate the development of hypotension, if it does not already exist, in patients with RVI, and anticipate the need for aggressive fluid volume administration. As such, identification of RVI and large-bore IV access is necessary prior to nitrate administration in cases of RVI.

11. Describe the procedure and lead placement for acquiring a 15-lead ECG. p. 266

The procedure for placing leads and acquiring a 15-lead ECG is as follows:

1. Run the initial 12-lead ECG as usual.
2. Place an electrode pad on the midclavicular line at the fifth intercostal space on the right side of the patient.
   a. This will be lead V4R.
3. Place an electrode pad in the fifth intercostal space, midscapular line.
   a. This will be lead V8.
   b. This lead aligns with V4 on the front of the patient's chest.
4. Place an electrode between V8 and the spine in the same intercostal space.
   a. This will be lead V9.
5. Remove the electrode wires for leads V4, V5, and V6.
6. Attach the V4 wire to the V4R lead placement.
7. Attach the V5 wire to the lead V8 placement and the V6 wire to the lead V9 placement.
8. Run a second 12-lead ECG with the new lead placements.
9. Clearly label the second 12-lead ECG to reflect the new leads.
   a. V4 as V4R
   b. V5 as V8
   c. V6 as V9

Case Study

Your team has been called to transport a 64-year-old male patient from a small rural emergency department to the area cardiac center, a transfer of approximately 45 miles by ground. The patient drove himself to the ED after 14 hours of epigastric "pressure" and nausea. The ED nurse, still appearing a bit shaken, tells you that the patient had a sudden V-fib cardiac arrest while being evaluated, and was quickly defibrillated into a perfusing rhythm. Subsequent lab studies and 12-lead ECG found the patient to be suffering an inferior wall myocardial infarction. He is being transferred to the cardiac center for emergent cardiac catheterization. He received aspirin therapy, and is on an amiodarone drip to prevent the return of the ventricular arrhythmia.

Your patient, Jose, is a slightly obese retired police officer who presents on the ED stretcher in no obvious distress. He is alert but is not able to recall any of the past day's events. He tells you that he is comfortable, with the exception of feeling like he just "went 12 rounds with Tyson." He further elaborates that he is feeling fatigued and sore "all over." He currently denies any chest or epigastric pain or pressure. He has no shortness of breath or nausea. Physical exam findings show that his skin is warm and dry, breath sounds are clear in all fields, heart has a regular rate and rhythm without murmurs or

96 CRITICAL CARE PARAMEDIC

©2007 Pearson Education, Inc.
Critical Care Paramedic

extra sounds, abdomen is soft and nontender without masses, and all extremities have strong pulses. His vital signs are: respiratory rate of 12, heart rate of 78 beats per minute, and blood pressure 110/74.

While en route to the cardiac center, Jose tells you that the pressure is returning and he is beginning to feel some nausea. His vital signs remain unchanged. Because you are concerned about extension of the MI, you perform an ECG using the standard 12 leads and another with V8, V9, and V4R leads. As you suspected, you see ST segment elevations in leads II, III, and aVF, as well as in V4R, indicating an inferior wall MI with a right ventricular infarct. Knowing that this patient will be sensitive to nitrates and other vasoactive drugs, you decide to discuss the presentation with your medical control before you administer any medications. While you're on the phone, you have your partner put up a liter bag of normal saline on the second saline lock that you established before leaving the ED, reassess the patient's lung sounds, and get the dopamine out of the medication cabinet. Since your ETA to the receiving facility is now less than 5 minutes, your medical control physician feels it is best not to administer any medications unless the patient has significant changes. Within 10 minutes, the patient is on the cath table being prepped for the procedure.

DISCUSSION QUESTIONS

1. What are the clinical implications of a right ventricular infarct?
2. How is a right ventricular infarct diagnosed?
3. What is the procedure for obtaining a 15-lead ECG?

Content Review

MULTIPLE CHOICE

_____ 1. To monitor lead MCL-1 with a standard 3-lead ECG monitor, the care provider should move the _____ lead from its normal position to _____.
  A. black, the fourth intercostal space midclavicular line
  B. red, the fourth intercostal space right of the sternum
  C. white, the fifth intercostal space left of the sternum
  D. green, the fifth intercostal space midscapular line

_____ 2. With the leads of a 3-lead ECG monitor properly placed to monitor MCL-1, the monitor should be placed to read lead:
  A. I.   C. III.
  B. II.   D. IV.

_____ 3. The benefits of lead MCL-1 include all of the following except:
  A. P waves may be easier to visualize.
  B. the lead looks at the ventricles.
  C. bundle branch blocks are easy to identify.
  D. artifact is reduced, making analysis of the ECG easier.

_____ 4. To monitor lead MCL-6 with a standard 3-lead ECG monitor, the care provider should move the _____ lead from its normal position to _____.
  A. black, the fourth intercostal space midclavicular line on left side
  B. white, the sixth intercostal space left of sternum
  C. red, the fifth intercostal midaxillary on left side
  D. green, the fifth intercostal space midscapular line on right side

_____ 5. The benefits of lead MCL-6 include all of the following except:
  A. bundle branch blocks are easy to identify.
  B. a better view of the right ventricle is obtained.
  C. the lead looks at the ventricles.
  D. it may be used with dressing in place, or trauma on anterior chest wall.

_____ 6. Which of the following combination of ECG findings places a patient at high risk for complete heart block?
A. sinus pause and a first-degree heart block
B. fascicular block and multifocal atrial tachycardia
C. atrial fibrillation and a bundle branch block
D. bradycardia and sinus arrest

_____ 7. A left-anterior hemiblock involves the:
A. left anterior hemi-fascicle of the bundle branch system.
B. left anterior hemi-fascicle of the Bundle of His.
C. anterior hemi-fascicle of the left bundle branch system.
D. anterior bundle branch of the left hemi-fascicle.

_____ 8. A left-posterior hemiblock involves the:
A. posterior bundle branch of the left hemi-fascicle.
B. left anterior hemi-fascicle of the bundle branch system.
C. left anterior hemi-fascicle of the Bundle of His.
D. posterior fascicle of the left bundle branch system.

_____ 9. Which of the following statements regarding the clinical significance of hemiblock is true?
A. Mortality rate is four times higher for patients having an MI with a hemiblock than those without hemiblock.
B. In the setting of AMI, hemiblock can indicate distal coronary artery occlusion.
C. The patient is at high risk for complete heart block.
D. Hemiblock renders the patient "preload dependent."

_____ 10. Which 3 ECG leads are utilized when using the Rapid Axis and Hemiblock Chart?
A. II, V1, and aVL
B. I, II, and III
C. III, V3, and aVR
D. II, III, and aVF

_____ 11. Which of the following statements regarding bundle branch blocks is false?
A. Left bundle branch block makes interpretation of the ST segment difficult.
B. The presence of a bundle branch block increases the risk of complete heart block.
C. Right bundle branch blocks are associated with higher mortality rates than left bundle branch blocks.
D. Bundle branch blocks can develop secondary to myocardial infarction, congenital defects, and ischemic tissue.

_____ 12. You have just evaluated the QRS complex of a suspect ECG rhythm utilizing the "turn signal criteria" and have shaded in a triangle that points "up." According to the criteria, an upward triangle indicates the presence of a:
A. left-posterior hemiblock.
B. left-anterior hemiblock.
C. left bundle branch block.
D. right bundle branch block.

_____ 13. Which of the following ECG findings is not suggestive for ventricular tachycardia?
A. a predominantly negative QS complex in MCL-2
B. a predominantly positive QS complex in MCL-1
C. a predominantly negative QS complex in MCL-1
D. a single, upright peak (steeple sign) in MCL-1

_____ 14. Wolff-Parkinson-White syndrome is caused by:
A. electrolyte imbalance.
B. an accessory conduction pathway.
C. decreased PaO_2.
D. increased cardiac workload.

_____ 15. The disappearance of P waves and the appearance of sine waves on the ECG suggests:
A. hyperkalemia.
B. left bundle branch block.
C. hypocalcemia.
D. right ventricular infarction.

_____ 16. Hyperkalemia is defined as a serum potassium greater than:
A. 3.5 mEq/L.
B. 5 mEq/L.
C. 6.5 mEq/L.
D. 8 mEq/L.

_____ 17. Common causes of hypokalemia include:
A. acidosis, renal failure, and medication or supplement OD.
B. renal failure, vomiting, and diarrhea.
C. vomiting, diarrhea, diuretics, and gastric suctioning.
D. dysrhythmia, muscle weakness, and digitalis toxicity.

_____ 18. The management of hyperkalemia centers around:
A. administering potassium, replacing intravascular volume, and correcting cardiac dysrhythmia.
B. correcting cardiac dysrhythmia, replacing intravascular volume, and dialysis.
C. airway, breathing, and circulation.
D. stabilizing the myocardial membrane, promoting an intracellular shift of potassium, and promoting potassium excretion.

_____ 19. All of the following medications are used in the treatment of hyperkalemia except:
A. insulin and glucose.
B. albuterol.
C. calcium.
D. amiodarone.

_____ 20. Patients with right ventricular infarction (RVI) are at particular risk for hypotension with the administration of nitrates because:
A. they are at high risk of complete heart block.
B. they are "preload dependent."
C. their compensatory mechanisms are insufficient.
D. they are at high risk for bradycardia.

_____ 21. Typical signs of right ventricular infarct include:
A. JVD, clear lungs sounds, and hypotension.
B. crackles, hypertension, and peripheral edema.
C. cool, pale, diaphoretic skin and hypertension.
D. JVD, crackles, and hypotension.

_____ 22. ECG findings that are suggestive for right ventricular infarct include ST segment elevation in:
A. II, III, and aVF.
B. V1-V6.
C. III and aVR.
D. MCL-1 and MCL-6.

_____ 23. A stable 44-year-old female being transported to a regional cardiac center for ablation develops an unstable tachycardia during transport. She complains of chest pain and dizziness as you place the patient on O_2 12 lpm via a nonrebreather mask and note that your IV access is still patent. The patient's vitals are: HR = 190, BP = 62/38, RR = 20 and shallow, and SpO_2 = 92 percent on 15 lpm. A 12-lead ECG reveals a tachycardia with a PR interval of 80 ms and the presence of delta waves in V1-V6. Based on the clinical presentation, the most appropriate treatment would be:
A. administration of amiodarone IV.
B. administration of procainamide IV.
C. administration of adenosine IV.
D. immediate cardioversion.

_____ 24. During ground transport to your tertiary care facility, your 52-year-old patient develops chest pain and nausea. He describes the pain as a dull aching in his neck and left shoulder. You note that his skin is pale and cool, lung sounds are clear, and there is no JVD present. His vitals are: HR = 108 and regular, RR = 20 and regular, BP = 102/70, and SpO_2 = 98 percent on a nasal cannula. Your cardiac monitor shows sinus tachycardia. An 18 g IV is in place and is patent, with a 1,000 mL bag of normal saline with a macrodrip set hanging. Based on the patient's clinical condition, which of the following would be the best course of immediate action?

A. Place the patient on oxygen 15 lpm via a nonrebreather mask and administer sublingual nitrates.

B. Administer sublingual nitrates and obtain additional large-bore IV access.

C. Place the patient on oxygen 15 lpm via a nonrebreather mask and obtain a 15-lead ECG.

D. Administer IV nitrates and prepare a dopamine infusion should hypotension occur.

_____ 25. You are called to transport a 72-year-old male patient in acute renal failure to a regional care facility for evaluation and dialysis. Upon arrival at the sending facility, you are informed that the patient has a serum potassium of 6.6 mEq/L, and the ECG shows sinus tachycardia with frequent PVCs and tall, peaked T waves. The patient's skin is cool and dry, lung sounds are clear, and he is not producing urine. His vitals are: HR = 98 and irregular, BP = 142/100, RR = 18 and regular, and SpO_2 = 99 percent on 2 lpm via nasal cannula. Based on the clinical status of the patient, which of the following would be the most appropriate management?

A. Administration of calcium, insulin, glucose, sodium bicarbonate, a beta blocker, and kayexalate

B. Administration of calcium, insulin, glucose, a beta blocker, furosemide, and kayexalate

C. Administration of calcium, lidocaine, insulin, glucose, albuterol, and furosemide

D. Administration of insulin, glucose, sodium bicarbonate, a beta blocker, and kayexalate

11

Critical Care Pharmacology

Review of Chapter Objectives

Upon completion of this chapter, the student should be able to:

1. Discuss why it behooves the critical care paramedic to have a solid understanding of a drug's mechanism of action. p. 273

It is impossible to memorize every particular about every drug's pharmacodynamics, especially those drugs that are infrequently used. Understanding a drug's mechanism of action, rather than just rote memorization of its actions, is necessary to truly understand its indications, contraindications, and side effects, and to be able to determine which drug will be best suited to treat the particular patient you are dealing with at the time. The only information you should be memorizing is a drug's dose, and there is no shortcut to memorizing doses; you have to dedicate yourself to it, spend time, and make an effort.

2. Define the role of critical care pharmacology. p. 274

While practicing critical care transport medicine, the paramedic will enjoy the benefit of an expanded formulary, and have medicinal agents far above and beyond the typical ACLS agents utilized in the prehospital environment. The ongoing (not just emergent) management of cardiovascular, neurological, pulmonary, and infectious disease is now within the scope of practice of the critical care paramedic. As such, critical care pharmacology forces the paramedic to start to think not only about the acute care of patients, but also about the continued care as well.

3. Understand the difference between pharmacodynamics and pharmacokinetics. p. 275

Pharmacodynamics is the study of how a drug interacts with the body to cause its effects. In other words, pharmacodynamics considers how a drug accomplishes what it does. Does it cross the blood-brain barrier? Does it bind with a receptor? Is it an agonist or an antagonist? These are some of the questions asked when pharmacodynamics are considered.

Pharmacokinetics is the study of how a drug is absorbed, distributed, biotransformed (metabolized), and excreted; in other words, how a drug is transported into and out of the body. Pharmacokinetics addresses questions such as, "Can a drug be ingested and absorbed through the intestinal mucosa, or does it have to be administered intravenously?" "Does it circulate as a free molecule in the blood plasma, or is it transported bound to a blood protein?" "Is it metabolized in the liver, decreasing its bioavailability, and is it excreted by the kidney?"

4. Describe the factors that can affect the administration of critical care pharmacologic agents.
5. Understand how derangements in normal cellular activity may influence the response that medications exert on the body. **p. 275**

Influences on drug actions that determine its effectiveness include the metabolic, hemodynamic, and elimination capabilities of the patient. Metabolic derangements may delay the breakdown of a drug, increasing its half-life and time of effect. Conversely, fever or other hyperdynamic states may increase drug biotransformation, effectively decreasing its half-life.

The hemodynamic status of a critically ill patient is often significantly altered, and as end-cell perfusion is decreased, the ability to transport a drug to the cellular receptor sites is delayed. Onset of action can be delayed in instances of hypotension and/or peripheral hypoperfusion. In addition, altered hemodynamics, specifically hypotension and shock, may limit effective elimination of a drug when organs such as the kidneys are hypoperfused.

Case Study

Your patient is a 68-year-old male with a diagnosis of bilateral pneumonia. He is being transferred from a small rural ED to a community medical center for admission. He has a history of hypertension and was resuscitated from a sudden cardiac death two years ago. After his cardiac arrest, he had an automated implantable cardioverter defibrillator (AICD) placed. He admits to a long history of heavy drinking with at least "a six-pack" a day for several years. His medications include sotolol 120 mg every 12 hours, hydrochlorothiazide 25 mg each day, and zolpidem 12.5 mg at bedtime. He is complaining of mild shortness of breath on your arrival, but is otherwise without complaint. He is on oxygen at 3 lpm via nasal cannula, and is just finishing a nebulized albuterol treatment as you arrive. He received 500 mg each of IV azithromycin and levofloxacin about 20 minutes ago, and the IV now has normal saline infusing at 150 mL/hr.

Physical assessment shows that his skin is warm and moist; breath sounds are slightly diminished in the bases with light crackles bilaterally; heart sounds are irregular, but without extra sounds; and his abdomen is soft and without tenderness. His vital signs are: temperature 39 °C, respiratory rate 20 breaths per minute, heart rate 108 bpm, blood pressure 110/68, and SpO_2 95 percent with the oxygen. The cardiac monitor shows an irregular sinus tachycardia with approximately 4 unifocal premature ventricular complexes per minute.

While en route to the receiving hospital, the patient suddenly becomes unresponsive, pulseless, and apneic. The ECG shows a wide bizarre tachyarrhythmia that appears irregular, but seems to have a repeating pattern. The patient's AICD discharges and the patient converts back to a sinus rhythm, but, before you can assess the patient's perfusion status, the tachyarrhythmia returns. The patient is again unresponsive, pulseless, and apneic, and you recognize the arrhythmia as torsades de pointes. You instruct your partner to begin CPR while you draw up 2 grams of magnesium to administer IV. With continued CPR and two more discharges of the patient's AICD, the rhythm converts to a sinus tachycardia at 110 beats per minute with strong radial pulses and a BP of 112/66. The patient now has adequate respiratory effort and is becoming more responsive. The patient's condition stabilizes and you arrive at the destination hospital without any further incident.

Later while discussing the case with your medical director, you learn that the patient's previous medical history and medication use, combined with the choice of medications to treat his respiratory infection, were probably responsible for the patient's cardiac arrest.

DISCUSSION QUESTIONS

1. What factors can affect the administration of critical care pharmacologic agents?
2. Why is it important for the critical care paramedic to have a solid understanding of a drug's mechanism of action?
3. What are some ways in which alterations in normal cellular activity may influence the body's response to medications?

Content Review

Note: Refer to the emergency drug cards for answers to some of the following questions.

MULTIPLE CHOICE

_____ 1. _____ is the study of how a drug interacts with the body to cause its effects.
- A. Pharmacokinetics
- B. Pharmacodynamics
- C. Half-life
- D. Bioavailability

_____ 2. _____ is the study of how a drug is absorbed, distributed, biotransformed, and excreted.
- A. Pharmacokinetics
- B. Pharmacodynamics
- C. Half-life
- D. Bioavailability

_____ 3. Which of the following is least likely to influence the effect a drug has on the body?
- A. fever
- B. acidosis
- C. hypotension
- D. hypertension

_____ 4. The extent to which a drug is in a free, unbound state and capable of exerting an action is its:
- A. half-life.
- B. toxicity.
- C. bioavailability.
- D. pharmacokinetics.

_____ 5. Drugs that affect myocardial contractility are termed:
- A. chronotrophs.
- B. inotrophs.
- C. dromotrophs.
- D. antihypertensives.

_____ 6. Antihypertensive agents are used for their ability to:
- A. reduce myocardial workload.
- B. reduce afterload.
- C. increase myocardial oxygen demand.
- D. improve end-organ perfusion.

_____ 7. All of the following are desirable effects of vasopressor agents except:
- A. increased venous capacitance.
- B. increased afterload.
- C. increased distal capillary bed perfusion.
- D. increased blood pressure.

_____ 8. Generally speaking, most antidysrhythmic agents act to:
- A. prolong the refractory period of myocardial cells.
- B. block calcium ion channels.
- C. block sodium ion channels.
- D. prolong the depolarization time of myocardial cells.

_____ 9. Cardioprotectants are utilized post-myocardial infarction because they reduce all the following except:
- A. infarction size.
- B. mortality.
- C. risk for re-infarction.
- D. coronary artery vasospasm.

_____ 10. Fibrinolytic agents exert their effect by:
- A. preventing the synthesis of coagulation factors.
- B. converting plasminogen to plasmin.
- C. preventing new clots from forming.
- D. inhibiting glycoprotein IIb/3a receptors.

_____ 11. Depolarizing neuromuscular blocking agents are particularly desirable as a primary paralytic in RSI because they have a:
  A. rapid onset of action and a long half-life.
  B. long onset of action and a long half-life.
  C. rapid onset of action and a short half-life.
  D. long onset of action and a short half-life.

_____ 12. Sedatives and hypnotics are not commonly utilized to:
  A. treat ICU psychosis.
  B. alleviate the anxiety and stress of transport.
  C. facilitate intubation.
  D. treat pain.

_____ 13. With regard to IV antibiotic therapy, the critical care paramedic's role will be to:
  A. determine which patients will receive IV antibiotics.
  B. monitor IV antibiotic administration during transport.
  C. determine the proper dosage of antibiotic to be administered.
  D. initiate IV antibiotic therapy.

_____ 14. H_2 receptor blockers are commonly administered to critical care patients in an effort to:
  A. prevent ulcer formation.
  B. prevent nausea.
  C. increase myocardial oxygen supply.
  D. decrease peripheral vascular resistance.

_____ 15. The administration of antiemetic medications can help reduce the risk of all of the following except:
  A. increased intrathoracic and intracranial pressure.
  B. aspiration.
  C. compartment syndrome.
  D. electrolyte imbalances.

_____ 16. Which of the following medications does not have vasodilatory effects?
  A. nesiritide   C. fenoldopam
  B. nitroprusside   D. fosphenytoin

_____ 17. Overadministration of which of the following medications can result in hypertension?
  A. enalapril   C. hydralazine
  B. phenylephrine   D. inamrinone

_____ 18. Which of the following should not be used to treat a patient with known severe hyper-responsive airways disease?
  A. inamrinone   C. phenytoin
  B. propranolol   D. nimodipine

_____ 19. Which of the following medications would not be given to an ICU patient to help prevent stress ulcers?
  A. nimodipine   C. famotidine
  B. cimetidine   D. ranitidine

_____ 20. Which of the following is considered a first-line agent for the treatment of hypertension secondary to toxemia of pregnancy?
  A. clonidine   C. dobutamine
  B. phenylephrine   D. hydrazaline

_____ 21. Which of the following medications is classified as an ace inhibitor?
  A. enalapril   C. inamrinone
  B. esmolol   D. enoxaparin

_____ 22. Which of the following descriptions contains an incorrect adult dose?
  A. esmolol: 500 mcg/kg bolus over 1 minute followed by a maintenance infusion of 50 mcg/kg/min that can be increased every 5–10 minutes to a maximum infusion rate of 300 mcg/kg/min
  B. phenylephrine: 1–1.8 mg/min until BP stabilizes, then 4–6 mg/min infusion for maintenance
  C. eptifibatide: 180 mcg/kg bolus, followed by maintenance infusion of 2 mcg/kg/min for 72–96 hrs (or until hospital discharge)
  D. fentanyl: 25–200 mcg slow IV push over 1–2 minutes

_____ 23. You have determined that your patient with CHF requires a medication that will increase cardiac contractility. Which of the following will provide that effect?
  A. metoprolol   C. enalapril
  B. diltiazem   D. milrinone

_____ 24. Clopidogrel and enoxaparin are both classified as:
  A. glycoprotein IIb/IIIa inhibitors.   C. anticoagulants.
  B. anti-platelet agents.   D. fibrinolytics.

_____ 25. You are transporting a patient who was treated at an outlying facility for acute coronary syndrome and is now being transferred to a cardiac center for PCTA. Which of the following medications are most likely to be infused during transport?
  A. heparin and tirofiban   C. aspirin and clopidogrel
  B. warfarin and reteplase   D. nicardipine and abciximab

_____ 26. Which of the following medications is matched with its correct classification?
  A. nimodipine: calcium channel blocker
  B. terbutaline: sympathomimetic
  C. vecuronium: nondepolarizing neuromuscular blocking agent
  D. meperidine: narcotic agonist

_____ 27. Which of the following medications is incorrectly paired with its action?
  A. fentanyl: narcotic analgesic
  B. etomidate: decreases GABA activity in cerebrum to induce hypnotic effects
  C. lorazepam: increases GABA activity in CNS to induce sedation and muscle relaxation
  D. flumazenil: GABA receptor antagonist reverses benzodiazepine effects

_____ 28. Which of the following antibiotics should you consider discontinuing during transport if the patient develops nausea, vomiting, or diarrhea?
  A. clindamycin   C. vancomycin
  B. fluconazole   D. gentamicin

_____ 29. Which of the following medications is not an antiemetic?
  A. prochlorperazine   C. promethazine
  B. ondansetron   D. cimetidine

_____ 30. Which of the following medications does not have hypotension as a contraindication?
  A. bumetanide   C. succinylcholine
  B. furosemide   D. nesiritide

Interpretation of Lab and Basic Diagnostic Tests

Review of Chapter Objectives

Upon completion of this chapter, the student should be able to:

1. **Discuss the importance of laboratory and basic diagnostic testing in critical care transport.** p. 328

   As a critical care paramedic, you will encounter diagnostic test results on just about every interfacility transport you take part in. Because these tests provide valuable information about the patient, you must have a basic understanding of the common lab tests that are routinely encountered. Diagnostic and laboratory tests frequently play a large role in patient care, helping the health care team decide such things as patient hemodynamic status, ventilator parameters, medication use, and destination facility.

   Diagnostic tests can be divided into three general categories: laboratory tests, imaging studies, and physiological tests. There may be significant overlap between these categories, and some require formal interpretation by a physician (X-rays, CT scans) while others do not (BGA, electrolyte panel).

2. **Describe how normal laboratory values are established.** p. 328

   Normal reference values are usually established based on a large number of lab tests conducted over several years and then published periodically in the *New England Journal of Medicine*. There are two commonly used statistical methods of determining what "normal" values are: the Gaussian distribution method and the percentile ranking system. The Gaussian distribution method takes all collected data, determines the mean, and then considers all values greater than about 2 standard deviations from the mean (average) outside of "normal" values. In doing so, about 95 percent of the tested population is considered normal and the remaining 5 percent (who fell outside the 2 standard deviation cutoff point) are considered abnormal. The percentile ranking system ranks all collected data and determines the median (the value in the middle, different from the average!). The median is the 50th percentile for that lab test, and all other values are compared to the 50th percentile value.

   Local laboratories will confirm the normal values in their own local populations and will, when appropriate, alter the normal reference range to better represent local variations from the norm. In addition, since pregnant women and children often deviate from the norm, this should be considered when evaluating their data. The major physiological variables that affect normal reference values are sex and age.

3. **Define the terms** *specificity* **and** *sensitivity* **as they pertain to medical testing.**   p. 329

Specificity is a measure of how well a test detects a disease without yielding a false positive result. In other words, it's the probability that the test will give a negative result in patients who do not have the disease. A test that is 100 percent specific will detect a disease in 100 percent of individuals who have it; few tests are 100 percent specific. A test with high specificity has few false-positives.

Sensitivity is the degree to which a test detects a disease without yielding a false-negative result; no test is 100 percent sensitive. A test with high sensitivity has few false-negatives.

4. **List the elements of a complete blood count and discuss what any abnormal readings may indicate.**   p. 331

A complete blood count (CBC) measures hemoglobin, hematocrit, white blood cells (WBC), red blood cells (RBC), mean corpuscular volume (MCV), mean corpuscular hemoglobin (MCH), mean corpuscular hemoglobin concentration (MCHC), red blood cell distribution width (RDW), platelet count, and platelet volume.

The hemoglobin component of a CBC measures the amount of hemoglobin present in the blood. Normal values for men are 13–18 g/dL, and for women, 12–16 g/dL. High values are commonly found in smokers; low values can result from anemia, blood loss, and overhydration.

Hematocrit is a measure of the percentage of RBCs in the plasma. Normal values for men are 37–49 percent, and for women, 36–46 percent. High values can occur secondary to dehydration and polycythemia; low values can result from overhydration, anemia, and blood loss.

The WBC count measures the number of WBCs per cubic millimeter of blood. Normal values for men and women are 4,500–11,000/mm^3. Infection, leukemia, and steroid use can raise values, while viral infection and immunodeficiency can lower values.

The RBC count measures the number of RBCs per cubic millimeter of blood. Normal values are 4.5–5.3 million/mm^3 for men, and 4.1–5.1 million/mm^3 for women. High values can be caused by polycythemia and high altitude, and low values can result from bone marrow suppression or some other abnormal loss or suppression of erythrocytes.

The MCV measures RBC size, which is normally 78–100 μm^3 in men, and 78–102 μm^3 in women. High values occur with folic acid deficiency, vitamin B$_{12}$ deficiency, and alcoholism. Low values occur with iron-deficiency anemia and lead poisoning.

The MCH measures the amount of hemoglobin present in one RBC, normally 25–35 pg. A high MCH can occur with folic acid and vitamin B$_{12}$ deficiency, and low MCH can occur with iron-deficiency anemia and thalassemias.

MCHC measures the proportion of each cell occupied by hemoglobin, normally between 31–37 percent. As with MCH, high values can occur with folic acid and vitamin B$_{12}$ deficiency, and low values can occur with iron-deficiency anemia and thalassemias.

RDW, calculated from the MCV and RBC, correlates with the degree to which the red blood cell size differs, an aid in differentiating different types of anemia. Normal values are between 11.5–14 percent, and high values can indicate iron deficiency or thalassemia minor.

5. **List the elements of a coagulation panel and discuss what any abnormal readings may indicate.**   p. 334

Coagulation studies measure the effectiveness of anticoagulant medications, identify increased risk of hemorrhage, and identify increased risk of thrombus formation. Prothrombin time (PT), partial thromboplastin time (PTT), and International Normalized Ratio (INR) are often utilized for such evaluations.

PT measures the effectiveness of coumarin-type anticoagulant medications, such as warfarin (Coumadin), which act on prothrombin (factor II), produced by the liver. Changes in other factors (V, VII, X) can cause an abnormal PT. Normal PT values are 11.2–13.2 seconds, and high values can result from liver cirrhosis, vitamin K deficiency, and disseminated intravascular coagulation (DIC). Low PT is insignificant.

PTT detects coagulation disorders in the intrinsic pathway of the coagulation cascade, and is commonly used to monitor heparin therapy. Normal values for PTT are between 22.1 and 34.1 seconds, and an elevated value suggests a bleeding disorder or excessive heparin administration. Low PTTs are insignificant.

An INR is used to report the PT in a more standardized form, comparing the PT to a pre-established control. In persons not on coagulation therapy, the control and PT are equal, resulting in an INR ratio of 1.0. With warfarin therapy, INR should be between 1.5–2.5 (the time for blood to coagulate should be 1.5 to 2.5 longer in a patient on warfarin than in a patient not taking warfarin).

6. Describe calculation of the International Normalized Ratio (INR).   **p. 334**

Recall that PT results are used to monitor the effectiveness of coumarin-type medications. The reporting of PT in seconds can be problematic in determining the effectiveness of these medications because the PT time varies depending on the type of reagent used. INR adjusts for the variability in the type of reagents used for the PT, comparing the PT to a pre-established control. In a normal patient not on anticoagulants, the PT and control should be the same, resulting in a ratio of 1.0. With coumarin-type medication therapy, the goal is to maintain an INR of 1.5–2.5.

7. Discuss the significance of the D-dimer assay.   **p. 335**

The term "D-dimer" refers to the degradation products of cross-linked fibrin, which are created during fibrinolysis (clot lysis); as such, the D-dimer assay test measures the amount of fibrin degradation that is occurring. It is useful in diagnosing disseminated vascular coagulation (DIC), pulmonary embolism, abruptio placenta, and deep venous thrombosis. In such situations, clots are forming and subsequently being lysed (although not fast enough!), elevating the D-dimer serum level.

8. Describe why electrolytes are measured in milliequivalents per liter.   **p. 336**

Electrolytes are measured in milliequivalents per liter (mEq/L) instead of milligrams per liter (mg/L) because mg units only measure the weight of the chemical element, not chemical activity. The standard of equivalents is based on how many grams of an element or compound interact with 1 gram of hydrogen in solution. As a result, 1 mEq of one element or compound has the same amount of chemical activity as 1 mEq of another element or compound. For example, 23 mg of sodium (Na^+), 36 mg of chloride (Cl^-), 39 mg of potassium (K^+), and 30 mg of bicarbonate (HCO_3^-) all constitute 1 mEq. So, we know that 23 mg of Na^+ has the same amount of chemical activity as 39 mg of K^+, as 23 mg of $Na^+ = 1$ mEq $= 39$ mg of K^+. Now, milligrams and grams can be used to measure the amount of electrolytes in a diet or medication, but the mEq amount of an electrolyte must be determined to consider the effects on physiology. To illustrate this point, consider Na^+ both in your diet and in electrolyte physiology. Look at the nutritional information label on a food item and you will note that the amount of Na^+ in the food item is offered in mgs: When considering serum Na^+ levels, we refer to values in mEq.

9. Describe the anion gap, how it is calculated, and is its clinical significance.   **p. 336**

Within the serum, it is necessary to maintain a state of chemical electrical neutrality between the cations and anions present. When the cations (Na^+ and K^+) and anions (Cl^- and HCO_3^-) in the serum are measured, a difference, or gap, of 14 mEq is present. This 14 mEq represents the unmeasured anions such as phosphates, sulfates, and organic acids. When there is an increase in organic and inorganic acids, as in states of acid-base balance, the anion gap is affected, and herein lies its clinical importance: understanding how the four different types (metabolic and respiratory acidosis and alkalosis) of acid-base balance affect both the anion gap and the individual serum electrolytes that make up the anion gap can help identify the specific etiology of acidosis in a patient and drive patient management.

10. List the elements of an electrolyte panel and discuss what any abnormal readings may indicate.   **p. 336**

An electrolyte panel determines serum sodium (Na^+), potassium (K^+), chloride (Cl^-), bicarbonate (HCO_3^-), magnesium (Mg^{++}), calcium (Ca^{++}), and phosphate (HPO_4^-).

Sodium
Measures: Sodium
Normal value: 135–145 mEq/L

High values: Dehydration, excess saline administration, exchange transfusion with stored blood, impaired renal function

Low values: Overhydration, sodium loss (vomiting, diarrhea, sweating, GI suctioning), increased renal sodium loss (diuretics, DKA, Addison's disease, renal disease)

Potassium
Measures: Potassium

Normal value: 3.5–5 mEq/L

High values: Renal failure, excess K^+ replacement, massive tissue damage, associated with metabolic acidosis

Low values: Diuretics, inadequate intake, large steroid doses, associated with metabolic alkalosis

Chloride
Measures: Chloride

Normal value: 100–108 mEq/L

High values: Increased Na^+ level, decreased HCO_3^- levels, renal failure

Low values: Vomiting, gastric suction, diarrhea, and diuretic use

Bicarbonate
Measures: Bicarbonate

Normal value: 24–30 mEq/L

High values: Base excess, metabolic alkalosis, loss of gastric contents, diuretic use

Low values: Base deficit, metabolic acidosis, consumption of bicarbonate, loss of bicarbonate, and increase in serum chloride level

Magnesium
Measures: Magnesium

Normal value: 1.4–1.9 mEq/L

High value: Hypermagnesemia

Low value: Hypomagnesemia

Calcium
Measures: Calcium

Normal value: 4.3–5.3 mEq/L

High values: False rise due to dehydration, hyperparathyroidism, malignant tumors, immobilization, thiazide diuretics, and vitamin D intoxication

Low values: Hypoparathyroidism, chronic renal disease, pancreatitis, massive blood transfusions, severe malnutrition, false decrease due to low albumin levels

Free calcium
Measures: Ionized calcium

Normal value: 4.3–5.3 mEq/L

High values: Hyperparathyroidism, metastatic bone tumor, multiple myeloma, Paget's disease, sarcoidosis, tumors producing a PTH-like substance, vitamin D intoxication

Low values: Hypoparathyroidism, malabsorption, osteomalacia, pancreatitis, renal failure, rickets, and vitamin D deficiency

Phosphate
Measures: Phosphate

Normal values: 1.8–2.6 mEq/L

High values: Hyperparathyroidism, renal failure, increased growth hormone, vitamin D intoxication

Low values: Hypoparathyroidism, diuresis, malabsorption/malnutrition, carbohydrate loading, and antacid abuse

©2007 Pearson Education, Inc.
Critical Care Paramedic

11. **List the elements of a renal function panel and discuss what any abnormal readings may indicate.**   p. 337

A renal function panel measures the blood urea nitrogen (BUN), creatinine, and BUN/creatinine ratio. Other less frequently utilized renal tests include the creatinine clearance rate, serum osmolality, and uric acid.

BUN
Normal: 8–25 mg/dL
High levels: Renal disease, renal damage, dehydration, shock, CHF, GI bleeding, high protein diets
Low level: Overhydration, increased ADH secretion

Creatinine
Normal:
       Men: 0.6–1.4 mg/dL
       Women: 0.6–1.1 mg/dL
High values: Renal disease, nephrotoxic medications
Low values: Low muscle mass, muscle atrophy

BUN/creatinine ratio
Normal ratio: = 10:1
Ratio > 10:1
       Meaning: Extrinsic renal disease
       Causes: Decreased renal perfusion, increased urea load
Ratio < 10:1
       Meaning: Renal disease
       Causes: Chronic renal failure, decreased urea load, inhibited creatinine secretion, dialysis

12. **Describe the importance of blood glucose testing in modern emergency care.**   p. 340

Glucose, along with proteins and fats, are important fuel sources for the body, and glucose is the only fuel source used by the brain. When glucose is unavailable, altered mental status and loss of consciousness, the familiar effects of hypoglycemia, ensue. Just as important is the fact that the catabolization of protein and fats leads to ketone production and acidosis, which can complicate the hemodynamic status of an already physiologically challenged, critical care patient.

13. **List the elements of a lipid panel and discuss what any abnormal readings may indicate.**   p. 340

Elements of a lipid panel include cholesterol, triglyceride, high-density lipoprotein (HDL), low-density lipoprotein (LDL), and very-low-density lipoprotein (VLDL) levels.

Cholesterol
Normal:
       Desirable: < 200 mg/dL
       Borderline high: 200–239 mg/dL
       High: ≥ 240 mg/dL
High levels: Cause often unknown, dietary, hereditary, pregnancy, pancreatic problems
Low levels: Hyperthyroidism, severe liver damage, and malnutrition

Triglycerides
Normal:
       Desirable: < 150 mg/dL
       Borderline high: 150–190 mg/dL
       High: 200–499 mg/dL
       Very high: ≥ 500 mg/dL
High levels: Dietary, hereditary, pregnancy, pancreatitis, and alcohol abuse
Low levels: Malnutrition, medications

HDL

Normal:

> *Positive Cardiac Risk Factor:*
> > HDL < 35 mg/dL
> > > Total cholesterol to HDL ratio:
> > > > Men > 5.0
> > > > Women > 4.5
> *Negative Cardiac Risk Factor:*
> > HDL > 60 mg/dL

High levels: Moderate alcohol intake, exercise, and weight loss

Low levels: Diabetes mellitus, menopause, and obesity

LDL

Normal: < 160 mg/dL

High levels: High-fat diet, hyperthyroidism, nephrotic syndrome, diabetes mellitus, and familial lipid disease

Low levels: Advanced liver disease, malnutrition

VLDL

Normal: 10–31 mg/dL

High levels: Diabetes, obesity, and hepatic oversecretion

14. List the five most frequently used cardiac markers.   p. 342

The five most frequently used cardiac markers are creatine kinase (CK or CPK), lactate dehydrogenase (LD or LDH), myoglobin, troponin, and B-natriuretic peptide (BNP).

15. Detail the timing of cardiac marker elevations after a myocardial infarction.   p. 342

Creatine kinase (CK or CPK)

- First enzyme to elevate after acute myocardial infarction
- Increases in 90 percent of infarctions
- Begins to rise 4 to 6 hrs after onset of infarction
- Peaks at 24 hrs
- Returns to normal in 3 to 4 days

Lactate dehydrogenase (LD or LDH)

- Increases in more than 90 percent of infarctions
- Begins to rise 24 hrs after infarction
- Peaks in 3 days
- Returns to normal in 8 to 9 days

Myoglobin

- Myoglobin rapid assay kits allow for testing in the critical care and ED setting
- Rises 2 hrs after infarction
- Peaks in 6 to 8 hrs
- Returns to normal in 20 to 36 hrs

Troponin

- Troponin I is the form most frequently assessed.
- Troponin rapid assay kits allow for testing in the critical care and ED setting
- Rises 4 to 6 hrs after infarction
- Peaks in 12 to 16 hrs
- Stays elevated for up to 10 days

16. Discuss the importance of isoenzymes in CK and LDH testing. p. 342

When considering CK and LDH serum levels during evaluation of AMI, it is necessary to evaluate the isoenzyme of each marker that is specific for myocardial tissue. Specifically, the CK-II (MB) and LDH1 isoenzymes are specific for myocardial injury, and are evaluated during the assessment of AMI. In general terms, CK elevation, for example, just tells the clinician that muscle tissue—maybe skeletal, maybe smooth, maybe myocardial muscle—was injured. Elevation of CK-II tells the clinician that the myocardium was injured.

17. List the elements of a liver function panel and discuss what any abnormal readings may indicate. p. 344

Elements of a liver function panel include total bilirubin, indirect bilirubin, direct bilirubin, alkaline phosphatase (ALP), Gamma-glutamyl transferase (GGT), ammonia, alanine transaminase (ALT), aspartate transaminase (AST), aldolase, amylase, and lipase.

Total bilirubin
Measures: Total bilirubin
Normal value: 0.1–1.0 mg/dL
High value: See indirect and direct
Low value: No clinical significance

Indirect bilirubin
Measures: Indirect unconjugated bilirubin
Normal value: 0.1–1.0 mg/dL
High value: Sickle cell disease, autoimmune disease, hemorrhage, drug toxicity
Low value: No clinical significance

Direct bilirubin
Measures: Conjugated bilirubin
Normal value: 0.0–0.4 mg/dL, mean = 0.1 mg/dL
High value: Obstructive jaundice, gallstones, congenital biliary tract abnormalities, and medications
Low value: No clinical significance

ALP
Measures: Alkaline phosphatase
Normal value: Men: 45–115 Units/L. Women: 30–100 Units/L
High value: Bone abnormality, liver abnormality, and eclampsia
Low value: Scurvy, genetic defects, excessive vitamin D intake

GGT
Measures: Total gamma-glutamyl transferase
Normal value: Men: 1–94 Units/L. Women: 1–70 Units/L
High value: Liver disease, alcohol use
Low value: No clinical significance

Ammonia
Measures: Ammonia
Normal value: 18–80 mcg/dL
High value: Liver failure, Reye's syndrome
Low value: No clinical significance

ALT
Measures: Alanine transaminase
Normal value: Men: 10–55 Units/L. Women: 7–30 Units/L
High value: Severe hepatitis, cirrhosis, and mononucleosis
Low value: Liver failure

AST

Measures: Aspartate transaminase
Normal value: Men: 10–40 Units/L. Women: 9–25 Units/L
High value: Myocardial infarction, hepatitis
Low value: Liver failure

Aldolase

Measures: Aldolase
Normal value: 0–7 Units/L
High value: Muscular disorders
Low value: No clinical significance

Amylase

Measures: Amylase
Normal value: 53–123 Units/L
High value: Pancreatitis, pancreatic trauma
Low value: Pancreatic destruction

Lipase

Measures: Lipase
Normal value: 3–19 Units/L
High value: Pancreatitis, pancreatic trauma
Low value: No clinical significance

18. **Describe the role of serologic testing in critical care transport.**   p. 344

Serologic testing is a broad area of laboratory analysis that includes blood banking, identification of antibodies against infectious disease, and autoimmunity studies. Serologic tests can be either specific or nonspecific depending on the test and method employed.

Blood banking includes tests that are routinely performed prior to the administration of blood, and are extremely important, as transfusion reactions can be fatal. These tests include ABO typing, Rh factor determination, direct Coombs' test, and the indirect Coombs' test. In addition, donor blood is routinely tested for the presence of infectious diseases such as HIV, cytomegalovirus, mononucleosis, syphilis, and hepatitis A, B, and C virus.

ABO typing determines which of the four blood groups—A, B, AB, or O—is represented in a sample. Recall that the blood group refers to the antigens present on the red blood cell (RBC) membrane. Rh factor testing determines if the RBCs in a sample contain the Rh antigen. The direct Coombs' test, also called the RBC antibody screen, is used to screen blood for cross matching, check for hemolytic reactions, and assess for hemolytic disease of the newborn. It detects antibodies attached to the RBC surface that may cause cellular damage. The indirect Coombs' test is used to detect various free circulating antibodies present in the blood serum, and to prevent transfusion reactions to incompatible blood caused by minor blood-type factors.

19. **Discuss the importance of accurate blood banking in emergency care.**   p. 345

Accurate blood banking is important in all areas of medicine in order to avoid such unpleasantries as anaphylaxis, transmission of infectious disease, hemolytic reactions, and transfusion reactions.

20. **Describe common endocrine function tests encountered in critical care transport.**   p. 346

Common endocrine function tests include serum cortisol, thyroid-stimulating hormone (TSH), L-thyroxine (Total T_4), triiodothyronine (T_3), and free thyroxine (Free T_4).

Cortisol

Measures: Adrenocortical function
Normal value: 5–25 mcg/dL

High value: Cushing's syndrome, pituitary tumors
Low value: Addison's disease

TSH
Measures: Thyroid-stimulating hormone
Normal value: 0.5–5.0 µU/mL
High value: Thyroid failure, pituitary tumor
Low value: Hyperthyroidism, pituitary failure

T$_3$
Measures: Triiodothyronine
Normal value: 60–181 ng/dL
High value: Hyperthyroidism
Low value: Hypothyroidism

Total T$_4$
Measures: L-thyroxine
Normal value: 4.5–10.9 mcg/dL
High value: Hyperthyroidism
Low value: Hypothyroidism

Free T$_4$
Measures: Free thyroxine
Normal value: 0.8–2.7 ng/dL
High value: Hyperthyroidism
Low value: Hypothyroidism

21. Briefly describe how bacteria are identified and isolated.   **p. 347**

Bacteria are classified as to whether or not their cell wall absorbs a Gram stain (gram-negative or gram-positive), their shape (round, rod, spiral = cocci, bacilli, and spirilla, respectively), and whether they are aerobic or anaerobic. In addition, various biochemical tests can be used to identify bacteria.

22. List the elements of a urinalysis and discuss what any abnormal readings may indicate.   **p. 347**

Elements of a urinalysis include pH, specific gravity, protein, glucose, ketones, bilirubin, nitrites, leukocyte esterase, urobilinogen, casts, white blood cells (WBCs), and red blood cells (RBCs). A microscopic evaluation is required to determine the presence of casts, RBCs, and WBCs, which are reported as the number visible per high-powered field.

pH
Measures: Acidity of the urine
Normal value: 5–9, mean = 6
High value: UTI, bicarbonate use
Low value: Acidosis

Specific gravity
Measures: Concentration of the urine
Normal value: Adult: 1.001–1.035. Child: 1.001–1.018
High value: Dehydration, increased ADH secretion
Low value: Overhydration

Protein
Measures: Presence of protein in the urine
Normal value: Negative
High value: Renal disease, preeclampsia/PIH
Low value: No clinical significance

Glucose

Measures: Presence of sugars in the urine
Normal value: Negative
High value: Diabetes, stress
Low value: No clinical significance

Ketones

Measures: Presence of ketones in the urine
Normal value: Negative
High value: Malnutrition, DKA, dieting
Low value: No clinical significance

Nitrites

Measures: Presence of nitrites in the urine
Normal value: Negative
High value: UTI
Low value: No clinical significance

Leukocyte esterase

Measures: Presence of leukocyte esterase in the urine
Normal value: Negative
High value: UTI
Low value: No clinical significance

Bilirubin

Measures: Presence of bilirubin in the urine
Normal value: Negative
High value: Liver disease
Low value: No clinical significance

Urobilinogen

Measures: Presence or urobilinogen in the urine
Normal value: 0.1–1.0 Ehrlich Units/dL
High value: Hepatic insufficiency
Low value: No clinical significance

Casts

Measures: Presence of hyaline casts in the urine
Normal value: Variable, very few present
High value: Cancer
Low value: No clinical significance

WBCs

Measures: Presence of WBCs in the urine
Normal value: < 4–5 per HPF
High value: Infection, leukemia, steroid use
Low value: No clinical significance

RBCs

Measures: Presence of RBCs in the urine
Normal value: < 2–3 per HPF
High value: Trauma, infection, and kidney stones
Low value: No clinical significance

23. Discuss the importance of toxicological testing in critical care transport. p. 347

Toxicological testing is useful in the realm of critical care transport to both measure the serum levels of therapeutic medications, and to screen for illicit substances, such as opiates, benzodiazepines, THC, cocaine, amphetamines, barbiturates, and other substances.

24. Discuss the role of diagnostic imaging in medicine and briefly describe the following:

X-rays p. 349

X-rays are the primary examination tool for bones and are considered a screening exam for the chest. Tissue density determines the film exposure to X-rays; bone is most dense, allowing the least amount of film exposure, creating white on film. Conversely, air, being the least dense, allows the most film exposure, creating black on film. Contrast is used to make tissues more visible in the GI/GU tract.

Fluoroscopy p. 349

X-ray and contrast media are used for real-time imaging that is displayed on the screen while the fluroscope is on.

CT (CAT) scanning p. 349

A CT scanner uses focused X-rays to examine body tissue, and a computer enhances the interpretation. Sequential images, or "cuts," are displayed on the computer screen, allowing for detailed examination.

Ultrasonography p. 349

Sound waves are transmitted through body tissue. More dense tissue reflects waves back to the transducer, and a computer interprets tissue density based on the wave return. The image is then displayed on screen for interpretation.

Nuclear medicine p. 349

A radioisotope is injected into the patient and its movement is recorded using a nuclear medicine camera.

Magnetic resonance imaging (MRI) p. 349

MRI does not utilize ionizing radiation as does an X-ray. Rather, a strong magnetic field introduced around the patient causes water molecules in the tissues to align along the field. When the magnetic field is turned off, the water molecules return to their original orientation, allowing a computer to interpret tissue densities based on water movement. MRI is excellent for tissue that contains water, such as nervous tissue, joints, and organs. MRI is poor for tissue containing little water, such as bone.

Positron emission tomography (PET) p. 349

PET scanning produces information on organ function.

25. Describe common physiological tests encountered in medicine. p. 349

Common physiological tests include pulmonary function testing, arterial blood gas analysis, stress testing, specialized electrocardiographic imaging, and numerous others.

26. List the elements of an arterial blood gas panel and discuss what any abnormal readings may indicate. p. 350

Elements of an arterial blood gas (ABG) include pH, $PaCO_2$, PaO_2, HCO_3^-, SaO_2, and Hgb.

pH
Measures: Blood acidity
Normal value: 7.35–7.45
High value: Alkalosis
Low value: Acidosis

PaCO₂

Measures: Partial pressure of carbon dioxide in the blood
Normal value: 35–45 mmHg
High value: Respiratory acidosis, hypoventilation
Low value: Respiratory alkalosis, hyperventilation

PaO₂

Measures: Partial pressure of oxygen in the blood
Normal value: 80–100 mmHg
High value: Over-oxygenation, hyperventilation
Low value: Hypoxia, hypoventilation

HCO₃⁻

Measures: Bicarbonate ion concentration in the blood
Normal value: 24–30 mEq/L
High value: Base excess, metabolic alkalosis, and bicarbonate ingestion
Low value: Base deficit, metabolic acidosis, increased serum chloride

SaO₂

Measures: Hemoglobin oxygen saturation
Normal value: 95–100 percent
High value: No clinical significance
Low value: Hypoxia, hypoventilation

Hgb

Measures: Blood hemoglobin concentration
Normal value: 12–18 g/dL
High value: Dehydration, polycythemia
Low value: Overhydration, anemia, and hemorrhage

Using ABGs to determine cause of acid-base disturbance

Respiratory acidosis
- pH < 7.35
- Increased $PaCO_2$
- Increased HCO_3^-

Respiratory alkalosis
- pH > 7.45
- Decreased $PaCO_2$
- Decreased HCO_3^-

Metabolic acidosis
- pH < 7.35
- Decreased HCO_3^-
- Decreased $PaCO_2$

Metabolic alkalosis
- pH > 7.45
- Increased HCO_3^-
- Decreased $PaCO_2$

Case Study

Case #1

Your team is called to transfer a 74-year-old man from a small community three-bed ED to the regional medical center ICU for admission. The patient has a long-standing history of insulin-dependent diabetes and was intubated by EMS for decreased mental status. The patient has the

©2007 Pearson Education, Inc.
Critical Care Paramedic

following labs: hemoglobin/hematocrit 17 g/dL and 48 percent, white blood cells 16.5 M/mm^3 with 24 percent bands, potassium 5.8 mEq/L, chloride 76 mEq/L, sodium 155 mEq/L, HCO$_3^-$ 10 mEq/L, and blood glucose 860 mg/dL.

Case #2

Your patient is a 22-year-old female who was the sole occupant of a one-vehicle MVC in which the vehicle left the road and struck a tree at a high rate of speed. EMS had difficulty securing her airway, and the rural ED provider on duty suspects she aspirated a great deal of blood before she was finally able to be intubated. In the ED, a chest tube was inserted for a right hemopneumothorax and exam showed midfacial injuries consistent with a Le Fort 3 fracture. Chest X-ray now shows that the pneumothorax has almost completely resolved, and that the ET and chest tubes are in proper position. The patient has been unresponsive to pain since arrival at the ED, and remains so; however her pupils are equal and reactive to light. Her ABG results showed pH = 7.50, PaO$_2$ = 250 mmHg, PaCO$_2$ = 11 mmHg, HCO$_3^-$ = 21 mEq/L. The patient is to be transported for 45 minutes by ground to the area trauma center, and the ED provider insists that you hyperventilate this patient en route, despite the lack of evidence of rising ICP.

Case #3

You are called to a community ED to transfer a patient to the regional cardiac center for cardiac catheterization. Your patient has been pain free for the past two days since being placed on the medical floor. While flipping through the chart, you notice that your patient's heparin drip was increased from 800 to 1,000 Units/hr the day before, but that the last PTT/INR in the chart was drawn over 48 hours ago. The results were 110 seconds and 2.0, respectively.

DISCUSSION QUESTIONS

1. What is the importance of laboratory and basic diagnostic testing in critical care transport?
2. In general, what are the differences between laboratory tests, medical imaging, and physiological testing?
3. What are normal reference values and how are they established?
4. For each of the above cases, what concerns do the presented laboratory values raise for safe patient transfer?

Content Review

MULTIPLE CHOICE

_____ 1. Which of the following is not one of the three general categories of diagnostic tests?
   A. physiological tests
   B. laboratory tests
   C. electrolyte tests
   D. imaging studies

_____ 2. Which distribution method takes all collected data, determines the mean, and then considers all values greater than about two standard deviations from the mean outside of "normal" values?
   A. statistical system
   B. percentile ranking system
   C. Gaussian distribution method
   D. standard deviation model

_____ 3. Which of the following statements regarding specificity is true?
   A. A test with high specificity has few false-positives.
   B. Specificity is the degree to which a test detects a disease without yielding a false-negative result.
   C. Many tests have 100 percent specificity.
   D. A test with high specificity has few false-negatives.

_____ 4. Which of the following statements regarding sensitivity is true?
   A. A test with high sensitivity has many false-negatives.
   B. Sensitivity is the degree to which a test detects a disease without yielding a false-negative result.
   C. Few tests are 100 percent sensitive.
   D. A test with high sensitivity has few false-positives.

_____ 5. What is the advantage of an International Normalized Ratio (INR) over a prothrombin time (PT)?
   A. An INR compares the PT to a control, allowing a more accurate interpretation of coagulation time.
   B. An INR can be determined more rapidly than a PT.
   C. PT does not take into account a patient's blood type.
   D. A PT can only be used on patients on coumarin-type medications.

_____ 6. Which of the following lab tests is used to monitor heparin therapy?
   A. PTT   C. INR
   B. PT   D. coumarin-type tests

_____ 7. Which of the following lab tests is used to monitor warfarin therapy?
   A. PTT   C. INR
   B. PT   D. coumarin-type tests

_____ 8. A D-dimer assay measures:
   A. the electrical differences between measured ions in the blood serum.
   B. liver enzymes.
   C. direct bilirubin.
   D. the degradation products created during clot lysis.

_____ 9. Why is it necessary to measure serum electrolytes in milliequivalents per liter (mEq/L) instead of milligrams per liter (mg/L)?
   A. Mg/L are too large a unit for practical serum measurement.
   B. Measuring electrolytes in mEq/L recognizes the biotransformation that occurs after the ingestion of electrolytes.
   C. Measuring electrolytes in mEq/L allows for the measuring and comparing of the chemical activity of electrolytes.
   D. Mgs are used to measure weights of elemental electrolytes.

_____ 10. The anion gap measures:
   A. phosphorous, sulfur, and organic acids.
   B. unmeasured anions in the blood serum.
   C. 14 mEq of cations.
   D. the electrical difference between all charged ions in the blood serum.

_____ 11. The clinical importance of the anion gap is that it can:
   A. determine the need for electrolyte management.
   B. identify genetic abnormalities.
   C. aid in the identification of the specific etiology of acid-base balance disturbances.
   D. identify specific electrolyte disturbances.

_____ 12. Which of the following is paired with an incorrect normal value?
   A. sodium: 1.4–1.9 mEq/L   C. chloride: 100–108 mEq/L
   B. potassium: 3–5 mEq/L   D. bicarbonate: 24–30 mEq/L

_____ 13. _____ is the most prevalent cation in the intracellular fluid, and _____ the most prevalent cation in the extracellular fluid.
   A. Sodium, calcium   C. Calcium, potassium
   B. Potassium, sodium   D. Sodium, potassium

_____ 14. Dehydration can result in an increase of which of the following lab values?
   A. magnesium, sodium, and chloride
   B. bicarbonate, magnesium, and calcium
   C. calcium, free calcium, and phosphate
   D. sodium, calcium, and chloride

_____ 15. Which of the following laboratory tests is paired with an incorrect normal value?
   A. BUN: 8–25 mg/dL
   B. creatinine: men: 0.6–1.4 mg/dL, women: 0.6–1.1 mg/dL
   C. creatinine clearance rate: 1.2–1.5 mL/min/m^2 BSA
   D. BUN/creatinine ratio: Normal ratio = 10:1

_____ 16. A patient with chronic renal failure who has missed dialysis can be expected to have:
   A. an increased BUN, increased creatinine, and decreased BUN/creatinine ratio.
   B. a decreased BUN, increased creatinine, and increased BUN/creatinine ratio.
   C. a decreased BUN, decreased creatinine, and decreased BUN/creatinine ratio.
   D. a decreased BUN, decreased creatinine, and increased BUN/creatinine ratio.

_____ 17. Which of the following laboratory tests is paired with an incorrect normal value?
   A. cholesterol: Desirable level is less than 200 mg/dL.
   B. triglycerides: Desirable level is less than 500 mg/dL.
   C. HDL: Total cholesterol to HDL ratio should be greater than 5.0 for men, and greater than 4.5 for women.
   D. LDL: 160 mg/dL

_____ 18. The five most frequently used cardiac markers are:
   A. creatine kinase (CK or CPK), low-density lipoprotein (LDL), myoglobin, troponin, and B-natriuretic peptide (BNP).
   B. creatinine kinase (CK or CPK), lactate dehydrogenase (LD or LDH), myoglobin, troponin, and B-natriuretic peptide (BNP).
   C. creatine kinase (CK or CPK), lactate dehydrogenase (LD or LDH), myoglobin, troponin, and B-natriuretic peptide (BNP).
   D. creatine kinase (CK or CPK), lactate dehydrogenase (LD or LDH), hemoglobin, troponin, and B-natriuretic peptide (BNP).

_____ 19. Pancreatitis or a pancreatic trauma would most likely result in:
   A. increased ALT and increased AST.
   B. decreased total bilirubin and increased indirect bilirubin.
   C. increased amylase and increased lipase.
   D. increased amylase and decreased ammonia.

_____ 20. Liver failure would most likely result in:
   A. decreased ALT, decreased AST, increased ammonia, increased GGT, and increased ALP.
   B. decreased direct bilirubin, decreased indirect bilirubin, decreased total bilirubin, decreased AST, and decreased ALT.
   C. decreased amylase, decreased lipase, decreased GGT, and decreased ALP.
   D. increased amylase, increased AST, decreased ALP, and decreased AST.

_____ 21. _____ is used to determine the type of blood group antigen present on the red blood cell membrane.
   A. Direct Coombs' test   C. Rh factor test
   B. Indirect Coombs' test   D. ABO typing

_____ 22. Addison's disease would most likely result in an:
   A. increased serum TSH.   C. increased serum aldolase.
   B. decreased serum cortisol.   D. decreased serum ammonia.

_____ 23. Hyperthyroidism would most likely result in:
    A. decreased TSH, decreased T_3, decreased total T_4, and decreased free T_4.
    B. increased TSH, increased T_3, decreased total T_4, and decreased free T_4.
    C. increased TSH, increased T_3, increased total T_4, and increased free T_4.
    D. increased TSH, decreased T_3, increased total T_4, and decreased free T_4.

_____ 24. All of the following can be used to aid in the identification of bacteria except:
    A. color.
    B. shape.
    C. gram staining.
    D. whether or not they are aerobic or anaerobic.

_____ 25. Which of the following components of a urinalysis are usually not present in the urine of a normal, healthy person?
    A. pH, occult blood, urobilinogen, bilirubin, casts, RBCs, and WBCs
    B. RBCs, WBCs, glucose, and ketones
    C. glucose, ketones, occult blood, nitrates, leukocyte esterase, and bilirubin
    D. protein, glucose, occult blood, urobilinogen, and ketones

_____ 26. Which of the following imaging studies is considered a screening exam for the chest?
    A. MRI
    C. ultrasonography
    B. CT scan
    D. X-ray

_____ 27. A D-dimer assay can be expected to show increased levels after:
    A. aeromedical transport.
    C. RSI.
    B. administration of a fibrinolytic.
    D. intravenous access.

MATCHING

Match the laboratory test with its components.

_____ 28. Endocrine function tests

_____ 29. Coagulation panel

_____ 30. Arterial blood gas panel

_____ 31. Renal function panel

_____ 32. Complete blood count (CBC)

_____ 33. Lipid panel

_____ 34. Liver function panel

_____ 35. Urinalysis

_____ 36. Electrolyte panel

_____ 37. Blood banking

  A. Hemoglobin, hematocrit, white blood cells (WBCs), red blood cells (RBCs), mean corpuscular volume (MCV), mean corpuscular hemoglobin (MCH), mean corpuscular hemoglobin concentration (MCHC), red blood cell distribution width (RDW), platelet count, and platelet volume

  B. Prothrombin time (PT), partial thromboplastin time (PTT), and International Normalized Ratio (INR)

  C. Sodium (Na^+), potassium (K^+), chloride (Cl^-), bicarbonate (HCO_3^-), magnesium (Mg^{++}), calcium (Ca^{++}), and phosphate (HPO_4^-)

  D. Blood urea nitrate (BUN), creatinine, and BUN/creatinine ratio. Other less frequently utilized tests include the creatinine clearance rate, serum osmolality, and uric acid.

©2007 Pearson Education, Inc.
Critical Care Paramedic

E. Cholesterol, triglyceride, high-density lipoprotein (HDL), low-density lipoprotein (LDL), and very-low-density lipoprotein (VLDL) levels

F. Total bilirubin, indirect bilirubin, direct bilirubin, alkaline phosphatase (ALP), Gamma-glutamyl transferase (GGT), ammonia, alanine transaminase (ALT), aspartate transaminase (AST), aldolase, amylase, and lipase

G. Serum cortisol, thyroid-stimulating hormone (TSH), L-thyroxine (Total T_4), triiodothyronine (T_3), free thyroxine (Free T_4)

H. ABO typing, Rh factor determination, direct Coombs' test, indirect Coombs' test

I. pH, specific gravity, protein, glucose, ketones, bilirubin, nitrites, leukocyte esterase, urobilinogen, casts, white blood cells (WBCs), red blood cells (RBCs)

J. pH, $PaCO_2$, PaO_2, HCO_3^-, SaO_2, and Hgb

13 Introduction to Trauma

Review of Chapter Objectives

Upon completion of this chapter, the student should be able to:

1. **Describe some of the main points regarding the epidemiology of trauma in the United States.** p. 359

   The following bulleted points summarize the main points of trauma epidemiology in the United States:

   - Trauma is the leading cause of death in the United States for all persons under the age of 44
     - Fifth leading cause of death overall
     - Leading cause of death in children
   - 150,000 deaths annually in the United States
     - 400 deaths per day—50 of these are children
     - 90,000 secondary to unintentional injury—remainder result from violence
   - Motor vehicle crashes (MVCs) most common cause of death in the United States
     - 1 in 70 Americans will die in an MVC
     - 500,000 hospitalizations per year
     - 50 percent of MVCs involve alcohol
   - Firearms second most common cause of death

2. **Discuss the costs of modern trauma care.** p. 359

   Annually, about 1.5 million persons require hospitalization for trauma, but survive to be discharged. Of these, tens of thousands of people are left with temporary or permanent debilitating injury. In 1994, the cost of such injuries was $224 billion for medical costs, rehabilitation costs, and lost wages. In addition to direct costs in terms of dollars spent, trauma costs can also be considered in years of productive life lost (YPLL), a figure calculated by subtracting the age at death from 65, the average age of retirement.

3. **Describe the history of trauma care and trauma systems in the United States.** p. 361

   Historically, trauma has been viewed differently than disease in the United States; unlike disease, trauma was considered unavoidable or accidental. As a result, little was done prior to the 1960s to organize trauma care, and there was a lack of development of a system's approach to trauma care. The development of trauma care in the United States paralleled the growth of EMS, and was greatly aided in 1966 by the publication of a white paper by the National Academy of Science and the National Research Council entitled, *Accidental Death and Disability: The Neglected Disease of Modern Society*. This landmark paper increased medical and public awareness of the magnitude of the trauma epidemic and significantly influenced Congress to pass the Highway Safety Act in 1966. The act required each state to develop highway safety programs and suggested funding for EMS development. In 1973, the Emergency Medical Services Systems Act, which offered funding and a detailed outline for the development of EMS systems, passed. The Trauma Care Systems Planning and Development Act of 1990 provided additional funding and guidance for the development of trauma systems at a time when federal funding had significantly decreased.

The military approach to trauma hugely influenced the civilian approach, which recognized that rapid surgical intervention for seriously injured patients resulted in a decreased mortality. As a result, trauma systems in Maryland and Illinois mirrored the military's Medivac system, setting the stage for the development of the concepts of "golden hour" and one "rapid transport." In 1960, the University of Maryland developed the first dedicated, civilian, trauma-specific care in the United States, and the first trauma unit was opened at Cook County Hospital in Chicago, Illinois, in 1966. Illinois once again set the example for the rest of the United States when, in 1971, it developed the first statewide trauma system in Illinois. Maryland followed in 1977, setting the stage for the development of trauma systems across the United States.

4. Describe the basic structure of a regional trauma system in the United States. p. 362

The four levels of trauma center accreditation as outlined by the American College of Surgeons (ACS) are Level I, Level II, Level III, and Level IV. Level I trauma centers offer comprehensive trauma care from initial evaluation to rehabilitation, and offer specialty services such as burn and neurological units. Level I trauma centers must have a predetermined number of operating rooms, resuscitation areas, and ICU beds. Yearly patient quotas must be met, and Level I trauma centers are usually located at teaching hospitals.

Level II trauma centers can manage most trauma patients but lack some surgical subspecialties that prevent them from obtaining Level I status.

Level III trauma centers are often located in community hospitals and are capable of providing initial resuscitation and stabilization, but they lack specialties and ICUs.

Level IV trauma centers are typically rural health care facilities where the goal is rapid transport from the facility to a tertiary care facility.

5. Discuss the categories for trauma facilities in the United States and the characteristics and limitations of each. p. 362

The American College of Surgeons' Committee on Trauma publishes guidelines and provides accreditation of regional trauma centers, as do most states. Numerous components must be considered when developing a regional trauma system: one of the central ideas is that enough serious trauma cases must be available in order to maintain a high level of expertise among the specialists at the receiving trauma centers.

The four levels of trauma center accreditation as outlined by the American College of Surgeons (ACS) are:

Level I: Offers comprehensive trauma care from initial evaluation (and often transport) to rehabilitation. Can manage any type of patient and offers many specialized services, such as burn, neurologic, and cardiovascular surgical subspecialists. Level I centers must maintain a predetermined number of available operating rooms, resuscitation areas, and ICU beds. They remain active in planning and research and are usually located at university medical centers. An important point is that a Level I center must receive a predetermined number of severe trauma patients annually.

Level II: Can appropriately manage most seriously injured patients, but lacks some surgical subspecialties. A Level II facility may not focus as much on research and education as a Level I facility, but still must adhere to rigorous staff educational and credentialing requirements.

Level III: Often located in community hospitals, these centers provide expert initial resuscitation and stabilization but lack much of the surgical specialty and intensive care services that are available at the larger centers.

Level IV: This designation has been implemented to help guide the very rural center in developing standardized plans for the initial management and rapid transfer of the trauma patient.

©2007 Pearson Education, Inc.
Critical Care Paramedic

6. **Discuss the importance of injury prevention in modern society.** p. 363

Death from trauma follows a trimodal distribution. The first group, approximately 50 percent of all trauma deaths, die immediately or within several minutes of injury. The second group, representing about 30 percent of all trauma deaths, die within the first 4 hours after their injury. The third group, about 20 percent of trauma deaths, die within 2 weeks of their injury. The take-home point is that 50 percent of trauma patients will die on scene. These victims can only be saved by preventing the injury in the first place.

7. **Discuss the application of the Haddon Matrix to trauma prevention programs.** p. 363

The most notable influence on changing the concept that trauma occurred from random, uncontrollable "accidents" was William Haddon, the first director of the National Highway Traffic Safety Administration (NHTSA). He refined and sold the idea that illness and injury result from interactions between an agent (i.e., a car), the environment (i.e., a wet road), and a host (i.e., the driver of car). His Haddon Matrix, the idea that disease transfer is predictable and can be prevented by manipulating the agent, environment, and host behavior, has become the classic illustration of the method of communicable disease and has been widely used in the development of disease-prevention programs. When considering energy transfer instead of disease transfer, the matrix can be applied to injury prevention, though implementation is difficult.

Injury prevention can be active or passive. Active prevention requires the host to engage in actions likely to reduce the risk of an exposure to an insult; buckling a seatbelt and wearing a helmet when operating a motorcycle are examples. The problem with active prevention is that it requires effort on behalf of the host, who, more often than not, proves unreliable unless mandated by law and threatened with a penalty.

Passive prevention measures do not require action from the host; examples are the placement of airbags in cars and improved road design. Passive measures are more reliable than active measures because they are inherent in the design of the environment.

8. **Describe the utility and basis for common trauma scoring systems.** p. 364

Trauma scoring systems are usually meant to serve either as a triage tool or as a method of stratifying injury severity for research purposes. Scoring systems meant for field use as triage tools must be valid and accurate, yet easy to use. Some of the trauma scoring systems used in the prehospital and critical care environments include the Glasgow Coma Scale (GCS), Trauma Score (TS) and Revised Trauma Score (RTS), Pediatric Trauma Score (PTS), Abbreviated Injury Scale (AIS), Injury Severity Score (ISS), and the Trauma and Injury Severity Score (TRISS) method.

The GCS, first published in 1974, provides an objective analysis of a patient's level of consciousness and cerebral function. It considers three parameters: eye opening, verbal response, and motor response. Each parameter is graded on a numerical scale, and rapidly determines trends in the patient's neurological status. Many references suggest that trauma patients with a GCS < 13 should be evaluated at a Level I or II trauma center.

The TS considers the GCS along with four additional parameters: respiratory rate, respiratory expansion, systolic blood pressure, and capillary refill. It scores patients from 1–16 points, with those patients scoring 12 or less requiring a trauma center. The TS was revised in 1989 and morphed into the RTS. The parameters respiratory expansion and capillary refill were dropped, and patients scored between 0 and 12, with 11 or less requiring specialized trauma care. The RTS considers three parameters: respiratory rate, systolic blood pressure, and the GCS.

The PTS is a version of the RTS modified to consider pediatric physiology. Parameters considered include patient size, airway status, systolic blood pressure, CNS status, skeletal system, and the cutaneous system. The AIS was developed jointly by the American Medical Association, American Association for Automotive Medicine, and the Society of Automotive Engineers. It details the types and severity of injuries suffered in MVCs, and includes assessment of the head and face, chest, neck, spine, abdomen and pelvic organs, pelvis and extremities, and the integument. The ISS is retrospectively calculated using AIS data, and is used by trauma registries for data collection and research purposes. The TRISS method combines patient age and data from the RTS and ISS to indicate overall severity and survivability of injuries. It is primarily used by trauma registries and is impractical for clinical use.

9. Describe the physics and biomechanics of trauma. p. 367

Trauma occurs secondary to the introduction of energy into the human body in a quantity sufficient to cause physical damage to body cells and tissue. While kinetic, thermal, electrical, and radiological are all types of energy that can cause injury and death, kinetic energy, by far, results in the most number of deaths in the United States.

Kinetic energy is the energy of an object in motion, and is related to an object's mass and velocity by the equation: $KE = (M \times V^2) \div 2$. While mass does have an influence on KE, note that velocity is squared, doubling an object's weight results in a doubling of the KE. Doubling an object's velocity results in a four-fold increase in the KE, giving credence to the old saying "speed kills!" Recall from your paramedic education that Newton's first law, his law of inertia, states that an object in motion will tend to stay in motion until acted upon by an outside force. This seemingly mundane law of physics takes on especially serious consequences when the "object in motion" is a human torso and the "outside force" acting on it is a steering wheel being struck at 60 mph, the speed at which the unrestrained driver is moving forward after hitting an immovable bridge abutment. Newton's second law (summarized by the equation $F = MA$, or MD for deceleration) can help one appreciate how a rapid deceleration, say from 60 mph to 0 over the two feet that the patient moves forward as the vehicle crumples, can result in the introduction of tremendous amounts of force into the human body, especially the unrestrained one.

In addition to the laws of motion, the biomechanics of trauma should always be considered. The events of an impact (vehicle, body, organ, and secondary collisions), type of impact, path of penetrating objects, effects of blasts, and objects and surfaces struck should all be evaluated to help form a mechanism of injury (MOI) that can be reported to other members of the health care team. The MOI considers the physical cause of the injury and assesses how energy was introduced into the body, suggesting which organs and systems may be affected. As such, the MOI can help direct assessment and treatment.

10. Describe the initial assessment and priorities during resuscitation of the trauma patient. p. 368

The initial assessment and priorities during resuscitation of the trauma patient are no different for the critical care paramedic than they are for any other clinician, and are universal and clear in the prehospital setting:

1. Safety of the rescuer(s)
2. Safety of the victim(s)
3. Management of airway and/or respiratory system compromise
4. Management of life-threatening hemorrhage
5. Protection/prevention of actual or potential spinal cord injury
6. Rapid transport to an appropriate facility
7. Maintenance of body temperature
8. Pain control
9. Other concerns specific to the situation

The critical care paramedic will, however, often find herself performing interfacility transports that do not have some of the more dynamic variables typical of the prehospital environment, but that often require therapies or interventions not usually performed in the field.

11. Describe general considerations for transport of a severely traumatized patient. p. 369

General considerations for the transport of a patient with severe trauma begin with the airway and breathing. Decisions such as whether or not to intubate, to perform RSI, and the type of airway to be utilized all need to be made prior to the initiation of transport, and ventilator settings determined and set. Circulatory status should be stabilized as much as possible prior to transport, and the procurement of blood products and the preparing of IV infusion pumps accomplished.

Patient packaging should center on keeping the patient immobilized, warm, and secure, and time should be spent ensuring that the patient is packaged neatly. Monitor leads, IV lines, oxygen tubing, ventilator circuits, and such, should be in order, and IV ports, easily accessible. Finally, ensure that the receiving facility is the appropriate one for the patient, and make contact early to alert the staff and provide them with adequate time to prepare needed resources.

Case Study

Pacing around the command post at the edge of the landing zone (LZ), you glance at your watch again, watching the last 30 seconds of your patient's "golden hour" tick away. Unfortunately, nothing can be done about it, as you haven't even seen the patient yet. The landing zone in which you are located is in an overgrown field approximately 100 miles from the hospital at which you are based. Your team has been called to a state forest area for a hunter that has been shot. The patient was accidentally shot by a member of his hunting party at a remote camp, which is over 3 miles from the LZ and 8 miles from the nearest road. The patient is being carried to the LZ by a mountain rescue team with whom you have been in contact with via radio.

The patient, a 66-year-old man, sustained a gunshot wound to the abdomen at close range from a hunting rifle and has lost a significant amount of blood. The EMTs with the rescue team are administering oxygen and IV fluids to the patient and advise you that their ETA to the LZ is approximately 5 minutes. After discussing the patient with your partner and the pilot, it's agreed that you will transport the patient to a Level II trauma center which is only a 10-minute flight away. Although your base hospital is a Level I trauma center and your original destination, due to the delay in extrication you decide that the patient should be transported as soon as possible to the closest facility capable of managing his wounds.

While the pilot starts the helicopter's engines and updates your communications center, you and your partner meet the rescue team at the edge of the woods to begin your assessment. The patient is alert and complaining of lower-left, abdominal pain which radiates to his left leg. Although obviously in pain, he is speaking well and is clearly maintaining his own airway without much effort. An assessment of his breathing shows a respiratory rate of 20 and slightly labored, with clear and equal breath sounds bilaterally. The patient is already on high-flow, high-concentration oxygen by mask, and that is left in place. During your assessment of the circulatory system, you note a large, blood-soaked trauma dressing in place over the lower abdominal area that is secured with triangular bandages. The medic on the rescue team tells you that the dressing is the third to be soaked, and that the patient has had a total of 3 liters of normal saline IV so far. The patient has a thready, radial pulse at approximately 144 beats per minute, and his skin is cool and clammy. Your partner tells you that she cannot auscultate a blood pressure, but palpates a BP of around 70 systolic. While your partner establishes a second large-bore IV line to allow the transfusion of 2 units of O negative blood, you continue your assessment. Examination of the wound shows an approximately 1.5 cm, circular, open wound low in the left, lower quadrant. Light pressure on the pelvic wings elicits left-sided pain, raising your concern for skeletal involvement. There are no visible exit wounds, and the patient can move and feel both lower extremities, but has no palpable pedal pulses. Placing a new trauma dressing over the wound, you then place bulky dressings over it and tightly secure it all with a bed sheet as a cravat. After binding the pelvis in the same manner, the patient is "hot loaded" into the aircraft.

As the helicopter climbs into the air you contact the receiving facility, which was made aware of the patient via your communications center, to give a report. There is no significant change in the patient's condition during your short flight. On later follow-up with the facility, you learn that the patient suffered a myocardial infarction during surgery to repair an iliac artery laceration. He later expired in the surgical intensive care unit.

DISCUSSION QUESTIONS

1. What are the categories for trauma facilities in the United States and the characteristics and limitations of each?
2. What are the components of the initial assessment and management of the major trauma patient?

Content Review

MULTIPLE CHOICE

_____ 1. Which of the following statistics about trauma in the United States is true?
   A. It is the leading cause of death overall.
   B. It is the leading cause of death in children.
   C. There are over 500,000 deaths annually secondary to trauma.
   D. One in seven Americans will die in an MVC.

_____ 2. All of the following Acts of Congress helped further the development of EMS and trauma systems in the United States except the:
   A. Trauma Care Systems Planning and Development Act.
   B. Emergency Medical Services Systems Act.
   C. Highway Safety Act.
   D. Accidental Death and Disability Act.

_____ 3. Which institution developed the first dedicated, civilian, trauma-specific care in the United States?
   A. Cook County Hospital in Chicago, IL
   B. St. Vincent's Medical Center in New York, NY
   C. St. Krost Center for Emergency Care in Toledo, OH
   D. University of Maryland in Baltimore, MD

_____ 4. Which state operated the first statewide trauma network in the United States?
   A. Maryland   C. New York
   B. Illinois   D. California

_____ 5. What level trauma center can provide expert initial resuscitation and stabilization, but lacks much surgical specialty and intensive care?
   A. Level I   C. Level III
   B. Level II   D. Level IV

_____ 6. What percentage of patients die immediately, or within minutes of their injury?
   A. 20 percent   C. 40 percent
   B. 30 percent   D. 50 percent

_____ 7. The former NHTSA director whose "matrix" illustrated the preventability of trauma deaths was:
   A. William Haddon.   C. James Crowley.
   B. John Madden.   D. Theodore Adams.

_____ 8. An example of active injury prevention is:
   A. the securing of a seatbelt.
   B. the reengineering of a hairpin turn in a road.
   C. the placing of airbags in automobiles.
   D. buying auto insurance.

_____ 9. Passive measures of injury prevention are more reliable than active measures because they are inherent in the design of the environment.
   A. True
   B. False

_____ 10. All of the following statements regarding the mechanism of injury (MOI) are true except:
  A. the MOI can help direct assessment and treatment.
  B. the MOI considers the physical cause of the injury.
  C. the MOI indicates how energy was introduced into the body.
  D. the MOI is the most important determining factor when deciding if a patient requires the services of a trauma center or not.

_____ 11. Which of the following is given the least priority during the initial assessment and resuscitation of the trauma patient?
  A. safety of the victim(s)   C. splinting of extremities
  B. maintenance of body temperature   D. pain control

_____ 12. A trauma patient with a hemorrhage who presents with tachycardia, a normal BP, and decreased peripheral pulses would be considered to be in which class of shock?
  A. Class I   C. Class III
  B. Class II   D. Class IV

_____ 13. The least important general consideration for the transport of a patient with severe trauma is to determine:
  A. whether or not to intubate prior to transport.
  B. the need for administering blood or blood product.
  C. if all equipment such as IV infusion pumps, hemodynamic monitors, IV bags, and such, are secured and arranged in an orderly fashion.
  D. if the first responding EMTs who were on scene will be available to report to the physician at the receiving hospital.

MATCHING

Match the scoring system to its description

14. Injury Severity Score (ISS)   _____

15. Abbreviated Injury Scale (AIS)   _____

16. Pediatric Trauma Score (PTS)   _____

17. TRISS Method   _____

18. Trauma Score (TS)   _____

19. Revised Trauma Score (RTS)   _____

20. Glasgow Coma Scale (GCS)   _____

  A. Provides an objective analysis of a patient's level of consciousness and cerebral function by considering three parameters: eye opening, verbal response, and motor response

  B. Scores patients 1–16 points by considering the GCS along with four additional parameters: respiratory rate, respiratory expansion, systolic blood pressure, and capillary refill

  C. Scores patients 0–12 by considering three parameters: respiratory rate, systolic blood pressure, and the GCS

  D. A modified version of the RTS. Parameters considered include patient size, airway status, systolic blood pressure, CNS status, skeletal system, and the cutaneous system

  E. Details the types and severity of injuries suffered in MVCs, and includes assessment of the head and face, chest, neck, spine, abdomen and pelvic organs, pelvis and extremities, and the integument

  F. Retrospectively calculated using AIS data, and used by trauma registries for data collection and research purposes

  G. Combines patient age and data from the RTS and ISS to indicate overall severity and survivability of injuries. It is primarily used by trauma registries and is impractical for clinical use

14 Neurologic Trauma

Review of Chapter Objectives

Upon completion of this chapter, the student should be able to:

1. Understand the mechanism underlying the progression of secondary injuries after central nervous system (CNS) trauma. **p. 374**

Secondary injury to the CNS can occur in the first few hours and days after injury as a result of edema, loss of autoregulatory function, and histopathological changes. Let's consider the brain and spinal cord separately.

Secondary injury of the brain can be thought of in terms of systemic events and intracranial events. Systemic events that contribute to secondary brain injury are hypotension, hypoxia, hypercapnia, and anemia. Hypotension (systolic BP < 90 mmHg), in instances of head injury and increased intracranial pressure (ICP), can result in inadequate cerebral perfusion pressures (CPP) and resultant ischemia and infarction. Systemic hypoxia (PaO_2 < 60 mmHg) and hypercapnia ($PaCO_2$ < 40 mmHg) can further hamper oxygen delivery to the brain, hypoxia via inadequate arterial oxygen content, and hypercapnia by its vasodilatory effect on cerebral vasculature. Anemia (Hct < 30 percent), caused by blood loss, can reduce the oxygen-carrying capacity of the blood, reducing the amount of oxygen delivered to the injured brain tissue. Intracranial events that contribute to secondary brain injury begin with local inflammation; neuronal insult promotes the production of free radicals, free iron, and excitatory neurotransmitters, resulting in edema, increased ICP, decreased cerebral perfusion, and ischemia. In addition, the rather compact cranial vault does not allow for much displacement of brain tissue, and local pressure can herniate or crush brain tissue far from the injury site up against the cranium or intracranial structures, such as the tentorium cerebelli.

Secondary injury mechanisms for the spinal cord are the same as those for the brain. In addition, the blood supply to the spinal cord is not very substantial, and can be easily disrupted by trauma to blood vessels or local swelling and edema. The majority of secondary injury to the spinal cord is caused by ischemia.

Cerebral edema can be subdivided into two etiological categories, vasogenic and cytotoxic. Vasogenic edema occurs when failure of the tight junctions between the endothelial cells of the capillaries that form the blood-brain barrier allow transvascular leakage of blood proteins (albumin) into the cerebral parenchyma. An osmotic gradient is formed, and fluid shifts from the intravascular space to the interstitium. Vasogenic edema eventually resolves as edema fluid is reabsorbed into the ventricular system or vascular space. Cytotoxic edema is an intracellular process resulting from cell membrane sodium-potassium (Na^+/K^+) pump failure. Normal pump activity relies on the adequate delivery of oxygen to ensure aerobic respiration and ATP production; ATP being the "fuel" the pump utilizes. If cerebral blood flow (CBF) is reduced to less than about 40 percent of baseline, anaerobic metabolism occurs, ATP production suffers, and pump failure occurs. With pump failure, Na^+ accumulates in the cell, creating a hypertonic, intracellular environment that creates an osmotic gradient that draws water into the cell; edema results.

2. **Develop neurologic assessment skills.** p. 375

The development of a comprehensive neurological assessment can be facilitated by utilizing the following guidelines and considerations.

Conscious patient

- Can the patient open his eyes, and does he regard the examiner and track the examiner's movements?
- Assess extraocular movement:
  Nystagmus
  Gaze restriction
- Assess for visual field deficit—peripheral vision
- Assess for visual changes
- Subjective complaints (including, but not limited to):
  - Spots
  - Blurred vision
  - Diplopia
  - Floaters
  - Flashing lights
  - Loss of vision
- Assess facial symmetry
- Assess for tongue deviation, bilateral rise of soft palate
- Assess CAO status
- Assess speech for clarity
- Assess for pronator drift
- Assess for cerebellar ataxia
- Assess motor strength of extremities
- Assess for paresthesias or other sensory abnormalities

Unconscious patient

- If the patient is unresponsive, has she received NMBAs and/or sedation?
- Assess for presence of spontaneous respirations
- If the patient's eyes are open
  - Gaze preference
  - Disconjugate gaze
  - Repetitive eye movements
  - Notable patterns of movement
- Assess for blink reflex
- Assess for cornel reflex
- Assess for seizure activity
- Assess response to pain
- Assess for presence of Babinski reflex
- Assess for clonus
- Assess for CSF drainage

3. **Identify diagnostic tests and imaging used in the treatment of CNS-injured patients.** p. 376

Diagnostic tests and imaging used in the treatment of CNS-injured patients includes:

- Radiographs (X-rays)
- Computed tomography (CT) scan

- Magnetic resonance imaging (MRI)
- Lumbar puncture
- Electroencephalogram (EEG)

4. Discuss the role of autoregulation in the maintenance of normal cerebral perfusion pressure and cerebral blood flow. p. 379

Autoregulation is the ability of an organ to maintain a constant blood flow despite changes in perfusion pressure. Specifically, cerebral autoregulation is the ability of the brain to maintain a constant cerebral blood flow (CBF) despite changes in the cerebral perfusion pressure (CPP). Optimal CBF is maintained by the cerebral vasculature's ability to dilate and constrict in response to changing physiological conditions. For example, hypotension, acidosis, and hypercarbia cause cerebral vasculature dilation, and hypertension, alkalosis, and hypocarbia cause cerebral vasculature constriction. Another way of considering the maintenance of CBF is by looking at it from a CPP perspective; if CPP decreases (say, during an episode of hypotension), vasodilation occurs to improve CBF. Conversely, if CPP increases (say, during an episode of hypertension), vasoconstriction occurs to decrease CBF. At normal intracranial pressures (ICP), CBF is maintained at a constant level at mean arterial pressures (MAP) of 60 to 150 mmHg. In other words, the brain's autoregulatory system is able to keep cerebral blood flow steady over a 90 mmHg-swing in pressure.

CPP can be thought of as the pressure gradient across the brain. This pressure gradient must be kept intact to push blood up to and through the brain. A normal CPP is about 80–90 mmHg, and a CPP below 60 or above 160 mmHg results in poor cerebral perfusion. CPP is equal to the mean arterial pressure (MAP) minus the intracranial pressure (ICP). So, a reduction in MAP (as in hypovolemic shock) or an increase in ICP (as in head injury) can overcome the autoregulatory system and result in a reduction of CPP and cerebral perfusion.

Normal ICP is < 10 mmHg, and values from 10–20 mmHg are considered elevated. An ICP > 20 mmHg for more than a few minutes is associated with increased mortality, and ICPs > 40 mmHg are considered severe and life threatening. Increases in ICP, without increases in MAP, result in decreased CPP and decreased CBF, illustrating the importance of maintaining adequate blood pressure in trauma patients with closed head injuries and elevated ICP.

5. Identify the basic concepts of intracranial pressure (ICP) monitoring, as well as equipment and techniques utilized. p. 384

ICP monitoring can aid in the management of the head-injured patient, helping in the determination of management and assessing the effects of treatment. Monitors are inserted by a neurosurgeon, and are frequently monitored and maintained by critical care transport teams. Some of the specific types of ICP monitoring devices in use include ventriculostomy, fiber-optic bolts, and subarachnoid screws.

Ventriculostomy, the insertion of a catheter through a burr hole drilled through the skull and into one of the ventricles of the brain, is generally regarded as the standard for ICP monitoring. It also, however, has the greatest risk of complications. The ventricular catheter is usually placed in the ventricle on the patient's nondominant side, tunneled under the scalp for a short distance, and is then connected to a pressure transducer that produces an ICP waveform on a monitor. The transducer is placed at the level of the external auditory meatus (EAM), which is equal to the level of the lateral ventricles in the brain (this is the same principle that applies to placing a pulmonary artery catheter transducer at the phlebostatic axis). An extraventricular drain (EVD) is used with ventriculostomy. Advantages of EVD include the ability to drain cerebral spinal fluid (CSF) for sampling, or to reduce ICP. Disadvantages of EVD include a high risk of infection, difficulty in insertion when the ventricles are displaced by compression, and catheter occlusion, dislodgement, and breakage. In addition, CSF leakage may occur around the catheter, and the transducer requires frequent attention with respect to location and recalibration.

Fiber-optic bolts are inserted directly into the brain parenchyma and interpret pressure in the brain tissue, recording and displaying the pressure as a waveform on a monitor. Advantages of fiber-optic bolts include the fact that they are easy to place, have a low risk of infection, do not require leveling at the EAM, and are more accurate than other types of ICP monitoring devices. Disadvantages of fiber-optic bolts include the inability to recalibrate the device after insertion, their increasing inaccuracy with time, and the fact that they do not allow for CSF draining or sampling.

A subarachnoid screw is a hollow screw or bolt that is inserted through a hole drilled in the skull and through a hole cut in the dura mater, coming to rest in the subarachnoid space. Advantages of the screw include quick, easy placement, and the fact that there is no parenchymal penetration. Disadvantages include the fact that subarachnoid screws are less accurate devices, require frequent leveling, and do not allow for CSF drainage.

6. Discuss the role of pharmacologic agents in reducing intracranial pressure in the management of head- and spinal-injured patients. p. 392

Pharmacological agents employed to reduce intracranial pressure in the head-injured patient include mannitol, hypertonic saline, and barbiturates. Mannitol, an osmotic diuretic, creates an increased osmotic gradient between the intravascular space and the interstitial space, thereby drawing fluid out of the cerebral tissue, decreasing cerebral edema and, consequently, ICP. It is considered a first-line agent in the treatment of cerebral hypertension, and is administered at a dose of 1 g/kg every 6 hrs. Care should be taken to administer mannitol through an in-line filter to prevent the infusion of precipitate, as the drug can crystallize at room-to-low temperatures.

Hypertonic saline, another osmotic diuretic, reduces ICP. In addition, it decreases epithelial inflammation, further increasing cerebral blood flow. Hypertonic saline has the added benefit of increasing mean arterial pressure without the large volumes required of isotonic saline solutions.

The use of barbiturates to induce coma is a technique that is considered dated, its efficacy has been questioned, and it carries the high risk of deleterious side effects that typically accompany prolonged coma. Perhaps the most directly deleterious side effect is a reduction in mean arterial pressure, a condition that can be disastrous in instances of increased ICP. Vasopressors are often required to correct the hypotension that accompanies barbiturate coma, in order to maintain MAP and CPP. Barbiturate coma effectively eliminates all motor and sensory nerve responses, including reflexive and cranial nerve function.

Case Study

Even though the weather is clear, you seem to have trouble visualizing the landing zone. According to the GPS coordinates, you should be almost on top of it. Suddenly, beyond the edge of a small hill, the scene comes into view. As the pilot begins a high recon orbit, and your partner speaks to the LZ coordinator via radio, you think about the most recent patient update from the scene. The teenage driver of a compact car crossed the center line and struck a tractor-trailer head on. The patient is reportedly unresponsive, and is still being extricated at the time of the update.

Upon arrival, you are updated by the paramedic in charge. She tells you that your patient is an 18-year-old female who is unresponsive, has significant mid-facial trauma, and is still trapped in the vehicle. Although there is full access to her upper torso, both legs are caught under the dash and steering wheel, and the fire department is having a great deal of difficulty pulling the dash up enough to extricate her. After donning protective equipment provided by the fire department rescue squad, you approach the car to begin your assessment. Sitting in the driver's seat, which has been reclined, is your patient—a small, white female whose airway and spinal precautions are being managed by two EMTs from the fire department. The patient has a cervical collar in place, and although she appears to be breathing adequately on her own, bloody secretions are being suctioned almost continuously from her oropharynx. She is responsive only to deep pain, has a large stellate laceration on the left side of her face, and has so much swelling that you are unable to open her eyelids to assess her pupils. Her chest wall is stable with clear breath sounds. There is a seatbelt mark over the left shoulder. Her abdomen is soft and her pelvis is stable. Both lower extremities are caught under the dashboard. Her right arm shows no evidence of trauma, but the mid-upper, left arm is swollen and slightly deformed. Her right arm has a 16-gauge IV of normal saline infusing well. Her vital signs are: respirations 22 and irregular, heart rate 65 with a bounding radial pulse, and blood pressure 155/88. Because of her airway concerns and the potential need for neurological resuscitation, you elect to immediately secure the patient's airway via intubation. After administering 100 mg of Lidocaine IV and a defasciculating dose of vecuronium, etomidate is given as an induction agent, followed by succinylcholine to induce paralysis. Once paralyzed, the patient is intubated without difficulty; $EtCO_2$ monitoring confirms placement of the tube in the trachea.

Shortly after the patient's airway is secured, her lower extremities are disentangled and she is rapidly extricated and secured to a long spine board. Examination of the patient's legs shows no deformities or crepitus, but does reveal multiple, small lacerations and swelling of both legs distal to the knees. Once the patient is moved into the helicopter, the head of the backboard is propped up. The transport ventilator is attached, and the tidal volume is set to maintain an $EtCO_2$ of 30–35 mmHg in an effort to help decrease intracranial pressure. Reassessment of her vital signs shows a heart rate of 58 with pulses still bounding at the radial artery, and a blood pressure of 184/104. Due to indications of continuing increases in intracranial pressure, you decide to administer mannitol. Your partner administers an IV push of 50 mg of mannitol through an in-line filter, and a propofol infusion is started to maintain temporary sedation. During the flight, the patient remains stable and has no further signs of increasing ICP. As the aircraft is on final approach at the trauma center helipad, your reassessment shows a heart rate of 64, strong and regular at the radial artery, and a blood pressure of 170/98, very positive changes that you hope reflect a trend toward improvement. As the skids touch down on the pad, your partner shuts off the propofol infusion to allow for a better assessment by the neurosurgeon on arrival at the ED. After a quick assessment in the trauma room, the patient, still on your stretcher, is moved directly to the radiology suite for a CT scan. Once off your stretcher, the monitors and ventilators are switched over to hospital equipment and you return to the ED to restock your equipment.

Later in the shift you learn that the patient had, among lesser injuries, a large, left, subdural hematoma that required surgical evacuation.

DISCUSSION QUESTIONS

1. What is the role of autoregulation in the maintenance of normal cerebral perfusion pressure and cerebral blood flow?
2. What are some nonpharmacological interventions to reduce intracranial pressure in the management of head trauma patients?
3. What are some pharmacological interventions to reduce intracranial pressure in the management of head trauma patients?

Content Review

MULTIPLE CHOICE

_____ 1. Secondary brain injury is a term that describes:
   A. the injury that occurs to brain parenchyma at the time of a traumatic event.
   B. the shearing of neuronal axons as the brain shifts in the cranium during injury.
   C. changes that evolve over hours-to-days after the initial brain injury.
   D. microscopic injury to the brain that is not easily identified on CT scan or MRI.

_____ 2. All of the following contribute to secondary brain injury except:
   A. ischemia.   C. hypoxia.
   B. hypotension.   D. hypercapnia.

_____ 3. Vasogenic edema occurs when:
   A. failure of the sodium-potassium pump results in the intracellular accumulation of sodium and the formation of edema.
   B. capillary cells leak their contents into the cerebral parenchyma.
   C. excessive vasodilation secondary to hypercapnia results in fluid leakage into the brain tissue.
   D. loosening of the tight junctions between capillary epithelial cells allows for the leakage of proteins and fluid into the cerebral parenchyma.

4. Which of the following can result with failure of the sodium-potassium pump?
    A. Increased intracellular potassium and hypokalemia
    B. Increased intracellular sodium and cellular edema
    C. Decreased intracellular sodium and dehydration
    D. Decreased ATP production and edema

5. Cerebral perfusion pressure is the:
    A. ability of the arterial system within the brain to adjust to changes in systemic pressure.
    B. measurement of brain perfusion.
    C. pressure required to perfuse the brain.
    D. difference between the mean arterial pressure and cerebral blood flow.

6. The practice of permissive hypotension in the treatment of multisystem trauma that includes closed head injury is potentially dangerous because:
    A. disturbances in autoregulation make it challenging to maintain a low systolic blood pressure.
    B. increased intracranial pressure requires a decreased cerebral blood flow to lessen developing edema.
    C. an adequate, mean arterial pressure is necessary to overcome any increased intracranial pressure and ensure cerebral perfusion.
    D. hypocapnia can cause excessive cerebral vasoconstriction, decreasing cerebral blood flow and worsening ischemia.

7. A cerebral perfusion pressure of _____ in an adult is suggestive of hypoperfusion.
    A. 40 mmHg   C. 60 mmHg
    B. 50 mmHg   D. 70 mmHg

8. Which of the following statements about neurons is false?
    A. Of all the cells in the body, neurons are among the most sensitive to hypoperfusion.
    B. Neurons require enormous amounts of oxygen and glucose for proper functioning.
    C. Neurons have little reserve to compensate for an interruption of substrate delivery.
    D. Like all body cells, neurons are capable of anaerobic metabolism during periods of hypoperfusion.

9. Autoregulation is unable to compensate for a cerebral perfusion pressure of < _____ or > _____.
    A. 60 mmHg, 160 mmHg   C. 40 mmHg, 160 mmHg
    B. 60 mmHg, 140 mmHg   D. 40 mmHg, 140 mmHg

10. If cerebral perfusion pressure rises:
    A. cerebral vasoconstriction occurs to increase cerebral blood flow.
    B. cerebral vasoconstriction occurs to lower cerebral blood flow.
    C. cerebral vasodilation occurs to increase cerebral blood flow.
    D. cerebral vasodilation occurs to decrease cerebral blood flow.

11. Hypercapnia results in:
    A. cerebral vasodilation, decreased cerebral blood flow, and decreased intracranial pressure.
    B. cerebral vasoconstriction, increased cerebral blood flow, and increased intracranial pressure.
    C. cerebral vasodilation, increased cerebral blood flow, and increased intracranial pressure.
    D. cerebral vasoconstriction, decreased cerebral blood flow, and decreased intracranial pressure.

12. In accordance with (the) _____, a volume expansion of the brain parenchyma will result in a decreased volume of intracranial blood and cerebral spinal fluid.
    A. Monroe-Kellie hypothesis   C. cerebral perfusion pressure
    B. Monroe Doctrine   D. autoregulation

©2007 Pearson Education, Inc.
Critical Care Paramedic

_____ 13. Normal ICP:
   A. is 15 mmHg.
   B. ranges from 0–10 mmHg.
   C. ranges from 5–15 mmHg.
   D. is 20 mmHg.

_____ 14. The damage caused by a rise in intracranial pressure is determined by all of the following except the:
   A. amount of pressure.
   B. duration of elevation.
   C. speed at which the elevation occurs.
   D. cause of intracranial pressure.

_____ 15. Transient elevations in intracranial pressure can occur in normal individuals with coughing or sneezing.
   A. True
   B. False

_____ 16. Which type of herniation occurs when diffuse or midline lesions push the diencephalons downward through the tentorial hiatus?
   A. tentorial herniation
   B. central tentorial herniation
   C. subfalcine herniation
   D. tonsillar herniation

_____ 17. Which type of herniation occurs when the midline of the brain is pushed under the falx cerebri?
   A. uncal herniation
   B. central tentorial herniation
   C. subfalcine herniation
   D. tonsillar herniation

_____ 18. Which of the following terms best describes hydrocephalus?
   A. the excessive accumulation of cerebrospinal fluid in the brain
   B. the accumulation of blood in the brain
   C. dehydration of the brain parenchyma
   D. a mass effect that can lead to elevations in intracranial pressure

_____ 19. Which external landmark corresponds with the level of the lateral ventricles within the brain?
   A. external auditory meatus
   B. ear lobe
   C. pupils
   D. first cervical vertebrae

_____ 20. Which of the following is the most commonly used intracranial pressure-monitoring device?
   A. ventriculostomy
   B. fiber-optic bolt
   C. extraventricular drain
   D. subarachnoid screw

_____ 21. Which of the following procedures allows for sampling of the cerebral spinal fluid?
   A. subarachnoid screw
   B. fiber-optic bolt
   C. ventriculostomy
   D. tentorialostotmy

_____ 22. The intracranial pressure waveform represents:
   A. the intracranial pressure created by accumulated blood, cerebral spinal fluid, or masses in the brain parenchyma.
   B. the arterial pulse.
   C. the transmission of the systolic pulse through the choroid plexus into the brain parenchyma.
   D. the pulsations created by the cardiovascular system, transmitted by the choroid plexus through cerebral spinal fluid into the brain parenchyma.

_____ 23. Which of the following is the highest component in a normal intracranial pressure waveform?
   A. P_1
   B. P_2
   C. P_3
   D. P_4

_____ 24. Which of the following components of the intracranial pressure waveform tends to rise as brain compliance is impaired?
A. P_1
B. P_2
C. P_3
D. P_4

_____ 25. Which of the following statements regarding an extraventricular drain setup is false?
A. The catheter, after exiting the skull, is tunneled under the scalp for a short distance and sutured in place.
B. A three-way stopcock is used to connect the catheter, transducer, and drainage system.
C. An IV fluid bag can be attached to the system to allow for flushing of the lines to prevent occlusion from debris.
D. The transducer, always kept level with the external auditory meatus, lays in-line between the stopcock and pressure monitor.

_____ 26. A patient whose extraventricular drain is being maintained in an open position is going to be moved from a hospital bed to your transport stretcher. Which of the following should be done prior to moving the patient to prevent complications with the drain?
A. The transducer should be rezeroed.
B. The collection bag should be placed at a level lower than the external auditory meatus.
C. The drain should be turned to the closed position during the transfer.
D. The extraventricular drain should be disconnected from the ventriculostomy catheter.

_____ 27. In order to record an accurate intracranial pressure:
A. the transducer must be maintained at the level of the external auditory meatus.
B. the drain must be closed.
C. a monitor must be hooked up to the system.
D. all of the above.

_____ 28. In the event that there is an absence of a waveform on the intracranial pressure monitor, all of the following should be done except:
A. ensure that the transducer is leveled properly.
B. ensure that the transducer is zeroed properly.
C. briefly lower the collection burette to determine the presence of cerebral spinal fluid drainage.
D. ensure that the three-way stopcock is turned off to the collection burette.

_____ 29. The most important thing to rule out if you identify a grossly abnormal intracranial pressure value is:
A. a full collection bag.
B. pathological change.
C. catheter occlusion.
D. transducer malfunction.

_____ 30. Which of the following statements regarding the surgical management of head trauma is false?
A. A hemicraniectomy, the excision of a lobe of the brain, is used to reverse the effects of edema in accordance with the Monroe-Kellie hypothesis.
B. Subdural hematomas are generally evacuated through burr holes.
C. Intraparenchymal hemorrhages tend to be inoperable.
D. Nondisplaced skull fractures are generally not operated on.

_____ 31. Suctioning the airway can result in increased intracranial pressure and should be avoided in the head-injured patient.
A. True
B. False

_____ 32. With regard to blood glucose levels, a head-injured patient should be kept in:
A. a hypoglycemic state.
B. a normoglycemic state.
C. a hyperglycemic state.
D. none of the above. Glycemic state is of no importance in the head-injured patient.

140 CRITICAL CARE PARAMEDIC

_____ 33. In an attempt to reduce intracranial pressure, a patient with a head injury should be ventilated:
   A. at a rate of 30/min.
   B. at a rate of 20/min.
   C. to a PCO_2 of 30–35 mmHg.
   D. to a PO_2 of 100 percent.

_____ 34. Which of the following statements regarding mannitol is false?
   A. It is an osmotic diuretic.
   B. It should be administered with an in-line filter.
   C. Administration can result in dehydration.
   D. It is commonly administered in doses of 50–100 mg/kg IV.

_____ 35. In addition to its osmotic properties, hypertonic saline aids in improving cerebral blood flow by:
   A. decreasing capillary endothelial cell inflammation.
   B. inducing neurohormonal responses to brain injury.
   C. suppression of the immune system.
   D. lowering mean arterial pressure.

_____ 36. How may the administration of norepinephrine aid in the treatment of increased intracranial pressure?
   A. Cerebral vasoconstriction reduces cerebral blood flow, decreasing intracranial pressure.
   B. The increased force of myocardial contractions results in a more prominent intracranial pressure waveform.
   C. Increased mean arterial pressure increases cerebral perfusion pressure.
   D. Increased systolic blood pressure decreases cerebral blood flow.

_____ 37. This syndrome is typified by ipsilateral motor weakness and loss of light touch, vibratory, and position sense, and contralateral loss of pain and temperature sensation.
   A. anterior cord syndrome
   B. Brown-Sequard syndrome
   C. central cord syndrome
   D. autonomic dysreflexia

_____ 38. Which of the following imaging exams is preferred for identifying ligamentous injury to the spinal column?
   A. MRI
   B. CT scan
   C. radiograph
   D. ultrasound

_____ 39. The most commonly utilized medication for the treatment of spinal cord injury is:
   A. mannitol.
   B. furosemide.
   C. diphenhydramine.
   D. methylprednisolone.

_____ 40. An episode of autonomic dysreflexia may be triggered by:
   A. a decrease in sympathetic tone.
   B. spinal cord injury.
   C. a full, distended urinary bladder.
   D. bradycardia.

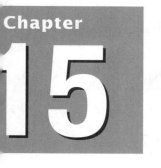

Thoracic Trauma: Assessment and Management

Review of Chapter Objectives

Upon completion of this chapter, the student should be able to:

1. Identify common and life-threatening thoracic injuries based on anatomy and mechanism of injury.   **p. 402**

A thorough clinical assessment, an appreciation of anatomy, and an understanding of the mechanism of injury (MOI) involved can help with the identification of specific intrathoracic injuries. For example, a known MOI of blunt force trauma to the lower, left rib cage; the presence of pain and crepitus with palpation to the left rib cage; and decreased lung sounds on the left side should suggest a pneumothorax to even the newest paramedic. Perhaps a more challenging assessment would be the suggestion of pericardial tamponade after finding a stab wound to the left lateral sternum, hypotension, and JVD.

2. Explain the physiology of ventilation.   **p. 403**

Ventilation is the act of moving air into and out of the lungs. For ventilation to occur, several structures and systems need to be intact, including chemoreceptors, baroreceptors, the brain stem, nerve pathways, respiratory muscles, the pleural cavity, and the chest wall. Central chemoreceptors in the medulla detect pH changes in the cerebral spinal fluid, and peripheral chemoreceptors in the aortic arch and carotid bodies detect changes in arterial pH, CO_2, and O_2. Increased CO_2 and decreased pH and O_2 results in increased respiratory rate and ventilation. Afferent fibers leaving the aortic and carotid bodies reach the respiratory center in the medulla by traveling within cranial nerves X (vagus) and IX (glossopharyngeal), respectively. Baroreceptors, also located in the carotid and aortic bodies, affect the respiratory center as well. Specifically, when blood pressure falls, respiratory rate increases, and when blood pressure rises, the respiratory rate decreases. Based on input from the chemoreceptors and baroreceptors, the respiratory centers in the medulla (and pons also, technically!) initiate respiration and send the signals via the phrenic nerve (to the diaphragm) and spinal nerves (to the other respiratory muscles). Within the pons, the apneustic and pneumotaxic centers adjust the output of the respiratory signals emanating from the medulla, and, in effect, control the strength and duration of each breath. During periods of heavy breathing (tidal volumes > 1,000 mL) the Hering-Bruer reflex, relying on sensory input from stretch receptors in the lungs, influences the effects of the apneustic centers. There are two parts to the Hering-Bruer reflex: the inhalation reflex and the exhalation reflex. The inflation reflex relies on stretch receptors in the bronchial smooth muscle to influence the cessation of inhalation as the lungs reach their maximum volume. The deflation reflex relies on receptors in the alveolar walls to signal when adequate deflation has occurred, stimulating the respiratory center to begin another inhalation. Both reflexes are active during periods of heavy breathing and forced

during periods of normal breathing. Specifically, the apneustic center increases the
_ _ _ation, and the pneumotaxic center inhibits the apneustic influence after about 2 sec-
_ _ _ for passive or active exhalation. Signals are sent to the respiratory muscles, which con-
_ _ _result in a flattening of the diaphragm and a lifting, up and out, of the chest wall. This
_ _ _es intrathoracic volume, decreases intrathoracic pressure relative to the outside environment,
_ _ allows air to move from the area of high pressure (outside) to the area of low pressure (inside) the
_ _ ngs. In order for the lungs to move outward with the chest wall (and allow for adequate ventilation), the visceral pleura, parietal pleura, and intrapleural space must all be intact.

3. **Integrate the relationship between anatomy, kinematics, and assessment
   findings to identify specific thoracic injuries.** p. 403

Tension pneumothorax

A tension pneumothorax can develop at any time from a closed or open pneumothorax. MOIs may
include blunt trauma, penetrating trauma, barotrauma (especially in patients who are being ventilated), and, on rare occasions, from a spontaneous pneumothorax. Air enters the pleural space and
accumulates, increasing intrapleural pressure and further deflating the injured lung, resulting in increasing difficulty in breathing and hypoxia. As air progressively accumulates and intrapleural pressure continues to increase on the injured side, the mediastinum is pushed to the uninjured side,
kinking the vena cava and restricting venous return to the right side of the heart. Decreased venous
return leads to reduced cardiac output and hypotension, and kinking of the vena cava results in a
back-up of blood and engorgement of the jugular veins manifested as JVD (this may not be present
if the patient is hypovolemic). Lung sounds on the injured side, originally diminished, may now be
absent, and impeded lung expansion on the uninjured side secondary to the mediastinal shift may
result in decreased lung sounds there, also. Increasing difficulty in breathing, tachypnea, tachycardia, and hypotension eventually give way to respiratory, and then cardiovascular, collapse. Tracheal
deviation, a very late sign of tension pneumothorax, is typically appreciated on chest radiograph,
but can be quite difficult, if not impossible, to identify on the physical exam as the upper trachea
(which we can see and palpate) shifts markedly less than does the lower trachea contained within
the thorax. This brings up a good point: You should never see a radiograph of a tension pneumothorax, as it is a clinical diagnosis that does not, and should not, require a chest radiograph.

Hemothorax

MOIs suggestive of hemothorax include blunt and penetrating trauma resulting in intrathoracic
bleeding, and nontraumatic causes include lung cancer or leaking, AV malformations. Injuries to
smaller blood vessels in the thorax tend to be self-limiting, while injuries to larger vessels can be devastating, leading to hypovolemic shock and death. Clinical indications depend on the amount of
blood loss suffered, with classic signs of hemorrhagic shock (tachycardia, tachypnea, diaphoresis,
and decreased BP) predominating, along with decreased lung sounds on the affected side. With larger
amounts of blood loss, dullness to percussion may be appreciated, and very large accumulations of
blood may result in mediastinal shift, interference with the ipsilateral lung expansion, and decreased
breath sounds on the unaffected side.

Pneumothorax

With perforation of the parietal (which accompanies perforation of the chest wall) or visceral
pleura, loss of the negative intrapleural pressure occurs and lung collapse follows. MOIs for pneumothorax include penetrating trauma, blunt trauma, and barotrauma (again, common in ventilated patients), but they can also result from an iatrogenic or spontaneous etiology. Typical signs
and symptoms include dyspnea, tachypnea, tachycardia, grunting, and decreasing SpO_2.

Flail chest

Flail Chest is defined as the presence of three or more ribs fractured in two or more places, typically involving the anterior or lateral ribs, and is usually the result of blunt trauma. The classic
sign of a flail chest is paradoxical chest wall motion, which, though classic, is not as common as
pain with palpation and respiration, difficulty breathing, tachypnea, tachycardia, and decreased
SpO_2.

Pericardial tamponade

Pericardial tamponade can result from both blunt and penetrating trauma, as the pericardium has a rather unique ability to seal defects resulting from penetrating trauma, allowing blood to accumulate within the intraplural space. Hemodynamic effects of tamponade depend on two things: the amount of fluid in the intrapleural space and the speed at which the fluid accumulates. Large amounts (up to 2 L) of fluid can be tolerated if the accumulation is slow, but as little as 150–200 mL of fluid that accumulates rapidly can have profound effects. The fluid that most often accumulates in cases of trauma is, of course, blood. As accumulating blood prevents proper expansion of the ventricles during diastole, ventricular preload is decreased, resulting in decreased cardiac output and hemodynamic compromise. Signs and symptoms of shock are typical early in the progression of tamponade; later signs include JVD, diminished or muffled heart sounds, and hypotension. Additional signs include pulseless paradoxous and increased distension of the neck veins during inspiration (Kussmaul sign).

Myocardial rupture

Myocardial rupture, one of the more lethal of all intrathoracic injuries, is most often the result of significant blunt force trauma to the chest. The typical presentation for patients presenting with myocardial rupture is cardiac arrest.

Myocardial contusion

Myocardial contusion is most often the result of blunt force trauma to the chest that causes the myocardium to strike against adjacent anatomy, usually the sternum and spinal column. Typical MOIs include MVCs, falls, and blows to the chest. Actual bruising of the myocardium can range from small areas of microhemorrhage to large areas of necrosis, and the potential for hemodynamic compromise is related to the size of the contusion. Signs and symptoms include chest pain, shock from reduced cardiac output (result of rhythm disturbance or injured tissue), rhythm disturbances, and ST segment changes on 12-lead ECG.

Aortic rupture

Aortic rupture can occur secondary to penetrating or blunt mechanisms, particularly instances of rapid deceleration. Up to 90 percent of patients who experience traumatic aortic rupture die immediately, so the most common presentation will be cardiac arrest. However, for the 10 percent or so who survive the initial injury, signs and symptoms include severe chest and midscapular back pain, dyspnea, tachypnea, tachycardia, systemic hypotension (upper extremity hypertension is a possibility), and other signs and symptoms of shock.

Pulmonary contusion

Pulmonary contusions are commonly seen in instances of blunt force trauma, and are always present to some degree with more severe injuries such as flail chest. Penetrating trauma can also result in pulmonary contusion to the area surrounding the penetration, especially with high-velocity objects, as energy is introduced into the surrounding tissue. Typical clinical findings include dyspnea, tachypnea, tachycardia, pain, and decreased SpO_2.

Diaphragmatic rupture

Diaphragmatic rupture occurs secondary to blunt or penetrating trauma to the lower thorax or abdomen that creates a defect in the diaphragm, allowing the herniation of abdominal contents into the thorax. As a result, lung expansion is compromised; abdominal organs may become strangulated, hypoxic, and ischemic; and intestinal obstruction may occur. Clinical signs can vary, and range from severe distress to a complete lack of symptoms. Pain in the abdomen or chest with radiation to the shoulder is not uncommon. Auscultation of the lung fields may reveal diminished air movement or bowel sounds in the thorax, though paralytic ileus accompanying intestinal insult will result in no production of sounds. Other signs include dyspnea, tachypnea, tachycardia, and decreased SpO_2.

Tracheobronchial rupture

The majority of tracheobronchial injuries result from sudden deceleration and shearing forces, though penetrating trauma can certainly result in injury also. Signs and symptoms include chest pain, pain with respiration, dyspnea, hemoptysis, and developing hypoxia. Leakage of air into surrounding tissue can result in the formation of subcutaneous emphysema, and pneumothorax and tension pneumothorax are possible.

Esophageal rupture

Esophageal perforation most commonly occurs with penetrating trauma, but can occur from blunt MOIs as well. Signs and symptoms can be vague, but include substernal pleuritic chest pain, neck or chest pain that worsens with swallowing, subcutaneous emphysema, dysphagia, and fever.

4. **Describe general treatment modalities for the following thoracic injuries:**

Tension pneumothorax   p. 404

First and foremost, the development of a tension pneumothorax must be promptly identified and decompressed via needle thoracostomy (needle decompression). After decompression, adequate airway, ventilation, and oxygenation should be assured, and may be accomplished with treatment as simple as high-flow, high-concentration oxygen via a nonrebreather mask for conscious and breathing patients, or endotracheal intubation and mechanical ventilation for patients who can't protect their airway or who have inadequate respirations. The insertion of a thoracostomy tube (chest tube) may be required to ensure adequate re-expansion of the pneumothorax and/or to remove blood from the thoracic cavity. The patient should also be assessed for the need for volume replacement.

Hemothorax   p. 405

Since airway management and ventilation are a priority, it is important to ensure and keep a patent airway and to assure proper ventilation and oxygenation. Tube thoracostomy (chest tube insertion) may be performed to both evaluate for the presence of blood and air, and to remove them. If greater than 1,000 mL of blood is removed via a thoracostomy tube, it should be clamped, and constant evaluation for ventilatory compromise performed. Blood loss into the thorax can be significant, and fluid volume resuscitation may be necessary. Consider the need for the administration of blood and blood products if large replacement volumes are necessary.

Pneumothorax   p. 410

Assure that the airway is patent and that the patient is breathing properly and achieving adequate ventilation and oxygenation; if not, make it so! At the very least, every patient with a pneumothorax should get 100 percent high-flow, high-concentration oxygen via a nonrebreather mask. In addition, open pneumothoracies should be sealed with a bandage, commercial or a self-made dressing, that prevents the entrance of air from the outside environment, but lets accumulating intrathoracic air escape. The need for fluid volume resuscitation should be evaluated for, as pneumothoracies and hemothoracies frequently coexist.

Flail chest   p. 412

Patients who are *in extremis* with flail chest should be promptly intubated and ventilated with 100 percent high-flow, high-concentration oxygen; CPAP is another possible treatment modality that may be effective. After securing the airway and providing ventilation, the flail segment should be secured with the use of trauma dressings or a small pillow.

Pericardial tamponade   p. 413

Treatment for hemodynamically significant pericardial tamponade centers on ensuring airway control, oxygenation and ventilation, and improving ventricular filling pressures. Improving filling pressures can be initially accomplished with the administration of fluid volume or with pericardiocentesis. Definitive treatment includes surgical repair of the defect and/or the formation of a pericardial window with constant drainage.

Myocardial rupture   p. 415

As with all emergencies, secure the airway, ventilate, and oxygenate adequately. Surgical repair of the defect is essential, though medical therapy may be utilized to stabilize a patient for the short term during transport. Vasodilators may be employed in an attempt to decrease afterload, and insertion of an intra-aortic balloon pump may be useful to increase cardiac output in cases of papillary muscle or ventricular-septal defect. Rapid volume administration to increase preload, and inotropic medication to increase cardiac output, may be helpful in cases of ventricular wall rupture for short-term stabilization on the way to surgery.

Myocardial contusion   p. 416

Patients with myocardial contusion are treated essentially the same as patients with ACS: ABCs, oxygen, large-bore IV access, and the administration of antidysrhythmics, if warranted.

Aortic rupture   p. 415

Basic trauma resuscitation centering on the ABCs should occur while a patient with an aortic rupture is transported promptly to a facility that can perform surgical repair. Without prompt surgical repair, death is unpreventable.

Pulmonary contusion   p. 416

Adequate oxygenation and ventilation are extremely important in the treatment of pulmonary contusion, and positive pressure ventilation and endotracheal intubation is necessary if a patient's PO_2 is less than 60 mmHg on room air, or 80 mmHg on supplemental oxygen. Fluid administration should be restricted to reduce pulmonary edema unless it is absolutely needed for resuscitation.

Diaphragmatic rupture   p. 417

Management of diaphragmatic rupture is primarily supportive in nature, with attention paid to airway, breathing, and circulation while en route to surgical care.

Tracheal and bronchial rupture   p. 417

A potentially devastating injury, tracheal or bronchial rupture requires aggressive airway management that usually includes endotracheal intubation, preferably below the level of airway disruption, if possible. Tube thoracostomy is commonly performed. A persistent, high-volume air leak through the chest tube is suggestive for tracheobronchial injury, if not already identified.

Esophageal perforation   p. 418

After assuring that the ABCs are attended to, naso- or orogastric tube insertion and the administration of antibiotics are generally all that is required prior to definitive surgical care.

5. **Identify and differentiate between patients who require stabilization and rapid transport versus on-the-scene assessment and management.**

As a member of a critical care transport team, you will have additional skills, medications, and procedures to aid in the stabilization of hemodynamically unstable patients: advanced airway maneuvers, rapid sequence intubation, the use of blood and blood products, and chest tube insertion. However, the basic rule of trauma that you learned in paramedic school remains the same. Any hemodynamically unstable patient with a devastating injury that you cannot control requires rapid transport to a trauma center for surgery rather than on-scene attempts at assessment and management. Aortic rupture, myocardial rupture, and massive hemothorax are examples of injuries that will ultimately prove unmanageable in the field and require surgical intervention. In such situations, it is prudent to initiate rapid transport and assess and treat while en route rather than remain on scene. Aeromedical critical care transport, especially with rotor-winged aircraft, may hamper this approach, as space is sometimes limited, and some assessment and treatment must take place prior to transport. Every case and situation is unique, and must be evaluated by the critical care team.

6. **Discuss ongoing maintenance care for chest tubes and the various drainage systems that may be present.**   p. 407

Maintenance of a chest tube and drainage system starts immediately after the chest tube has been placed; all connections should be taped in place, and the chest tube secured to the chest wall with sutures (silk sutures tend to grip the chest tube better than nylon, which can slip on the surface of the tube). In addition, an occlusive dressing of petroleum-impregnated gauze (with Y-cut running from the middle of one side to the center) should be applied where the tube enters the chest wall. Cover with two or more gauze pads (also with Y-cut) and then secure with cloth adhesive tape, cutting the tape so that three strips are available at one end: the two outside strips to secure to the gauze and patient's skin, and the middle piece to wrap around and secure the tube. Additional, uncut strips of cloth tape can be used to further anchor the gauze in place along its sides.

After securing the tube, ensure that there are no kinks in the system components. Clamping of the chest tube should be avoided unless specifically indicated. Maintain the appropriate fluid levels in both the underwater seal chamber as well as the suction chamber.

Case Study

It is a bright day and unseasonably warm for January. The sun reflecting off the snow is so bright that it hurts your eyes, even though your helmet has a tinted visor. You've been called to a large, mountain recreation area approximately 85 miles from the Level I trauma center where your program is based, for a patient who struck a tree and has chest injuries. The aircraft lands near the lower ski lodge in an area that is always roped off and kept clear of snow just for this purpose. Meeting a medic from the ski patrol at the edge of the LZ, you are updated on the patient. The patient was skiing on a closed trail and struck a small tree at high speed. There was no loss of consciousness, but the patient is complaining of difficulty breathing.

Entering the first aid room in the lodge, your "view from the door" tells you that your patient is in trouble. The patient is a teenage male who is sitting up, but leaning to the right side and gasping for air. He is conscious, but appears extremely anxious and doesn't respond to questions. His skin is pale and he is holding his right arm and left hand against his right chest wall. He is on oxygen via a nonrebreather mask, but his SpO_2 is only 86 percent. The ski patrollers tell you that the patient has a large, swollen, tender area on the right anterior chest wall. Initially, he complained of mild trouble breathing, but his respiratory distress has been getting markedly worse. His last vital signs were: respirations 36 and labored, pulse 144 and weak at the radial, and blood pressure 90/72 mmHg. While you continue your assessment, your partner attaches monitor leads and prepares to establish IV access. The patient's airway is clear and self-maintained. The patient is expending a great deal of effort breathing and has significant jugular venous distension. Listening to the chest, you note that the patient has markedly diminished breath sounds on the right side and that there is a large hematoma on the right chest wall. Suspecting a tension pneumothorax, you prep the right upper chest wall with a splash of povidone-iodine solution. You then insert a 14-gauge IV catheter over the third rib into the second intercostal space in the midclavicular line. With a small shower of blood and a long soft hiss of air, the patient's respiratory status improves dramatically. Respirations decrease to 22 per minute and are less labored, and his heart rate decreases to 128 bpm, and a radial pulse is easily palpable. The SpO_2 improves to 92 percent and the patient is now able to speak in short sentences. Since the patient is still experiencing difficulty breathing and remains hypoxic on high-flow, high-concentration oxygen, you decide to intubate him for transport. While you discuss the expected plan of care with the patient and get consent, your partner draws up medications and prepares a chest tube tray. After securing the airway with rapid sequence intubation, you note that the area of hematoma clearly bulges out with each squeeze of the BVM. Palpating the area, you feel a depression on exhalation and a small area of subcutaneous emphysema contained within the borders of the swelling. While your partner secures the flail segment with tape and a bulky dressing, you make a sterile prep of the area around the fifth intercostal space in the midaxillary line. After anesthetizing the skin and subcutaneous tissues of the intercostal area and over the fifth rib, you make a 3-cm incision into the pleural space. As a small rush of air and a gush of blood escapes, you insert your index finger into the wound to dislodge any pleural adhesions and palpate the lung tissue to confirm entry into the pleural space. Certain of the proper location, you advance a 24 French thoracostomy tube into the pleural space until the last hole is well within the chest wall. Attaching the tube to the tubing of the pleural drainage unit, you note a small amount of blood draining into the collection chamber, and a few bubbles in the water seal with each ventilation. After suturing the tube into place, you apply an occlusive dressing to the area over and around the wound and over the catheter that you used to decompress the chest. You then attach the suction port of the drainage unit to your portable suction, adjusting the bypass valve to 20 cm/H_2O and verify that there is gentle, rolling bubbling in the suction bypass chamber. Reassessment of vital signs shows a heart rate of 102 bpm, sinus tachycardia on the monitor, a blood pressure of 100/88, SpO_2 95 percent on 100 percent FiO_2, and a respiratory rate of 10 breaths per minute via the transport ventilator.

With the patient's condition stabilized, you fully immobilize him and begin transport to the trauma center while assuring that the tube remains patent and that the drainage unit continues to function properly en route. Transport is uneventful, and after transferring the patient to the stretcher in the main trauma room, you give a full report to the attending MD in charge of the trauma service.

DISCUSSION QUESTIONS

1. What are the general treatment modalities for the following thoracic injuries?
   a. Closed, open, and tension pneumothorax
   b. Hemothorax
   c. Flail chest
2. What are the transport considerations for chest tubes and pleural drainage systems?

Content Review

MULTIPLE CHOICE

_____ 1. _____ of deaths from trauma are directly due to thoracic injury.
   A. 20 percent   C. 30 percent
   B. 25 percent   D. 35 percent

_____ 2. Rapidly developing tachycardia, tachypnea, and hypotension with absent lung sounds on the right side in a patient with a stab wound on the right midaxillary line between ribs 5 and 6 are most likely due to:
   A. pericardial tamponade.   C. pneumothorax.
   B. cardiac contusion.   D. tension pneumothorax.

_____ 3. You have just identified a developing tension pneumothorax in a patient with a gunshot wound to the left chest, midclavicular at the nipple line. You note that the patient is obtunded, gasping for breath at 18/min and shallow, and has no radial pulse. The most appropriate, immediate treatment would be:
   A. administration of 100 percent high-flow, high-concentration oxygen via nonrebreather mask.
   B. assisted ventilations with a BVM and 100 percent high-flow, high-concentration oxygen.
   C. endotracheal intubation.
   D. needle thoracostomy.

_____ 4. Which of the following represents a proper placement site for a needle thoracotomy?
   A. 2nd intercostal space, midclavicular line
   B. 1st or 2nd intercostal space, midclavicular line
   C. 4th or 5th intercostal space, midaxillary line
   D. 2nd or 3rd intercostal space, midaxillary line

_____ 5. Clinical exam findings including decreased breath sounds on the injured side of the thorax, decreased SpO_2, and dullness to percussion on the injured side are most likely the result of:
   A. pneumothorax.   C. hemothorax.
   B. tension pneumothorax.   D. pulmonary contusion.

_____ 6. Priorities in the management of massive hemothorax include all of the following except:
   A. needle decompression.   C. administration of 100 percent oxygen.
   B. tube thoracostomy.   D. fluid volume replacement.

_____ 7. Tube thoracostomy is indicated in all of the following injuries except:
    A. pneumothorax.
    B. cardiac tamponade.
    C. hemothorax.
    D. tension pneumothorax.

_____ 8. Chest tubes are indicated in all cases of pneumothorax.
    A. True
    B. False

_____ 9. Chest tube insertion is performed utilizing sterile technique.
    A. True
    B. False

_____ 10. Chest tube insertion requires that the patient be properly sedated so as to experience no discomfort during the procedure.
    A. True
    B. False

_____ 11. During tube thoracostomy, the patient should be placed:
    A. lateral recumbent, injured side up.
    B. supine.
    C. in the Trendelenburg position.
    D. in a 30–60° reverse Trendelenburg position.

_____ 12. Which of the following is not typically performed during tube thoracostomy?
    A. A scalpel is used to make a 3- to 4-cm transverse incision over the inferior aspect of the rib below the insertion site.
    B. A curved hemostat is used to puncture the intercostal muscles and pleura, then a finger is inserted over the clamp into the thoracic cavity.
    C. Digital examination of the intrapleural space is performed.
    D. The thoracostomy tube is inserted superiorly and posteriorly no more than 5 cm beyond the last hole of the tube.

_____ 13. After thoracostomy tube insertion and drainage system attachment, evaluation and maintenance of the tube and drainage system include all of the following except:
    A. suturing and/or taping the chest tube to the chest wall.
    B. maintaining adequate fluid levels in the drainage system chambers.
    C. clamping the chest tube.
    D. assessing the amount of bubbling in the suction chamber.

_____ 14. An absence of fluctuations in the fluid level in the drainage (long) tube of the underwater seal chamber indicates:
    A. that a "closed" system exists.
    B. that the lung has re-expanded or the chest tube is occluded.
    C. the presence of increased respiratory effort due to obstruction or atelectasis.
    D. chest tube dislodgement

_____ 15. "Stripping" a chest tube is considered an appropriate method for removing visible clots or obstructions.
    A. True
    B. False

_____ 16. Management of an open pneumothorax is most likely to include:
    A. the application of an occlusive dressing secured on all sides.
    B. tube thoracostomy.
    C. pericardiocentesis.
    D. needle decompression.

_____ 17. Paradoxical chest wall movement is a clinical finding associated with:
    A. flail chest.
    B. tension pneumothorax.
    C. pneumothorax.
    D. rib fractures.

©2007 Pearson Education, Inc.
Critical Care Paramedic

_____ 18. Patients with flail chest are likely to have concomitant injuries.
   A. True
   B. False

_____ 19. Immediate treatment for flail chest includes:
   A. assisting spontaneous ventilations with positive-pressure ventilations.
   B. needle thoracostomy.
   C. pericardiocentesis.
   D. tube thoracostomy.

_____ 20. A patient has sustained a stab wound to the left of his sternum and now presents with signs and symptoms of shock, distended neck veins, and clear and equal lung sounds bilaterally. Which of the following injuries is most likely the cause of his shock?
   A. tension pneumothorax   C. myocardial contusion
   B. aortic dissection   D. pericardial tamponade

_____ 21. Beck's triad includes:
   A. flat jugular veins, hypotension, and muffled heart sounds.
   B. hypotension, flat jugular veins, and pulsus paradoxus.
   C. JVD, muffled heart sounds, and hypotension.
   D. pulsus paradoxus, JVD, and muffled heart sounds.

_____ 22. The presence of Beck's triad suggests which of the following traumatic injuries?
   A. cardiac contusion   C. pneumothorax
   B. pericardial tamponade   D. tracheobronchial rupture

_____ 23. Pulsus paradoxus is:
   A. a fall in diastolic BP > 15 mmHg during normal inspiration.
   B. a fall in systolic BP > 15 mmHg during normal inspiration.
   C. a rise in systolic BP > 15 mmHg during normal exhalation.
   D. a fall in diastolic BP > 15 mmHg during normal exhalation.

_____ 24. The management of pericardial tamponade involves all of the following except:
   A. ensuring a patent airway, ventilation, and oxygenation.
   B. improving ventricular filling pressures.
   C. fluid volume administration.
   D. needle thoracostomy.

_____ 25. Which of the following is not typical procedure during pericardiocentesis?
   A. The patient is placed in a reverse Trendelenburg position.
   B. The needle is inserted using a subxiphoid approach at a 30° angle.
   C. Negative pressure is applied on the syringe until fluid or blood is aspirated.
   D. Continuous cardiac monitoring is performed throughout the procedure.

_____ 26. Radiographic findings suggestive of aortic dissection include all of the following except:
   A. depression of the left mainstem bronchus.   C. right-sided pneumothorax.
   B. widening of the superior mediastinum.   D. loss of the aortic shadow.

_____ 27. Which of the following is not a clinical sign associated with myocardial contusion?
   A. cardiac dysrhythmia   C. muffled heart sounds
   B. ST segment abnormalities   D. decreased cardiac output

_____ 28. Management of myocardial contusion includes all of the following except:
   A. IV fluid administration.
   B. administration of antidysrhythmics.
   C. pericardiocentesis.
   D. administration of 100 percent high-flow, high-concentration oxygen.

_____ 29. A patient who has suffered blunt force trauma to his lateral chest wall resulting in fractured ribs is most likely to have also suffered a:
A. myocardial contusion.
B. pulmonary contusion.
C. tension pneumothorax.
D. esophageal rupture.

_____ 30. Management of pulmonary contusion includes all of the following except:
A. cardiac monitoring.
B. correction of acid-base imbalances.
C. aggressive airway management, ventilation, and oxygenation.
D. aggressive fluid volume resuscitation.

_____ 31. A patient presents CAO in distress after sustaining blunt force trauma to the lower, left thorax and upper, right abdomen. The patient complains of chest and abdominal pain radiation to his shoulder, and of dyspnea. Clinical exam reveals decreased breath sounds to the left base and a scaphoid left abdomen. The patient has most likely suffered a:
A. diaphragmatic rupture.
B. pneumothorax.
C. tension pneumothorax.
D. aortic rupture.

_____ 32. You are transporting a conscious and hemodynamically stable male patient to the regional trauma center after he sustained a pneumothorax secondary to a stab wound to the chest. While en route, the patient complains of an onset of chest pain and dysphagia, and you note the presence of subcutaneous emphysema on his upper chest. Lung sounds have not changed, nor have vital signs. Of the following, which is the most likely cause of the patient's changing clinical picture?
A. tension pneumothorax
B. cardiac tamponade
C. esophageal perforation
D. pulmonary contusion

16 Abdominal and Genitourinary Trauma

Review of Chapter Objectives

Upon completion of this chapter, the student should be able to:

1. **Describe the anatomy and physiology of the organs and structures that are of concern in abdominal trauma.**
p. 423

The abdominal cavity is divided into three spaces: the peritoneal space, the retroperitoneal space, and the pelvic space. Organs and structures located within the peritoneal space include the stomach, the proximal duodenum, ascending colon, transverse colon, sigmoid colon, liver, gallbladder, and the spleen. Retroperitoneal organs include the kidneys, ureters, distal duodenum, descending colon, and the pancreas. The urinary bladder, rectum, and urethra are located in the pelvic space. In the female, the ovaries and fallopian tubes are also located in the pelvic cavity.

The peritoneal space is lined with a serous membrane, the parietal peritoneum, which is continuous with the visceral peritoneum covering the abdominal organs. The portions of the digestive tract located within the peritoneal space are suspended by the mesentery, which is continuous with both the visceral and parietal membranes. The mesentery acts as both a conduit for the rich, abdominal vascular network and as a supportive structure for the digestive tract, preventing the movement and entanglement of the intestines. The greater omentum lies over, and conforms to, the abdominal viscera, and its rich supply of adipose tissue provides padding, protection, and insulation to the underlying structures. The lesser omentum lies in the space between the liver and stomach, providing an access route for blood vessels entering the liver, and providing support for the stomach.

Abdominal components of the digestive tract include the very distal esophagus, stomach, small intestine (duodenum, jejunum, and ilium), large intestine (colon), and rectum. The majority of the stomach lies in the upper, left quadrant of the abdomen, immediately inferior to the diaphragm, between the level of vertebrae T7 and L3. The stomach has a rich vascular supply consisting of the left gastric artery, and branches of the splenic and common hepatic arteries. These arteries, together, comprise the three branches of the celiac artery, which itself branches off the abdominal aorta. Gastric juice consists of the secretions of chief cells and parietal cells, which are located in the gastric glands of the stomach walls. Parietal cells secrete hydrochloric acid, and chief cells secrete pepsinogen. Chyme exits the stomach through the pyloric sphincter and enters the small intestine, where further digestion, and up to 90 percent of nutrient absorption, will take place.

The small intestine is located in every abdominal quadrant and takes up the majority of space in the peritoneal cavity. It is frequently injured when the abdomen is subjected to traumatic insult. The main divisions of the small intestine are the duodenum, jejunum, and ilium. The duodenum reenters the peritoneal cavity just before its transition with the jejunum. The jejunum is the site of the bulk of digestion and absorption within the small intestine. The most distal segment of the small intestine is the ilium; the ileocecal valve at its terminus regulates the flow of material into the first segment of the large intestine, the cecum.

The large intestine, from its beginning at the ileocecal valve, runs a horseshoe-shaped route around the small intestine to its terminus at the anus. It is responsible for the resorption of water, electrolytes, and some vitamins from the intestinal contents. The colon is further divided into the ascending, transverse, and descending colon.

The accessory organs of the digestive tract include the liver, gallbladder, and pancreas. The liver lies in the upper, right quadrant of the abdomen within the peritoneal cavity and is the largest organ in the abdominal compartment. As such, it is frequently the recipient of traumatic forces. The inferior rib cage provides some bony protection to the liver. The falciform ligament bisects the liver, dividing it into the left and right lobes, and anchors the liver to the posterior and anterior abdominal walls. The inferior margin of the falciform ligament thickens to form the ligamentum teres, which is actually the remnant of the fetal umbilical vein. The liver is encapsulated in a tough, fibrous layer that is, itself, covered with a layer of visceral peritoneum. The hepatic artery provides the liver's enormous blood supply, which is about 25 percent of cardiac output. Venous return occurs via the hepatic vein, which deposits blood into the inferior vena cava. In addition to a rich arterial supply, the liver receives all venous blood exiting the digestive system through the hepatic portal vein. The hepatic portal vein, hepatic artery, nerves, lymphatic structures, and the hepatic bile ducts pass through the hilus. The liver's functions can be divided into three categories: metabolic regulation, hematologic regulation, and bile synthesis and secretion.

The gallbladder is located on the posterior surface of the liver and stores and concentrates bile produced in the liver prior to secretion into the duodenum. When needed, bile exits the gallbladder through the cystic duct, which joins the common hepatic duct from the liver to form the common bile duct that terminates at the duodenum. The pancreatic duct shares this terminus, and the hepatopancreatic sphincter controls the secretion of bile and pancreatic juice into the duodenum.

The pancreas is a retroperitoneal structure. Its head is tucked into the C-shaped fold of the duodenum, and its body and tail extend back into the abdominal cavity toward the spleen, coming to a point at, and adhering to, the posterior abdominal wall. The pancreatic duct carries digestive enzymes and buffers secreted by the pancreas to the duodenum. The pancreas also secretes insulin, glucagons, and somatostatin from specialized cells located in the islets of Langerhans. As such, it has both endocrine and exocrine functions.

The spleen lies in the upper, right abdominal quadrant, sitting just inferior to the diaphragm, and protected by the inferior margin of the left rib cage. The spleen removes abnormal blood cells from circulation and stores B and T cells that combat antigens detected in the circulating blood. As such, the spleen receives a significant blood supply via the splenic artery. Approximately 5 percent of circulating blood volume is filtered through the spleen every minute. The splenic vein returns blood to the inferior vena cava. Blood vessels, nerves, and lymphatic structures entering and exiting the spleen travel through the hilus.

The abdomen has a rich vascular network. The abdominal aorta travels inferiorly along the left, lateral spinal column, bifurcating in the pelvis at the level of the sacrum to form the common iliac arteries. Numerous branches of inferior and superior mesenteric arteries, themselves branches of the aorta, supply the bowel with blood. The mesenteric, splenic, gastroepiploic, and gastric veins all join the hepatic portal vein to divert venous blood flow from the bowel, spleen, and stomach to the liver, prior to deposition in the inferior vena cava.

2. **Discuss and differentiate the pathophysiology of specific abdominal injuries.**   p. 428

Liver

The liver, being the largest solid organ in the abdomen, is extremely vulnerable to both blunt and penetrating mechanisms of injury. The liver's tough, fibrous outer capsule often "fractures" when injured. The liver's significant blood flow and its dense vascular anatomy combine to contribute to severe hemorrhage and hemodynamic instability when the liver is injured. About 80 percent of liver injuries are secondary to penetrating trauma, with blunt trauma being responsible for the remaining 20 percent.

Liver injuries are categorized according to the American Association for the Surgery of Trauma (AAST) Liver Injury Scale, on which they are assigned a grade of I–VI. Grade I and II injuries are subcapsular hematomas that are nonexpanding and represent less than 50 percent of surface area, or are lacerations of the capsule that are, at most, bleeding lightly with a depth of less than 3 cm or a length of less than 10 cm. Grade III injuries start to get more serious, and include hematomas involving greater than half of the liver surface area and lacerations deeper than 3 cm. Grade IV–VI injuries are increasingly more severe, with a grade VI resulting in total avulsion of the liver from the hepatic artery and vein.

Gallbladder

Due to the protected location of the gallbladder, injuries to it, the bile duct, and the cystic duct almost never present as isolated injuries. Factors that predispose individuals to biliary injury include gallbladder distension and alcohol abuse. Penetrating trauma is a common cause of gallbladder injuries, but compression injuries sustained when it is crushed between the liver and spine account for the majority of trauma. Due to a lack of signs and symptoms, diagnosis of biliary injury on clinical grounds only can prove quite challenging, if at all possible.

Spleen

The spleen is the second most commonly injured abdominal organ in blunt trauma, with motor vehicle collisions the most frequent mechanism of injury. Mechanisms sufficient to cause splenic injury can be so unimpressive that a patient may have no recall of a "traumatic" incident, with most cases presenting within 2 to 3 weeks of injury.

Splenic injuries are categorized according to the American Association for the Surgery of Trauma (AAST) Spleen Injury Scale, on which they are assigned a grade of I–V. Grade I injuries include small subcapsular hematomas and shallow capsular lacerations. Grade II injuries include hematomas involving up to 50 percent of surface area, and capsular lacerations up to 3 cm and hemorrhaging. Grade III injuries are subcapsular hematomas covering greater than 50 percent of surface area or are expanding, and lacerations greater than 3 cm or involving trabecular blood vessels in the spleen parenchyma. Grade IV injuries include ruptured, hemorrhaging, interparenchymal hematomas and deep laceration resulting in devascularization of greater than 25 percent of the spleen. Grade V injuries are those that completely shatter or devascularize the spleen.

Stomach

Stomach injury secondary to blunt trauma is an extremely rare event. Most often, gastric rupture occurs when a full stomach is subjected to a compressive force. The stomach is injured much more frequently in penetrating injuries. Gunshot and stab wounds typically involve other structures in the perigastric area, including the colon, liver, spleen, small intestine, pancreas, and omentum. In addition, stomach contents, including digestive enzymes and partially digested chyme, can spill into the peritoneal cavity resulting in gastrointestinal contamination and possible infection, autodigestion, and eventual peritonitis.

Duodenum

The duodenum is well protected and, as a result, accounts for a rather low 3 to 5 percent of all abdominal injuries. Because of its intimacy with other organs, duodenal injuries almost never occur in isolation. Other organs commonly injured in decreasing frequency include the liver, pancreas, small intestine, and colon. Duodenal rupture is usually contained within the retroperitonal space, and patients often initially present asymptomatic. A high index of suspicion based on appreciation of mechanism of injury is usually required to suspect duodenal injury.

Jejunum and ilium

Overall, penetrating trauma accounts for the vast majority of small bowel injury. Blunt trauma most often results in injury to the proximal jejunum and terminal ileum as the small bowel is torn away from the ligament of Trietz and the cecum, which are well anchored. Mesenteric vasculature is often involved, contributing to hemorrhage. In addition, bowel contents, including digestive enzymes and partially digested chyme, can spill into the peritoneal cavity resulting in gastrointestinal contamination and possible infection, autodigestion, and eventual peritonitis. Bowel evisceration occurs when the abdominal wall is violated, allowing abdominal contents, most often mesentery and small bowel, to protrude through. Slashing injuries secondary to assault with a knife or other sharp object are frequent causes of injuries that result in evisceration.

Pancreas

With the pancreas located in a protected location deep within the peritoneal cavity, pancreatic trauma is uncommon. The majority of pancreatic injury is secondary to penetrating trauma. A common mechanism of blunt trauma occurs when the midbody of the pancreas is crushed against the vertebral column by the application of a crushing force to the anterior chest, as when a driver of a car collides with a steering wheel. The majority of patients with pancreatic insult have injury to an additional abdominal organ; the three organs most likely to be injured with the pancreas are the liver, stomach, and major abdominal vascular structures. In addition to the threat of hemorrhage, disruption of the exocrine pancreas tissue can lead to the leaking of digestive enzymes within the retroperitoneal space and subsequent autodigestion of surrounding tissue.

Large intestine

The colon and rectum account for a very small percentage of all intra-abdominal injuries, and the majority of injuries to these structures are secondary to penetrating trauma. Gunshot wounds are the most frequent cause of colon and rectal injury, with stab wounds accounting for a small percentage. Blunt force trauma accounts for 3 to 10 percent of all traumatic colorectal injuries. Colorectal trauma is often complicated by the introduction of fecal material into the abdominal or pelvic compartments, resulting in peritonitis and sepsis. Mortality from colon injury is between 2 to 12 percent.

Vascular injuries

The abdominal cavity and viscera are rich in large vascular structures that circulate a significant quantity of blood. As such, injury to abdominal vascular structures is associated with some of the highest mortality rates of abdominal injuries. Individually, injuries to the aorta have a 50 to 70 percent mortality; iliac artery, 40 to 53 percent; inferior vena cava, 30 to 53 percent; portal and splenic veins, 40 to 70 percent; and iliac vein 38 percent. Almost all of abdominal vascular injuries occur secondary to penetrating trauma. Blunt trauma can occur to abdominal vasculature in a variety of ways. The mobile small bowel and colon often avulse branches off the fixed superior mesenteric artery when subjected to rapid deceleration and manipulation. Aortic injuries can occur when the aorta is crushed against the spine by pressure applied to the abdomen from a seatbelt. In such cases, the intimal layer of the aorta may be lacerated, resulting in thrombus formation. As the abdominal compartment is able to expand and accommodate a significant amount of blood, outward evidence of massive internal bleeding can be occult; the care provider must suspect intra-abdominal bleeding secondary to mechanism of injury and clinical exam findings suggesting developing hypovolemic shock.

3. **Discuss imaging and laboratory studies available to aid in the identification of intra-abdominal injury.**   p. 432

Imaging Studies

Laporatomy

Laparotomy is considered the "gold standard" therapy for intra-abdominal injury as it allows an unparalleled assessment of the abdomen and retroperitoneum, is definitive, and allows for immediate injury repair. Laparotomy is usually reserved for those patients who present with hemodynamic instability, penetrating abdominal injury, peritoneal findings, gross blood in the abdomen, intraperitoneal free air, and CT findings that suggest the necessity for surgical repair. In hemodynamically stable patients, less invasive methods of assessing the abdomen such as CT, sonography, and diagnostic peritoneal lavage (DPL) are usually considered.

Critical care teams (unless they staff a physician) do not normally perform laparotomy, though they are likely to transport a patient that has undergone emergent laparotomy for abdominal trauma. In such a case, the CCTT should be expected to receive a report on injuries diagnosed, repair procedures performed, and any other information that the surgeon feels is important for the team to be aware of.

Diagnostic Peritoneal Lavage (DPL)

Diagnostic peritoneal lavage (DPL) involves the insertion of a catheter into the peritoneal cavity to assess for the presence of blood; it has an impressive history of 97 percent accuracy.

The procedure is performed by inserting a catheter into the peritoneal space by either the open or closed technique. In the open technique, a small incision is made through the abdominal fascia, muscle, and peritoneum just below the umbilicus, and then a catheter is passed through. In the closed method, a catheter is used to puncture the fascia, muscle, and peritoneum, and the catheter is advanced off the needle via the Seldinger technique, much like initiating an IV. The open technique is preferred, as it minimizes the risk of injury to the abdominal contents. Once the catheter is in place, a syringe is used to attempt aspiration of any gross blood. Aspiration of 10 mL of blood is considered positive, and the patient will often receive explorative laparotomy. If no blood is aspirated, 1L of NS is infused into the peritoneal cavity, allowed to diffuse for 5–10 minutes, and then removed. This can often be accomplished by simply lowering the IV bag to the floor, allowing gravity to aid. The fluid is then inspected in a laboratory, and considered positive if there are greater than 100,000 RBC/mm^3 for blunt trauma or 5,000 RBC/mm^3 for gunshot wounds; greater than 500 WBC/mm^3 if bile or an amylase greater than serum amylase are present; or if bacteria, fecal matter, or food particles are present.

While DPL is rapid and sensitive, it is not specific. All a DPL really reveals is that there is blood in the abdomen; the site and severity of the hemorrhage remains unknown. It has often been lamented that DPL results in the identification of minor, normally inoperative injuries that result in unnecessary laparotomies. In addition, while DPL enjoys a relatively low complication rate of 0.9 to 2.4 percent, it is not without the potential for complications, is not able to determine if a patient is continuing to bleed, and is not sensitive for retroperitoneal hemorrhage.

The role of DPL in critical care transport is limited, as the technology for peritoneal fluid evaluation has not caught up with CCTT requirements for small, light, easily portable units. The critical care paramedic could be trained to perform DPL in the field, thereby having the 50-mL sample ready for evaluation promptly at the time of arrival. However, it is more likely that a critical care transport team may be asked to finish a lavage that was started prior to their arrival. In cases of transport from a facility that has performed a DPL, knowledge of the results could aid in decision making prior to, and during, transport.

Sonography

Focused assessment with sonography for trauma (FAST) is an ultrasound assessment designed to detect blood in the pericardium or abdomen secondary to traumatic injury. It is quickly becoming an important tool in the emergency department because, as the acronym implies, the study is fast (performed in 3 to 4 minutes by experienced examiners), accurate (96 to 98 percent accuracy at detecting fluid in the peritoneal cavity), inexpensive, without complications, and repeatable as often as warranted.

The FAST exam involves the assessment of four areas of a supine patient:

- The pericardium is assessed for fluid via a sagittal view from the subxiphoid area.
- A sagittal view of the abdomen from the right midaxillary line between the 11th and 12th rib is used to evaluate the hepatorenal space, or Morrison's pouch, for blood.
- A sagittal view of the abdomen from the left midaxillary line between the 10th and 11th rib is used to assess the spleen and kidney and assess the splenorenal space for blood.
- A coronal view superior to the pubis symphysis is utilized to assess the pelvis for blood.

FAST can be considered an initial diagnostic modality to rule out hemoperitoneum performed during the secondary exam, after the ABCs have been secured. FAST does have its limitations, chief among them an inability to reveal small amounts of blood (< 200 mL).

It has been shown that the level of accuracy of the exam is independent of the level of the practitioner performing the study. Ultrasound technicians produce results equal to those of ED physicians and trauma surgeons. This suggests that with proper training and frequent use, it could be adapted to the critical care transport environment with success.

Due to recent advances in technology, ultrasound is now a very real possibility in CCT, as handheld U.S. units are now readily available and arguably affordable. It has been shown that while helicopter CCTTs can be successfully taught to adequately perform FAST assessments in the field, they are often unable to perform a true, complete exam secondary to time restraints, limited personnel, and a dynamic environment.

Computed tomography

Computed tomography (CT) provides an excellent modality to screen for specific abdominal injury in the stable trauma patient who may not require operative management of his intra-abdominal injuries. It is also indicated in patients with altered sensorium secondary to pharmacologic or traumatic etiologies. However, the more critically injured a patient is, the greater the danger of delays introduced by CT. In unstable patients, greater emphasis should be placed on immediate DPL or direct transport to the operating room for laparotomy. The availability of the new, more advanced helical or spiral CT changes this equation somewhat, as study times with these scanners can be as low as 5 minutes, thus reducing the risk of worsening hemodynamic instability during the exam.

CT's great advantage over DPL is that it allows for a specific diagnosis, particularly in solid organ injuries, allowing for a greater number of intra-abdominal trauma patients to be managed nonoperatively. In addition, it can, unlike DPL, diagnose retroperitoneal injuries. CT does, however, tend to miss injuries that do not result in the introduction of blood or other fluids into the abdominal cavity. Injuries to the pancreas, diaphragm, empty urinary bladder, mesentery structures, and small bowel are often underdiagnosed.

Evaluation of a CT requires the services of a radiologist to identify the finer injury patterns that can appear on CT. CCTT members can, however, be taught how to identify frank blood and obvious organ insult on a CT result, allowing for a better understanding of patient pathology and a patient's particular needs with regard to transport and management.

X-Ray

While every abdominal trauma patient should receive a pelvic and chest X-ray, they are of limited use in patients with blunt abdominal trauma. A radiograph can detect free air in the abdomen and diaphragmatic rupture, but it cannot detect hemoperitoneum, hollow organ injury, solid organ injury, or vascular injury. There is limited use though in penetrating trauma to rule out the presence of a missile. At best, common radiograph findings in abdominal trauma can be suggestive for abdominal and genitourinal injuries, but not definitive. Fractured ribs can raise the index of suspicion for liver, spleen, and renal injury, while pelvic fractures may be suggestive of urinary and vascular injuries.

Laboratory Studies

ABG

Serum pH indicates the acid-base status. Metabolic acidosis with a high lactate indicates that anaerobic metabolism is taking place secondary to tissue hypoperfusion. In other words, your patient is in shock, regardless of the blood pressure. In addition, PO_2 and PCO_2 are invaluable information to help determine the oxygenation and ventilation status of your patient.

A venous blood gas (VBG) can be obtained rapidly, and can determine pH, but not PO_2 or PCO_2. It is as reliable as an ABG in pH determination.

Blood chemistry

It is important to remember that most blood chemistry changes that occur secondary to abdominal trauma do not occur acutely. Rather, numerous hours, and even days, are required for many values to change.

A liver function test, consisting of an ASP (SGOT), GTT/Alkaline phosphatase, and ALT (SGPT) may be elevated in liver trauma or incidences of "shock liver." Particularly in crushing injuries, there can be a transient increase in serum bilirubin secondary to the lyses of red blood cells. Bilirubin will not be elevated in acute liver trauma, but will rise at a rate of approximately 0.8–1.0 mg per day in liver failure.

The serum lactate is a good indicator of the perfusion status of tissue, especially tissue in the GI tract. An elevated lactate indicates that VO_2, the rate of oxygen uptake by tissues from the microcirculation, does not meet the metabolic demand.

Serum amylase and lipase are not reliable indicators for pancreatic trauma. A rising serum amylase and lipase indicate a need for further, more sensitive studies of the pancreas. In cases of normal serum amylase after blunt trauma, there is a 95 percent likelihood of no injury to the pancreas. In small bowel injury, serum amylase will rise independent of lipase.

Low or decreasing serial hemoglobin/hematocrit (H&H) values after a traumatic mechanism of injury to the abdomen are an indication of intra-abdominal bleeding. It is unlikely that a low H&H is secondary to pre-existing, unidentified anemia, and serial change strongly suggests insult.

A leukocyte above 15,000 units/L is considered suggestive of, but not diagnostic for, traumatic injury when a mechanism of injury has been identified. Any stress on the body, physical or psychological, can result in an elevated WBC count, so it's extremely nonspecific, and has questionable value. In addition, the WBC count could have been elevated prior to the traumatic event.

An HCG screen to rule out pregnancy should be performed on every female trauma patient of childbearing age to rule out pregnancy.

BUN/creatinine will gradually increase in patients who have sustained renal trauma and have limited or no kidney function.

A finger stick, or similarly rapid glucose determination, should be made on every patient as soon as the ABCs have been addressed, as traumatic events often occur secondary to hypoglycemia.

Urinalysis

Evaluation of the urine for blood is required in trauma patients to assess for hematuria secondary to GU insult. Determination of gross blood can be made clinically by direct observation of the urine after catheterization. Urine reagent strips are useful for a rapid assessment of the urine.

Sublingual capnometry

Sublingual capnometry is an emerging assessment modality that is gaining support in the trauma and critical care environments and may possibly enter the transport arena in the future. An electrode is placed under the tongue to evaluate the sublingual PCO_2. As the sublingual mucosa is embryologically and anatomically continuous with the intestinal mucosa, evaluation of the sublingual PCO_2 is, in effect, an evaluation of the gut PCO_2. As the gut is among the first tissue to be affected by decreasing tissue perfusion, monitoring of its PCO_2 can alert the care provider very early in the development of shock. Of special interest in abdominal trauma, insult to the bowel results in increased PCO_2. Sublingual capnometry can therefore help identify subclinical cases of blunt abdominal trauma.

4. Discuss the management of intra-abdominal injury.   p. 440

After securing the airway and ensuring proper ventilation, the patient's circulatory status should be addressed. Initiation of large-bore peripheral access is appropriate, but the establishment of two sites is more desirable. Ideally, and especially in cases of developing or severe hypovolemic shock, central venous access should be established. Note that the external jugular (as opposed to the internal jugular) vein is considered a peripheral and not a central site for IV access due to its smaller lumen diameter. A venous blood sample should be obtained immediately after successful venous cannulation.

Recent trends in volume resuscitation suggest that providers should avoid the blind administration of 1–2 L of a crystalloid solution that was the standard of care for hypotensive trauma patients. The critical care paramedic should endeavor to achieve a blood pressure of about three-quarters of the patient's normal blood pressure via the administration of 250 cc fluid boluses of a crystalloid solution until a BP of 75–80 mmHg is obtained. The emerging practice of permissive hypotension does not suggest that the administration of large volumes of crystalloid should never occur. Many trauma patients lose large volumes of blood that must be replaced rapidly to even reach any threshold of hemodynamic stability, and in such cases administration of 2–3 L of crystalloid may be warranted to keep systolic BP at 75–80 mmHg.

The administration of whole blood or packed RBCs should be considered whenever the need for significant volume replacement exists. While there is no clear point at which the literature suggests transitioning from fluid to blood, it is acceptable (if not prudent), to start administration as soon as it is obvious that a patient has lost large quantities of blood volume. Ideally, typed and cross-matched blood should be administered, but type-specific or O blood is more often administered in the acute emergency.

Placement of a Foley catheter should occur prior to transport after urethral injury has been ruled out to allow for the monitoring of urine output, color, and consistency. After addressing airway, breathing, circulation, and immobilization needs, few other true treatments for abdominal injuries exist. A bowel evisceration is treated by covering the exposed bowel with a moist, sterile dressing. Penetrating objects in the abdomen should be treated like all penetrating objects; they should not be removed, but secured in place and kept stable during transport.

5. Describe the anatomy and physiology of the organs and structures that are of concern in genitourinary trauma. p. 441

The kidneys play a major role in fluid and electrolyte regulation, urine formation, waste product removal, red blood cell production, and homeostasis. The kidneys, each about 4 inches in length, are located in the retroperitoneal space lateral to the spinal column between the 12th thoracic and 3rd lumbar vertebrae. The left kidney typically sits a bit higher in the abdominal cavity than does the right. A layer of collagen fibers called the renal capsule covers the outer surface of the kidney. Some of these collagen fibers extend out and attach with the renal fascia, which itself is connected posteriorly to the deep fascial layers surrounding the abdominal muscles of the posterior abdominal wall. Between the renal capsule and the renal fascia is a layer of adipose tissue. Together, the renal capsule, adipose layer, and renal fascia serve to suspend and protect the kidneys.

The kidneys receive 20 to 25 percent of total cardiac output via the renal artery, a branch of the abdominal aorta. The renal vein returns blood to the inferior vena cava. All blood vessels, lymphatic structures, and the ureters travel through the hilus when entering or exiting the kidney.

The ureters drain urine from the kidney, and proceed inferiorly in the retroperitoneal cavity into the pelvic cavity where they enter the bladder on its posterior side. The urinary bladder is an expandable, muscular reservoir for urine located in the pelvic cavity. Its exact position differs in men and women due to differences in reproductive anatomy. In men, the inferior urinary bladder sits between the rectum and symphysis pubis; in women, it sits inferior to the uterus and anterior to the vagina. When full, the urinary bladder distends and can extend well into the lower abdominal quadrants. The urethra exits the bladder at the neck, and travels to the terminus of the external genitalia. The female urethra is about 1–1.5 inches in length and terminates at the vaginal vestibule. The male urethra is about 7–8 inches in length and terminates at the tip of the penis. In the male, the urethra is divided into three parts: the prostatic urethra, the membranous urethra, and the penile urethra. The prostatic urethra passes through the prostate gland, the membranous urethra travels through the urogenital diaphragm, and the penile urethra travels the length of the penis.

The female reproductive system consists of the ovaries, fallopian tubes, uterus, and vagina. The ovaries are small, paired organs that are located near the lateral walls of the pelvic cavity that are secured in place in the pelvic cavity by the suspensory and ovarian ligaments. The two primary functions of the ovaries are the production of ova and the secretion of hormones.

The fallopian tube is a hollow, muscular tube about 5 inches in length. It is divided into three parts: the infundibulum, the ampulla, and the isthmus. The most distal part of the fallopian tube, the infundibulum, has a number of finger-like projections termed fimbriae, whose wave-like motion creates a current in the intra-abdominal fluid of the pelvic cavity that encourages the released ovum to travel into the fallopian tube. The ovum then travels through the ampulla and isthmus, which opens up into the uterus.

The nongravid uterus is a small, hollow, pear-shaped organ about 3 inches long and 2 inches wide that lies on the superior aspect of the urinary bladder, anterior to the rectum. It is held in place in the pelvic cavity by the uterosacral, the broad, and the round ligaments, and receives a rich blood supply provided by the uterine artery. It is divided into four parts: the superior fundus, the body, the isthmus, and the inferior cervix. The uterus serves as the "organ of pregnancy," providing protection and support for a developing fetus.

The cervix houses the cervical canal, which enters into the vaginal canal, an elastic, muscular tube that extends about 3 inches to the vestibule of the external genitalia. The vagina receives its blood supply via the vaginal artery, a branch of the uterine artery. The vagina is the birth canal, and is able to stretch and accommodate the fetus as it is expelled from the uterus during labor. In addition, it is a passageway for menstrual blood flow, and receives the penis during sexual intercourse.

The male reproductive system consists of the testes, epididymis, ductus deferens, seminal vesicle, ejaculatory duct, prostate gland, urethra, and penis. The testes are the site of sperm production and hang in the scrotum. The testes and its blood vessels, nerves, lymphatic structures, and ductus deferens are all enclosed in the spermatic cord, a tough layer of fascia, muscle, and connective tissue that descends into the scrotum from the pelvic cavity through the inguinal canal.

Immature sperm develop in the epididymis, located on the posterior aspect of the testes. The epididymis is a coiled, twisted tube that is up to 7 feet long. It transitions into the ductus deferens, which travels through the spermatic cord, joining with the ejaculatory duct. The ejaculatory duct connects the seminal vesicles, located on the inferior surface of the urinary bladder, with the urethra. The seminal vesicles secrete seminal fluid, which accounts for about 60 percent of the volume of semen. The urethra then travels the length of the penis to the outside environment.

The penis is a tubular organ that conducts urine from the bladder to the outside environment, and introduces semen into the female vagina during sexual intercourse. The majority of the body of the penis consists of the erectile tissue: the corpus spongiosum and the corpus cavernosa. Blood supply to the penis and the erectile tissue occurs via the dorsal artery.

6. Discuss and differentiate the pathophysiology of specific genitourinary injuries. p. 443

The kidneys are moderately well protected, suspended in an adipose layer within the retroperitoneum, and protected by the 11th and 12th ribs. The vast majority of renal trauma is secondary to blunt force trauma. Injury to the kidney can be graded according to the AAST Renal Injury Scale. Grade I injuries include surface contusions and subcapsular hematomas. Grade II injuries include lacerations no deeper than 1 cm, while Grade III injuries are those deeper than 1 cm with hemorrhage or collection-system rupture. Grade IV injuries include those lacerations extending through the collection system, and those resulting in vascular pedicle injury. Grade V injuries include shattered and devascularized kidneys.

Renal contusions (Grade I and II injuries) include subcapsular hematomas, small surface lacerations, and parenchymal bruising. CT evidence of microextravasation of contrast material into the renal parenchyma suggests parenchymal bruising, and a flattening of the renal cortex suggests subcapsular hematoma.

Renal lacerations are divided into two categories: those that extend into the corticomedullary junction or collecting system (Grade IV), and those that don't (Grade III). The risk of extreme hemorrhage and associated injuries increases significantly with Grade IV injuries. CT studies will reveal extravasation of contrast material into the perirenal area or disruption of the renal outline.

Renal ruptures are associated with severe hemorrhage and shock. CT findings include extravasation of contrast material into the perirenal area, severe renal lacerations, and possible renal fragmentation. Rupture that involves the renal pelvis will result in the introduction of urine into the perirenal space.

Ureteral injuries are rare. They are often the result of penetrating trauma that transects the ureter. Blunt force injury as a result of hyperflexion of the spine results in ureteral rupture at, or just below, the ureteropelvic junction. Cavitation forces from the passing of a bullet through the pelvic cavity can result in microvascular thrombosis and, over days, necrosis and perforation.

Bladder rupture can be intraperitoneal or extraperitoneal. An intraperitoneal bladder rupture is most often the result of a full bladder and blunt force trauma to the abdomen. Pressure on the full bladder ruptures the bladder dome, spilling urine into the peritoneal cavity. CT or cystogram will reveal extravasation of urine into the bowel above the bladder. Extraperitoneal bladder ruptures are associated with pelvic fracture and occur most often at the bladder neck. CT and cystogram findings include extravasation of contrast material into the pelvic tissue, often described as "flamelike" due to the pattern it produces.

In males, injuries to the urethra can be divided into those that occur to the posterior urethra (prostatic and membranous) and to the anterior urethra (penile). Posterior urethra injuries are associated with pelvic fractures and additional abdominal, thoracic, and head injuries. Anterior injuries often result secondary to penile fractures and direct force to the penis (falls, straddle injuries). Female urethral injury is rare, and most often occurs secondary to direct pelvic trauma and fractures. Extravasation of contrast material into the surrounding tissue revealed on CT and cystogram are diagnostic for urethral injury.

Overall frequency of scrotal injury is low, most likely due to its mobility. Blunt trauma is the most common cause of scrotal injury, with direct blow and impingement against the symphysis pubis the most common mechanisms. Scrotal tissue can also be avulsed secondary to shearing forces. Injury can result in blood accumulation and engorgement of the scrotum, and the testicles themselves can be avulsed, contused, crushed, or dislocated into the inguinal canal.

Penile injuries include penile fractures, hematomas, lacerations, avulsions, and degloving injuries. Vacuum cleaner injuries can cause extensive damage to both the glans and urethra. Penile fractures occur when an erect penis experiences excessive compressive force resulting in extreme bending, fracturing the engorged corpus cavernosum and injuring the surrounding tissue. A loud, cracking sound is often audible and remembered by the patient. Urethral injury or occlusion due to swelling and developing hematoma are possible concomitant injuries.

Injuries to the female reproductive structures are rare, but most often involve the external genitalia, vagina, and uterus. Ovarian and fallopian tube injuries are extremely uncommon due to their small size and mobility. When injuries do occur to these structures, they most often include contusions, hematomas, and devascularization injuries. In addition, ovaries, as solid organs, can fracture or shatter. Penetrating trauma is the most frequent cause of injury to the uterus. Devascularization injuries can result secondary to blunt trauma that results in severe movement of the uterus and disruption of its vasculature.

Injuries to the external genitalia occur as a result of straddle injuries, aggressive consensual sex, sexual assault, and rape. Injury types include hematomas, lacerations, and avulsions.

7. **Discuss imaging studies available to aid in the identification of genitourinary injury.**   p. 447

Cystography

A retrograde cystogram can be useful in the diagnosis of urethral or bladder injury. In this study, approximately 300–500 mL of contrast media is infused into the urethra and serial radiographs are performed. Any extravasation of contrast from the urethra or bladder indicates perforation.

X-rays

Plain X-rays cannot detect renal injury or function, so they are of limited value in the assessment of the GU patient. X-rays can discover fractures of ribs 10–12, which should increase the index of suspicion for renal trauma.

Computed tomography

Spiral CT with contrast is the imaging modality of choice for the diagnosis of kidney injury, and is able to show enough detail to allow accurate grading of the renal injury. It is important to evaluate the BUN/creatinine prior to the administration of contrast dye to ensure uncomplicated renal elimination. A CT cystogram can be performed much like a radiographic one.

Sonography

Sonography has no real role in the evaluation of genitourinary trauma. Numerous conditions make adequate imaging of anatomical structures difficult, and the test reveals nothing regarding renal function.

Case Study

"This has got to be the worst storm of the year," you think as the ambulance pulls into the emergency department ambulance parking area. There is a steady wind blowing out of the northeast and occasional gusts buffet the side of the rig with enough force to feel the sway. It is not a day that you would have picked for a 50-mile emergency transfer, but that's what you're here for.

Your ground transport team has been called to transport a trauma patient from this rural emergency department to the regional trauma center for surgical evaluation. Normally this patient would be flown, but the storm has grounded all air assets for the foreseeable future and, as is the case with all trauma patients, time is of the essence. Your patient is a 32-year-old male who was the driver of a car that hit a tree that had blown down across the road on a blind corner. He was brought into the emergency department by EMS, complaining of abdominal pain. The ED physician tells you that the patient has complained of right, upper quadrant and right-sided chest pain since arrival. He had no loss of consciousness, is not experiencing any respiratory difficulties, and has remained hemodynamically stable since EMS arrival. A CT scan of the chest and abdomen shows single fractures of the seventh, eighth, and ninth ribs on the right side, with a small underlying pulmonary contusion and a right lobe intrahepatic hematoma thought to be from a Grade IV liver laceration. The patient's doctor tells you that the spine has been cleared and, other than the obviously serious intra-abdominal injury, the patient escaped the crash with relatively few other injuries. The patient's nurse advises you that the patient's vital signs are: respirations 20 and regular with an SpO_2 of 95 percent on 2 lpm oxygen by nasal cannula, heart rate 102 and regular, showing sinus tachycardia on the monitor, and blood pressure of 106/84. There is no blood in his urine and his hematocrit on arrival was 33 percent. He has one IV site infusing normal saline at 100 mL/hr. While you begin your assessment, your partner works on establishing another site.

Your patient presents lying in mid-Fowler's position on the ED stretcher, alert and oriented, but in mild distress. His skin is pale, but warm and dry. Breath sounds are slightly diminished on the right, but otherwise clear to auscultation bilaterally. The right chest wall and right, upper quadrant of the abdomen have a continuous large ecchymotic patch, which the patient is obviously guarding with his right arm. The patient's abdomen is slightly distended, but feels soft with very light palpation. You defer checking deep palpation due to the fact that it will not add anything significant to your assessment and could actually worsen any hemorrhage by disrupting formed clots. As you finish your assessment, your partner tells you he has a good line of normal saline established with a large-bore catheter. Advising him to set the line at a "keep open" rate, you both gently transfer the patient over to your ambulance stretcher to begin transport.

During your transport you have noticed a gradual trending of the patient's BP downward and his heart rate upward. With approximately 20 minutes left in the transfer, you note that the patient's heart rate is 118 and his blood pressure is 92/60. The patient remains alert and you elect to change his oxygen over to a nonrebreather mask even though his respirations remain at 20 and his SpO_2 continues to be 94 to 95 percent. Updating the trauma center via radio, you are advised to monitor the patient's condition at this time and not to bolus with IV fluids unless the systolic BP falls below 80 mmHg.

The patient remains stable for the rest of the transport and you arrive at your destination without further deterioration. In the ED trauma room, you again gently transfer the patient over and give a report to the nurse. When finished, you find the chief surgical resident who is already leafing through the transfer paperwork and give her a report, asking to be updated on how the patient makes out. Later, you learn that the patient did indeed have a Grade IV liver laceration that was managed with embolization in the angiography suite, and is now doing quite well.

DISCUSSION QUESTIONS

1. What are the various imaging studies that are available to assist in the evaluation of abdominal trauma?
2. What are some general considerations for the management of patients with abdominal trauma?
3. What are the various imaging studies that are available to assist in the evaluation of genitourinary trauma?
4. What are some general considerations for the management of patients with genitourinary trauma?

Content Review

MULTIPLE CHOICE

_____ 1. The three spaces that make up the abdominal cavity are the:
  A. peritoneal space, retroperitoneal space, and pelvic cavity.
  B. peritoneal space, abdominal space, and pelvic cavity.
  C. abdominal space, retroabdominal space, and peritoneal space.
  D. thorax, abdomen, and pelvis.

_____ 2. The three layers of serous membrane that line the peritoneal space and cover and suspend the abdominal organs are the:
  A. mesentery, omentum, and greater omentum.
  B. omentum, greater omentum, and mesentery.
  C. parietal peritoneum, visceral peritoneum, and mesentery.
  D. parietal pleura, visceral pleura, and mesentery.

_____ 3. Which of the following is not a retroperitoneal organ?
  A. kidney   C. pancreas
  B. distal duodenum   D. ascending colon

_____ 4. The _____ lies over the abdominal viscera, providing protection, padding, and insulation to the underlying structures.
  A. lesser omentum   C. parietal peritoneum
  B. greater omentum   D. visceral peritoneum

_____ 5. The stomach receives its vascular supply from three branches of which artery?
  A. hepatic artery   C. celiac artery
  B. splenic artery   D. gastric artery

_____ 6. Which organ occupies the most space in the abdomen?
  A. small intestine   C. stomach
  B. liver   D. large intestine

_____ 7. The divisions of the large intestine, in order, from proximal to distal, are the:
  A. rectum, ascending colon, transverse colon, descending colon, sigmoid colon, and cecum.
  B. ascending colon, transverse colon, descending colon, sigmoid colon, cecum, and rectum.
  C. cecum, ascending colon, transverse colon, descending colon, sigmoid colon, and rectum.
  D. cecum, descending colon, transverse colon, ascending colon, sigmoid colon, and rectum.

_____ 8. Which ligament bisects the liver, anchoring it to the anterior and posterior abdominal walls?
  A. ligamentum teres   C. hepatic ligament
  B. broad ligament   D. falciform ligament

_____ 9. The liver receives about what percent of total cardiac output?
  A. 15 percent   C. 25 percent
  B. 20 percent   D. 30 percent

_____ 10. Functions of the liver include:
  A. metabolic regulation, bile synthesis and secretion, and hematologic regulation.
  B. bile synthesis, hematologic detoxification, and glucose storage.
  C. metabolic regulation, bile synthesis and secretion, and antibody synthesis.
  D. hematologic regulation, detoxification, and red blood cell germination.

_____ 11. The gallbladder is connected to the duodenum via the:
   A. common bile and hepatic ducts.
   B. hepatic and cystic ducts.
   C. cystic and common bile ducts.
   D. common bile duct only.

_____ 12. The pancreas extends back and adheres to the posterior abdominal wall.
   A. True
   B. False

_____ 13. How much blood volume is filtered through the spleen?
   A. 5 mL/kg/min
   B. 5 percent of circulating volume/min
   C. 25 percent of cardiac output
   D. 25 mL/kg/min

_____ 14. Numerous branches of the _____ arteries, themselves branches of the aorta, supply the bowel with blood.
   A. gastric and hepatic
   B. inferior and superior mesenteric
   C. renal and hepatic
   D. celiac and mesenteric

_____ 15. The kidneys receive about _____ of total cardiac output.
   A. 5 to 10 percent
   B. 20 to 25 percent
   C. 15 percent
   D. 50 percent

_____ 16. All of the following are roles of the kidneys except:
   A. antibody formation.
   B. red blood cell production.
   C. regulation of fluid and electrolytes.
   D. waste product removal.

_____ 17. The urinary bladder's location differs in men and women because of differences in:
   A. height.
   B. weight.
   C. physiology.
   D. reproductive anatomy.

_____ 18. Which of the following statements about the uterus is false?
   A. The uterus receives its blood supply from the uterine artery.
   B. The uterus lies on the inferior aspect of the urinary bladder, anterior to the rectum.
   C. Divisions of the uterus include the fundus, body, isthmus, and cervix.
   D. The uterus is held in place by the broad, uterosacral, and round ligaments.

_____ 19. The abdominal organs most frequently injured in blunt trauma, in order of highest frequency to lowest, are the:
   A. liver, spleen, kidneys, and small intestine.
   B. liver, spleen, small intestine, and large intestine.
   C. spleen, liver, small intestine, and large intestine.
   D. liver, spleen, large intestine, and small intestine.

_____ 20. The spermatic cord encloses (the):
   A. testes, blood vessels, lymph structures, and ductus deferens.
   B. blood vessels, lymph structures, epididymis, and seminal vesicle.
   C. testes, blood vessels, epididymis, and seminal vesicle.
   D. seminal vesicle, ejaculatory duct, prostate gland, and urethra.

_____ 21. The abdominal organs most frequently injured from gunshot wounds, in order of highest frequency to lowest, are the:
   A. liver, spleen, small intestine, colon, and diaphragm.
   B. small intestine, stomach, pancreas, and large intestine.
   C. small intestine, mesenteric structures, liver, colon, and diaphragm.
   D. stomach, liver, small intestine, large intestine, spleen, and diaphragm.

_____ 22. A renal injury that involves a $\frac{1}{2}$-cm deep laceration of the renal cortex not resulting in urinary extravasation would be considered what grade on the AAST Spleen Injury Scale?
   A. Grade I
   B. Grade II
   C. Grade III
   D. Grade IV

23. Intraperitoneal bladder rupture is most often the result of:
    A. blunt force trauma to the abdomen and a full bladder.
    B. penetrating trauma to the back.
    C. pelvic fractures.
    D. spinal column injury.

24. CT or cystogram findings of extraperitoneal bladder rupture can be described as:
    A. "waterfall-like."   C. "wave-like."
    B. "flame-like."   D. "open-book."

25. A liver injury involving a hematoma covering greater than one-half the liver surface area would be considered what grade on the AAST Liver Injury Scale?
    A. Grade I   C. Grade III
    B. Grade II   D. Grade IV

26. Which of the following predisposes individuals to biliary injury?
    A. alcoholism and ulcers
    B. pancreatitis and gallbladder distension
    C. use of lap belt only, and cirrhosis
    D. alcoholism and gallbladder distension

27. Up to 80 percent of splenic injuries that occur secondary to blunt trauma present within:
    A. 1 to 4 hours after injury.   C. 24 to 48 hours after injury.
    B. 2 to 24 hours after injury.   D. 2 to 3 weeks of injury.

28. A splenic laceration resulting in devascularization of 50 percent of the spleen would be considered what grade on the AAST Spleen Injury Scale?
    A. Grade II   C. Grade IV
    B. Grade III   D. Grade V

29. Abdominal organ injuries that almost never occur in isolation include all of the following except:
    A. liver.   C. stomach.
    B. duodenum.   D. pancreas.

30. The most common cause of small bowel injury occurs secondary to blunt force trauma.
    A. True
    B. False

31. The most common injuries to the small bowel sustained from blunt force injuries are:
    A. compression injuries to the jejunum and duodenum.
    B. injuries sustained by the proximal jejunum and terminal ileum as they are torn away from the ligament of Trietz and the cecum.
    C. bowel wall contusions and perforations resulting in the spilling of bowel contents into the abdominal peritoneum.
    D. tears from shearing forces generated by compression.

32. The three organs or structures most likely to be injured with the pancreas are the:
    A. liver, stomach, and spleen.
    B. small intestine, liver, and stomach.
    C. liver, stomach, and abdominal vascular structures.
    D. aorta, small intestine, and liver.

33. The most common cause of colon and rectal injuries is/are:
    A. stab wounds.   C. blunt force trauma.
    B. gunshot wounds.   D. MVCs.

34. Injury to which abdominal vascular structure has the greatest mortality?
    A. aorta   C. inferior vena cava
    B. iliac artery   D. iliac vein

35. Outward evidence of massive intra-abdominal hemorrhage may be occult because:
   A. blood travels down into the pelvis and remains hidden from exam.
   B. local tissue swelling can tamponade bleeding.
   C. physical manifestation can take hours to days to develop.
   D. the abdominal compartment is able to expand and accommodate a significant amount of blood.

36. Which of the following is considered the "gold standard" imaging study for assessment of the abdomen and retroperitoneum?
   A. CT scan
   B. X-ray
   C. laparotomy
   D. ultrasound

37. Saline that is infused into the abdomen during DPL is removed, assessed, and considered positive if:
   A. there are more than 100,000 WBC/mm^3 for penetrating trauma.
   B. there are more than 5,000 RBC/mm^3 for blunt trauma.
   C. there are more than 500 WBC/mm^3.
   D. bile or serum amylase is present.

38. _____ involves the insertion of a catheter into the peritoneal cavity to access for the presence of blood.
   A. Laparotomy
   B. DPL
   C. Ultrasound
   D. Cystogram

39. The acronym FAST stands for:
   A. Fast Assessment with Sonography for Trauma.
   B. Focused Assessment with Sonography for Trauma.
   C. Fast Abdominal Sonographic Trauma exam.
   D. Focused Abdominal exam with Sonography for Trauma.

40. Which of the following areas is NOT assessed during a FAST exam?
   A. subdiaphragmatic space
   B. hepatorenal space
   C. splenorenal space
   D. pelvis

41. Advantages of utilizing a CT scan for the evaluation of abdominal injuries include all of the following except:
   A. CT allows for the specific diagnosis of solid organ injuries.
   B. injuries to the pancreas, diaphragm, empty urinary bladder, and small bowel are easily diagnosed.
   C. CT can diagnose retroperitoneal injuries.
   D. CT avoids the need for the perforation of, or incision through, the peritoneum.

42. Abdominal X-rays are a useful tool in the diagnosis of specific abdominal injuries.
   A. True
   B. False

43. You are preparing a patient with a liver laceration for transfer and are given her lab results that have just been sent to the ED. You note that metabolic acidosis is present and that her lactate is high, indicating that:
   A. supportive measures to this point have been adequate.
   B. she is hemodynamically stable.
   C. tissue hypoperfusion is present.
   D. an insulin infusion is required.

44. Which of the following statements about a liver function test in abdominal trauma is false?
   A. Bilirubin will be elevated in acute liver failure.
   B. Crushing injuries can result in a transient increase in serum bilirubin.
   C. Bilirubin will rise at a rate of approximately 0.8–1.0 mg per day in liver failure.
   D. A liver function test consists of an ASP (SGOT), GTT/alkaline phosphatase, and ALT (SGPT).

_____ 45. What does an elevated serum lactate indicate?
   A. The rate of oxygen uptake by tissues from the microcirculation does not meet the metabolic demand.
   B. The patient is pregnant.
   C. The patient is in renal failure.
   D. The patient is in liver failure.

_____ 46. In small bowel injury, serum amylase and lipase will:
   A. remain unchanged.
   B. serum amylase will rise and serum lipase will remain unchanged.
   C. serum lipase will rise and serum amylase will remain unchanged.
   D. both rise.

_____ 47. Which of the following is indicative of intra-abdominal bleeding after abdominal injury?
   A. high or increasing serial hemoglobin and hematocrit
   B. increasing serial hematocrit and decreasing hemoglobin
   C. increasing serial hemoglobin and decreasing hematocrit
   D. low or decreasing serial hemoglobin and hematocrit

_____ 48. BUN/Creatinine levels can be expected to gradually increase in patients who have sustained:
   A. liver injury and shock.
   B. small bowel injury with necrosis.
   C. renal injury and decreased renal function.
   D. pancreatic injury with leaking of autodigestive enzymes.

_____ 49. A 24-year-old female has suffered blunt force abdominal trauma and has suspected liver, stomach, and small bowel injury. A HCG screen should be ordered to rule out:
   A. pregnancy.
   B. hepatic injury.
   C. renal injury.
   D. bowel injury.

_____ 50. An elevated leukocyte level is considered specific for traumatic injury.
   A. True
   B. False

_____ 51. Sublingual capnometry is particularly useful in abdominal trauma because:
   A. liver injury often results in metabolic acidosis, which is identified early with sublingual capnometry.
   B. systemic hypoperfusion is more easily identified.
   C. it easily identifies the subclinical systemic hypoperfusion typical of bowel trauma.
   D. insult to the bowel results in local elevations of visceral PCO_2, allowing for identification of subclinical cases of blunt abdominal trauma.

_____ 52. Routine treatment of abdominal trauma includes all of the following except:
   A. central venous catheterization.
   B. venous and arterial blood sampling.
   C. administration of 1–2 L of fluid volume.
   D. placement of a Foley catheter.

_____ 53. All of the following are advantages of Foley catheter insertion prior to transport except:
   A. it is a route for drug administration.
   B. a Foley allows for the accurate measurement of urine output.
   C. urine color and consistency can be monitored.
   D. it prevents the need for manual voiding of the bladder during transport.

_____ 54. A Foley catheter can be utilized to assess for urethral injury.
   A. True
   B. False

_____ 55. You have determined that your patient is suffering from a significant intra-abdominal hemorrhage. Which of the following would be the most ideal to use for volume replacement?
A. crystalloid solution
B. crystalloid solution with packed RBCs
C. type-O blood
D. typed and cross-matched blood

_____ 56. Permissive hypotension is the practice of:
A. not treating a patient's hypotension.
B. administering enough fluid volume to maintain a BP of 75–80 systolic.
C. administering one 20 mL/kg fluid challenge only.
D. administering 2–3 L of crystalloid solution to maintain hypotension.

_____ 57. Cullen's sign can be described as:
A. periumbilical bruising.
B. retroperitoneal bruising.
C. referred pain to the left shoulder secondary to diaphragmatic irritation.
D. bruising to the flank.

_____ 58. Kehr's sign can be described as:
A. periumbilical bruising.
B. retroperitoneal bruising.
C. referred pain to the left shoulder secondary to diaphragmatic irritation.
D. bruising to the flank.

_____ 59. Assessment of the gastrourinary system often occurs concurrently with assessment of the:
A. thorax.   C. airway.
B. abdomen.   D. extremities.

_____ 60. Fractures to the posterior aspects of ribs 11 and 12 may suggest injury to what organ?
A. Liver   C. Kidneys
B. Spleen   D. Stomach

_____ 61. The classic triad associated with bladder rupture is:
A. muffled heart sounds, tachycardia, and hypotension.
B. abdominal pain, hematuria, and tachycardia.
C. positive cystogram, abdominal pain, and a positive FAST exam.
D. abdominal pain, inability to void, and gross hematuria.

_____ 62. The best imaging modality available for the diagnosis of renal injury is:
A. cystography.   C. X-ray.
B. CT scan.   D. sonography.

_____ 63. A disproportionate increase in serum urea compared to creatinine is suggestive for:
A. bladder rupture.   C. urethral occlusion.
B. renal injury.   D. urinary retention.

17 Face/Ear/Ocular/Neck Trauma

Review of Chapter Objectives

Upon completion of this chapter, the student should be able to:

1. **Describe basic facial, neck, ocular, and auditory anatomy and physiology.** p. 453

Soft tissue of the face

The soft tissue of the face consists of a layer of highly vascularized and innervated skin over a layer of multiple facial muscles. Two major arteries are the facial and the temporal, and both vessels are branches of the external carotid artery. Numerous smaller arteries, branches of the ophthalmic artery which itself originates at the internal carotid artery, supply blood to the soft tissue around the bridge of the nose, orbitals, and central forehead. Innervation of the face is supplied by cranial nerves V and VII. The trigeminal nerve (CN V) provides sensory function to the face and controls the muscles of mastication. The trigeminal nerve divides into three main branches, each supplying sensation to a specific area of the face. The facial nerve (CN VII) controls lacrimation, salivation, and the facial muscles.

Specific salivary glands include the parotid, sublingual, and submandibular glands. Salivary secretion is controlled by the autonomic nervous system. Parasympathetic stimulation results in increased secretion and copious saliva production, while sympathetic stimulation results in the secretion of smaller volumes of highly concentrated saliva.

The parotid gland lies over the ramus of the mandible, just superior to the angle of the mandible, anterior to the auditory canal, and inferior to the zygomatic arch. Another paired gland, the sublingual gland, is located on the floor of the oral cavity at the base of the tongue. The submandibular gland, also paired, lies inferior to the angle of the mandible.

The lacrimal glands are located bilaterally in the superolateral orbital area, and are divided into superior and inferior regions. These glands secrete lacrimal fluid, which moistens and lubricates the globe of the eye. Lacrimal fluid exits the gland through multiple lacrimal ducts and flows into the lacrimal sac. The lacrimal sac drains into the nasal cavity via the nasolacrimal duct.

Bones of the face

Collectively, the skull is made up of 22 bones, 8 of which form the cranium and 14 of which form the face. The cranium is made up of the ethmoid, sphenoid, frontal, parietal, occipital, and temporal bones, and serves to protect the brain. The facial bones include the vomer, mandible, and paired maxillary, palatine, nasal, inferior conchae, zygomatic, and lacrimal bones. These bones provide minimal protection for the airway as well as attachment points for the muscles that control facial expressions and the manipulation of food.

The mandible, the second largest facial bone behind the paired maxillary bones, is the most mobile of the facial bones. This bone is divided into the horizontal body and the ascending ramus, which transition at the mandibular angle. The condylar process of the mandible articulates with the mandibular fossae of the temporal bone at the temporomandibular joint (TMJ).

Seven cranial and facial bones articulate to form the orbital complex that house and protect each eye. The maxillary bone forms the inferior rim and floor, the zygomatic bone forms the lateral rim and wall, and the frontal bone forms the superior rim and wall of each orbit. Proceeding lateral to medial across the posterior wall of the orbit, the zygomatic bone articulates with the sphenoid bone, which constitutes the majority of the posterior wall. The ethmoid bone articulates with the lacrimal bone and the orbital process of the palatine bone to complete the posterior and medial walls of the orbit. Numerous foramens, fissures, and canals are located in the orbit to allow the passage of nerves and blood vessels.

The bones that form the nasal cavities and the paranasal sinuses are collectively known as the nasal complex. The perpendicular plate of the ethmoid bone and the vomer form the nasal septum, which serves as the medial border of the left and right nasal cavities. Portions of the frontal bone, ethmoid bone, and sphenoid bone form the superior border of each cavity. Portions of the maxillary, lacrimal, and ethmoid bones define the lateral borders. The inferior border consists of the maxillary and palatine bones. The inferior, middle, and superior nasal conchae occupy the central portion of the nasal cavity. The bridge of the nose is formed by the paired nasal bones, which articulate with the maxillary bone. The soft tissue and cartilage of the nose enclose the vestibule, which opens to the outside environment through the nares.

The paranasal sinuses are air-filled chambers continuous with the nasal cavities and located within the frontal, ethmoid, sphenoid, and maxillary bones. These sinuses lighten the skull; produce mucus, which flows into the nasal cavity; and produce resonance during phonation. The frontal sinuses, ethmoid sinuses, and maxillary sinuses are all connected to the nasal cavities by a passageway, or meatus.

The ear and auditory function

The ear is commonly divided into three anatomical regions: the external ear, the middle ear, and the inner ear. The external ear, comprised of the auricle, or pinna, and the external auditory canal, collects and directs sound waves to the tympanic membrane, or eardrum. The tympanic membrane is a thin, delicate membrane that vibrates when hit by sound waves, and separates the external ear from the middle ear. The pinna, the twisting path and narrowness of the external auditory canal, and the presence of hairs and wax all provide protection for the tympanic membrane. The middle ear communicates with the nasopharynx via the auditory tube, or eustachian tube. This conduit allows for equalization between the middle ear chamber and the atmospheric pressure of the external ear canal. The middle ear contains the auditory ossicles, three delicate bones that transmit vibrations of the tympanic membrane to the vestibulocochlear complex located in the inner ear. The vestibulocochlear complex is made up of the vestibular complex and the cochlea. The vestibular complex consists of the semicircular canals and the vestibule, which provide information regarding the body's orientation in space and equilibrium. The cochlea houses the auditory sensory receptors and provides the sense of hearing. The vestibulocochlear complex is housed within the temporal bone, receives its blood supply from the vertebrobasilar system, and is innervated by the vestibulocochlear nerve, CN VIII.

The eye

In addition to the boney orbital, the eyelids, eyelashes, and lacrimal apparatus all protect the ocular surface. Frequent blinking of the eyelids keeps the surface of the eye well lubricated and free of debris. Reflexive blinking by irritation of the eyelashes and the soft tissue of the eyelids protects from minor trauma. The conjunctiva is a mucus membrane covering the inner surface of the eyelid and the anterior sclera that serves to keep the eye surface moist. The lacrimal apparatus, consisting of the lacrimal gland, lacrimal ducts, lacrimal sac, and the nasolacrimal duct, produces tears, distributes them across the eye surface, and facilitates tear removal. The cornea is dependent on lacrimal secretions for lubrication as well as oxygenation. Without proper function of the lid and lacrimal apparatus, the cornea can dehydrate, become hypoxic, and suffer ischemia or infarction.

The eye shares the orbit with a number of structures including the extrinsic eye muscles, blood vessels, cranial nerves, and a mass of orbital fat that provides padding and insulation to the globe. The wall of the globe can be divided into three distinct layers, or tunics: the outer fibrous tunic, the middle vascular tunic, and the inner neural tunic. The hollow interior of the eye is divided into the anterior and posterior cavities.

The outer layer of the eye, the fibrous tunic, consists of the sclera and the cornea. The sclera serves as the attachment site for the six extrinsic eye muscles. The transparent cornea is continuous with the sclera, and covers both the pupil and the iris. Having no vascular supply, the cornea is dependent on the constant washing of lacrimal fluid over its surface for oxygenation.

The middle layer of the eyeball wall, the vascular tunic, contains the iris, which is the colored, muscular portion that controls the diameter of the pupil and therefore the amount of light entering the eye. The ciliary body attaches to the peripheral posterior aspect of the iris, and the ciliary muscles connect to the lens via the suspensory ligaments, holding the lens in place behind the iris and centered on the pupil.

The retina, or neural tunic, is the innermost layer of the eye wall. It consists of a pigmented layer and a neural layer that act together as the photoreceptive organ of the eye. The optic disc is the area where the optic nerve and central retinal vein leave the eye, and the central retinal artery enters the retina. As no photoreceptors are located in the optic disc, light striking this area goes unnoticed, resulting in a blind spot in the field of vision.

The ciliary body and lens divide the eye into the anterior and posterior cavities. The anterior cavity's borders are the cornea anteriorly, the lens posteriorly, and are further divided into the anterior and posterior chambers, separated by the pupil. Aqueous humor, a clear fluid in the anterior cavity, circulates freely between the anterior and posterior chambers through the pupil. The posterior cavity is the larger of the two, encompassing all of the area behind the lens, and is filled with a clear, gelatinous fluid known as vitreous humor.

The muscles and cranial nerves that control eye movement and vision are discussed in the next section, cranial nerves.

The cranial nerves

Cranial nerves I–VIII all play a role in sensory or motor function of the face and associated structures.

- CN I, the olfactory nerve, is responsible for the sense of smell.
- CN II, the optic nerve, carries visual information from the eye to the diencephalon.
- CN III, the oculomotor nerve, innervates the intrinsic and four of the six extrinsic eye muscles.
- CN IV, the trochlear nerve, innervates one of the six extrinsic eye muscles, the superior oblique.
- CN V, the trigeminal nerve, has both sensory and motor functions. As suggested by the name, the trigeminal is divided into three major branches, the ophthalmic, maxillary, and mandibular, which exit the cranium at different sites. The ophthalmic branch has purely sensory functions, innervating the nasal cavity and sinuses, various intraorbital structures, and the skin of the forehead, eyebrows, upper eyelids, and portions of the nose. The maxillary branch, also purely sensory, innervates the lower eyelids, cheek, upper lip, and portions of the nose. Deeper divisions of the maxillary branch innervate the teeth, gums, portions of the pharynx, and the palate. The mandibular branch has both motor and sensory functions. The motor components innervate the muscles of mastication, while the sensory components innervate the anterior portion of the tongue, the mandible, gums, and teeth, as well as the skin of the temple region.
- CN VI, the abducens nerve, innervates the lateral rectus, one of the six extrinsic eye muscles that control eye movement.
- CN VII, the facial nerve, has both sensory and motor functions. The nerve provides sensory information to taste receptors on the distal two-thirds of the tongue, while the motor component innervates the lacrimal, submandibular salivary, and sublingual salivary glands, as well as the muscles of facial expression.
- CN VIII, the vestibulocochlear nerve, also known as the acoustic or auditory nerve, is a sensory nerve that is divided into the vestibular and cochlear branches. The vestibular branch relays information regarding movement, position, and balance from the sensory receptors in the inner ear to the medulla oblongata and eventually, the cerebellum. The cochlear branch relays auditory information from the cochlea in the inner ear to the medulla.

- CN IX, the glossopharyngeal nerve, has both sensory and motor functions. Afferent nerve fibers relay sensory information from the proximal one-third of the tongue, the soft palate, and the pharynx to the medulla. The carotid sinus branch relays information from the carotid sinuses and bodies. Efferent motor nerve fibers innervate the parotid gland and the muscles involved in swallowing.

The pharynx

The pharynx connects the nose, throat, and mouth to one another, and is divided into three sections: the superior nasopharynx, the oropharynx, and the inferior laryngopharynx. Important structures in the nasopharynx include the superior, middle, and inferior concha. The nasal cavity has a significant vascular supply. Anteriorly, the anterior and posterior ethmoid arteries converge to form Kesselbach's plexus. Blood is supplied to the posterior nasal cavity by the spenopalatine artery.

The oropharynx is separated from the nasopharynx by the soft palate, and extends inferiorly to the level of the hyoid bone. The laryngopharynx extends from the hyoid bone inferiorly to the entrance to the esophagus.

The oral cavity and dentition

The oral cavity borders include the oropharynx posteriorly, the lips anteriorly, the hard and soft palates superiorly, the floor of the mouth anteriorly, and the cheeks laterally. The tongue is, of course, the most obvious structure in the oral cavity, and receives blood supply via the lingual artery. The parotid, sublingual, and submandibular ducts open into the oral cavity, and their respective glands secrete copious amounts of saliva when activated by the parasympathetic nervous system.

An adult normally has 32 teeth, with equal distribution between the upper and lower dental arches. Specifically, each arch contains 2 central incisors; 2 lateral incisors; 2 cuspids, or *canines*; 4 bicuspids, or *premolars*; and 6 molars. In a perfect set of teeth, all occlusal surfaces of the teeth on the upper dental arch match up with their counterparts on the lower arch. Many adults will normally exhibit some degree of malocclusion.

The neck

Systems represented within the neck include the cardiovascular, musculoskeletal, central nervous, respiratory, digestive, and endocrine. The major vascular structures located in the neck are the carotid arteries and the jugular veins. The common carotid arteries originate from the brachiocephalic artery on the right and the aorta on the left. They ascend deep in the neck tissue parallel to the trachea before bifurcating at the level of the larynx, forming the external and internal carotid arteries. The carotid sinuses and bodies are located at the carotid bifurcation. The internal carotid arteries enter the skull through the carotid canals located in the temporal bones and, along with the vertebral arteries, deliver blood to the brain. The internal jugular vein descends lateral to the common carotid artery. Both structures, along with the vagus nerve, are housed in a fascial layer known as the carotid sheath. This sheath is but one of many planes created by the deep cervical fascia, and provides compartmentalization of the major vascular structures of the neck, limiting external blood loss and reducing the risk of exsanguination should the integrity of any of the vessels be compromised. The external jugular veins descend superficial to the sternocleidomastoid muscle, and drain blood from the face, scalp, and cranium into the subclavian vein posterior to the clavicle.

The two major airway structures located in the neck are the larynx and the trachea. The larynx, located prominently in the superior anterior neck at the level of CIV/CV to CVI, consists of the thyroid and cricoid cartilages, and houses the vocal cords, corniculate and arytenoid cartilages, and the epiglottis. The cricothyroid, or intrinsic ligament, connects the inferior thyroid to the superior cricoid. Cricotracheal ligaments attach the inferior cricoid to the first C-shaped cartilaginous ring of the trachea located at the level of CVI.

The anterior esophagus is connected to the posterior trachea by the annular ligament; hence, the two structures are located in close proximity for their entire traverse of the neck. The posterior esophagus lies immediately anterior to the spinal column.

The cervical spine, consisting of the seven cervical vertebrae, is wholly located within the neck and serves to support the head and neck, provide a passageway for the spinal nerves that enter and exit the spinal cord, and protect the spinal cord.

Additional structures of importance in the neck include the thyroid gland, parathyroid glands, cranial nerves IX and X, and the cervical and brachial plexus. The thyroid gland manufactures, stores, and secretes thyroid hormone. It is located inferior to the thyroid cartilage and anterior to the trachea. Two main lobes lie lateral to the trachea and are connected by a small bridge of thyroid tissue called the isthmus. The gland is afforded a significant blood supply from the superior and inferior thyroid arteries. The carotid sinus branch of the glossopharyngeal nerve, CN IX, traverses the neck as do numerous branches of the vagus nerve as it spreads out to destinations in the pharynx, carotid bodies and sinuses, diaphragm, heart, lungs, and abdominal viscera, among others. The cervical plexus originates bilaterally from spinal nerves CI–CV, and branches innervate muscles in the neck and account for the entire innervation of the diaphragm via the phrenic nerve. The brachial plexus originates bilaterally from spinal nerves CV–T1 and innervates the pectoral girdle and arm on their respective side.

Numerous muscles in the neck serve to hold up and allow movement of the head, assist in respiration if needed, and, to some degree, protect deep vital structures such as blood vessels located underneath. The sternocleidomastoid originates at the sternal end of the clavicle and the manubrium, and inserts at the mastoid of the skull. It is an important landmark for procedures such as subclavian and internal jugular vein catheterization. In addition, the neck can be divided into the anterior and posterior triangles using the sternocleidomastoid. The platysma is a thin, superficial muscle layer located just below the subcutaneous tissue. It effectively covers the neck, originating just inferior of the clavicles in the deep fascia of the upper chest, extending across the neck, and inserting on the mandible and the fascia at the corner of the mouth. Any penetrating trauma that violates the platysma should raise concern for potential damage to the deeper vital structures of the neck.

The neck can be divided into anatomical zones, discussed in objective 2, and also into the anterior and posterior triangles. The anterior triangle is the area bordered by the body and sternal head of the sternocleidomastoid, the mandible, and the midline of the neck. The posterior triangle is the area bordered by the body and clavicular head of the sternocleidomastoid, the middle third of the clavicle, and the trapezius muscle.

2. **Describe the anatomical zones of the neck.** p. 467

To aid in the evaluation and management of penetrating neck injuries, the anterior neck is divided into three zones.

- Zone I extends from the clavicle to the cricoid cartilage.
  - Structures include: subclavian vessels, innominate veins, common carotid arteries, jugular veins, aortic arch, trachea, esophagus, lung apices, and cervical spine and cord
- Zone II extends from the cricoid cartilage to the angle of the mandible.
  - Structures include: carotid arteries, vertebral arteries, jugular veins, pharynx, larynx, trachea, esophagus, and cervical spine and cord
- Zone III extends from the angle of the mandible to the base of the skull.
  - Structures include: carotid arteries, jugular veins, trachea, esophagus, cervical spine and cord, and cranial nerves IX, X, XI, and XII

3. **Discuss and differentiate the pathophysiology of specific facial, neck, ocular, and auditory injuries.** p. 467

Pathophysiology of facial injuries

Soft-tissue injuries
The rich, vascular supply of the facial soft tissue and scalp ensure that even minor lacerations will bleed impressively at times. This rich, vascular supply also allows for rapid wound healing and reduces the incidence of infection. While it is uncommon for facial lacerations to hemorrhage significantly enough to result in hemorrhagic shock, insult to a major vessel such as the facial or temporal artery can result in shock if bleeding is not controlled adequately. Facial lac-

erations, avulsions, incisions, and even contusions can result in damage to underlying structures such as cranial nerves, salivary glands, and lacrimal glands that can be identified during a proper physical exam.

Remember that in addition to shearing, torsional, and frictional forces, compressive forces via blunt force trauma can result in lacerations to soft tissue. Particular attention must be paid to ensure that there is not a more serious underlying internal injury. In particular, contusions, abrasions, and hematomas should alert the provider that blunt forces were involved, and that assessment for underlying injury must take place. Common underlying injuries can include fractures and internal hemorrhaging.

Penetrating trauma may also result in a seemingly benign facial insult, and must always be considered when evaluating soft-tissue injuries. Low-velocity gunshot wounds to the face can have a minimal superficial presentation, but extensive internal tissue destruction. Stab wounds typically do not result in the extensive internal tissue destruction typical of gunshot wounds. While it is not as common as blunt force trauma, penetrating trauma to the face is associated with a higher incidence of life-threatening airway compromise than is blunt force trauma. In addition, penetrating trauma to the inferior tissue of the face may extend internally into Zone III of the neck, and include structures such as the internal carotid, external carotid, and vertebral arteries.

Unless it compromises the airway, all penetrating objects are left in place to be removed by a surgeon. Impaled objects frequently impinge or even lacerate arteries, veins, and nerves, and it is not uncommon for an impaled object to tamponade bleeding. Movement or removal of the object can result in further damage to underlying structures and/or severe hemorrhaging.

Human and animal bites to the face can result in extensive tissue destruction and hemorrhaging. Bite wounds to the cheek can be especially extensive and hemorrhage considerable, potentially compromising the airway. Human bites are of particular concern, and even seemingly minor bites can result in infection and tissue deformity. Without proper care, severe complications and even death can occur secondary to animal, and especially human, bites.

Facial fractures

Due to their prominent location, the nasal bones are the most commonly fractured facial bones, followed by the mandible and zygoma. All of these bones require relatively little force to fracture and frequently present as isolated injuries. Bones that require much more force to fracture include the components of the supraorbital ridge and the ramus of the mandible. Any injury to these structures necessitates the ruling out of concomitant, potentially life-threatening injuries including closed, head, and cervical spine injury.

Nasal fractures often involve only the cartilaginous septum. If the insult is sufficient to fracture the underlying nasal bones and deeper nasal structures such as the ethmoid bones, significant hemorrhaging can occur if the rich vascular supply of the nasal conchea is disrupted. In such cases, airway obstruction is of concern. In addition, rupture of the cribriform plate of the ethmoid bone can result in basilar skull fracture and torn meninges, exposing the subarachnoid space. Since developing septal hematomas can result in decreased blood flow and avascular septal necrosis, they should be drained.

The most common sites of mandibular fractures, in descending order of occurrence, are the body, condyle, angle, symphysis, ramus, and coronoid process. Fractures to the symphysis region, the midline of the mandible between the central incisors, are of particular concern as they can result in glossoptosis and subsequent airway compromise, especially when a patient is supine on a spine board.

Temporomandibular joint dislocation occurs when the condylar process of the mandible disarticulates from the mandibular fossae of the temporal bone. Blunt trauma is a common cause, but it can also occur secondary to yawning or seizures.

Zygoma fractures are most often the result of blunt force trauma secondary to assault, motor vehicle collisions, and sports injuries. The most common type of zygoma fracture is a simple fracture of the arch. Isolated zygomatic arch fractures are not a serious life threat. The less common and more serious tripod fracture involves the disarticulation of the zygomatic-frontal suture, fracture of the arch, and fracture of the infraorbital rim. In addition, fractures may extend into the orbital rim.

Maxillary fractures are classified according to the Le Fort system of classification. A Le Fort I maxillary fracture is a transverse fracture just superior to the apices of the teeth, through the maxillary sinus and across the nasal septum. It allows movement of the maxilla when the upper

©2007 Pearson Education, Inc.
Critical Care Paramedic

teeth are grasped and manipulated. A Le Fort II maxillary fracture, the pyramid fracture, extends superiorly through the infraorbital rims to an apex above the bridge of the nose. It allows movement of the maxilla, infraorbital rims, and nose when manipulated, but not the eyes. A Le Forte III maxillary fracture, the craniofacial dysjunction fracture, is the most serious of the Le Forte fractures. This fracture includes the zygomatic arches, frontozygomatic suture, sphenoid bone, and nasal bone. Simply stated, the facial skeleton is separated from the skull, allowing for movement of most of the facial structures, including the eyes, when manipulated. Significant force, up to 100 times the force of gravity, is required to fracture the midface, and significant, potentially life-threatening trauma to other systems can be present.

Injuries to the face can result in concomitant dentition injury. Teeth can fracture, chip, and be avulsed from the mandible or maxilla. In addition, cases of teeth intruding into the nasal cavity and maxillary sinus after facial trauma have been reported. Care must be taken to account for all teeth, when possible, to reduce the risk of aspiration. All missing teeth should be considered aspirated until proven otherwise. If possible, intact teeth should be properly cared for, as they can be re-implanted with a high likelihood of success.

Orbital blowout fractures result when a direct blow to the orbit results in an instantaneous increase in intraorbital pressure and subsequent rupture of the orbital floor. Specifically, the maxillary and zygoma bones are most often fractured, but any of the bones comprising the orbit can be involved. In addition, direct blows to the orbital rim can also result in a blowout fracture.

Superior orbital fissure syndrome can occur when an orbital fracture involving the superior orbital fissure compresses the oculomotor and ophthalmic branch of the trigeminal nerves. A much more serious variant of this injury, apex syndrome, involves the optic nerve.

Pathophysiology of ear and auditory injuries

External ear injury

The pinna, due to its exposed position in the head, is frequently subjected to trauma. Because of the limited blood supply to the cartilaginous framework of the pinna, it does not hemorrhage significantly when lacerated or avulsed. Lack of vasculature can also contribute to necrosis should the perichondrium be sheared from the underlying cartilage, as the cartilage is dependent on the perichondrium for its blood supply. The external ear canal, due to its narrow, winding path, and location in the skull, is not often subjected to the forces of trauma, and serves to protect the tympanic membrane.

Ruptured tympanic membrane

Injuries to the tympanic membrane occur either as a result of direct injury, such as when an object is introduced into the external ear canal and pushed up against the membrane, or indirect injury, as when rapid changes in pressure rupture the membrane. Explosions, blows to the pinna, and barotraumas from diving are common causes of tympanic membrane rupture. In addition, impact to the anterior mandible can transmit forces through the condyles sufficient enough to fracture the temporal bone and rupture the tympanic membranes. Though isolated tympanic injuries are not life threatening and frequently heal themselves, evaluation in an emergency department is appropriate. The tympanic membrane can also be ruptured in cases of basilar skull fracture. Patients with otorrhea and hemorrhagic otorrhea secondary to any insult to the head should be considered to have a basilar skull fracture until proven otherwise.

Auditory trauma

Due to their location in the inner ear, protected by the temporal bone, injuries to the vestibulocochlear complex are uncommon. When they do occur, they are frequently associated with cranial injury. Less frequently, disruption of the apparatus can occur secondary to violent shaking or shearing forces, resulting in physical damage or dislocation of the vestibulocochlear complex or the vestibulocochlear nerve, CN VIII.

Pathophysiology of ocular injuries

Eyelid lacerations

Though injuries to the eyelid may seem unimpressive, they can include injury to the lacrimal apparatus, tarsal plate, levator muscle, and even the globe itself, and should be evaluated by an ophthalmologist. Isolated lid injuries should undergo ophthalmological repair within 24 hours of insult to preserve normal lid function and harmony with the lacrimal apparatus.

Conjunctival injuries

A subconjunctival hemorrhage can occur when blunt trauma injures the blood vessels within the conjunctiva. In addition, traumatic asphyxiation, sneezing, coughing, vomiting, or any other maneuver that results in increased pressure can cause rupture of the conjunctival blood vessels. While potentially impressive, subconjunctival hemorrhage is not a serious injury, but does suggest that insult has occurred and additional injuries may be present.

Corneal injuries

Corneal abrasions are the most common eye injury evaluated in the emergency department. Possible foreign bodies include dust, dirt, glass, and metal. Contact lenses, if left in too long, can also cause corneal abrasions, and often have a bacterial component to the insult as well. It is important that the critical care paramedic ensure that all unconscious patients who are undergoing interfacility transfer have had contact lenses removed. Diagnosis of corneal abrasion is made with the application of fluorescein and illumination with an ultraviolet or Wood's lamp.

Hyphema

A hyphema is a collection of blood in the anterior chamber, and is often the result of blunt trauma to the globe. The bleeding is most commonly a result of torn vessels of the peripheral iris but can also result secondary to lens and retina detachment. The condition is more easily appreciated with the patient sitting upright, as blood will pool dependently in the inferior anterior chamber. With the patient lying supine, blood may not be recognized as readily as it disperses throughout the anterior chamber. Small hyphemas may not be recognized easily, and identification of microhyphemas requires the use of a slit lamp. Hyphema is a potential threat to a patient's vision, and evaluation by an ophthalmologist is required.

Ocular globe rupture

Globe rupture is a serious injury with a high risk for loss of vision, and is always considered a serious ophthalmalogical emergency and always requires surgical intervention. Posterior chamber injury and loss of vitreous humor is associated with a higher frequency of vision loss than of injuries to the anterior chamber. Luckily, the orbit provides a significant amount of protection to the posterior globe. Globe rupture should be suspected whenever there is a history of penetrating or significant blunt trauma. Common penetrating objects include writing instruments, fishhooks, knives, darts, and needles. In addition, any patient who suffers acute eye injury while in the presence of heavy machinery, a power saw, metal grinders, metalworking, or any other situation of high-energy, metal-to-metal contact should be considered high risk for globe insult.

Ocular avulsion

In severe maxillofacial trauma, enucleation of the globe from the orbit may occur. Loss of vision can be avoided and depends on the extent of injury, as well as the quality of care. The tearing and shearing forces associated with an ocular avulsion often result in significant damage to the major blood vessels and optic nerve, in which case loss of vision is assured. Care must be taken in such circumstances to control active hemorrhaging and rule out additional, potential life-threatening injuries.

Traumatic retinal detachment

Traumatic retinal detachment occurs most often as a result of blunt trauma and is considered a surgical emergency. In retinal detachment, the outer, pigmented layer of the retina separates from the inner, neural layer. There are three mechanisms by which this can happen. First, increased intraocular pressure from blunt force trauma can tear the retina and force vitreous humor from the posterior chamber into the defect, resulting in a dissection-like injury between the layers. Second, tractional retinal detachment can occur when adhesions form between the vitreous humor and the retina, and mechanical forces within the globe secondary to blunt or penetrating trauma separate the layers of the retina, with or without tearing it. Third, blood can escape from damaged vessels, separating and filling the retinal layers.

Pathophysiology of neck injuries

The critical care paramedic will find it useful to classify neck injuries according to the anatomical zones affected. This will not only aid in providing a clear, comprehensible verbal and written report to the receiving facility, but can also help the paramedic anticipate injuries based on known anatomy within the zones.

Injuries to Zone I are associated with high mortality because they can involve the great vascular structures of the chest, the inferior larynx and trachea, as well as intrathoracic structures such as the lungs. Injuries to Zone II commonly involve the carotid arteries and airway structures, and are readily identifiable owing to the exposed nature of this area of the neck. Zone III injuries often involve the internal and external carotid arteries, the vertebral artery, and the cranial nerves.

Any wound that obviously penetrates the platysma should immediately increase the index of suspicion for underlying injury to the deeper structures of the neck. This is an injury that will most likely be explored surgically.

Vascular neck injuries

The vascular structures of the neck are commonly injured in penetrating neck trauma, and laceration of the carotid arteries or internal jugular veins can result in rapid loss of significant amounts of blood and the development of hemorrhagic shock. In addition, insult to the carotid arteries can decrease cerebral perfusion and cause cerebral hypoxia and ischemia, and an expanding hematoma can occlude blood vessels and compromise the airway. Injury to the common carotid artery occurs in 11–13 percent of all penetrating neck trauma. Laceration of the jugular vein can also result in the development of an air embolism as venous pressure drops below atmospheric pressure during deep exhalation.

While not as common as penetrating trauma, blunt trauma can also be associated with significant arterial injury. Mechanisms of injury that result in hyperextension, hyperflexion, hyperrotation, and direct blows to the neck should alert the critical care paramedic to the possibility of vascular injury. Specific carotid and vertebral artery injuries include pseudoaneurysm and dissection.

Laryngotracheal injuries

Laryngotracheal injuries include edema and swelling of the soft tissue, thyroid and cricoid cartilage fracture, hyoid bone fracture, and laryngotracheal disruption. "Clothesline" injuries can occur as a result of striking stationary ropes, cords, or wires while operating vehicles such as bicycles, ATVs, or motorcycles. In addition, strangulation or hanging can cause similar insult.

Conversely, penetrating trauma to Zones I and II resulting in laryngotracheal injury are seldom occult. Clinical exam findings include obvious airway defect, dyspnea, hemoptysis, air bubbling from the wound, and subcutaneous emphysema.

In cases of both blunt and penetrating trauma, deformity of the normal anatomical landmarks can make oral intubation difficult even for the most experienced provider, and these situations often require the use of a surgical airway. Tracheostomy rather than cricothyrotomy may be the airway of choice, as a cricothyrotomy attempt may worsen existing trauma.

Neurological injuries

Direct injury to nerves located outside of the spinal cord is the most common etiology of neurological deficits secondary to neck trauma. Of particular concern are two injuries that are potentially life threatening: injuries to the phrenic nerves and to the recurrent laryngeal nerves. The paired phrenic nerves provide all of the innervation to the diaphragm, and insult to one can cause a marked insult to normal respiration. Insult to both phrenic nerves, however unlikely, would result in paralysis of the diaphragm. The paired recurrent laryngeal nerves provide innervation allowing for opening of the vocal cords. Insult results in vocal cord paralysis and airway obstruction secondary to a closed glottic opening. In addition, injuries to the deep cervical and brachial plexus can occur.

Thyroid injuries

Of all the structures in the neck, the thyroid gland is one of the most exposed and is very susceptible to injury. Of primary concern would be the potential for significant hemorrhage secondary to laceration of the superior and inferior thyroid arteries. Although rare, thyrotoxicosis secondary to thyroid trauma can occur, and should be considered in any patient with injury to the thyroid or surrounding tissues and presenting with the clinical manifestations associated with thyrotoxicosis.

Pharynx and esophagus injuries

Due to their deep, protected location in the neck, pharyngeal and esophageal injuries are fairly uncommon, and are most often the result of penetrating neck trauma. Esophageal injuries are often difficult to identify clinically, and are often overlooked during the initial assessment. However, due to the close to 100 percent mortality if treatment is delayed 24 hours, it is imperative that these injuries are identified quickly.

4. **Discuss the assessment and management of the patient with a facial injury.**   p. 477

Assessment

The ears, nose, and mouth should be assessed for the presence of blood or fluid. The mouth should be more closely inspected for teeth, secretions, or blood in the oropharynx, and suctioning provided, as necessary. The oral cavity should be inspected for malocclusion, lacerations, avulsions, penetrating injury, bone fragments, foreign bodies, and compound fractures.

A systematic inspection and palpation of the boney structures of the midface should reveal the majority of facial fractures. The entire face should be palpated for loss of integrity, crepitus, subcutaneous air, and pain.

Orbital fractures can be identified by loss of integrity of the infraorbital rim, loss of symmetry between the orbitals, and periorbital anesthesia. In addition, enophthalmos, restriction of extraocular movement, or diplopia may be present. X-ray findings consistent with orbital fracture include the "hanging teardrop" and "open bomb-bay door" signs resulting from the herniation of orbital fat and displacement of orbital bone into the maxillary sinus, respectively. Air/fluid levels may also be appreciated in the maxillary sinus. An orbital blowout fracture may present with restricted upward gaze and diplopia secondary to entrapment of the inferior rectus muscle. Entrapment of the infraorbital nerve can result in anesthesia of the maxillary teeth and upper lip. Enophthalmos may be appreciated, though it may prove difficult to discern secondary to local tissue swelling. Superior orbital fissure syndrome commonly results in paralysis of the extraocular muscles, ptosis, and periorbital anesthesia. In addition to the findings consistent with superior orbital syndrome, patients with Apex syndrome will also experience decreased visual acuity or blindness. Any patient with these syndromes requires immediate ophthalmic evaluation and intervention to prevent permanent vision loss.

Maxillary fractures are classified according to the Le Fort system of classification. A Le Fort I maxillary fracture is a transverse fracture just superior to the apices of the teeth, through the maxillary sinus and across the nasal septum. It allows movement of the maxilla when the upper teeth are grasped and manipulated. A Le Fort II maxillary fracture, the pyramid fracture, extends superiorly through the infraorbital rims to an apex above the bridge of the nose. It allows movement of the maxilla, infraorbital rims, and nose when manipulated, but not the eyes. A Le Fort III maxillary fracture, the craniofacial dysjunction fracture, is the most serious of the Le Fort fractures. This fracture includes the zygomatic arches, frontozygomatic suture, sphenoid bone, and nasal bone. Simply stated, the facial skeleton is separated from the skull, allowing for movement of most of the facial structures, including the eyes, when manipulated.

Zygoma fractures can be identified by the presence of a flattened cheek, lateral subconjunctival hemorrhage on the affected side, and infraorbital anesthesia. If the displaced zygoma impinges the master muscle or coronoid process, trismus or limited range of motion can occur. Additional signs and symptoms include subconjunctival hemorrhage, infraorbital anesthesia, difficulty opening the mouth, and flattening of the midface over the fracture site. X-ray is adequate for the interpretation of arch injuries, while tripod injuries are best evaluated with CT scanning.

Nasal fractures to the bony or cartilaginous structures can be readily identified by asymmetry, deformity, and pain. Nasal fractures often involve only the cartilaginous septum, resulting in deformity, swelling, pain, and minor hemorrhage. If the insult is sufficient to fracture the underlying nasal bones and deeper nasal structures such as the ethmoid bones, significant hemorrhaging can occur if the rich vascular supply of the nasal conchea are disrupted. Presence of cerebral spinal fluid rhinorrhea can be difficult to appreciate, but is indicative of basilar skull fracture. The need for nasal films can be described as controversial.

Mandibular fractures can be identified clinically by the presence of malocclusion, instability, and immobility of the mandible. The tongue-blade test can be a useful technique for detecting mandibular fractures that are not readily apparent on initial inspection. The examiner instructs the patient to bite down forcefully on a tongue blade inserted between the teeth. The examiner then twists the blade, attempting to break it. The patient with a fractured mandible will experience pain and reflexively open his mouth. A positive tongue blade test is extremely sensitive for mandibular fracture.

TMJ dislocation presents with a mandible deviated away from the side of a unilateral dislocation, or jutting forward in the case of bilateral dislocation. While the condition is often painful, it seldom results in airway compromise. Treatment is relocation under conscious sedation by a physician.

Management

Airway management is obviously of primary concern in the management of a patient with facial trauma, and is discussed in detail in objective 7.

Although patients rarely develop shock secondary to facial hemorrhage, care should be taken to control any bleeding with a pressure dressing. Clamping of wounds with hemostats should be avoided, as inadvertent damage to facial nerves or salivary ducts may occur. Pinching the upper nasal cartilage together often easily controls nasal hemorrhage. In rare cases, packing of the anterior or posterior nasal cavity may be necessary for severe bleeds, but care must be taken not to pack the cranium as well. A Foley catheter inserted into the nasal cavity and filled with saline is often used in such circumstances. Le Fort fractures that are hemorrhaging significantly can be reduced with gentle inferior traction in an attempt to control bleeding. Patients should be encouraged not to swallow any blood, as it can lead to gastric irritation and vomiting, further complicating airway status. Very often, conscious and alert patients are able to suction their airway themselves if given a rigid tip suction device and instructions on its use.

Unless it interferes with airway control, any impaled object in the face, neck, or eye should be immobilized in place. This can be accomplished in any number of ways, and some creativity is sometimes required when patients are impaled with unusually shaped objects. More often than not, penetrating objects can be stabilized with bulky dressings placed, and secured, around the object.

5. **Discuss the assessment and management of the patient with an ocular injury.**   p. 478

Assessment

The periorbital area should be inspected for ptosis, lacerations, swelling, deformity, or any dysfunction. Palpation of the orbital rims should be performed to evaluate for crepitus, loss of integrity, or periorbital anesthesia.

The external eye and anterior chamber should be inspected for penetrating objects, foreign bodies, signs of infection, flattening, protrusion, lacerations, hemorrhage, hyphema, and any other sign of trauma.

Pupil assessment is best performed in a slightly underlit environment. They should be assessed for symmetry, shape, accommodation, and reaction to light. Anisocoria is pupil variance greater than 1 mm and is normal in some individuals.

Visual acuity in both eyes should be evaluated in all patients that are conscious and alert. Near or distance charts should be utilized when practical, assessing for the smallest line readable for each eye while the other is covered. Uncorrected vision should be tested first, followed by corrected vision. If the patient's corrective lenses are not available, a pinhole occluder can be utilized in conjunction with a near card. If the patient's vision is diminished to the point of not being able to discern an acuity card, have the patient count fingers that you hold up. Record the farthest distance at which the patient can discern your fingers. If this fails, test the patient's ability to detect motion by waving your hands 1 to 2 feet in front of his eyes. If the patient cannot detect hand motion, test for light perception by turning off all lights and illuminating the eye with a penlight.

Evaluation of the six extraocular muscles and the cranial nerves that innervate them can be performed by having the patient move her eyes through all six positions of gaze. Disconjugate gaze, diplopia, or limitation in motility should be recorded.

An ophthalmoscope can be utilized to magnify and visualize the anterior and posterior cavities of the eye, allowing for evaluation of the retina, optic nerve, and macula. Dilation of the pupils makes the visualization of these structures easier.

Corneal abrasions result when a foreign body scratches the corneal epithelium resulting in significant pain, lacrimation, sensation of tearing, and photophobia. Most patients will report a foreign body sensation, and sympathetic movement of the affected eye under a closed lid will often result in increased pain.

It is important for the critical care paramedic to remember that globe rupture may initially be insidious, and not readily apparent. More often, decreased visual acuity, an irregular pupil, flattening of the globe, and subconjunctival hemorrhage or hyphema may be present. Careful inspection of the eye is of the utmost importance when attempting to identify globe rupture.

Retinal detachments may have no outward signs, and diagnosis by the critical care paramedic is often made after considering the mechanism of injury and symptoms. Symptoms include seeing flashes of light, curtain-like shadows in the peripheral vision, dimmed or filmy vision, and black spots.

6. **Discuss the assessment and management of the patient with a neck injury.**   p. 478

Inspect and palpate the neck and note any lacerations, asymmetry, swelling, pulsating masses, subcutaneous emphysema, and tracheal deviation. Pay particular attention to the area of Zone III under the mandible, the posterior triangle, and the inferior aspect of Zone I, as these areas are often passed over, and injuries overlooked, with devastating consequences. Remember that penetrating injuries to Zone I can result in thoracic injury, and a chest film can be useful to rule out pneumothorax, hemothorax, and pneumomediastinum. Cervical spine films must be evaluated in all patients with neck injury. Assess for foreign bodies, fractures, subcutaneous air, soft-tissue injury, hematoma, tracheal disruption or deviation, and retropharyngeal thickening.

Specific carotid artery injuries include pseudoaneurysm and dissection, resulting in hematoma formation, neurological deficits, bruits, ipsilateral Horner's syndrome, and pulse deficits. Because 25 to 50 percent of patients with carotid injury secondary to blunt trauma initially present with no external signs of trauma, an appreciation for the mechanism of injury is essential in such cases. Similar injury to the vertebral arteries presents clinically with hemiparesis, diplopia, nystagmus, vertigo, and dysarthria.

Clinical findings of laryngotracheal injuries include dysphonia, hoarseness, dysphagia, dyspnea, pain, and hemoptysis. Clothesline, hanging, and strangulation injuries can be overlooked due to their unimpressive initial presentation, but these patients are at high risk for developing total airway occlusion secondary to swelling and edema of the surrounding tissues. Developing hoarseness is an ominous sign of impending airway occlusion. Conversely, penetrating trauma to Zones I and II resulting in laryngotracheal injury are seldom occult. Clinical exam findings include obvious airway defect, dyspnea, hemoptysis, air bubbling from the wound, and subcutaneous emphysema.

7. **Understand the importance of airway maintenance in the initial management of the patient with facial and/or neck trauma.**   p. 480

The most common cause of death from maxillofacial trauma is obstruction of the upper airway secondary to posterior displacement of the tongue into the hypopharynx. The modified jaw thrust, simple chin lift, and suctioning of the oropharyngeal cavity are often sufficient to open up the airway and keep it clear. Care must be taken not to manipulate the cervical spine if cervical injury is suspected.

If simple airway maneuvers are not sufficient to open the airway, an oropharyngeal airway can be inserted. Use of a nasopharyngeal airway is contraindicated in cases of suspected fracture of the cribriform plate. Frequent suctioning of the airway is often required in maxillofacial trauma, and particular care should be paid to patients who are immobilized in a supine position on a backboard.

Distortion of the soft tissue and bony structures of the face can make achieving a proper mask seal difficult. A flail mandible not only makes mask seal difficult, but may allow the tongue to fall into the posterior hypopharynx, thereby obstructing the airway as well. In neck injuries, air dissecting into the surrounding tissue and facial compartments can quickly distort airway anatomy and make ventilation, as well as recognition of laryngeal structures, difficult, if not impossible.

Developing airway compromise should be suspected if worsening dyspnea, tachypnea, cyanosis, agitation, altered mental status, loss of consciousness, accessory muscle use, nasal flaring, subcutaneous emphysema, or hoarseness are noted. In such cases, endotracheal intubation should be considered.

Endotracheal intubation is frequently required to ensure adequate oxygenation and ventilation. Orotracheal intubation is preferred over nasotracheal intubation in most cases because of the risk of basilar skull fracture in this population of patients. In-line cervical spine stabilization should be held in those patients identified to be at risk for cervical spine injury. Numerous tools, such as the Viewmax™, fiber-optic stylettes, and the gum elastic bougie, can facilitate intubation of the difficult airway. In addition, advanced techniques such as retrograde intubation can be utilized in situations where routine endotracheal intubation is difficult or impossible.

Rapid-sequence intubation in patients with severe maxillofacial or neck injury is not without significant risk. Failure to intubate a paralyzed patient can be further complicated by failure to adequately ventilate with a BVM due to distortion of normal facial anatomy. This population of patients are prime candidates for facilitated intubation, in which sedation with benzodiazepines, barbiturates, droperidol, or other induction agent is administered to increase the likelihood of successful intubation without rendering the patient paralyzed and apneic. Whether RSI or sedation is used, a backup method of securing the airway in case of failed intubation must be prepared. Options for backup include alternative (rescue) airways such as the endotracheal CombiTube® or surgical airway.

Surgical airway options for the patient with maxillofacial trauma include needle cricothyrotomy, surgical cricothyrotomy, and tracheostomy. Severe neck trauma that includes the larynx may result in the deformation of landmarks, effectively excluding cricothyrotomy as an option. In such cases, tracheostomy is the airway of choice.

8. Discuss the assessment and management of the patient with an auditory injury. **p. 482**

The critical care paramedic cannot effectively treat auditory injuries to the middle and inner ear. These often require thorough evaluation and treatment by an otolaryngologist. In cases where injury results in otorrhea or hemorrhage, external application of sterile gauze dressing is warranted, but packing of the external ear canal is not suggested. Care should be taken to ensure that water or other fluids are not allowed to enter the ear canal. Common signs of tympanic membrane rupture include hearing loss and otorrhea.

Case Study

As the helicopter begins its descent toward the landing zone, you think to yourself how much different the place looks without snow. Your team has been called to a remote ski area that you came to know well last winter due to frequent calls for traumatized skiers. There has not been a transfer out of that general area for weeks, so you were surprised that today, a hot day in the middle of August, you received a call for a trauma patient at the top of the ski slope.

Your dispatcher advised you that you would be picking up a worker who has fallen approximately 25 feet from a lift tower to the ground. The patient is a 26-year-old male who is conscious, but who has severe facial injuries. The medics on the ground are finding it nearly impossible to maintain an open airway. You meet the rescue team's medic at the edge of the LZ, and get an update. The patient reportedly slipped while working at the top of the tower, striking a metal cross arm brace on the way to the ground. The fall was witnessed by coworkers and they report a loss of consciousness of approximately 3 minutes. The patient is able to follow most commands and has been hemodynamically stable since the rescue team arrived 15 minutes ago. You are told the patient has severe midfacial injuries and an obvious fracture of the right humerus, but otherwise is without obvious injuries.

Arriving at the patient's side, you introduce yourself. The patient is sitting up, inclined forward on a spine board. He is wearing a cervical collar, leaning on his left arm facing the ground, and intermittently spitting out long strings of blood and saliva. He looks directly up at you for a few seconds when you talk to him, but then returns quickly to the same position in which you found him. When he looks up, you note that his eyes do not seem to line up completely, and that his right eye seems to protrude somewhat. His right, upper lip and infraorbital area have a large stellate laceration and his midface seems sunken. Looking sheepish, the medic from the rescue team tells you that they tried to fully immobilize and package the patient before your arrival, but that the patient could not tolerate being supine. You reassure the team that their care for the patient so far has been just fine. While your partner sets up the intubation equipment, you complete the initial assessment. Although the patient's airway has a large amount of bleeding, loose tissue, and broken teeth, it is adequately maintained in the patient's current position. His respiratory rate is 20 per minute, lungs are clear, and the SpO_2 is 95 percent with blow-by oxygen. There are no tender areas of the chest wall and there is no evidence of trauma. The patient has a strong radial pulse of 116 beats per minute and the cardiac monitor shows a sinus tachycardia. Other than the blood in the oropharynx, there is no sign of external hemorrhage. As your partner works on establishing IV access, you continue your assessment. The patient's pupils are reactive to light, but his right eye is clearly pushed forward and he is unable to follow extraocular movements. Bone is visible through the laceration on his face but there is minimal bleeding. His face has the "dished in" appearance typical of a Le Fort III fracture. You note a small amount of bloody discharge from both nostrils and the left ear. The right arm is immobilized in a vacuum splint and has strong distal pulses. All other extremities are without evidence of significant trauma. The abdomen is soft, nontender, and is without evidence of trauma. The pelvis is stable and nontender.

As you finish your assessment, your partner advises you that she has gotten the patient's consent and is ready to attempt intubation. While the rescue team medic holds the patient's head, you administer etomidate as an induction agent and assist the medic in laying the patient back on the board. The patient struggles to sit up once, but quickly loses consciousness and no longer attempts to rise. You quickly administer succinylcholine as the paralyzing agent, and then take over C-spine stabilization from below, opening the front of the cervical collar while doing so. Once paralysis is complete, your partner makes an attempt at intubation. After suctioning, digitally removing tissue and teeth, and suctioning again, she exclaims, "I see it!" and easily passes the endotracheal tube. After confirming the tube by auscultation and $EtCO_2$ monitor, it is secured with a tube-holding device. Midazolam and vecuronium are administered for continued sedation and paralysis.

As the rescue team finishes packaging the patient, you advise the pilot that you are ready to go. Once back in the aircraft, the patient is placed on the transport ventilator, his wounds are dressed, and IV ceftriaxone is administered for prophylaxis. The flight to the trauma center is uneventful and your patient arrives without change.

DISCUSSION QUESTIONS

1. What are the general assessment and management concerns for patients with facial injuries?
2. What are the general assessment and management concerns for patients with ocular injuries?

Content Review

MULTIPLE CHOICE

_____ 1. Innervation of the face is supplied by:
   A. the facial nerve.
   B. cranial nerves V and VI.
   C. the facial and trigeminal nerves.
   D. cranial nerve VII.

_____ 2. Blood supply to the soft tissues of the face is supplied by:
   A. the facial, ophthalmic, and temporal arteries.
   B. the vertebral and carotid arteries.
   C. the internal carotid artery.
   D. the parotid and salivary arteries.

©2007 Pearson Education, Inc.
Critical Care Paramedic

_____ 3. The facial bones of the skull include the:
   A. facial, vomer, mandible, zygomatic, and lacrimal bones.
   B. lacrimal, zygomatic, palatine, and vomer bones.
   C. parietal, sphenoid, ethmoid, mandible, and zygomatic bones.
   D. maxillary, mandible, zygomatic, nasal, and sphenoid bones.

_____ 4. The three branches of the trigeminal nerve are the:
   A. superior, middle, and inferior divisions.
   B. vestibulocochlear, glossopharyngeal, and trochlear divisions.
   C. anterior, posterior, and lateral divisions.
   D. ophthalmic, maxillary, and mandibular divisions.

_____ 5. The specialized glands that secrete fluid to moisten and lubricate the surface of the eye are the:
   A. lacrimal glands.   C. salivary glands.
   B. parotid glands.   D. lacrimal papillae.

_____ 6. Which of the following statements about the vestibulocochlear complex is false?
   A. It is made up of the vestibular complex and the cochlea.
   B. It consists of the semicircular canals and the cochlea.
   C. It provides information regarding the body's equilibrium and orientation in space.
   D. It is located in the middle ear.

_____ 7. The tympanic membrane:
   A. secretes wax to help protect the external ear.
   B. separates the external ear from the middle ear.
   C. is innervated by CN VII.
   D. connects the middle ear to the pharynx.

_____ 8. The retina:
   A. is the photoreceptive organ of the eye.
   B. controls the diameter of the pupil.
   C. is dependent on the constant washing of lacrimal fluid over its surface.
   D. lies between the sclera and the cornea.

_____ 9. Aqueous humor:
   A. circulates freely between the anterior and posterior cavities through the pupil.
   B. is contained within the anterior chamber.
   C. circulates freely between the anterior and posterior chambers through the pupil.
   D. is contained within the posterior cavity.

_____ 10. The posterior cavity:
   A. encompasses all of the area behind the pupil.
   B. is filled with a clear, gelatinous fluid called vitreous humor.
   C. is divided into the anterior and posterior chambers.
   D. all of the above.

_____ 11. Ocular motility is controlled by _____ extrinsic eye muscles.
   A. 4   C. 6
   B. 5   D. 7

_____ 12. The extrinsic eye muscles are innervated by CNs:
   A. II, IV, and VI.   C. III, IV, and V.
   B. II, III, and IV.   D. III, IV, and VI.

_____ 13. Sense of smell is provided by CN:
   A. I.   C. III.
   B. II.   D. IV.

_____ 14. Which cranial nerve relays sensory information from the proximal one-third of the tongue?
   A. CN III   C. CN VII
   B. CN V   D. CN IX

_____ 15. Blood supply to the anterior nasal cavity is provided by the _____ , and the posterior nasal cavity is supplied by the _____.
   A. anterior olfactory artery, posterior olfactory artery
   B. facial artery, Kesselbach's plexus
   C. ethmoid arteries, sphenopalatine artery
   D. Kesselbach's plexus, ethmoid arteries

_____ 16. In an adult, each dental arch normally contains:
   A. 2 lateral incisors, 2 canines, 2 bicuspids, 4 premolars, and 6 molars.
   B. 2 central incisors, 2 lateral incisors, 2 cuspids, 4 bicuspids, and 6 molars.
   C. 2 anterior incisors, 2 lateral incisors, 2 cuspids, 6 bicuspids, and 6 molars.
   D. 2 incisors, 2 anterior cuspids, 2 lateral cuspids, 4 bicuspids, and 6 molars.

_____ 17. The carotid sheath houses the:
   A. internal jugular vein, common carotid artery, and the vagus nerve.
   B. external jugular vein, external carotid artery, and the vagus nerve.
   C. internal jugular vein, internal carotid artery, and the vagus nerve.
   D. internal jugular vein, internal carotid artery, and the phrenic nerve.

_____ 18. The external jugular vein:
   A. descends superficial to the sternocleidomastoid muscle and drains into the common jugular vein.
   B. drains blood from the brain into the superior vena cava.
   C. runs parallel and posterior to the sternocleidomastoid muscle.
   D. descends superficial to the sternocleidomastoid muscle and drains into the subclavian vein.

_____ 19. Blood supply to the brain is provided by the:
   A. carotid arteries.   C. carotid and vertebral arteries.
   B. vertebral arteries.   D. cranial artery.

_____ 20. The cranial nerves that completely traverse the neck include:
   A. VII and X.   C. VII and IX.
   B. IX and X.   D. IX, X, XI, and XII.

_____ 21. The phrenic nerve originates:
   A. in the brain stem.
   B. from the brachial plexus.
   C. from the cranial nerves I–V.
   D. from the spinal nerves TI–TV.

_____ 22. The platysma is:
   A. a thin muscle that covers the anterior neck.
   B. a fascial layer that covers the anterior neck.
   C. the layer of subcutaneous tissue between the clavicles and mandible.
   D. a spinal nerve that innervates the diaphragm.

_____ 23. Zone I of the anterior neck extends:
   A. from the clavicle to the cricoid cartilage.
   B. from the cricoid cartilage to the angle of the mandible.
   C. from the angle of the mandible to the base of the skull.
   D. from the clavicle to the angle of the mandible.

_____ 24. Zone II of the anterior neck extends:
   A. from the clavicle to the cricoid cartilage.
   B. from the cricoid cartilage to the angle of the mandible.
   C. from the cricoid cartilage to the base of the skull.
   D. from the clavicle to the angle of the mandible.

_____ 25. Zone III of the anterior neck extends:
  A. from the clavicle to the cricoid cartilage.
  B. from the cricoid cartilage to the angle of the mandible.
  C. from the clavicle to the angle of the mandible.
  D. from the angle of the mandible to the base of the skull.

_____ 26. The anterior triangle of the neck is the area bordered by the:
  A. body and clavicular head of the sternocleidomastoid, the mandible, and the trapezius muscle.
  B. body and clavicular head of the sternocleidomastoid, the middle third of the clavicle, and the trapezius muscle.
  C. body and sternal head of the sternocleidomastoid, the mandible, and the midline of the neck.
  D. body and sternal head of the right and left sternocleidomastoid and the mandible.

_____ 27. The carotid arteries, jugular veins, trachea, and lung apices are all present in neck zone(s):
  A. I.   C. I, II, and III.
  B. I and II.   D. II and III.

_____ 28. Infection occurs in approximately what percentage of human bites?
  A. 5 percent   C. 10 percent
  B. 5 to 10 percent   D. 10 to 15 percent

_____ 29. The most commonly fractured facial bones, in descending order, are the:
  A. mandible, zygoma, and supraorbital ridge.
  B. supraorbital ridge, nasal bones, and mandible.
  C. nasal bones, mandible, and zygoma.
  D. nasal bones, zygoma, and mandible.

_____ 30. Fracture of the cribriform plate of which of the following bones can result in basilar skull fracture?
  A. nasal   C. sphenoid
  B. ethmoid   D. temporal

_____ 31. The most common type of zygoma fracture is a:
  A. simple fracture of the arch.   C. bipod fracture.
  B. tripod fracture.   D. complex fracture of the arch.

_____ 32. Temporomandibular joint dislocation occurs when:
  A. the ramus of the mandible disarticulates from the condylar process of the temporal bone.
  B. the body of the mandible disarticulates from the condylar process of the temporal bone.
  C. the coronoid process of the mandible disarticulates from the mandibular process of the temporal bone.
  D. the condylar process of the mandible disarticulates from the mandibular fossae of the temporal bone.

_____ 33. A Le Fort II maxillary fracture can be best described as a fracture that:
  A. extends superiorly through the infraorbital rims to an apex above the bridge of the nose.
  B. includes the zygomatic arches, frontozygomatic suture, sphenoid bone, and nasal bone.
  C. transverses just superior to the apices of the teeth, through the maxillary sinus and across the nasal septum.
  D. extends just superior to the apices of the teeth and forms an apex above the bridge of the nose.

_____ 34. Avulsed teeth can be reimplanted with a high likelihood of success if properly cared for.
  A. True
  B. False

_____ 35. Paralysis of the extraocular muscles, ptosis, and periorbital anesthesia are characteristic of:
     A. apex syndrome.
     B. a blowout fracture.
     C. superior orbital fissure syndrome.
     D. increased intraorbital pressure.

_____ 36. Which of the following syndromes results from insult to the trigeminal and optic nerve?
     A. superior orbital fissure syndrome
     B. Apex syndrome
     C. blowout syndrome
     D. enophthalmos syndrome

_____ 37. The portion of the ear exposed outside the head is the:
     A. external ear canal.
     B. auditory ossicle.
     C. cochlea.
     D. pinna.

_____ 38. Common signs of tympanic membrane rupture include:
     A. hearing loss and rhinorrhea.
     B. muffled hearing and hemorrhagic otorrhea.
     C. basilar skull fracture and rhinorrhea.
     D. hearing loss and otorrhea.

_____ 39. Isolated lid injuries should undergo ophthalmological repair within how many hours of insult?
     A. 6
     B. 12
     C. 14
     D. 48

_____ 40. Rupture of the conjunctival blood vessels can occur secondary to:
     A. traumatic asphyxiation.
     B. coughing.
     C. sneezing.
     D. all of the above.

_____ 41. Diagnosis of corneal abrasion is made:
     A. based on symptoms only.
     B. with fluorescein and illumination with a Wood's lamp.
     C. with a slit lamp.
     D. all of the above.

_____ 42. A hyphema is a:
     A. collection of blood in the anterior chamber.
     B. collection of blood in the anterior cavity.
     C. collection of blood in the posterior cavity.
     D. collection of blood in the posterior chamber.

_____ 43. A hyphema can best be appreciated with the patient positioned:
     A. sitting up.
     B. supine.
     C. prone.
     D. reverse Trendelenburg.

_____ 44. Diagnosis of microhyphema requires:
     A. use of fluorescein and illumination with a Wood's lamp.
     B. laboratory analysis of lacrimal fluid for red blood cells.
     C. use of a slit lamp.
     D. all of the above.

_____ 45. Any patient who experiences acute eye injury while operating heavy machinery should be considered high risk for:
     A. hyphema.
     B. ocular avulsion.
     C. corneal abrasion.
     D. ocular globe injury.

_____ 46. Enucleation is the:
     A. presence of blood in the anterior chamber.
     B. scratching of the corneal surface.
     C. traumatic removal of the ocular globe from the orbit.
     D. detachment of the retina from the neural layer.

_____ 47. Traumatic retinal detachment occurs when:
A. the pigmented layer of the retina separates from the inner neural layer.
B. the photosensitive layer of the retina detaches from the optic nerve.
C. the peripheral layer of the retina separates from the ocular ciliary muscles.
D. the retina fractures.

_____ 48. Retinal detachment can occur when:
A. increased intraocular pressure tears the retina and forces vitreous humor from the posterior chamber into the defect, resulting in a dissection-like injury between layers.
B. adhesions form between the vitreous humor and the retina and mechanical forces within the globe separate the layers of the retina with or without tearing it.
C. blood escapes from damaged vessels, separating and filling the retinal layers.
D. all of the above.

_____ 49. Symptoms of retinal detachment include:
A. ocular pain.   C. hyphema.
B. light flashes.   D. all of the above.

_____ 50. Laceration of the jugular vein can result in _____ as venous pressure drops below atmospheric pressure during deep exhalation.
A. JVD   C. the development of an air embolism
B. pulsus paradoxus   D. hypotension

_____ 51. Injury to vascular structures in the neck can occur secondary to:
A. blunt trauma.   C. hyperflexion.
B. hyperextension.   D. all of the above.

_____ 52. Clinical exam findings of ptosis, facial anhidrosis, and papillary miosis are known collectively as:
A. Horner's syndrome.   C. Cullen's sign.
B. Wernike's syndrome.   D. Apex syndrome.

_____ 53. Clinical findings of neurologic defects, ipsilateral Horner's syndrome, and hematoma formation on the lateral neck are indicative of:
A. spinal cord injury.   C. carotid artery injury.
B. vertebral artery injury.   D. jugular vein injury.

_____ 54. Clinical findings of diplopia, nystagmus, vertigo, dysarthria, and hemiparesis are indicative of:
A. carotid artery injury.   C. jugular vein injury.
B. spinal cord injury.   D. vertebral artery injury.

_____ 55. Injury to all of the following nerves or structures can result in interruption of normal breathing except:
A. CN I.   C. the brachial plexus.
B. the phrenic nerve.   D. the laryngeal nerve.

_____ 56. Injury to the thyroid may result in:
A. thyrotoxicosis.   C. both A and B.
B. severe hemorrhage.   D. none of the above.

_____ 57. Pharyngeal and esophageal injuries are very common and most often the result of blunt force trauma.
A. True
B. False

_____ 58. Radiographic findings consistent with orbital fracture include all of the following except:
A. the "hanging teardrop" sign.
B. the "open bomb-bay door" sign.
C. air/fluid levels in the maxillary sinus.
D. the presence of vitreous humor in the posterior orbital.

_____ 59. The "hanging teardrop" signs on radiograph result from the:
   A. herniation of orbital fat into the maxillary sinus.
   B. displacement of orbital bone into the maxillary sinus.
   C. presence of air in the maxillary sinus.
   D. all of the above.

_____ 60. A radiograph is an adequate imaging modality for the evaluation of a tripod injury to the zygomatic arch.
   A. True
   B. False

_____ 61. The clinical finding of malocclusion is most likely a result of which of the following?
   A. zygoma fracture   C. mandibular fracture
   B. orbital fracture   D. ocular globe injury

_____ 62. When assessing visual acuity, which of the following should be tested first?
   A. uncorrected vision   C. lateral vision
   B. corrected vision   D. none of the above

_____ 63. The use of an ophthalmoscope allows visualization of the:
   A. optic nerve.   C. retina.
   B. macula.   D. all of the above.

_____ 64. Injury to which of the following neck zones can result in pneumothorax?
   A. Zone I   C. Zone III
   B. Zone II   D. None of the above

_____ 65. Which of the following cannot be appreciated on radiograph of the neck?
   A. tracheal injury   C. nerve injury
   B. soft-tissue injury   D. cervical spine injury

_____ 66. Which of the following airway options should be considered in a patient with severe laryngeal trauma that has resulted in the distortion of landmarks, making endotracheal intubation impossible?
   A. needle cricothyrotomy   C. tracheostomy
   B. surgical cricothyrotomy   D. none of the above

Burns and Electrical Injuries

Review of Chapter Objectives

Upon completion of this chapter, the student should be able to:

1. **Describe the epidemiology, including incidence, mortality/morbidity, and risk factors, for thermal burn injuries.** **p. 490**

   The epidemiology, incidence, morbidity, mortality, and risk factors for thermal burn injuries can be summarized in the following bulleted points:

   - Burn injuries: the fourth leading cause of traumatic death (all age groups) in the United States
     - Second leading cause of death in children under 12 years of age
   - 1.25–2 million in United States treated annually
     - 50,000 hospitalized
     - 3 to 5 percent of injuries considered life-threatening
   - 68 percent of burns occur in the home
     - 24 percent in the industrial environment
   - Inhalation injuries present in 20 to 50 percent of patients admitted to burn centers
     - Present in 60 to 70 percent of patients who die in burn centers
   - Those at risk include:
     - Elderly
     - Infirm
     - Young
     - High-risk occupations
   - Extremes of age contribute to morbidity and mortality
     - > 50 years, < 2 years
     - Age in years + percent TBSA burned = Probability of mortality

2. **Describe the effects of heat according to Jackson's theory of thermal wounds.**

   Zone of coagulation **p. 490**
   Suffering the most damage, the zone of coagulation is characterized by the rupture of cell membranes, the denaturing of proteins, and coagulation. The injury is considered a third-degree burn if it penetrates the dermis.

   Zone of stasis **p. 491**
   The zone of stasis surrounds the zone of coagulation, and is an area characterized by decreased blood flow and injured cells that may or may not survive. Tissue necrosis often occurs 24 to 48 hours post burn.

Zone of hyperemia p. 491

The zone of hyperemia is the most peripheral part of the injury, containing injured cells that typically recover within 7 to 10 days. The term "hyperemia" refers to the increased blood flow experienced by this area of the wound.

3. **Describe techniques used to identify and establish priorities for treatment of the burn patient.** p. 493

The initial assessment and management of the burn patient is no different than with any other trauma patient, and follows the ABCDE approach. Emphasis is placed on stopping the burning process immediately, securing the airway, initiating volume replacement therapy (see objective 7), and providing pain control early (see objective 8).

4. **Identify the techniques used for airway management and ventilation support of the burn patient.** p. 493

Advanced airway management should occur early in the burn patient, ideally before or at initial signs of distress. Assessment findings such as stridor, grunting, wheezing, crackles, or tachypnea suggest the need for prompt endotracheal intubation. A procedure unique to burn management, escharotomy, can be used to reverse the decreased compliance created when burned skin loses its elasticity. Escharotomy can be performed on the chest and neck in an effort to assist ventilation. Reduced compliance will result in the need for higher airway pressures in order to provide adequate ventilation, which can be kept to a minimum by increasing respiratory rate and decreasing tidal volume.

5. **Calculate the total percentage of body surface area involved using one or more of the following methods.**

"Rule of nines" (adult and pediatric) p. 497

With the "rule of nines," anatomic regions of the body are divided so that each represents approximately 9 percent of total body surface area (BSA). In the adult, the divisions are:

- Head and neck
- Upper posterior trunk
- Lower posterior trunk
- Upper anterior trunk
- Lower anterior trunk
- Right upper arm
- Left upper arm
- Left posterior leg
- Left anterior leg
- Right posterior leg
- Right anterior leg

The external genitalia represent the remaining 1 percent.

The divisions and percentages for pediatric patients are slightly different, allowing for variations between adult and pediatric anatomy. In the pediatric patient, the divisions and percentages are:

- Upper anterior trunk = 9 percent
- Lower anterior trunk = 9 percent
- Upper posterior trunk = 9 percent
- Lower posterior trunk = 9 percent
- Left leg = 14 percent
- Right leg = 14 percent
- Posterior head/neck = 9 percent
- Anterior head/neck = 9 percent
- External genitalia = 1 percent

"Rule of palms"
p. 497

Also called the "palmer method," this method of measuring the area of a burn is based on the fact that the size of a person's hand is equal to about 1 percent of his TBSA. Comparing the patient's palm size to the burn size can therefore produce an estimate for the total area injured.

Lund and Browder chart
p. 498

The Lund and Browder chart is commonly used in hospitals, and is a more accurate method for determining TBSA injured by a burn. The chart determines BSA burned while accounting for developmental differences in age.

6. Identify and describe the depth classifications of burn injuries.

Superficial burns (first degree)
p. 499

First-degree burns are described as injuries involving only the epidermis, and are characterized with red, inflamed skin that is painful to touch. They generally do not require prehospital interventions, and healing time is usually 5 days with no scarring.

Partial-thickness burns (second degree)
p. 500

Second-degree burns involve injury to both the epidermis and dermis, and are characterized with reddened areas, blisters, or open weeping wounds. They cause significant pain to the patient, as well as significant fluid loss with subsequent hypovolemic shock. Healing time is usually 30 days, with late hypertropic scarring and possibly contracture formation.

Full-thickness burns (third degree)
p. 500

Third-degree burns are described as injury involving the epidermis, dermis, and the subcutaneous tissue, and are characterized by a charred or leathery appearance. They are painless unless associated with second-degree burns that are painful. The patient suffering from third-degree burns will not have any capillary refill to the burned area, and the healing time will be extensive, with significant scarring.

Fourth-degree burns
p. 501

Fourth-degree burns are full-thickness burns that also penetrate the subcutaneous tissue, muscles, fascia, periosteum, or bone. They are usually caused by incineration-type exposure or electrical injury in which the heat is sufficient to destroy tissues below the skin.

7. Describe the various formulas used for burn resuscitation and the techniques required to initiate and monitor fluid resuscitation.
p. 503

The goal of fluid resuscitation in the burn-injured patient is to maintain adequate end-organ perfusion and avoid the complications of under- or overhydration. A Swan-Ganz catheter is useful to help monitor fluid status. There are many different formulas for determining fluid volumes to be administered, and they all emphasize that adequate resuscitation results in normal urine output, 0.5–1.0 mL/kg/hr in the adult and 1.0 mL/kg/hr in the pediatric patient. The most commonly used method for determining the amount of fluid volume to be infused in an adult patient is the Parkland formula. Total fluid to be administered over 24 hours is determined by the formula 4 mL × body weight in kg × percent TBSA burned. Half of the total volume is administered over the first 8 hours, and the remainder is administered over the next 16 hours. The starting point is considered the time of injury, not time of presentation, so it is possible for the patient to be significantly "behind" in fluid volume administration at the time of presentation. Warmed (38°C) crystalloid solutions such as lactated Ringer's or normal saline should be utilized.

Pediatric patients require larger fluid volume administration than do adults, and also require the concomitant administration of glucose. Maintenance fluid requirements for the pediatric patient can be determined as follows, using a glucose-containing solution such as D_5W:

- For the first 10 kg of body weight: 100 mL/kg over 24 hours
- For the second 10 kg of body weight: 50 mL/kg over 24 hours
- For each kg of weight above 20 kg: 20 mL/kg over 24 hours

The administration is titrated to maintain urine output of 1.0 mL/kg/hr.

Other patients who may require additional fluid administration include:

- Patients with associated injuries
- Patients with electrical injuries
- Patients who sustain inhalation injuries
- Patients in whom resuscitation is delayed
- Patients with pre-existing dehydration
- Patients with very deep burns (i.e., fourth degree)

8. Discuss the use of pharmacological agents for the management of pain associated with burn trauma. p. 505

In addition to analgesics, sedatives, such as benzodiazepines, are needed for procedural and background pain in patients who have experienced burn injury. Intravenous narcotic analgesics such as morphine and fentanyl, and benzodiazepines such as Versed, are widely used. In addition, inhaled nitrous oxide can be considered.

9. Describe the three types of airway injuries.

Carbon monoxide poisoning p. 507

Carbon monoxide (CO) interacts with deoxyhemoglobin to form carboxyhemoglobin (COHb) which is unable to carry oxygen. The hemoglobin-CO binding is only slowly reversible, allowing individuals exposed to low levels of CO to accumulate high COHb levels. As such, COHb levels should be determined in all patients who have been exposed to CO, no matter how insignificant the ambient concentrations seem to be. Owing to the fact that CO has an approximately 240 times greater affinity for hemoglobin than oxygen, the half-life of COHb is about 4 to 6 hours. This falls to about 90 minutes with the administration of 100 percent oxygen at 1 atm of pressure, and to about 30 minutes with the administration of 100 percent oxygen at 3 atm of pressure. The dysfunction of hypoxia-sensitive organs such as the brain can occur at CO saturations as low as 15 to 40 percent, and levels of 40 to 60 percent can result in obtundation and coma.

Inhalation injury above the glottis p. 508

Most thermal burns to the airway are confined to the anatomy above the glottis, a result of the effective heat exchanging capacity of the upper airway (remember, the upper airway filters, humidifies, and *warms* inspired air). Chemical burns are also possible. Severe injury can result in airway edema and obstruction, so deterioration should be anticipated. Upper airway edema can evolve over 12 to 24 hours post-injury.

Inhalation injury below the glottis p. 508

Inhalation injuries below the glottis are almost always the result of chemical exposure, though steam inhalation, inhalation of superheated air/smoke, and aspiration of scalding liquids are other possible causes. Lower airway burns result in increased blood flow that promotes edema formation, hypersecretion, bronchospasm, impaired immune defenses, airway mucosal ulcerations, and impaired ciliary activity. In addition, pulmonary edema can develop both secondary to increased pulmonary capillary permeability from the injury and secondary to hypoxia. The amount of damage is unpredictable in the first few hours post-insult, and patients should be closely monitored for up to 24 hours after exposure.

10. Understand why pediatric patients with circumferential burns to the thorax require special ventilatory considerations. p. 509

The eschar formation and loss of elasticity (when collagen burns, it loses its elasticity, shortens its fibers, and becomes rigid) that accompany a circumferential burn to the thorax increases the workload of breathing and can quickly deplete the glycogen stores of the pediatric patient. In such cases, escharotomy should be performed to decrease the work of breathing.

11. **Discuss the basic assessment findings and management findings for the following inhalation injuries.**

Carbon monoxide p. 507

Signs and symptoms of carbon monoxide poisoning include altered mental status, loss of consciousness, elevated carboxyhemoglobin, and hypoxia despite a normal SpO_2 and ABG. SpO_2 is normal because a pulse oximeter cannot tell the difference between O_2 bound to hemoglobin and CO bound to hemoglobin, and an ABG will be normal because CO poisoning does not affect the amount of O_2 dissolved in the serum, which is what an ABG measures. A venous blood sample to determine carboxyhemoglobin percentage—the test measures the percentage of hemoglobin present as carboxyhemoglobin, normal is < 2.5 percent in nonsmokers, and as high as 12 percent in heavy smokers—should be drawn. Management centers around securing an airway, providing ventilation and oxygenation with high-flow, high-concentration oxygen, 100 percent oxygen, and treatment in a hyperbaric chamber.

Supraglottic inhalation injury p. 508

Signs and symptoms of supraglottic inhalation injury include burns to the face, soot in the nares and oropharynx, singed facial hair, and signs of respiratory insult such as stridor, grunting, or tachypnea. Prompt intubation is the treatment of choice (rather than observation or medications) for any patient exhibiting any signs of upper airway deterioration. Prophylactic endotracheal intubation is warranted in those patients undergoing transport who stand an increased likelihood of developing airway-threatening edema. Fiber-optic bronchoscopy is often used to both facilitate intubation and to identify supra- and subglottic injury. 100 percent oxygen should be administered via the appropriate delivery device, and BVM ventilations or mechanical ventilation provided if endotracheal intubation has been performed. Eschar formation on the neck can accentuate pharyngeal edema, worsening the already compromised airway; a vertical escharotomy from the sternum to the chin can aid in maintaining a patent airway.

Subglottic inhalation injury p. 508

Subglottic inhalation injuries secondary to thermal sources will have signs and symptoms identical to supraglottic injury, and will also have lower respiratory signs such as wheezing, crackles, or decreased lung sounds. Like a supraglottic burn injury, a subglottic burn injury can evolve over time periods of up to 24 hours. Airway control decisions should be made early, with error on the side of endotracheal intubation and mechanical ventilation to ensure adequate oxygenation and ventilation. Airway resistance may be increased secondary to edema, debris (shed epithelium, or soot) in the airway, or bronchospasm. The goal of ventilation should be to utilize the lowest airway pressures necessary to provide sufficient ventilation and oxygenation. Airway pressures can be kept to a minimum by slightly increasing respiratory rate and decreasing tidal volume.

12. **Describe the anticipated signs and symptoms as well as management for the following burns.**

Eyes p. 509

Burns to the face should suggest the need for an eye exam as soon as possible (after potential life-threats have been addressed) as swelling of the eyelids may make examination impossible later. An evaluation for corneal injury, utilizing fluorescein, should be performed, and the eyes irrigated with copious amounts of water or saline in cases of chemical burns.

Ears p. 509

The ear canal and tympanic membrane should be examined as soon as possible, as swelling can make the ear canal inaccessible. The tympanic membrane should also be examined in patients that have sustained lightning strike or blast injuries. The ear canal should not be packed nor occlusive dressings applied.

Hands p. 509

In the evaluation of the affected hands, vascular and perfusion status should be performed immediately, and escharotomy performed if eschar is present and perfusion diminished. Evaluation of perfusion, sensory, and motor function should occur frequently to identify evolving injury and swelling. The injured hand should be elevated above the level of the heart to reduce swelling, and bandaging should be avoided so as not to interfere with reassessment or perfusion.

Feet   p. 510
Evaluation of burns to the feet should follow the same guidelines as burns to the hand, with emphasis on assessing perfusion and minimizing swelling.

Genitalia and perineum   p. 510
Foley catheter insertion should occur immediately to facilitate urethral patency in patients with burns involving the penis.

13. **Describe the specific assessment, management, and prognosis of burn patients with the following mechanisms of injury.**

Thermal burns   p. 501
Before clinical examination and treatment of burn injuries can proceed, the caregiver should stop the burning process if it has not already been done, and remove all clothes, belts, and jewelry. Assessment and management of thermal burns have already been covered extensively in objectives 3–11, and an outline of the management is offered in the following text for review. Specific questions regarding the history of the event can help suggest MOIs and direct assessment and care. Did the patient's clothes catch on fire? How long did it take to extinguish the flames? How were the flames extinguished? What was the MOI? Was there an explosion? Was there a house fire? Was there entrapment? See page 495 in the text for a complete list of questions to be considered in a patient with thermal burn wounds. The following laboratory tests are considered standard and should be assessed on every burn patient:

- Hematocrit and hemoglobin
- Electrolytes
- Blood urea nitrate (BUN)
- Urinalysis (UA)
- Chest radiograph
- Arterial blood gas (ABG) analysis

Management of the patient with thermal burns includes:

- Airway control and oxygenation
  - Administration of high-flow, high-concentration oxygen, 100 percent oxygen
  - Recognize the need for endotracheal intubation early
  - Escharatomy of chest and neck may be necessary
  - Ventilation
    - May require increased airway pressures
    - Increasing RR, decreasing TV may help keep pressures low
- Fluid resuscitation
  - Parkland formula
  - Guided by urine output
- Pain control
  - Goal is no pain
  - Generous use of analgesics
- Wound care
  - Prevent infection
  - Prevent hypothermia
- Tetanus immunization

Inhalation injury   p. 507
See objectives 9–11.

©2007 Pearson Education, Inc.
Critical Care Paramedic

Chemical burns to the eyes
p. 514

Chemical burns to the eyes commonly present with obvious burns about the face, swelling, pain, loss of or decreased vision, and spasm of the eyelid. Management consists of irrigation with copious amounts of water or saline. A device such as the Morgan lens or a nasal cannula can be used to limit waste of irrigation fluid and to better direct flow. While irrigating, care should be taken to ensure that runoff does not contaminate the other eye.

Electrical burns
p. 510

Of all burn injuries, electrical injuries can be the most difficult to assess as their small external injuries do not reflect the potential for devastating internal injuries. Questions that should be asked during the history that can aid in the determination of injury severity include: What kind of electricity was involved? What is the estimated voltage? What was the duration of contact? Was the patient thrown/did he fall? Was there loss of consciousness? Was CPR or defibrillation administered on scene?

Signs and symptoms indicating the possibility of significant electrical injury include:

- Loss of consciousness
- Paralysis or mummified extremity
- Loss of peripheral pulse
- Flexor surface burns (especially to antecubital, axillary, inguinal, or popliteal areas)
- Presence of myoglobinuria
- Serum creatine kinase (CK) levels above 1,000 international units
- Superior point of contact injury with very distal exit injuries (i.e., head/feet)

As with all patients, address life threats first in accordance with the ABCs. Cardiac arrest and dysrhythmia is a concern in electrical injury, and standard ACLS guidelines should be followed. Compartment syndrome, if present, should be managed with escharotomy or fasciotomy. Rhabdomyolysis requires the maintenance of an adequate glomerular filtration rate to prevent the glomerular accumulation of myoglobin and renal failure. Fluid administration should be titrated to achieve urine output of 75–100 mL/hr, and the administration of sodium bicarbonate (44 mEq in each L of lactated Ringer's) to maintain pH > 6.0 will aid in the removal of free myoglobin in the blood; alkalinization of the urine increases the solubility of myoglobin in the urine. Mannitol 0.5 mg/kg IV can also be used to promote diuresis.

Chemical burns
p. 513

A history of the event is especially important in chemical burns. Important questions to answer include: What was the agent? How did the exposure occur? What was the duration of contact? What decontamination occurred? Is there a Medical Safety Data Sheet? Was there an explosion?

Hydrofluoric acid burns are treated with copious irrigation and the application of calcium gel. Calcium gel can be created by mixing 1 amp calcium gluconate with 100 gm lubricating jelly. In addition, an IV calcium infusion can be initiated if severe pain persists.

Phenol burns are first treated with copious irrigation, then cleaned with 50 percent polyethylene glycol (PEG) or ethyl alcohol.

Tar burns first require irrigation with cold water to stop thermal burning, then the cooled tar is covered with a petroleum-based ointment and dressed in a manner to promote emulsification of the tar.

Anhydrous ammonia burns require copious irrigation until removal of the chemical odor is achieved.

The management of specific chemical and biological warfare agents cannot be addressed here, but general guidelines include first ensuring personal safety, followed by the isolation of the patient to prevent contamination of additional patients or surfaces. All contaminated clothing should be removed, visible residue brushed off, and copious irrigation used to remove remaining contaminants.

Radiation exposure
p. 516

Non-wartime methods of radiation exposure include exposure to, and contamination by, radioactive sources in laboratory or medical facilities, and industrial accidents. Radon gas, a breakdown product of uranium 238, is a major radiation exposure source for the general public, and is commonly found in basements where it leeches from the surrounding soil.

Acute radiation exposure occurs after whole-body irradiation, and presents after internal or external exposure to radiation over a short period of time. The signs and symptoms associated with radiation are related to the amount of radiation absorbed, expressed in units gray (Gy) or the rad, radiation absorbed dose (1 rad = 0.01 Gy). Mortality is about 50 percent for those patients receiving 4.5 Gy exposures, even with hospitalization and supportive care. The initial indicator of radiation exposure is a decreased absolute lymphocyte count that results from an exposure of about 3 Gy. For exposures greater than 3 Gy, a decreased peripheral granulocyte that reaches its lowest point 8 to 30 days post-exposure is common and diagnostic for this exposure level. With increasing exposure, thrombocytopenia and reticulocytopenia develop. GI symptoms occur in doses above 1 Gy because the higher the dose, the more immediate the onset. Mild nausea and vomiting are common with low doses, protracted nausea and vomiting with higher; the onset of fever and bloody diarrhea are ominous signs, often a harbinger of death. Hematopoietic syndrome can occur after a 2-day to 4-week latent period, and is characterized by leukopenia, thrombocytopenia, increased susceptibility to infection, fever, and petechial rash. CNS abnormalities are common ominous signs and typically occur immediately after exposure, indicating exposures in excess of 20 Gy. Specific signs and symptoms include headache, vertigo, tinnitus, sensory and motor dysfunction, and altered mental status. The combination of severe CNS and GI symptoms is indicative of significant exposure (in excess of 20 Gy) and is always fatal. Burns to the skin associated with penetrating radiation indicate significant exposure, and wound development and progression may be delayed.

Management of radiation exposure initially centers around decontamination and ensuring the safety of caregivers. A thorough history should be performed to ascertain the exact type of exposure and route of entry (internal versus external, whole versus partial body, topical versus inhalation versus ingestion), and the type of radioactive material involved. Patients with GI symptoms should have fluid volume and electrolytes replaced. Antiemetic agents can be administered for nausea but may prove ineffective. A chelating or blocking agent may be administered to prevent the GI absorption of ingested radioactive substances. In addition, the normal therapies for toxic ingestion (activated charcoal, gastric lavage, cathartics) may be useful. Laboratory tests that may be of help in acute cases of radiation exposure include a CBC to ascertain a leukocyte count. For those patients with fatal radiation doses, evidenced by fulminating GI and CNS symptoms, pain management and sedation should be considered to make the patient comfortable. Notifying the receiving facility early is of particular importance, as a predetermined radiation exposure plan will have to be put into effect.

14. Discuss the importance for assessing the concurrent signs of trauma in the burn patient. p. 517

In addition to a history, a full trauma exam should be performed on every burn-injured patient; evaluation of the history and MOI can help direct assessment and management. Circumstances surrounding the events leading to burn injury can include MVCs, falls from a height, explosions, assaults, and suicide attempts. Generally speaking, a burn patient found to be in shock most likely has an additional injury that is resulting in the hemodynamic compromise; shock secondary to burn injury takes time to develop.

15. Define the American Burn Association criteria/guidelines for patients requiring transport/treatment at a designated burn center. p. 517

American Burn Association recommendations for referral to burn center:

* Partial thickness burns greater than 10 percent TBSA
* Any burns involving the face, hands, feet, genitalia, perineum, or major joints
* Full-thickness burns in any age group
* Any electrical burns, including lightning injuries
* Any chemical burns
* Any inhalation burns

- Any pre-existing condition that may complicate management, prolong recovery, or affect mortality
- Any patient who has sustained concomitant trauma in which the burn injury poses the greatest immediate risk
  - If trauma poses the greatest risk then the patient should be evaluated and treated in a trauma center prior to transfer to the burn center's course of action in these patients
  - Burned pediatric patients in hospitals without qualified personnel or equipment to care for the child
  - Burn injury in patients who will require special social, emotional, and/or long-term rehabilitative intervention

16. Decide the proper mode of transportation of the burn patient to the designated burn center.   p. 519

There is no set criteria for determining what mode of transport is appropriate in each case that the health care team may encounter, but general considerations help drive the decision and are consistent with all trauma. For decisions of air versus ground transport, total travel time, pre-hospital time, and distance are factors that should be weighed. Crew configuration of the transport team can help drive the decision, based on the needs of the patient.

17. Discuss potential complications that the critical care paramedic should be cognizant of while transporting the burn patient.   p. 519

Perhaps the most serious complication that can occur during transport is deterioration of the airway. All patients with even the potential for airway burns are strong candidates for prophylactic intubation. All burn patients should receive 100 percent, high-flow oxygen via the appropriate delivery device. All intubated patients should receive $ETCO_2$ monitoring during transport to aid in the quick identification of a misplaced endotracheal tube.

Patients in the fluid-shift phase of the burn response can easily become intravascularly hypovolemic, adding to their hemodynamic instability. As such, the need for circulatory support during transport must be anticipated. Two large-bore IV's, or preferably a central venous catheter, should be placed prior to transport and warm IV fluids available for administration during transport. Fluid administration should be guided by a resuscitation formula, such as the Parkland, and urine output, determined by monitoring of the Foley catheter collection bag.

Burn patients are at increased risk for hypothermia, and efforts must be made to ensure that the patient cabin of the transporting vehicle is adequately heated. Unpressurized aircraft cabins (helicopters) are notorious for their tendencies to get significantly cold. Blankets, swathing, warm IV fluids, and thermal coverings should be considered along with the specific mode of transport to come up with a plan to prevent hypothermia.

It is possible that any pain medications administered prior to transport will wear off during transport. The transport team should anticipate the need for analgesics during transport and assure that they are readily available. Frequent assessment of the patient's pain will assist in assuring that the patient remains pain-free the entire transport.

Patients who have suffered electrical injuries are at high-risk for cardiac dysrhythmia. Ensure that a defibrillator is readily available, and consider monitoring the patient with "hands off" defibrillation pads during transport (if available), especially patients who have exhibited aberrant electrical activity prior to transport. This will not only decrease the time to defibrillation (or cardioversion, if appropriate!), but will allow proper placement of the pads in a non-emergent, more comfortable environment. Placing defibrillation pads on a patient who is secured to a stretcher in the back of a cramped patient compartment of a transport vehicle can prove difficult at times.

Case Study

Your critical care ground transport unit has been called for an ALS intercept of a BLS unit, to a scene call for a patient with burns. The fire department informs you that the patient was working in the basement of an abandoned school building that had a propane gas leak which layered out over the floor. When the patient started the wet/dry vacuum to clean up water from the floor, a spark from the switch must have ignited the gas. This caused a large flash that subsequently burned itself out. The patient extricated himself from the building and was kneeling on the lawn in front of the building when the fire department arrived. You find your patient lying on the stretcher in the back of the ambulance on high-flow, high-concentration oxygen via a nonrebreather mask. A report from the EMT in charge tells you that the patient has first-, second-, and third-degree burns of his face, anterior chest, and abdomen and thighs, as well as both arms and hands. He tells you that the patient's airway has been self-maintained without any evidence of burn trauma, and that he is breathing without difficulty.

You introduce yourself to the patient who is alert and oriented, and complaining of severe pain. The patient's eyebrows are singed, as well as the hair on the front his head. There are no singes, burns, or swelling noted in the patient's airway. You estimate the total body surface area burned to be almost 50 percent. Most of the burns appear to be partial thickness in nature, but at least 5 percent of the burns are full-thickness burns, including those on both hands.

Before your arrival, the BLS crew had removed the patient's clothing and jewelry and had covered him with a stretcher sheet that they soaked with normal saline. Although the patient reports that the pain decreased initially, it has now returned and is worse. Because the patient has critical burns and the nearest burn center is over 100 miles away, you ask your partner to call for one of your service's helicopters while you continue the initial assessment. Lung sounds are clear and the SpO_2 is 96 percent with the high-flow, high-concentration oxygen. A strong radial pulse is palpable at 110 beats per minute, and the cardiac monitor shows sinus tachycardia. Blood pressure is 100/60. The patient is moved to a dry stretcher, and blankets are placed over the wet dressing to preserve body heat and treat for shock. Since the helicopter's ETA is only 12 minutes by this time and the nearest ED is over 15 minutes by ground, you elect to wait on scene. You establish two large-bore IVs, one in each arm, both of which you suture in place. You would prefer to use an area with good access that was not burned, but none is readily available. Using the Parkland formula, you estimate that the patient should receive approximately 1,125 mL/hr of IV fluids during each of the next 8 hours. You program your infusion pump so that each line delivers a rate of 560 mL/hr of normal saline. You also administer 75 micrograms of fentanyl through the IV, which gives the patient significant relief from the pain. Once the helicopter arrives, you give a report to the flight crew and assist in loading the patient. As the aircraft disappears over the horizon, the fire captain asks if you would like to check out the scene. "Of course!" you say as you follow him into the building.

DISCUSSION QUESTIONS

1. What are the priorities for the treatment of burn patients?
2. What are the classifications used to describe burn wounds?
3. What formulas are most often used to estimate the fluid resuscitation requirements for burn patients?

Content Review

MULTIPLE CHOICE

_____ 1. The probability of mortality from a burn injury can be estimated using the formula:
   A. percent TBSA burned + patient's age in years.
   B. (percent TBSA burned ÷ degree of burn) + patient's age in years.
   C. patient's age in years × percent TBSA burned.
   D. (patient's age in years × degree of burn) + percent TBSA burned.

©2007 Pearson Education, Inc.
Critical Care Paramedic

_____ 2. According to Jackson's theory of thermal wounds, the burn zone characterized by limited inflammation and changes in blood flow is called the zone of:
   A. coagulation.
   B. stasis.
   C. hyperemia.
   D. hyphema.

_____ 3. The stage of the body's response to a burn characterized by the introduction of catecholamines into the bloodstream is termed the:
   A. emergent phase.
   B. fluid shift phase.
   C. hypermetabolic phase.
   D. resolution phase.

_____ 4. At which stage of the body's response to a burn is the patient at most risk for tissue edema and hypovolemia?
   A. emergent phase
   B. fluid shift phase
   C. hypermetabolic phase
   D. resolution phase

_____ 5. The increase in capillary permeability following a burn injury results in the leakage of all of the following from the intravascular space to the extravascular space except:
   A. proteins.
   B. electrolytes.
   C. plasma.
   D. blood cells.

_____ 6. Which of the following is the least important when considering a burn patient's medical history?
   A. age
   B. pre-existing disease
   C. family history of burns
   D. tetanus immunization status

_____ 7. According to the "rule of nines", burns covering the right arm, upper anterior and posterior trunk, and head would account for what percentage of TBSA?
   A. 27 percent
   B. 36 percent
   C. 45 percent
   D. none of the above

_____ 8. Which of the following methods for determining TBSA burned is the most accurate in a 6-year-old patient?
   A. rule of nines
   B. rule of palms
   C. Lund and Browder method
   D. Broselow tape

_____ 9. All of the following are major factors that determine the extent of damage from a burn except:
   A. heat source.
   B. temperature of the burning agent.
   C. thickness of the dermis.
   D. blood supply to the area burned.

_____ 10. Which burn results in injury to the dermis and epidermis and is characterized by blisters, reddened areas, and open and weeping wounds?
   A. first degree
   B. second degree
   C. third degree
   D. fourth degree

_____ 11. Which burn results in penetration to the muscles and bone?
   A. first degree
   B. second degree
   C. third degree
   D. fourth degree

_____ 12. Which of the following is of least importance in the initial care of a patient with severe burns?
   A. initiation of fluid volume resuscitation
   B. splinting of accompanying fractures
   C. insertion of a Foley catheter
   D. airway control

_____ 13. Generally speaking, endotracheal intubation should be performed at the earliest suggestion of potential airway compromise.
   A. True
   B. False

_____ 14. Assessment as to the effectiveness of fluid volume resuscitation is determined by:
   A. mean arterial pressure (MAP).
   B. urine output.
   C. level of consciousness.
   D. cardiac output.

_____ 15. How much fluid volume should be administered to a 220-pound, 34-year-old male who has sustained a 20 percent TBSA burn?
   A. 300 mL/hr
   B. 500 mL/hr
   C. 750 mL/hr
   D. 100 mL/hr

_____ 16. Ideally, fluid that is being administered to a burn patient should be warmed to how many degrees prior to administration?
   A. 38°C
   B. 40°C
   C. 43°C
   D. none of the above

_____ 17. Which of the following urine outputs indicates adequate fluid resuscitation for a 220-pound burn patient?
   A. 400 mL/hr
   B. 700 mL/hr
   C. 1,200 mL/hr
   D. none of the above

_____ 18. Which of the following urine outputs indicates adequate fluid resuscitation for a 44-pound pediatric burn patient?
   A. 10 mL/hr
   B. 22 mL/hr
   C. 34 mL/hr
   D. 44 mL/hr

_____ 19. A 20-kg pediatric patient with burns over 10 percent of her body would require the administration of how much _resuscitation_ fluid over 24 hours?
   A. 80 mL
   B. 88 mL
   C. 800 mL
   D. 8,000 mL

_____ 20. A 20-kg pediatric patient with burns over 10 percent of her body would require the administration of how much additional _maintenance_ fluid over 24 hours?
   A. 1,000 mL
   B. 1,250 mL
   C. 1,500 mL
   D. none of the above

_____ 21. All of the following are examples of patients who may require fluid administration beyond the normal recommendations except:
   A. patients with pre-existing cardiac disease.
   B. patients in whom resuscitation is delayed.
   C. patients with fourth-degree burns.
   D. patients with electrical injuries.

_____ 22. The use of wet sterile dressings should only be used in burn wounds less than _____ TBSA because of the risk of _____ .
   A. 5 percent, infection
   B. 10 percent, hypothermia
   C. 20 percent, hypothermia
   D. 10 percent, infection

_____ 23. All of the following are indications for escharotomy except:
   A. circumferential burns.
   B. cyanosis refractory to airway management.
   C. progressive decrease or absence of pulses.
   D. increased airway resistance.

_____ 24. The presence of "cherry red skin" is a common finding in carbon monoxide poisoning.
   A. True
   B. False

_____ 25. Pulse oximetry is a valuable tool in identifying carbon monoxide poisoning.
   A. True
   B. False

_____ 26. The PaO_2 of a patient with carbon monoxide poisoning, as determined by ABG analysis, will be:
A. normal.
B. low.
C. high.
D. any of the above, depending on the severity of the poisoning.

_____ 27. When a person inhales superheated air, the majority of heat exchange will occur in the:
A. pharynx and larynx.   C. mainstem bronchi.
B. trachea.   D. distal airways.

_____ 28. Edema secondary to facial burns can be minimized by:
A. the administration of an anti-inflammatory agent.
B. the administration of a diuretic.
C. the application of cold compresses.
D. elevating the head 30°.

_____ 29. Which of the following statements regarding the management of ocular burns is false?
A. Corneal injury should be evaluated by using fluorescein and a Wood's lamp.
B. Ophthalmic antibiotic ointment may be applied to prevent infection.
C. Steroid ointments may be applied to prevent edema.
D. Water or saline solution should be used to flush the eyes as soon as possible.

_____ 30. The tympanic membrane should be examined in all individuals burned in:
A. an explosion.   C. all of the above.
B. a lightning strike.   D. none of the above.

_____ 31. Burns involving the penis require prompt:
A. pain control.   C. insertion of a Foley catheter.
B. sedation.   D. escharotomy.

_____ 32. All of the following are indications of possible significant electrical burn injury except:
A. loss of consciousness.   C. myoglobinuria.
B. exit wounds on the extremities. D. CK > 1,000 international units.

_____ 33. AC electrical injuries tend to be more severe than DC current injuries.
A. True
B. False

_____ 34. The oxygen-carrying compounds that are released into the bloodstream during tissue destruction are:
A. rhabdomyolysis.   C. hemochromogens.
B. red blood cells.   D. hemoglobins.

_____ 35. Treatment of rhabdomyolysis includes all of the following except:
A. administration of sodium bicarbonate.   C. mannitol.
B. fluid resuscitation.   D. Solu-Medrol.

_____ 36. Categories of chemicals capable of causing cutaneous burns include:
A. alkalis.   C. carbonaceous compounds.
B. acids.   D. organic compounds.

_____ 37. Phenols, petroleum products, and creosote are examples of:
A. alkalis.   C. carbonaceous compounds.
B. acids.   D. organic compounds.

_____ 38. Which of the following lab results would be expected in a patient exposed to highly concentrated hydrofluoric acid?
A. low serum calcium   C. low serum sodium
B. high serum potassium   D. low serum potassium

_____ 39. Specific treatment for hydrofluoric acid burns includes:
  A. application of a petroleum-based ointment.
  B. application of topical calcium gel.
  C. washing of the burn with ethyl alcohol.
  D. application of petroleum gauze.

_____ 40. Specific treatment for phenol burns includes:
  A. application of a petroleum-based ointment.
  B. application of topical calcium gel.
  C. washing of the burn with ethyl alcohol.
  D. application of petroleum gauze.

_____ 41. Anthrax can be successfully treated with the antibiotic:
  A. ciprofloxacin.   C. penicillin.
  B. azrithromycin.   D. vancomycin.

_____ 42. All of the following are American Burn Association criteria for burn center referral except:
  A. the presence of comorbidities such as a history of heart failure.
  B. chemical burns.
  C. inhalation burns.
  D. patients who require special social, emotional, and/or long-term rehabilitative intervention.

_____ 43. Standard initial laboratory tests for burn-injured patients include all of the following except:
  A. an electrolyte panel.   C. ABG.
  B. BUN.   D. a cardiac marker panel.

_____ 44. Which of the following is not considered standard care for a 34-year-old male patient who has suffered 35 percent TBSA burns to his upper body?
  A. endotracheal intubation and mechanical ventilation
  B. fluid volume administration
  C. application of wet, sterile dressings
  D. neuromuscular blockade and sedation

©2007 Pearson Education, Inc.
Critical Care Paramedic

Chapter 19

Principles of Orthopedic Care

Review of Chapter Objectives

Upon completion of this chapter, the student should be able to:

1. **Describe the skeletal anatomy and physiology, using appropriate medical terminology.** p. 523

   The function of the skeletal system includes the provision of structure, the facilitation of movement, and the protection of internal organs. In addition, bone marrow is the site of red blood cell formation as well as a mineral (calcium, phosphorous, sodium, magnesium, carbonate) reservoir that controls mineral homeostasis.

   Bones are classified according to their size and shape; long, short, flat, and irregular bones. Joints are classified as: diarthrosis (movable), amphiarthrosis (slightly movable), or synarthrosis (nonmovable). Diarthrosis joints are further classified as enarthrosis (ball and socket), ginglymus (hinge), arthrodia (gliding), trochoid (pivot), and condyloid (saddle).

   The skeleton is divided into the axial (skull, spinal column, torso, pelvis) and appendicular (appendages). Muscles attached to the skeleton by tendons allow for movement. Ligaments attach bone to bone.

2. **Discuss the primary concerns regarding treatment of orthopedic injuries, including the following:**

   a. **Describe the differences in orthopedic injuries, including fractures, dislocations, and subluxations.** p. 524

      Dislocation is the displacement of a bone from its normal anatomical position. A subluxation is the partial or incomplete dislocation that has returned to its normal anatomical position. A fracture is the breaking of a bone, discussed in more detail in objective 3.

   b. **Describe fractures using current and correct medical definitions.** p. 524

      Fractures are specifically delineated into one of several types:
      - Open: The fractured bone is protruding through the skin—graded using the Gustilo grading system
      - Closed: The fractured bone does not break the skin—graded using the Tscherne method
      - Complete: The bone is broken completely through all layers
      - Incomplete: The fracture line does not extend through the entire bone
      - Displaced: The broken ends of the bone are no longer aligned
      - Greenstick: Part of the bone is broken along the length—most common in children whose bones have not fully calcified
      - Comminuted: The bone is fragmented into several small parts

- Segmental: Two complete fractures of the same bone that result in a free-floating segment
- Butterfly: A small portion of the bone breaks free, but there is no complete fracture
- Spiral: The fracture line extends circumferentially around the bone
- Hairline: A minute fracture, often difficult to see on a radiograph
- Occult: A fracture not visible on simple radiograph
- Epiphyseal: A fracture through the epiphysis of the bone
- Oblique: Breaks in a bone running across it at an angle other than 90 degrees
- Transverse: A break that runs across a bone perpendicular to the bone's long axis
- Fatigue: Breaks in a bone associated with prolonged or repeated stress
- Impacted: Breaks in a bone in which the bone is compressed on itself

c. Briefly discuss the pathophysiology of orthopedic injuries.   **p. 526**

Determining the mechanism of injury (MOI) is useful for anticipating injuries, which can be acute or chronic; acute fractures occur secondary to forceful impact, while chronic stress fractures occur secondary to prolonged introduction of forces. The force necessary to cause injury is dependent on several factors including the bone involved, any other concurrent forces, and any underlying pathology present.

d. Describe and demonstrate the proper assessment of the skeletal system.   **p. 527**

Prior to assessing the skeletal system, an initial assessment should be done first and any problems with the ABCs corrected and potential life-threats treated. The detailed assessment often reveals skeletal injury. The assessment should initially be focused on bones that can result in life-threats such as the femur, pelvis, spine tibia/fibula, and humerus. Signs of injury include deformity, contusions, abrasions, pain, lacerations, swelling, tenderness, instability, and crepitus. Imaging studies that can aid in the identification of skeletal injury include X-ray, CT, and MRI. Evaluation of vascular status can be accomplished by evaluating for the "Six Ps": pain, pallor, paralysis, paresthesia, pressure, and pulses. Sensation can be assessed by applying a light tactile stimulus following the dermatomes, and allowing the patient to report the sensation felt. Motor function can be tested by assuring that the patient can move the injured extremity, so long as doing so will not aggravate the injury. Assessment of reflexes is useful for the neurological evaluation of the unconscious patient; the superficial reflexes are easy for most health care providers to elicit, while the deep tendon reflexes require more practice at ascertaining. An evaluation of existing hardware should be performed. Splints should be checked to ensure that they are not overly constrictive and compromising circulation, and external fixating devices should be checked for tightness, rigidity, and stability. Assess the pin insertion sites for evidence of infection.

e. Discuss the proper treatment of orthopedic injuries.   **p. 530**

The treatment of orthopedic injuries is achieved by one of several methods including splinting, casting, external fixation, internal fixation, and amputation. Splinting, the most basic treatment, is a procedure in which the fractured bone is returned to normal alignment and then secured with a rigid splint. Splinting is used as a temporizing measure—up to 72 hours—until a more permanent solution is determined, such as surgery or casting. Splinting also allows the swelling that accompanies orthopedic injuries to abate somewhat prior to casting.

Casting is the application of a rigid material (typically fiberglass) placed over the realigned extremity. It is more permanent than a splint and is typically used for closed, simple fractures. Casts are usually applied 24 to 36 hours after injury to allow for the reduction of swelling that accompanies orthopedic injuries.

During reduction and realignment, the injury is corrected and the bones placed in normal position; this is a typical procedure for dislocation injuries that is relatively simple though there is great risk of complication if not performed correctly. Sedation and analgesia are required for patient comfort during the procedure.

External fixation is a procedure in which fractured bones are kept in alignment with fixation devices. The fracture is visualized under fluoroscopy, and pins, screws, and rods are inserted through the skin into the bone, fixing it in place. Indications for external fixation include open fractures, closed fractures with significant soft-tissue injury, and fractures complicated by infection.

Internal fixation is similar to external fixation in that reduction is performed and hardware placed, though the procedure is performed during surgery. Indications for internal fixation include displaced fractures, segmented fractures, comminuted fractures, and other complicated cases.

Amputation is considered a radical procedure that is reserved for those cases where repair is not possible, as in extensive trauma.

f. Identify the orthopedic injuries that are most likely to cause hemodynamic instability, and discuss the specific treatment considerations for each. p. 532

Pelvic fractures can result in life-threatening hemorrhage with blood losses of greater than 1,500 mL blood possible; these fractures sometimes remain unidentified until the patient is in stage IV shock. Pelvic fractures are classified according to the Tile Classification System:

- Type A: Stable
- Type B: Rotationally unstable, vertically stable
- Type C: Rotationally and vertically unstable

Pelvic fractures are typically stabilized with a bed sheet wrap, C-Clamp, or MAST in emergency situations.

Great force is required to fracture the femur, which can result in life-threatening hemorrhage of up to 1,500 mL blood. Femur fractures are typically stabilized with devices such as the Hare Traction Splint®, Sager Traction Splint®, Kendrick Traction Device®, MAST, or with rod insertion and gravity-induced traction. The proximal femur is referred to as the hip, and fracture usually requires open reduction and internal fixation: early fixation reduces morbidity and mortality. Hip fractures are usually described as intrascapular or extrascapular and the sub-classifications are as follows:

- Intracapsular fractures
  - Capital fractures
  - Subcapital fractures
  - Transcervical fractures
  - Basicervical
- Extracapsular fractures
  - Trochanteric fractures
  - Intertrochanteric
  - Subtrochanteric

C1 (Atlas) fractures usually result from axial loading of the spinal column. Perhaps unexpectedly, these fractures rarely result in neurological deficits. C1 fractures are commonly described as anterior arch fractures, posterior arch fractures, and Jefferson (burst) fractures. C2 fractures, commonly referred to as "hangman's fracture" (bilateral pedicle fractures to C2) can also occur. There are four types of traumatic spondylolisthesis of C2:

- Type I: Nondisplaced or less than 3 mm of C2/C3 translation, no angulation of the fracture fragments
- Type II: Translation of more than 3 mm with severe angulation and displacement
- Type IIA: Translation of more than 3 mm with severe angulation and no anterior displacement
- Type III: Severe angulation and translation, often with dislocation of the facets of the vertebral body

Other categories of vertebral fractures include avulsion, compression, facet joint, vertebral burst, and teardrop. An avulsion fracture typically occurs at the spinous process, and often requires nothing more than a soft cervical collar for support. Compression fractures occur when axial loading crushes the vertebrae, and treatment varies depending on the severity of the fracture. Facet joint fractures occur as a result of disruption of the supraspinous ligaments, interspinous ligaments, *ligamentum flavum*, and facet capsule. Burst fractures are comminuted fractures of the middle vertebral body, and spinal cord injury can occur secondary to bone fragments penetrating the spinal cord. Teardrop fractures are characterized by a displaced fracture of the antero-inferior corner of the superior vertebral body, segmental disc disruption, posterior ligament injury, and retropulsion of the proximal body into the neural canal. Treatment of burst and teardrop fractures is similar, and controversial. One approach advocates early and prompt reduction of the injury, despite the risk of furthering neurologic injury, while another advocates more detailed, prolonged assessment and performing surgical reduction only if doing so will not worsen any existing neurologic injury.

Thoracic vertebrae fractures have great potential for long-term neurological deficits, and are classified in much the same manner as cervical spine fractures according to the Denis system of fracture classification:

- Axial load injuries including compression and burst fractures
- Flexion-distraction injuries
- Fracture subluxation and/or dislocation

Primary treatment goals are protecting the spinal cord and preventing deformity and instability. The choice of surgical versus nonsurgical treatment depends on several factors including extent of injury, the presence of neurological deficits, cormorbid factors, and resultant deformity.

Owing to the large size of the lumbar vertebrae, the lumbar spine requires significant force to fracture. The Denis system has been extrapolated for use in describing lumbar fractures:

- Type A: involvement of both endplates
- Type B: involvement of the superior endplate
- Type C: involvement of the inferior endplate
- Type D: buckling of the anterior cortex with both endplates intact

Burst fractures of the lumbar spine are possible, though uncommon, and result from extreme hyperflexion of the spine. Treatment depends on the extent and degree of the fracture. Surgical intervention conditions include compromise of the spinal canal greater than 40 percent, kyphosis greater than 25 degrees, and the presence of neurological compromise.

Humerus fractures can result in significant hemorrhage (up to 750 mL of blood loss), and are classified by location and type of fracture (example: proximal oblique). Further classifications include:

- Proximal fractures
  - Nondisplaced
  - Two-part
  - Three-part
  - Four-part
- Distal fractures
  - Single-column
  - Bicolumn

Treatment of humerous fractures ranges from rigid casting for uncomplicated fractures to surgical repair with internal fixation for more severe injuries.

The primary concern in cases of rib fractures is injury to underlying pulmonary, cardiovascular, and abdominal anatomy. Careful evaluation (physical exam, imaging studies, lab studies) is necessary to rule out intrathoracic and abdominal injury. The treatment for the vast majority of rib fractures is limited to analgesia for pain.

In cases of amputation, it is important to remember that life takes precedence over limb and a proper evaluation of ABCs should be done before treatment of the limb is begun. Treatment of amputation involves stopping any active hemorrhaging and preparing the amputated part for transport:

- Clean the stump with Ringer's lactate
- Wrap the stump in moistened sterile gauze
- Place the amputated part in plastic bag

Transport the part in a container filled with ice, but do not place the part directly on the ice. A pulseless extremity can occur as a result of vascular damage secondary to bone fracture or dislocation; reduction or limb realignment may restore circulation. Reduction requires the use of analgesics and muscle relaxants, and requires judgment and skill.

Compartment syndrome is a potential complication of orthopedic injury, resulting from isolated fractures, crush injury, or internal hemorrhage. Injury results in changes in vascular permeability and a shift of fluid from intravascular to interstitial space increases pressure within isolated interfacial compartments. Early signs and symptoms are vague but late signs and symptoms include the "six Ps."

- Pain
- Pallor
- Paralysis

- Pulselessness
- Pressure
- Paresthesia

In the ICU and transport environment, pressure can be monitored via a transducer connected to a catheter placed in the affected compartment. Chronic compartment syndrome can be treated with rest, ice, elevation, nonsteroidal anti-inflammatory drugs, and physical therapy. In more severe, acute cases, surgical intervention is required to release pressure and promote perfusion.

3. Identify and discuss various pharmacologic agents utilized as supportive agents for orthopedic injuries, including antibiotics and analgesics.   **p. 538**

Various pharmacological agents are used to treat the inflammation, pain, infection, and thrombus formation that may accompany orthopedic injuries. Nonsteroidal anti-inflammatory agents (NSAIDs) decrease inflammation and decrease pain secondary to inflammation. Commonly used agents include ibuprofen, naproxen, ketoprofen, ketorolac, and aspirin. Special consideration groups include patients with ASA sensitivity, those with a history of peptic ulcer disease, renal failure/insufficiency, coagulopathies, congestive heart failure, or hypertension, and patients receiving angiotensin-converting enzyme (ACE) inhibitors.

Opiate analgesics are often used in conjunction with NSAIDs. Commonly used agents include morphine, hydrocodone, fentanyl, oxycodone, and hydromorphone. There is a potential for significant side effects with the use of these agents, including respiratory depression, hypotension, nausea and/or vomiting, ileus, sedation, and physical dependency with long-term use.

Antibiotics are used prophylactically in patients at high risk for infection (open fractures, extensive soft-tissue injuries, and multisystem trauma). Commonly used classes of agents include the cephalosporins, penicillins, penicillin derivatives, and sulfonamides. Commonly used agents include amoxicillin, cephalexin, cefazolin, gentamicin, and vancomycin.

Muscle relaxants reduce pain from muscle spasm secondary to fracture, and aid in the reduction of dislocation injuries. Commonly used agents includes Valium, Flexeril, and Soma. Significant side effects that can accompany the administration of muscle relaxants include hypotension, respiratory depression, and sedation.

Deep venous thrombosis (DVT) and pulmonary embolus are potential life-threatening complications of orthopedic injury and the invasive surgical procedures used to repair them. Commonly used anticoagulation agents include warfarin, heparin, low molecular weight heparin, and aspirin. The efficacy of anticoagulation therapy is determined by evaluating lab studies such as PT/PTT and INR.

4. Identify simple orthopedic injuries from radiographic images.   **p. 540**

While an exhaustive review on how to identify specific orthopedic injuries on radiograph is beyond the scope of this chapter, there are several basics in establishing a systematic approach to radiograph interpretation that can aid you in appreciating orthopedic fractures when they are present.

First, determine what body part you are looking at and the perspective shown on the radiograph (anterior-posterior, lateral, and so on). Considering the MOI and your physical exam findings may suggest what injuries you can expect to find, and which would be the highest priority. A systematic approach to the radiograph evaluation will enable the examiner to develop a routine, and ensure a thorough assessment. Observe the bones, noting the smoothness of the contours; any irregularities should raise suspicion for a fracture. The articulating areas of the joints should be assessed. Symmetry should be assessed by comparing both sides of a radiograph, if possible.

Case Study

Your critical care ground transport team has been called to a small, three-bed emergency department in a rural mountain town for the victim of a snowmobiling accident. The patient is being transferred for an orthopedic surgery consult. The physician assistant caring for the 19-year-old female advises you the patient was injured when the snowmobile she was riding slid off the side of a trail and rolled over her, trapping her leg underneath. The patient sustained a closed, midshaft femur fracture of her right leg and an open, midshaft humerus fracture of her right arm. She was wearing a helmet and, other than a few minor abrasions and contusions, the two fractures were the only injuries she sustained. She has received prophylactic IV antibiotics and her right arm was dressed and splinted in the position of function. The right leg is splinted only with pillows, and will need to be immobilized for transport.

The report from the nurse indicates that the patient's vital signs have been stable. The patient has received a total of 10 mg of morphine over the last hour, providing good pain relief. You introduce yourself to the patient and tell her what is likely to occur over the next few hours, advising her of the need to splint her leg. Due to the potential for these injuries to cause significant blood loss, you have your partner hang a liter of normal saline on the IV lock at an initial rate of 150 mL/hr. After applying a Sager® splint with 8 lbs of traction to the right leg, you gently transfer the patient to your stretcher. Although the patient had significant discomfort with splinting and with the move, now that she is settled on your stretcher she reports that her leg actually feels better that it did on the hospital cot. Before covering the patient with blankets, you attach the SpO$_2$ monitor probe to the little toe of the right leg to allow easy assessment of perfusion distal to the injury while en route. The patient receives frequent reassessments and neurovascular checks of her extremities distal to the injuries during transfer. She receives 4 mg of morphine for pain with good relief, but otherwise her condition remains stable and she arrives without change.

DISCUSSION QUESTIONS

1. What are the general assessment and management concerns for patients with orthopedic injuries?
2. What orthopedic injuries are most likely to cause hemodynamic instability, and what specific treatments can be performed to limit this effect?
3. What pharmacologic agents may be used as supportive therapy for orthopedic injuries?

Content Review

MULTIPLE CHOICE

_____ 1. Among older adults, the majority of fractures are caused by:
   A. MVCs.
   B. osteoporosis.
   C. falls.
   D. assaults.

_____ 2. Joints that are classified as movable are termed:
   A. diarthrosis.
   B. amphiarthrosis.
   C. synarthrosis.
   D. none of the above.

_____ 3. Joints that are classified as slightly movable are termed:
   A. amphiarthrosis.
   B. diarthrosis.
   C. synarthrosis.
   D. none of the above.

_____ 4. Joints that are classified as nonmovable are termed:
   A. diarthrosis.
   B. amphiarthrosis.
   C. synarthrosis.
   D. none of the above.

_____ 5. A movable pivot joint is classified as a _____ joint.
   A. condyloid
   B. trochoid
   C. synarthrosis
   D. enarthrosis

_____ 6. A movable hinge joint is classified as a _____ joint.
   A. arthrodia
   B. amphiarthrosis
   C. trochoid
   D. ginglymus

_____ 7. A ball and socket movable joint is classified as a _____ joint.
   A. amphiarthrosis
   B. synarthrosis
   C. enarthrosis
   D. condyloid

_____ 8. Functions of the skeletal system include all of the following except:
   A. production of white blood cells in the bone marrow.
   B. protection of organs.
   C. framework and attachment points for ligaments, tendons, and muscles.
   D. storage for such minerals as calcium, phosphorus, sodium, and magnesium.

_____ 9. The injury that results in the partial dislocation of a bone that spontaneously returns to its proper position is called a:
   A. fracture.
   B. simple fracture.
   C. dislocation.
   D. subluxation.

_____ 10. A fracture in which the bone has fragmented into several parts is termed:
   A. occult.
   B. displaced.
   C. comminuted.
   D. complete.

_____ 11. A fracture that involves the growth plate of a bone is termed:
   A. transverse.
   B. epiphyseal.
   C. greenstick.
   D. fatigue.

_____ 12. A _____ fracture results in a bone whose broken ends are not aligned.
   A. displaced
   B. comminuted
   C. greenstick
   D. complete

_____ 13. An _____ fracture results in fractured bone protruding through the skin.
   A. oblique
   B. impacted
   C. incomplete
   D. open

_____ 14. A fracture in which the bone is compressed on itself is termed a/an _____ fracture.
   A. occult
   B. spiral
   C. comminuted
   D. impacted

_____ 15. All fractures that are the result of gunshots, crushing forces, or agricultural machinery are classified as:
   A. Gustilo Type III.
   B. Tscherne Type II.
   C. Tscherne Type I.
   D. Gustilo Type IV.

_____ 16. The amount of force required to break a bone is determined by:
   A. underlying pathology.
   B. the bone involved.
   C. concurrent forces involved.
   D. all of the above.

_____ 17. The most often utilized imaging study for the identification of orthopedic injury is:
   A. CT.
   B. radiograph.
   C. MRI.
   D. ultrasound.

_____ 18. Which of the following fractures has the least potential for hemodynamic compromise?
   A. femur
   B. pelvis
   C. rib cage
   D. cervical spine

_____ 19. Which of the following is not one of the "6 Ps" that can aid in the evaluation of vascular status?
   A. pallor
   B. priaprism
   C. paresthesia
   D. paralysis

_____ 20. The reflex involving the L4, L5, and S1 spinal segments mediated through the deep peroneal nerve is the:
   A. deep peroneal reflex.
   B. deep tendon reflex.
   C. superficial reflex.
   D. deep reflex.

_____ 21. Dermatomes are:
   A. specific superficial reflexes that correlate with specific spinal nerve roots.
   B. areas of the skin (innervated by sensory nerves) that correlate with specific cranial nerves.
   C. areas of the skin (innervated by sensory nerves) that correlate with specific spinal nerve roots.
   D. specific superficial reflexes that correlate with specific cranial nerve roots.

_____ 22. The fracture classification system that classifies growth plate injuries is the:
   A. epiphysis system.
   B. Gustilo Classification system.
   C. Tscherne Classification system.
   D. Salter-Harris system.

_____ 23. In the Salter-Harris system of classifying growth-plate injuries, the likelihood of a permanent growth-plate deformity:
   A. decreases as the classification number decreases.
   B. increases as the classification number increases.
   C. increases as the classification number decreases.
   D. decreases as the classification number increases.

_____ 24. Splinting of a fracture:
   A. allows for the reduction of swelling prior to casting.
   B. is a temporizing measure only.
   C. all of the above.
   D. none of the above.

_____ 25. Casting of a fracture:
   A. occurs after realignment has peen performed.
   B. is used for simple fractures without infections or soft-tissue injuries.
   C. rarely occurs in the first 24–36 hours.
   D. all of the above.

_____ 26. All reductions are ideally performed after the administration of analgesics and muscle relaxants.
   A. True
   B. False

_____ 27. External fixation:
   A. requires open surgery for the placement of pins, rods, and screws to realign fractured bones.
   B. is indicated in open fractures, some closed fractures, and infected fractures.
   C. involves visualization of the fracture under fluoroscopy to assist in the application of a rigid, supporting framework held in place with pins and screws.
   D. both A and B.

_____ 28. ORIF is an acronym that stands for:
   A. Orthopedic Repair Involving Fluoroscopy.
   B. Open Reduction with Internal Fixation.
   C. Open Reduction Involving Fluoroscopy.
   D. Orthopedic Repair with Internal Fixation.

_____ 29. It is not uncommon for the repair of orthopedic injuries to be delayed for days.
   A. True
   B. False

_____ 30. Pelvic fractures can be classified according to the:
   A. Gustilo Classification system.
   B. Tscherne Classification system.
   C. Tile Classification system.
   D. Salter-Harris system.

_____ 31. Pelvic fractures can be stabilized with all of the following except a:
   A. bed sheet wrap.
   B. C-clamp.
   C. PASG.
   D. Sager splint.

_____ 32. According to the Tile Classification system, a pelvic fracture that is vertically stable but rotationally unstable is considered a:
A. Type A fracture.
B. Type B fracture.
C. Type C fracture.
D. Type D fracture.

_____ 33. Pressure changes associated with aeromedical transport can cause air expansion and possible injury with MAST/PASG and air splints.
A. True
B. False

_____ 34. A fracture to the proximal head of the femur is considered a "hip" fracture.
A. True
B. False

_____ 35. A femur fracture can result in the loss of almost 2,500 mL of blood.
A. True
B. False

_____ 36. The hip is a:
A. ball and socket joint consisting of the antebellum and the proximal femur.
B. ball and socket joint consisting of the acetabulum and the proximal femur.
C. ball and socket joint consisting of the acetabulum and the distal femur.
D. hinge joint consisting of the acetabulum and the proximal femur.

_____ 37. Hip fracture(s):
A. can be described as extracapsular or intracapsular.
B. incidence increases with age and doubles for every decade after age 50.
C. in ambulatory patients require open reduction and internal fixation.
D. all of the above.

_____ 38. A fracture to C1 resulting from a compression force can be described as a:
A. "hangman's fracture."
B. teardrop fracture.
C. Jefferson fracture.
D. all of the above.

_____ 39. Fracture to the C2 vertebral body with no neurologic deficit can be described as a:
A. "hangman's fracture."
B. teardrop fracture.
C. Jefferson fracture.
D. facet dislocation.

_____ 40. Facet joint fractures of the spinal column can occur as a result of disruption of the:
A. supraspinous ligaments.
B. interspinous ligaments.
C. facet capsule.
D. all of the above.

_____ 41. _____ are characterized by retropulsion of the proximal body into the neural canal, segmental disc disruption, posterior ligament injury, and a displaced fracture of the antero-inferior corner of superior vertebral body.
A. Posterior arch fractures
B. Teardrop fractures
C. Jefferson fractures
D. Facet dislocations

_____ 42. The primary imaging modality(ies) for identifying bone fractures include(s):
A. the radiograph.
B. CT.
C. MRI.
D. both A and B.

_____ 43. _____ lumbar spine fractures involve both the superior and inferior endplates.
A. Type I
B. Type II
C. Type III
D. Type IV

_____ 44. The most common humerus fracture seen in children is a:
A. bicolumn fracture.
B. single-column fracture.
C. supracondylar fracture.
D. distal humerus fracture.

_____ 45. The presence of rib fractures should lead to suspicion of concomitant injury to the:
A. lungs.
B. liver.
C. spleen.
D. all of the above.

46. Management of rib fractures most often consists of:
   A. open or closed fixation.
   B. administration of analgesics only.
   C. splinting with a rib belt.
   D. none of the above.

47. Which of the following should be performed first in a patient with an amputated extremity?
   A. initiation of rapid transport to a Level 1 trauma center
   B. assessment and management of airway, breathing, and circulation
   C. placing of the amputated part into a plastic bag and initiation of cooling by placing on ice
   D. placement of a central venous catheter and initiation of fluid volume replacement

48. Management of a pulseless extremity may include:
   A. reduction of a dislocation.
   B. realignment of a fracture.
   C. repositioning of the injured extremity.
   D. all of the above.

49. Easily reduced dislocations include those to the:
   A. elbow.
   B. knee.
   C. cervical vertebrae.
   D. both A and B.

50. Compartment syndrome should be suspected when:
   A. a patient complains of pain, paresthesia, or paralysis in an injured extremity.
   B. a patient complains of pressure or tightness in an injured extremity.
   C. the mechanism of injury results in crush injury, isolated fracture, and internal hemorrhaging in an extremity.
   D. all of the above.

51. NSAIDs administered for orthopedic injuries include:
   A. aspirin.
   B. ketorolac.
   C. oxycodone.
   D. both A and B.

52. The primary goal of NSAID therapy in orthopedic injury is:
   A. pain reduction through anti-inflammatory action.
   B. pain reduction through action at the mu receptors in the brain.
   C. mitigating infection through antimicrobial action.
   D. mitigating infection through anti-inflammatory action.

53. Medication combinations utilized to control pain associated with orthopedic injury include:
   A. antibiotics and NSAIDs.
   B. NSAIDs and muscle relaxants.
   C. NSAIDs and opiates.
   D. opiates and muscle relaxants.

54. Which of the following statements regarding anticoagulant therapy in the management of orthopedic injury is false?
   A. Anticoagulants are utilized to reduce the risk of DVT formation and pulmonary embolis.
   B. Aspirin, warfarin, and heparin are commonly utilized anticoagulants.
   C. PT/PTT and INR studies may be utilized to determine the effectiveness of anticoagulation therapy.
   D. All of the above.

55. A systematic review of a radiograph should include:
   A. determining the quality of articulating areas of joints.
   B. looking for variations in the smoothness and contours of bones.
   C. looking for symmetry between bilateral components.
   D. all of the above.

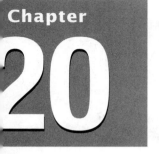

Special Patients: Pediatric, Geriatric, and Obstetrical Trauma

Review of Chapter Objectives

Upon completion of this chapter, the student should be able to:

1. **Discuss and detail the epidemiology of the following:**

   a. **Pediatric trauma patients**   **p. 545**

   The epidemiology of pediatric trauma can be summarized in the following bulleted points:
   - Injuries are the leading cause of death in children over one year of age.
     - Per year:
       - 25,000 deaths
       - 500,000 hospitalizations
       - 30,000 with permanent disability secondary to brain injury
       - 16 million emergency department visits
     - Trauma kills more children than all other diseases combined.
   - Falls are the single most common cause of injury in children
   - Motor vehicle collisions
     - Car-pedestrian
       - High morbidity/mortality
       - MOI differences from adult
     - Car-car
       - When child safety seats are used correctly, they are:
         - 71 percent effective in reducing infant deaths.
         - 54 percent effective in reducing toddler deaths.
   - Drowning and near-drowning
     - Drowning is the third leading cause of death in children between 0 and four years of age
       - 2,000 deaths annually in the United States
     - 20 to 25 percent of near-drowning survivors exhibit neurological deficits.
   - Penetrating injuries
     - Stab wounds and firearm injuries represent 10 to 15 percent of all pediatric trauma admissions.
       - Risk of death increases with age.
     - In the United States, homicide is the leading cause of death for young black males.
   - Burns
     - Leading cause of accidental death in the home for children over 14 years of age
       - About 500 deaths/year
       - 40,000 children injured
     - 70 percent of fire-related deaths occur secondary to smoke inhalation.
     - Scald burns (65 percent) and contact burns (20 percent) are the most common cause of hospitalization for burn-related injuries.

- Physical Abuse
  - 50,000 reports of suspected child abuse or neglect are made to Child Protective Services weekly.
    - An average of 2,450 children per day are found to have been victims of abuse or neglect.
    - In 2002, 2.6 million reports were filed concerning the welfare of about 4.5 million children.
  - In the United States, 4 children die per day as a result of abuse or neglect.

b. Geriatric trauma patients   **p. 565**

The epidemiology of geriatric trauma can be summarized in the following bulleted points:
- 35 million people in the United States are over 65 years of age.
  - The number of elderly has doubled over the past 40 years.
- Presently they represent about 13 percent of the total population
  - This number is expected to rise to 20 percent by 2030.
- The percentage of Americans over age of 85 years is increasing as well.
- Life expectancy is rising.
  - Maximum life span is now 100+ years.

c. Obstetrical trauma patients   **p. 572**

The epidemiology of obstetrical trauma can be summarized in the following bulleted points:
- Obstetric population makes up about 30 percent of EMS calls annually.
- Trauma is the number-one cause of morbidity and mortality in pregnant patients.
  - Accidental injuries occur in 6 to 7 percent of all pregnancies.
  - Penetrating trauma is responsible for 36 percent of all trauma deaths.

2. Examine important aspects of interaction with the critically ill child and family that will enhance interventions.   **p. 547**

Interaction between the health care team and the pediatric patient varies with the age of the patient and the emergency being treated. A consideration of the patient's emotional and physiological development is an important component of care, and a patient's family or caregivers should be considered part of the decision-making team.

The treatment of the pediatric patient begins with communication and psychological support that starts with your initial introduction and continues throughout transport and arrival at the receiving facility. For infants and toddlers, the parents will be the primary source of information for young patients, while older children are a capable source of information. In order to facilitate communication with, and a feeling of support in, your pediatric patient, the following guidelines should be followed:

- Treat all pediatric patients with respect.
- Allow pediatric patients to express opinions and ask questions.
- Listen.
- Understand that there are many methods of communication including:
  - Touch
  - Voice
  - Expression

Fear is a common response to injury for patients of any age, especially pediatric patients. It is important that as a health care provider you are familiar with the common fears and concerns of specific patient populations so that you are better able to alleviate fear, and in some cases, prevent it. Common fears of children include:

- Fear of being separated from the parents or caregivers
- Fear of being removed from a family place, such as the home, and never returning
- Fear of being hurt
- Fear of being mutilated or disfigured
- Fear of the unknown

To assist in helping a patient to understand the situation and procedures, use language and terminology that is appropriate for the patient's age, but be careful not to use "baby talk" with older children, who may be offended.

It is just as important to consider the concerns and fears of the parents or caregivers as it is those of the patient, and calming and informing the parents can often have as much of a calming effect on the situation as does calming and informing the patient. Suggested guidelines for communicating with parents or caregivers are as follows:

- Tell them your name and qualifications.
- Acknowledge their fears and concerns.
- Reassure them that it is all right to feel the way they do.
- Redirect their energies toward helping you care for the child.
- Remain calm and appear in control of the transport.
- Keep the parents or caregivers informed as to what you are doing.
- Don't "talk down" to them.
- Assure parents or caregivers that everything possible is being done for their child.

Allow one family member to travel with the patient, if the situation and mode of transport permit.

3. Analyze development aspects that necessitate the modification of physical assessment parameters and intervention techniques for the pediatric patient. p. 549

Children pass through many developmental stages on the way to adulthood, and your approach to the pediatric patient should be tailored to the patient's developmental level.

Newborns (first hours after birth) can be assessed using the APGAR scoring system, and treatment follows the inverted pyramid of care and the guidelines established by the Neonatal Advanced Life Support (NALS) curriculum.

Neonates (birth to one month) lose, then regain, about 10 percent of body weight in the first ten days of extrauterine life. Development during this stage centers around reflexes, and personality development also occurs. Common problems during the neonatal period include: jaundice, vomiting, respiratory distress, meningitis, and fever of unknown origin. Direct communication with the patient is impossible, but the neonate may respond to the mother or father, and may stare and smile at faces. The patient history is best obtained from the primary caregiver, and observation is important to pick up subtle clues as to patient disposition. The general approach to neonates includes keeping the patient warm, observing closely, and auscultating lung sounds early and/or when the patient is calm. Comfort techniques include having the caregiver hold the child and allowing the patient to use a pacifier.

Infants (one to five months) typically double their birth weight by five to six months of age. Development of muscle control occurs in a cephalocaudal direction, and the infants can follow the movements of others with their eyes. Their personality centers around caregivers. Common problems with this developmental group include: SIDS, vomiting, dehydration, meningitis, child abuse, and household accidents. Direct communication with the patient is similar to that of the neonate—impossible—but the infants may also respond to the mother or father, and may stare and smile at faces. The history is best obtained from the primary caregiver, and observation is important to pick up subtle clues as to patient disposition.

The general approach to the infant patient includes keeping the patient warm, close observation for subtle clues as to disposition, and opportunistic auscultation of lung sounds. Comfort techniques mirror those of the neonate; have the primary caregiver hold the child and encourage the use of a pacifier.

Infants in the age group of six to twelve months may stand or walk with assistance and are active, exploring their world with vigor. Their personality is more sophisticated, and they are able to readily express themselves and often exhibit anxiety toward strangers. Common problems during this developmental period include: FBAO, febrile seizures, meningitis, vomiting, diarrhea, dehydration, bronchiolitis, croup, airway obstructions, injuries from motor vehicle accidents, falls, child abuse, and poisoning. Again, the patient history is best obtained from the primary caregiver, and observation is important to pick up subtle clues as to patient disposition. During care, effort should be made to keep the patient warm, and to allow the patient time to become familiar with you, while sitting in the lap of a caregiver, if possible (though unlikely in the critical care setting). On conscious patients, perform a toe-to-head exam to acclimate the patient to the procedure. Avoid staring at the patient's face, if possible.

Toddlers (one to three years) experience great strides in gross motor development, and, as a result, always seem to be on the move. They tend to be braver, more curious, and stubborn, and will stray away from caregivers when comfortable, but will cling to the caregiver, if frightened. Language development begins, but toddlers are often better able to understand than to speak. Common problems include: febrile seizures, meningitis, vomiting, diarrhea, dehydration, bronchiolitis, croup, airway obstructions, injuries from motor vehicle accidents, falls, child abuse, and poisoning. While the majority of patient history is obtained from the caregiver, simple information may be obtainable from the toddler if you speak softly and ask simple, specific questions. Approach the patient slowly, and gain his confidence if the situation permits. Perform the physical exam in a toe-to-head order, and offer transitional objects, such as a blanket or toy, to ease stress. Whenever possible, avoid procedures on the dominant hand.

Preschoolers (three to five years) experience an increase in gross and fine motor development, and their language skills increase greatly, though they will refuse to speak if frightened. They have vivid imaginations, quick tempers, and a fear of mutilation. Common problems include: croup, asthma, epiglottitis, poisoning, ingestion of foreign bodies, injuries from motor vehicle accidents, burns, child abuse, drowning, febrile seizures, and meningitis. Most of the history will be obtained through communication with the patient; although the preschooler is able to provide information, his imagination and a distorted sense of time may interfere with facts. The general approach to patient care is to avoid baby talk, and avoid tricking or lying to the patient. Give the child choices, and involve the patient in the exam, whenever possible. The exam should start with the chest and end with the head.

School-age children (six to 12 years) tend to be active, and growth spurts can lead to clumsiness and injury. They are protective and proud of parents, and seek their attention. They value their peers, but also require familial support. Common problems include: drowning, bicycle accidents, falls, sports injuries, injuries from motor vehicle accidents, fractures, child abuse, and burns. School-aged children can provide history, though they may not want to incriminate themselves. During the physical exam, it is important to respect the patient's modesty and communicate honestly and openly.

Adolescence (13 to 18 years) begins with puberty at about age 13 for the male and 11 for the female. Adolescents can be physically similar to adults, and tend to be "body conscious" and concerned with physical appearance. They have a strong desire to be liked by their peers, and relationships with caregivers may be strained. Common problems include: mononucleosis, asthma, pregnancy, injuries from motor vehicle accidents, sports injuries, drug and alcohol problems, suicide gestures, and sexual abuse. Communication with the patient should be adequate enough to get a full and complete history; adolescents are good historians, though their perceptions may differ from those of their caregivers. Interview them away from their peers and parents, respect their privacy and modesty, and have the physical exam provided by a same-sex provider, if possible.

4. **Identify the components of the initial patient assessment that can be done during a visual examination of the pediatric patient.** p. 553

Elements to consider when forming a general impression include:

- Skin color
- Quality of cry or speech
- Interaction with surroundings
- Emotional state
- Response to the transport team
- Body tone and positioning

5. **List the pertinent information that the critical care paramedic should obtain from the sending facility regarding special patients.** p. 552

Pertinent information that should be obtained from the receiving facility includes, but is not limited to:

- Nature of illness/injury
- History of present illness

- Presence of fever
- Effects of illness/injury on patient behavior
- Bowel/bladder habits
- Urination frequency and output
- Presence of vomiting/diarrhea
- Treatment provided
- Effectiveness of treatment provided
- Nurse/physician notes
- Lab values
- Imaging studies
- Ventilator settings
- Transfer orders

6. Identify goals of therapy that maximize oxygen delivery and minimize oxygen demand in the pediatric patient.   **p. 554**

Proper positioning of the pediatric patient will help maintain a patent airway and maximize ventilation efficacy and oxygen delivery. Assure that the head is in line with the cervical spine, so as not to kink the narrow airway. A towel or other padding placed under the shoulders will help neutralize the hyperflexion and subsequent airway occlusion that occurs in children as a result of their large occiput. Use of BLS airway adjuncts such as an OPA or NPA will help remove the tongue (relatively large in the pediatric oropharynx) as a potential airway obstruction. In addition to BLS maneuvers, anxiety is a major source of increased oxygen demand, and anxiolytics or sedation may be appropriate to reduce stress and minimize oxygen demand.

7. Discuss the difference between oxygenation and ventilation.   **p. 555**

Oxygenation is a term used to describe the process of moving oxygen across the alveolar-capillary membrane and delivering it to the peripheral tissues. A pulse oximeter, which measures the percentage of hemoglobin bound to oxygen in the peripheral tissue, is used as a measuring device for the effectiveness of attempts at oxygenation. In addition, PO_2 can be measured to determine the effectiveness of oxygenation. Ventilation is the act of moving air into and out of the lungs, and the effectiveness of ventilation can be determined by assessing PCO_2 or $ETCO_2$; if ventilation is adequate, PCO_2 levels are normal; if inadequate, PCO_2 levels rise. As such, adequate ventilation can be thought of as ventilation that results in maintenance of a PCO_2 between 35–45 mmHg in a healthy person. It is important to realize that adequate oxygenation can occur with inadequate ventilation (especially with the administration of high flow 100 percent oxygen), resulting in an adequate pulse oximetry reading, but an accumulation of arterial carbon dioxide. For this reason, the ideal situation in all ventilated patients would be monitoring oxygenation via pulse oximetry and ventilation with $ETCO_2$, assuring that proper oxygenation *and* ventilation are being provided.

8. Identify normal values pertaining to the pediatric patient for the following:

a. Vital signs for infants and children   **p. 557**

Normal Pulse Rates (beats/min, at rest)

Newborn	100 to 180
Infant (0–5 months)	100 to 160
Infant (6–12 months)	100 to 160
Toddler (1–3 years)	80 to 110
Preschooler (3–5 years)	70 to 110
School Age (6–10 years)	65 to 110
Early Adolescence (11–14 years)	60 to 90

Normal Respiration Rates (breaths/min, at rest)

Newborn	30 to 60
Infant (0–5 months)	30 to 60
Infant (6–12 months)	30 to 60
Toddler (1–3 years)	24 to 40
Preschooler (3–5 years)	22 to 34
School Age (6–10 years)	18 to 30
Early Adolescence (11–14 years)	12 to 26

Normal Blood Pressure Ranges (mmHg, at rest)

	Systolic	*Diastolic*
Preschooler (3–5 years)	Average 98 (78 to 116)	Average 65
School Age (6–10 years)	Average 105 (80 to 122)	Average 69
Early Adolescence (11–14 years)	Average 114 (88 to 140)	Average 76

b. Continuous intracranial pressure   **p. 562**

Normal ICP ranges from 4–15 mmHg, with trends being more important than isolated values.

9. Discuss and apply the modified GCS for infants.   **p. 558**

Glasgow Coma Scale			
	> 1 year	*< 1 year*	
Eyes Opening	4 Spontaneously 3 To verbal command 2 To pain 1 No response	Spontaneously To shout To pain No response	
	> 1 year	*< 1 year*	

Best Motor Response	6 Obeys
	5 Localizes pain
	4 Flexion-withdrawal
	3 Flexion-abnormal
	  (decorticate rigidity)
	2 Extension
	  (decerebrate rigidity)
	1 No response
		Localizes pain
		Flexion-normal
		Flexion-abnormal
		  (decorticate rigidity)
		Extension
		  (decerebrate rigidity)
		No response	

	> 5 years	*2–5 years*	*0–23 months*

Best Verbal Response	5 Oriented and
	  converses
	4 Disoriented and
	  converses
	3 Inappropriate
	  words
	2 Incomprehensible
	  sounds
	1 No response
		Appropriate words
		  and phrases
		Inappropriate
		  words and phrases
		Cries and/or screams
		
		Grunts
		
		No response
			Smiles, coos, cries
			  appropriately
			
			Cries
			Inappropriate crying
			  and/or screaming
			Grunts
			
			No response

10. Identify the three components that influence the rise in intracranial pressure.   **p. 562**

The three influences on intracranial pressure are:

- Brain volume
- Blood volume
- Cerebrospinal fluid volume

11. Identify actions that are recommended to reestablish chest tube patency. p. 563

The following actions are recommended to reestablish chest tube patency:

- Attempt to alleviate the obstruction by repositioning the patient.
- If the clot is visible in the chest tube, straighten the tubing between the chest and drainage unit and raise the proximal end of the tube to enhance the effect of gravity.

12. Discuss system pathophysiology and organ system decline as it pertains to the geriatric patient in relation to the:

a. Respiratory system p. 566

Marked change begins after age 60. Pulmonary circulation is reduced by 33 percent, decreasing the amount of gas exchange at the alveolar-capillary membrane. A 50 percent reduction of tidal volume occurs secondary to reduced chest wall excursion and loss of muscle flexibility. Maximum respiratory capacity is reduced by up to 60 percent, and maximum oxygen uptake is reduced by up to 70 percent.

b. Cardiovascular system p. 567

Cardiac output is reduced by as much as 50 percent secondary to decreased heart rate and stroke volume. Additional factors such as medications, chronic dehydration, previous cardiac events, and increased systemic vascular resistance can also contribute to reduced cardiac output.

c. Renal system p. 568

A decrease in functioning nephrons of up to 40 percent, and a 50 percent decrease in renal blood flow can result in disruption of electrolyte balance, fluid balance, and blood pressure.

d. Nervous system p. 568

The aging process can result in the loss of up to 45 percent of brain cells because of injury, disease, or episodes of poor perfusion resulting in ischemia. The peripheral nervous system can suffer a loss of electrical conductivity along the nerve, resulting in a slowing of reaction time and a reduction in sensory function.

e. Musculoskeletal system p. 568

Degenerative diseases can affect bone, ligaments, cartilage, muscles, and the neuromuscular junction, making mobility difficult. It is not uncommon for the elderly to lose up to 35 percent of their muscle mass, and the loss of skin elasticity and the ability to repair the skin is greatly inhibited. Osteoporosis is manifest in the late 60s.

13. Discuss age-related changes in sensation in the elderly. p. 567

Age-related changes in sensation occur as a result of the degeneration of sensory and motor nerve fibers in the peripheral nervous system secondary to normal changes with aging and neuromuscular disease. Generally speaking, nerve impulse velocity decreases as a result of peripheral nerve demyelination. Recall that myelin is a lipid "wrapping" of insulation that surrounds a nerve and increases conduction velocity through that nerve (and, as lipids appear white, myelin is what makes the "white matter" of the brain, white). A decrease in myelin results in a decrease in conduction velocity from the peripheral nerves. As a result, sensory input such as sight, hearing, smell, taste, and pain are reduced.

In addition to the peripheral nervous system, changes to the central nervous system (CNS) can affect sensation, as well. Simply put, changes in mental functioning and CNS performance can add to the problems associated with a degradation of the peripheral nervous system described above. These changes include:

- Decreased blood flow to the brain
- Changes in the synaptic organization of the brain
- Decreased neurotransmitter production
- Accumulation of abnormal intracellular deposits
- Reduction in the total number of neurons
- Decreased size, weight, and volume of the cerebral cortex

14. Discuss considerations in trauma care of the elderly patient. p. 568

The elderly are at increased risk of trauma; contributing factors include: attenuating of reflexes, failing eyesight and hearing, and tissue fragility (skin, muscle, and bone). The geriatric population has an increased risk of head injury due to diminished brain volume resulting in a greater space between skull and brain tissue. Specifically, there is an increased risk of cerebral parenchymal injury and hemorrhage.

Cervical spine injury risk can be increased with osteoporosis, arthritic changes, and spondylolysis. Trauma care considerations for the elderly patient include:

- Past medical history that may have contributed to the traumatic event
- Careful monitoring of fluid administration
- Hypotension and hypovolemia are both very poorly tolerated
- Kidneys cannot compensate for fluid changes
- Organs are less tolerant of hypoxia and anoxia
- Airway management must be early and aggressive
- Possible need to modify immobilization to accommodate deformities

15. Discuss transport considerations and management of:

a. Pediatric patients p. 561

One of the first considerations regarding pediatric transport is the decision whether to utilize a specialized pediatric team or a general critical care transport team. A pediatric transport team would obviously be able to offer the highest level of care for the pediatric patient, but may not be immediately available or even logistically feasible because of distance. On the other hand, a general critical care transport service, while readily available, may lack the expertise with the pediatric population needed to effectively and efficiently care for the unstable or complicated pediatric patient. So, the advantage a transporting facility gains in the availability of a general critical care transport service may be offset by the inability of that service to provide adequate, specialized, pediatric care.

If transport is not a specialized pediatric transport team, the critical care team must ensure that they have all appropriate diagnostic and management equipment needed for all age groups, and the intimate knowledge to operate and troubleshoot such equipment. In addition, the crew must be familiar with the normal variations in lab values, diagnostic information, and vital signs of the various age groups, and have a resource, such as a color-coded resuscitation tape or reference guide, available for immediate referral.

Management considerations include airway maintenance and ventilation, fluid requirements, thermoregulation, blood glucose levels, nutritional requirements, and emotional care of the patient and family. Differences in airway anatomy place specific, well-known demands on the transport team with regard to airway control. Infants and children have the ability to sustain an increased respiratory rate for extended periods of time without fatigue, but when they do fatigue, they do so quickly. Therefore, decisions about definitive airway maintenance should be made prior to transport to avoid the additional difficulties of endotracheal intubation during transport. Ventilation parameters must be carefully determined and closely monitored to prevent barotrauma. Pediatric patients have a greater risk of dehydration; mechanisms of fluid loss include insensible loss via respiration, sweating, fever, shivering, and loss through the urine and stool, especially diarrhea. To establish fluid homeostasis, fluid intake must balance fluid loss; the insertion of a Foley catheter and monitoring of urine output will assist in establishing equilibrium. The transport team should strive for a urine output of no less than 1 mL/kg/hr. It is well established that early, aggressive, fluid resuscitation improves outcome in the pediatric patient with hypovolemic shock. In addition, neonates, infants, and children will require the administration of maintenance fluids based on body weight. IV access can be achieved via umbilical catheterization in neonates, by peripheral or central vasculature routes in older infants and children.

Inattention to thermoregulation can lead to both hypo- as well as hyperthermia, both of which can lead to increased fluid loss; hypothermia secondary to increased metabolic rate secondary to shivering, and hyperthermia secondary to sweating and increased metabolism.

©2007 Pearson Education, Inc.
Critical Care Paramedic

Transport personnel should strive to protect the patient from extremes in temperature; a neutral thermal environment is most desirable. Neonates are at particular risk of hypothermia as, while they are efficient at nonshivering methods of thermogenesis, they are unable to shiver and unable to voluntarily increase muscle activity to create heat, unable to increase metabolic rate, and inefficient at shunting blood from the periphery to their core. As such, they require particular attention with regard to thermal status.

All neonates require glucose administration during transport, as do most young pediatric patients. This can be achieved via the administration of glucose-containing solutions. In all infants at risk of hypoglycemia, blood glucose levels should be checked at least every two hours. The nutritional demands of the critically ill, pediatric and neonatal patient are complex, and determinations will be made by the transporting physician. Nutrition is preferred and is provided via the enteral rather than parenteral route, through a gastrointestinal tube. Drip feedings tend to be better tolerated than bolus feedings. A decision should be made prior to transport as to whether or not feeding will continue during transport.

Special attention should be given to the pediatric patient and his family to alleviate the emotional strain that often accompanies critical injuries or illness. Care should be taken by the transport team to gain the trust of the patient and the family. Specific emotional care of the patient is largely guided by the situation and the patient's developmental stage. Family members should be kept abreast of the current situation, provided all pertinent information, given the opportunity to ask questions and receive honest answers, and accompany the patient should circumstances allow it.

b. Geriatric patients   **p. 571**

Priorities of care in the elderly population are the same as for all other age groups, though one must consider age-related changes to the cardiovascular, respiratory, and renal systems that may affect care. Previous cardiac insults may contribute to hemodynamic instability in the geriatric, trauma patient secondary to decreased compensatory mechanisms. Higher than normal pressures may be required to ensure adequate perfusion of peripheral tissues and organs, though caution with fluid administration is required, as both hypo- and hypervolemia are poorly tolerated.

Respiratory changes that affect management of the elderly include decreased chest wall movement and vital capacity, and an increased incidence of pulmonary disease that can complicate trauma, decrease respiratory reserve, and increase the risk of barotrauma secondary to air trapping. In addition, dentures must be removed prior to airway management to prevent air compromise or obstruction.

Changes in the renal system result in a decreased ability to maintain acid/base and fluid balance. There is a risk of fluid overload, pulmonary edema, and the accumulation of toxins and medications.

During transport of the elderly patient, consider modifying positioning and immobilization to account for physical deformities accompanying advanced age. Special attention should also be paid to thermoregulation. Proper skin care for the elderly includes positioning and padding to prevent pressure necrosis, tearing, and bruising of skin.

c. Obstetrical patients   **p. 575**

The obstetrical patient should be transported in a position of comfort unless she is hypotensive, in which case she should be placed in a left lateral recumbent position at 20 to 30 degrees. This position should also be utilized in stable patients in whom supine hypotensive syndrome is appreciated. Hemodynamic monitoring is useful to determine fluid volume status, and restriction of fluids and/or administration of diuretics may be necessary when fluid volume overload or pulmonary edema is present.

16. Identify and discuss the physiological changes during pregnancy.   **p. 573**

The developing fetus is dependent on the maternal organ systems for the provision of nourishment and oxygen and the removal of metabolic waste. This places a significant strain on the mother, especially in the third trimester, and compensatory changes take place in maternal physiology. Systems affected in pregnancy include the cardiovascular, respiratory, reproductive, gastrointestinal, and urinary systems.

Changes in the cardiovascular and respiratory systems occur because the mother is, for all practical purposes, pumping blood, and breathing, for two. Blood flow to the placenta and uterus greatly reduces the volume available for systemic maternal circulation. In addition, fetal metabolism results in a decrease in the maternal PO_2 and an increase in PCO_2. As a result, renin and erythropoietin production increases, resulting in an increased blood volume and red blood cell production. Volume increase is more pronounced than red blood cell increase, resulting in the dilutional edema common in pregnancy. Toward the end of gestation, maternal blood volume has increased by 45 to 50 percent, resulting in an increased resting heart rate and increased cardiac output, and flow murmurs that may be appreciated on auscultation. In addition, slight decreases in peripheral vascular resistance result in a slight decrease in blood pressure during the first and second trimesters, which rises to prepregnancy levels during the third trimester, and intravascular fluid shifts into the intracellular space in dependent areas, especially the limbs, resulting in edema.

Although not a true physiological change, a transient decrease in venous return to the heart and subsequent hypotension can occur when the gravid uterus compresses the inferior vena cava (IVC), most often when the pregnant female is laid supine. This condition, supine hypotensive syndrome, can be avoided by placing the pregnant female in a left lateral recumbent position during transport, allowing the gravid uterus to displace to the left and away from the IVC located to the right of the spinal column.

Changes in blood chemistry also occur in the gravid female. Pregnancy results in a hypercoagulable state, secondary to an increase of clotting factors and a decrease in fibrinolytic activity, and an increase in platelet activation and venous stasis. As such, pregnant women have two components of Virchows triad, hypercoagulability and venous stasis. As a result, a pregnant female has an increased risk of DVT formation and a five-fold increase in risk of venous thromboembolism, which is the most common cause of maternal mortality in the United States. Trauma to a pregnant female provides the third component of Virchow's triad, vascular injury, further increasing the risk of thromboembolism. Other changes to blood chemistry include a decrease in hematocrit and an increase in WBC count.

A number of changes in the maternal respiratory system meet the increased needs for oxygen delivery and CO_2 removal. Maternal oxygen demand increases during pregnancy, and a 10 to 20 percent increase in O_2 consumption is typical. To help meet this demand, progesterone secretion results in the weakening of costal cartilage, allowing greater movement of the ribcage and a 35 to 40 percent increase in tidal volume. In addition, a mild increase in respiratory rate occurs; this, together with the increase in tidal volume, results in an increased minute volume. As a result, a mild, compensated respiratory alkalosis is often present, creating a greater CO_2 gradient between fetal and maternal circulation and greater CO_2 diffusion between the two.

For the critical care paramedic, the most obvious and significant change in the obstetric patient is the change in the reproductive system that occurs in the uterus. For the first 14 weeks of pregnancy, estrogen and progesterone influence uterine enlargement, after which time, the developing fetus stretches and enlarges the uterus to its full-gestational size of about 30 cm in length, 1,000 g in weight, and 5 L in volume. Considering that the nongravid uterus has a length of about 7.5 cm, a weight of about 60 g, and volume of 10 mL, this represents an enormous increase in both size and volume. By the end of gestation, the uterus receives about 15 percent of the maternal blood volume. Obviously, any insult to the uterus can result in significant, if not fatal, maternal blood loss.

The increased size of the uterus results in the compression and displacement of the abdominal organs, making the assessment of the abdomen challenging. In addition, peristalsis is slowed, delaying gastric emptying and making bloating and constipation common. Maternal nutritional requirements increase 10 to 30 percent during pregnancy as a result of fetal metabolic demands.

As a result of the increase in maternal blood volume and renal blood flow, glomerular filtration rate (GFR) increases by about 50 percent, accelerating the renal excretion of fetal metabolic waste. As a result of increased GFR, glucose may not be sufficiently reabsorbed in the proximal tubule, and subsequently, excreted in the urine. The resulting glucosuria may be normal, and not indicative of the development of gestational diabetes; as such, urine glucose is a poor indicator

©2007 Pearson Education, Inc.
Critical Care Paramedic

of serum glucose levels in a pregnant patient, and blood glucose levels should be obtained for a better appreciation of glucose control. Another consequence of increased GFR is a slight reduction in serum creatinine and BUN. Increased GFR, along with uterine compression of the bladder, results in increased urinary frequency in the gravid female.

17. Identify the most common post-traumatic condition that the critical care paramedic might encounter. p. 573

Placental separation after trauma (abrupto placentae) occurs in 1 to 5 percent of minor accidents and in up to 20 to 35 percent of major injuries. It is second only to the death of the mother as the most common cause of fetal demise. Maternal mortality from abruption is less than 1 percent, but fetal death ranges from 20 to 35 percent.

18. Discuss the effects of disruption of normal uterine and fetal physiology during critical care transport. p. 573

Uteroplacental insufficiency during transport will result in insult to fetal hemodynamic instability and will be evidenced by late or variable decelerations, accelerations in the absence of fetal movement, an absence of regular short- and long-term variability, and long-term changes in fetal heart rate baseline. Chapter 27 covers these issues in depth, and should be reviewed by the student.

Case Studies

Case #1

Your critical care ground transport unit has been called to an ALS intercept of a BLS ambulance. A seven-year-old boy was struck by a sport utility vehicle backing out of a driveway, and his abdomen was run over by the rear tire. He presents fully immobilized in the back of the ambulance. He is holding his abdomen, which is distended and has a large, linear, reddish purple patch over the majority of it. The child is conscious, crying loudly and incessantly, and does not follow commands. The child was in the care of a babysitter who is now hysterical. Local law enforcement is working with her to try to contact the parents. The EMT in charge tells you that he can't get any vital signs, with the exception of an apical pulse of 155 beats per minute.

Case #2

Your team has been activated for a scene call in which an elderly couple is entrapped in a compact car that left the road and struck a concrete drainage culvert. The driver was dead on arrival of EMS and his 80-year-old wife is just being extricated as you arrive. She denies any loss of consciousness. She complains of chest pain and pain in her left side. She reports a history of hypertension, for which she takes metoprolol, but denies any other medical history. Her chest wall is nontender with full equal breath sounds, but her abdomen is soft and diffusely tender. Her vital signs are respirations 20, heart rate 64, and blood pressure 94/60.

Case #3

Your critical care ground transport unit has been called to a small, rural emergency department for an OB transfer to the regional medical center. The patient is an 18-year-old, G_3P_2, at 28 weeks gestation, who was kicked in the lower abdomen by her boyfriend during a domestic dispute. She has mild tenderness of her uterine fundus and complains of crampy, lower abdominal pain. She has no vaginal bleeding or discharge, and fetal heart tones are heard at a rate of 144 beats per minute. Her respirations are 24, heart rate 100, and blood pressure 98/77. She presents lying supine on the ED stretcher.

DISCUSSION QUESTIONS

1. For each of the cases presented, discuss the unique challenges to the assessment and management of traumatic injuries presented by that particular special population.

Content Review

MULTIPLE CHOICE

_____ 1. According to the National Pediatric Trauma Registry, which of the following is the most common cause of injury in children?
A. bicycling accidents   C. MVCs
B. falls   D. auto-pedestrian accidents

_____ 2. Used correctly, child safety seats are _____ effective in reducing infant deaths in passenger cars.
A. 27 percent   C. 71 percent
B. 54 percent   D. 97 percent

_____ 3. The leading cause of accidental death in the home for children under 14 years of age is:
A. a fall from a height.   C. a burn injury.
B. physical abuse.   D. asphyxiation.

_____ 4. Resuscitation of a newborn:
A. follows the inverted pyramid and guidelines established in the neonatal advanced life support curriculum.
B. centers around airway control, oxygenation, and ventilation.
C. may include providing chest compressions.
D. includes all of the above.

_____ 5. A newborn with peripheral cyanosis, a pulse of 90 bpm, a slow and irregular respiratory pattern, and who has spontaneous movement and grimaces when stimulated would have which APGAR score?
A. 4   C. 6
B. 5   D. 7

_____ 6. A 22 kg neonate can be expected to lose 2 kg of birth weight by the end of his first month.
A. True
B. False

_____ 7. The same 22 kg neonate can be expected to weigh 44 kg by 6 months of age.
A. True
B. False

_____ 8. Muscle control in an infant develops in which direction?
A. from the extremities to the trunk   C. from head to tail
B. from the trunk to the extremities   D. from tail to head

_____ 9. Risk of foreign body airway obstruction first becomes significant in which developmental stage?
A. neonate   C. infant (6–12 months)
B. infant (1–5 months)   D. toddler

_____ 10. Significant motor development occurs during which developmental stage?
A. infant (1–5 months)   C. toddler
B. infant (6–12 months)   D. preschoolers

©2007 Pearson Education, Inc.
Critical Care Paramedic

_____ 11. During which developmental stage can a caregiver expect a patient to answer simple and specific questions?
A. infant (1–5 months)
B. infant (6–12 months)
C. toddler
D. preschoolers

_____ 12. The developmental stage at which a patient can be expected to be able to adequately provide his history is:
A. preschooler.
B. school age.
C. adolescent.
D. teenager.

_____ 13. The onset of puberty occurs about the age of _____ for females and age _____ for males.
A. 7, 13
B. 11, 13
C. 13, 18
D. 11, 18

_____ 14. Issues such as drug and alcohol abuse, suicide, and sexual abuse occur more frequently in which developmental stage?
A. preschooler
B. school age
C. adolescent
D. teenager

_____ 15. The three components of the pediatric assessment triangle include all of the following except:
A. mental status.
B. general appearance.
C. work of breathing.
D. circulation.

_____ 16. According to the pediatric assessment triangle, all of the following are elements to consider when forming an initial assessment of a pediatric patient except:
A. skin color.
B. interaction with surroundings.
C. emotional state.
D. auscultation of lung sounds.

_____ 17. Which of the following statements regarding the pediatric patient's airway is true?
A. The thyroid cartilage is the narrowest part of the upper airway.
B. A smaller, airway diameter results in less resistance to airflow during periods of airway edema.
C. The relatively large, pediatric tongue can be a cause of airway obstruction.
D. A large, frontal region on the pediatric skull can make opening the airway difficult.

_____ 18. Which of the following is a sign of inadequate oxygenation?
A. cyanosis
B. low SpO_2
C. altered mental status
D. all of the above

_____ 19. When auscultating the lungs of a pediatric patient, the stethoscope should be placed at the _____ to minimize transmitted breath sounds.
A. axillary area
B. nipple line
C. mid-clavicular line
D. suprascapular area

_____ 20. Tachypnea in the pediatric patient can indicate:
A. inadequate oxygenation.
B. fear.
C. pain.
D. all of the above.

_____ 21. _____ is the sound heard when an infant attempts to keep the alveoli open by building backpressure during expiration.
A. Stridor
B. Grunting
C. Apnea
D. Wheezing

_____ 22. Evaluation of breathing in the pediatric patient includes the assessment of:
A. skin color.
B. respiratory rate.
C. respiratory effort.
D. all of the above.

_____ 23. Urine output less than _____ in a pediatric patient is an indicator of poor renal perfusion.
A. 1 mL/kg/hr
B. 2 mL/kg/hr
C. 3 mL/kg/hr
D. 4 mL/kg/hr

_____ **24.** According to the pediatric Glasgow Coma Scale, a 6-month-old patient who opens her eyes and exhibits decorticate rigidity to pain and grunts during your exam would be scored a/an:

A. 5.
B. 6.

C. 7.
D. 8.

_____ **25.** According to the pediatric Glasgow Coma Scale, a 4-year-old patient who opens his eyes to verbal stimuli, localizes pain, and uses inappropriate words when communicating would be scored a/an:

A. 11.
B. 12.

C. 13.
D. 14.

_____ **26.** Because of the increased compliance of the pediatric chest wall:

A. blunt force trauma commonly results in fractured ribs.
B. tension pneumothorax occurs more frequently in children than in adults.
C. severe intrathoracic injury can be present without external signs of injury.
D. all of the above.

_____ **27.** The most commonly injured organ in children secondary to blunt trauma is the:

A. spleen.
B. liver.

C. lung.
D. heart.

_____ **28.** Intra-abdominal organ injury most often requires surgical intervention.

A. True
B. False

_____ **29.** A 2-year-old patient, weighing 15 kg, has been ejected from a car during an MVC rollover. You note that he is unconscious, requires an oral airway to keep his airway patent, and has a radial pulse with a BP of 90 mmHg by palpation. Physical exam reveals a contusion on his head, a penetrating chest injury, and a closed radius/ulna fracture. Using the pediatric trauma score for this patient would result in a score of:

A. 3.
B. 4.

C. 5.
D. 6.

_____ **30.** The number of American people reaching the age of 65 has been increasing because:

A. the mean survival rate of old persons is increasing.
B. medical care, nutrition, and disease control have improved since World War II.
C. there has been an absence of major wars and other catastrophes.
D. all of the above.

_____ **31.** It is estimated that by the year 2040, _____ of the population will be aged 65 or older.

A. 10 percent
B. 15 percent

C. 20 percent
D. 25 percent

_____ **32.** Age-related changes in the structure and function of organs:

A. modifies the threshold at which signs and symptoms of insult appear.
B. can affect the assessment and treatment of the elderly patient.
C. increases the probably of disease.
D. all of the above.

_____ **33.** Changes in the respiratory system that occur with age include all of the following except:

A. decreased tidal volume and increased respiratory rate that create a chronic respiratory alkalosis.
B. pulmonary circulation that is reduced by about 33 percent.
C. tidal volume that is reduced by as much as 50 percent.
D. reduced chest wall excursion and loss of muscle flexibility that leads to reduced tidal volume.

_____ 34. As a result of the normal cardiovascular changes associated with aging:
  A. hypotension is common.
  B. there is a greater risk of myocardial ischemia and stroke.
  C. there is less of a risk of significant bleeding from wounds.
  D. all of the above.

_____ 35. The aging process results in a number of changes to cardiovascular hemodynamic parameters including:
  A. afterload.   C. cardiac output.
  B. heart rate.   D. all of the above.

_____ 36. Cardiac output may be reduced in an elderly patient due to:
  A. decreased preload secondary to electrical conduction delays.
  B. decreased myocardial contractility secondary to a past MI.
  C. decreased afterload secondary to hypertension.
  D. all of the above.

_____ 37. Which of the following statements regarding renal function in elderly patients is false?
  A. Elderly patients can experience a 30 to 40 percent decrease in functioning nephrons.
  B. Renal blood flow can decrease as much as 50 percent in elderly patients.
  C. Elderly patients develop compensatory mechanisms to aid in the elimination of metabolic waste when renal function decreases.
  D. A direct result of decreased renal blood flow is electrolyte imbalance.

_____ 38. Elderly patients may lose up to 45 percent of their brain cells secondary to:
  A. disease.   C. intracellular plaque accumulation.
  B. strokes.   D. all of the above.

_____ 39. _____ is a disease characterized by decreased bone mass and deterioration of the bone microarchitecture.
  A. Osteoporosis   C. Arthritis
  B. Osteoarthritis   D. Acromegaly

_____ 40. Elderly patients are at increased risk of injury from trauma because of:
  A. decreased pain sensation.   C. fragile bones and tissues.
  B. slower reflexes.   D. all of the above.

_____ 41. Fluid administration should be carefully monitored in elderly patients because:
  A. hypotension and hypovolemia are poorly tolerated.
  B. the kidneys may not adequately compensate for fluid volume changes.
  C. hypervolemia may contribute to hypertension.
  D. both A and B.

_____ 42. During pregnancy, a mother's heart rate normally increases by about:
  A. 10 bpm.   C. 20 bpm.
  B. 15 bpm.   D. 25 bpm.

_____ 43. Cardiovascular changes that normally occur in the pregnant female include all of the following except:
  A. increased cardiac output.   C. increased heart rate.
  B. increased hematocrit.   D. hemodilution.

_____ 44. The onset of the signs and symptoms of shock can be delayed in pregnant females because of the _____ that normally occurs during pregnancy.
  A. hypervolemia   C. respiratory alkalosis
  B. tachycardia   D. hemodilution

_____ 45. Which of the following arterial blood gas analysis (ABG) abnormalities can be expected to be present in a female patient who is 30 weeks pregnant?
  A. mild respiratory alkalosis   C. decreased serum creatinine and BUN
  B. mild respiratory acidosis   D. mild metabolic acidosis

_____ 46. Which of the following physiological changes of pregnancy prevents the accumulation of metabolic waste as a result of an increase in baseline metabolic activity of the fetus and mother?
A. increased circulating blood volume
B. increased glomerular filtration rate
C. increased cardiac output
D. increased respiratory rate

_____ 47. Inferior vena cava syndrome (also known as supine hypotensive syndrome) can occur during the second and third trimesters, and results from:
A. hemodilution.
B. hemorrhage resulting in greater than 40 percent blood loss.
C. compression of the inferior vena cava by the gravid uterus.
D. the patient lying flat.

_____ 48. The pregnant female is at increased risk of deep venous thrombosis formation and pulmonary embolis secondary to:
A. the state of hypercoagulability that normally accompanies pregnancy.
B. disseminated intravascular coagulation.
C. the increase in circulating blood volume.
D. all of the above.

_____ 49. Which of the following lab values is not representative for what would be expected in a healthy, pregnant female?
A. PO_2 = 98 percent
B. PCO_2 = 35 percent
C. negative D-Dimer assay
D. all of the above

_____ 50. Which of the following is not an ECG change that is considered normal during pregnancy?
A. flat T waves in III, V_1, and V_2
B. inverted T waves in III, V_1, and V_2
C. Q waves in III and aV_F
D. Q waves in II and aV_R

_____ 51. The normal range for a fetal heart rate is:
A. 100–140 bpm.
B. 120–140 bpm.
C. 120–160 bpm.
D. 100–160 bpm.

_____ 52. Any fetus of _____ or greater weeks' gestation requires monitoring after a traumatic event.
A. 22
B. 23
C. 24
D. 25

_____ 53. Inferior vena cava syndrome can be corrected by:
A. tilting the patient 20 to 30° to the left.
B. manually displacing the uterus.
C. administering a fluid challenge.
D. both A and B.

©2007 Pearson Education, Inc.
Critical Care Paramedic

21 Pulmonary Emergencies

Review of Chapter Objectives

Upon completion of this chapter, the student should be able to:

1. Describe basic pulmonary anatomy and physiology.   p. 580

The respiratory system can be divided into the upper and lower airways, with the glottic opening being the transition between the two. In addition, the respiratory system can be considered in terms of function and divided into the conducting zone and the respiratory zone; the conducting zone extends from the entrance of the nasal and oral cavities to the terminal bronchioles of the lungs, and the respiratory zone, from the respiratory bronchioles to the individual alveoli, the functional unit of the lung and the site of gas exchange. The conducting zone, due to its lack of alveoli and inability to exchange gas, constitutes the anatomic dead space of the airway.

Although not a structure specific to the upper airway, the respiratory epithelium is a unique tissue structure that lines most of the respiratory tree. This specialized respiratory epithelium consists of goblet and psuedostratified, ciliated, columnar epithelial cells that line the respiratory tract in the nasal cavity, and extend from the trachea through the alveolar ducts. Goblet cells produce and secrete mucus that covers the exposed respiratory lumen. Cilia in the nasopharynx and lower respiratory tract sweep particulate material into the pharynx. This combination of goblet cells and ciliated epithelium form the mucociliary escalator.

The upper airway's primary function is to filter, warm, and humidify inspired, atmospheric air. Filtering is achieved by the coarse hairs that pack the nasal vestibule and extend across the external nares. Warming and humidification are accomplished by the nasal conchae (or turbinates), located in the nasal cavity, whose structure creates turbulent airflow over their warm, moist, mucus-covered surfaces.

The nose, mouth, and throat are all connected posteriorly by the pharynx, which is divided into the nasopharynx, oropharynx, and laryngopharynx. Occasionally, the term, hypopharynx, is used to describe the inferior portion of the pharynx, corresponding to the height of the epiglottis. Components of both the respiratory and the gastrointestinal tracts share the pharynx.

The larynx is a protective structure enclosing the glottis, which also serves as a filtering device of sorts; the epiglottis directs food into the esophagus and inspired air is allowed to enter the trachea via the glottic opening, or glottis. The larynx extends between the level of vertebrae C4 and C6. Three cartilaginous structures form the larynx: the thyroid cartilage, cricoid cartilage, and the epiglottis. Additional small cartilages located to the posterior surface of the larynx include two cuneiform cartilages, two corniculate cartilages, and two arytenoid cartilages.

The thyroid cartilage is the largest of the three; it forms the anterior and lateral walls of the larynx and is open posteriorly. It is commonly referred to as the Adam's apple. The cricoid cartilage is located inferior to the thyroid cartilage and attaches to the thyroid by means of the cricothyroid (or intrinsic) ligament. Unlike the thyroid cartilage, the cricoid is complete posteriorly. The inferior cricoid attaches to the first cartilaginous ring of the trachea via the cricotracheal (or extrinsic) ligament. The epiglottis has ligamentous attachments to the thyroid cartilage inferiorly and the hyoid bone superiorly; it covers the glottis during swallowing. Additional structures in the larynx include the arytenoids, corniculate and cuneiform cartilages, the vocal cords, and the glottis.

The trachea begins at about the level of C5–C6, and extends about 11 cm to its terminus at the carina, where it divides into the right and left main stem bronchi. It is a moderately flexible tube whose anterior and lateral walls consist of numerous C-shaped cartilaginous rings connected by intercartilaginous ,or annular, ligaments. This construction prevents the trachea from collapsing or overexpanding secondary to airway pressure changes. The posterior wall of the trachea is made up of a layer of smooth muscle termed the trachealis.

The trachea bifurcates at the carina to form the right and left mainstem, or primary, bronchi. Each primary bronchus enters the lung, along with the pulmonary vessels, lymph vessels, and nerves, through the hilus. Like the trachea, the primary bronchi are held open by cartilaginous rings.

The primary bronchi, after entering the lungs, divide to form the secondary bronchi and the tertiary bronchi, which have progressively lesser amounts of cartilaginous support. This cartilaginous support ends at the level of the terminal bronchi, and the first smooth muscle starts to appear in the walls of the terminal bronchioles, allowing autonomic control of the terminal bronchiole lumen diameter. Terminal bronchioles divide to form respiratory bronchioles, so named for the individual alveoli that start to appear on their outer wall. Respiratory bronchioles give way to alveolar ducts, alveolar sacs, and then, individual alveoli, the site of gas exchange in the lung.

The lungs contain approximately 300 million individual alveoli, each of which is almost completely enveloped in pulmonary capillaries. Gas exchange takes place across the alveolar-capillary membrane, which consists of three layers: the alveolar epithelial cell, the capillary endothelial cell, and the fused basil lamina of each in the interstitial space between them. At this level, the total distance separating the alveolar and capillary lumens is between 0.1 to 0.5 μm, allowing gas exchange to take place rapidly.

Three types of cells are present in the alveoli; Type I pneumocytes, Type II pneumocytes, and alveolar macrophages. The alveolar epithelium is made up primarily of a single layer of Type I alveolar cells; these cells are the ones that allow gas exchange. Interspersed among the Type I cells are Type II surfactant-producing cells. Pulmonary surfactant consists of an assortment of phospholipids that serve to decrease the surface tension of water in the alveoli, preventing alveolar collapse and atelectasis. Phagocytic alveolar macrophages roam the alveolar epithelium surface, cleaning up debris, such as dust or bacteria, which elude the respiratory defenses.

The lungs are located in the pleural cavity of the thorax, with the base of each resting on the diaphragm, and the apex of each extending superior to Zone 1 of the neck immediately superior to the first rib. The lungs are divided into distinct lobes separated by fissures; the left lung has two lobes, and the right lung, three. On the left lung, the oblique fissure separates the lung's superior and inferior lobes. On the right, larger lung, the horizontal fissure separates the superior and middle lobes, while the oblique fissure separates the middle and inferior lobes. The connective tissue of the root penetrates each lung into the parenchyma, branching often to divide each lobe into smaller and smaller compartments, called lobules. Each lobule receives a tributary of the bronchial tree, pulmonary artery, and pulmonary vein.

Each lung is covered with visceral pleura, which reflects with the parietal pleura which adheres to the inside surface of the chest wall. The pleura are serous membranes, that secrete pleural fluid to provide lubrication between the lung and chest wall as the two surfaces move over one another during the respiratory cycle. In addition, the pleural fluid helps to bind the two pleura together via the hydrostatic attraction of water molecules in the fluid. This attraction, along with the normal elasticity of the pulmonary tissue, creates a negative pressure between the two pleural layers (and also keeps the lung "attached" to the inside surface of the chest wall).

The pulmonary arteries enter the lungs at the hilus and branch with the bronchial tree so that each lobule receives its own pulmonary artery and vein. The pulmonary vein divides further to form the pulmonary capillaries, which surround and cover the alveolus. Gas exchange takes place across the alveolar-capillary membrane, and blood returns to the left atrium via the pulmonary venules and vein. In addition to their role in gas exchange, the pulmonary capillaries are the site of production of angiotensin-converting enzyme (ACE). The bronchial arteries supply arterial blood to the tissues of the bronchial tree, and venous blood flows into the pulmonary veins, mixing with the oxygen-rich blood leaving the alveoli and returning the left ventricle.

2. Define acute respiratory failure.   p. 588

Acute respiratory failure (ARF) can be defined as a state of inadequate gas exchange, and occurs when the respiratory system is unable to absorb oxygen and/or excrete carbon dioxide. ARF occurs as a result of many etiologies and may be the patient's primary problem, or as a secondary result of an existing disease process. ARF differs from chronic respiratory failure (CRF) in that it develops rapidly, not allowing adequate time for the normal compensatory mechanisms to alleviate the insult. However, ARF and CRF are not mutually exclusive of one another; ARF frequently develops as an exacerbation of a preexisting respiratory condition.

While ARF can be suspected based on purely clinical findings, the best method of diagnosing ARF is arterial blood gas (ABG) analysis. It is generally accepted that ARF exists when the following values exist on room air:

- $PaO_2 < 60$ mmHg
- $PaCO_2 > 50$ mmHg
- pH < 7.3

ARF can be categorized as a failure of oxygenation resulting in hypoxemia, a failure of ventilation resulting in hypercapnia, or both.

3. Discuss and differentiate the pathology of common respiratory diseases seen in the critical care environment.

a. Asthma   p. 597

Asthma is a chronic, inflammatory disorder of the lower airways characterized by hyper-responsiveness of the airways to various stimuli, inflammation and edema of the airways, and increased mucus production. Although this disorder is commonly reversible with proper medications, during the asthmatic episode these three pathophysiological changes serve to decrease the bronchiole lumen diameter, making it difficult for ventilation of the alveoli, and for gas exchange to take place. The airway inflammation accompanying asthma may be acute or chronic, and an acute episode usually follows a two-phased response. When an antigen is inhaled and presents in the lower airway, sensitized IgE antibodies trigger mast-cell degranulation in the airway submucosa, resulting in the release of chemical mediators. The release of these chemicals results in an inflammatory response that includes immediate bronchoconstriction and developing submucosal edema, vascular congestion, mucus production, and impaired mucociliary clearance. This first phase of an asthma attack typically occurs within the first 90 minutes of the introduction of an antigen. The second phase occurs about 3–4 hours later, and occurs secondary to invasion of the submucosa by eosinophils, platelets, lymphocytes, and leukocytes. These immune cells contribute further chemical factors that promote additional, sustained inflammation, mucus production, and edema. Chronic inflammation results in persistent submucosal cell damage and repair, resulting in microscopic airway changes including basement membrane thickening, hypertrophied airway smooth muscle, microvascular leakage, epithelial disruption, and increased numbers of goblet cells. Gross changes include the formation of mucus plugs in the large and small airways containing mucus, cellular debris, and immune cells.

Signs and symptoms include:
- Wheezing, tachypnea, dyspnea, cough
- Tachycardia, chest tightness
- Hyper-resonance to percussion, pulsus paradoxus
- Head bobbing, paradoxical breathing, combativeness, and altered mental status should be considered ominous signs, indicating that respiratory failure is imminent.

Labs and imaging:
- Continuous waveform capnography: "shark fin" appearance
- ECG: sinus tachycardia, right ventricular strain, right axis deviation, or early R-wave progression
- Spirometry: changes in PEFR and FEV_1
- Chest radiograph: may show hyperinflation of the lung fields, focal atelectasis, or appear normal

- ABG:
  - Acute asthma: $PaCO_2$ slightly lowered
  - Severe asthma: $PaCO_2$ elevated, $PaO_2 < 60$ mmHg
  - CBC: increased eosinophil count, leukocytosis may be present

b. Chronic obstructive pulmonary disease   p. 605

Chronic obstructive pulmonary disease (COPD) is a disease state characterized by airflow limitation that is not fully reversible. COPD is an umbrella term, covering the disease states of emphysema and chronic bronchitis. About 85 percent of patients with COPD suffer from chronic bronchitis, and 15 percent suffer from emphysema. Asthma is excluded from this classification because of its reversible nature. The condition is usually progressive and is associated with an abnormal inflammatory response in the lungs secondary to noxious gases and particles. Although tobacco smoking is the most critical risk factor for both the development and progression of COPD, asthma, exposure to ambient air pollution in the home and workplace, and respiratory infections are also key risk factors. The only proven genetic risk factor is α_1-antitrypsin deficiency ($<1\%$ of all cases).

Repeated exposure to noxious stimuli results in pathologic changes to the large and small airways. In the trachea, bronchi, and larger bronchioles, immune cells infiltrate the surface epithelium, resulting in edema. In addition, mucus-secreting glands and goblet cells become hypertrophic and secrete copious amounts of mucus, which cannot be removed due to destruction of the mucociliary escalator. In the smaller bronchioles, repeated injury and repair of the airway walls results in weakening and subsequent loss of recoil and collapse. In the alveoli, destruction of the walls between individual alveoli leads to the creation of enlarged terminal air spaces, called blebs, that contain far less surface area for gas exchange to take place across. In addition, pulmonary capillaries experience a thickening of their endothelial walls, further impeding gas exchange across the alveolar-capillary membrane.

These pathological changes lead to the characteristic physiological changes associated with the disease state. Early COPD is characterized by increased mucus secretion and decreased mucus elimination secondary to mucociliary escalator dysfunction. Late in the disease state, pulmonary hypertension develops secondary to the impedance of pulmonary blood flow through damaged pulmonary capillaries; this increased pulmonary pressure can lead to cor pulmonale. In addition, the increased pulmonary capillary impedance leads to diminished output from the pulmonary circulation that subsequently results in low-output from the left ventricle. Increased airway resistance, secondary to decreased mucus elimination and bronchiole collapse, leads to decreased alveolar ventilation and air trapping; hypoxemia and hypercapnia result. The likelihood of hypoxemia is further increased with the destruction of the alveolar membrane and thickening of the pulmonary capillary walls; a V/Q mismatch is created, and a right-to-left shunt results. As a result of chronic hypercapnia, COPD patients can develop a hypoxic drive.

The patient with pure emphysema will present slightly differently than the patient with pure chronic bronchitis, so we will consider the signs and symptoms of each separately. The critical care paramedic must remember, however, that a patient can have pathophysiological changes consistent with both diseases, and that the clinical findings of both may be present to some degree.

Chronic bronchitis: signs and symptoms:
- "Blue bloater" appearance
- Increased sputum production and expectoration
- Tachypnea, dyspnea, weakness, development of a productive cough
- Rhonchi, wheezing, diminished lung sounds

Emphysema: signs and symptoms:
- "Pink puffer" appearance
- Decreased lung sounds in all fields, diffuse wheezing
- "Silent chest" with evidence of hypoxemia, an ominous finding
- Increased anteroposterior chest diameter
- Tympany with percussion
- Purse-lipped breathing, accessory muscle use

Labs and imaging:
- Spirometry: changes in PEFR and FEV_1
- Chest radiograph: findings may include evidence of hyperinflation, including increased anteroposterior chest diameter, enlarged thoracic cage, increased width of the intercostal spaces, flattened diaphragm, increased pulmonary shadowing, and increased pulmonary parenchymal lucency
- ABG:
  - A PaO_2 of less than 60 mmHg or a SaO_2 of less than 90 percent on room air is suggestive for respiratory failure.
  - Ventilatory failure is suggested in those patients who present with a pH less than 7.30 or $PaCO_2$ greater than 70 mmHg.

c. Acute respiratory distress syndrome
p. 609

Clinically, acute respiratory distress syndrome (ARDS) is characterized by impaired oxygenation, rapidly progressive hypoxemia, the presence of diffuse bilateral infiltrates on chest radiograph, and decreased lung compliance following a known predisposing insult. Simply put, ARDS is the presence of pulmonary edema in the absence of depressed left ventricular function, or volume overload in the presence of a known insult.

ARDS is not a primary disease; rather, it is a complication that occurs when a disease or traumatic insult produces a severe and progressive systemic inflammatory response that ultimately involves the lungs. A wide and varying range of conditions is associated with ARDS; direct injuries, such as thoracic trauma, aspiration of gastric contents, or toxic gas inhalation result in direct damage to the lung epithelium. Indirect injuries include sepsis, pancreatitis, and major nonthoracic trauma.

Direct and indirect injuries result in a release of systemic activation of circulating neutrophils and macrophages. These activated cells become sticky and adhere to the pulmonary capillary endothelium, where they release proteases, oxygen metabolites, and leukotrines. These chemicals increase capillary permeability and allow neutrophilic invasion of the lung parenchyma, causing the inflammatory process to continue. The developing inflammation and capillary permeability result in the accumulation of interstitial and alveolar edema.

This initial accumulation of interstitial and alveolar edema causes a decrease in lung compliance, and blood flow to the lung is reduced. As a result of this diminished blood flow, platelets aggregate in the pulmonary capillaries, which may give rise to microthrombi that can obstruct the pulmonary capillaries and produce ischemic injury. In addition, the platelets are also a source of additional inflammatory mediators, which further damage the capillary membrane, increasing capillary permeability to plasma proteins. The movement of proteins into the interstitial space increases the interstitial osmotic pressure, drawing more fluid from the vascular space and causing pulmonary edema. As CO_2 dissolves more readily in water than does O_2, PaO_2 starts to diminish, and $PaCO_2$ remains normal or can decrease as respiratory rate increases and excess CO_2 is eliminated. As fluid accumulates in the alveolar space, pulmonary surfactant is washed from the alveoli epithelium surface, and pulmonary Type II surfactant-producing cells are damaged, resulting in atelectasis. As alveolar edema and atelectasis worsen, a V/Q mismatch occurs and a right-to-left shunt develops. Further injury to the lung results in fibrosis and CO_2 elimination is affected, resulting in hypercapnia. This late stage of ARDS is known as the fibroproliferative phase.

The end result of ARDS is naturally respiratory failure, yet only 10 to 40 percent of patients who develop ARDS subsequently die from respiratory failure. Many patients suffer mortality secondary to the original insult that resulted in ARDS.

Signs and symptoms:
- Tachypnea, progressing to hypoxemia and severe respiratory distress within 24 hours
- Rales upon auscultation
- Pertinent negatives in ARDS include:
  - Absence of JVD
  - S_3 heart sound
  - Signs of left ventricular failure or volume overload

Labs, diagnostics, and imaging:
- Chest radiograph: bilateral infiltrates
- Spirometry: $PaO_2/FiO_2 < 100$
- ABG:
  - Usually significant for hypoxia
  - Respiratory alkalosis may be present early in the disease from the initial tachypnea
  - Hypercarbia and respiratory alkalosis may develop late in the disease as blood gases become more deranged

d. Pneumonia   **p. 612**

Pneumonia is an infection of the alveoli and gas-exchanging units of the lungs, including the respiratory bronchioles, alveolar ducts, and alveolar sacs. Infectious agents causing pneumonia include bacteria, viruses, fungi, protozoa, or rickettsia. Common bacterial pathogens include *Streptococcus pneumoniae* (up to 70 percent of all cases of bacterial pneumonia), *Staphylococcus aureus*, *Pneumococcus*, *Haemophilus influenzae*, and *Pseudomonas*. Common viral causes include influenza virus types A and B, RSV, adenovirus, parainfluenza virus, rhinovirus, hantavirus, and cytomegalovirus. Very often, coinfection with bacterial and viral agents identified occurs. Atypical agents such as *Mycoplasma, Legionella, Chlamydia*, and SARS may also produce infection.

Numerous routes of infection exist and include the inhalation of infectious pathogens, the aspiration of oral or gastric contents, reactivation of a previous infection (common in immunocompromised individuals), and hematogenous seeding. Considering both the natural defenses and routes of infection, patients most at risk are those who have impaired mucociliary clearance, are at increased risk of aspiration, are immunocompromised, or have a risk of bacteremia.

Introduction of a pathogen into the airways distal to the respiratory bronchioles results in colonization and infection of the affected portion. The infection can spread throughout the lung, utilizing the bronchial tree and the pores of Kohn between adjacent alveoli. Some forms of pneumonia can elicit a severe inflammatory response resulting in the accumulation of immune cells, pathogenic material, cellular debris, pus, and fluid in the airway, while others will result in a less severe response and a much more subtle pathophysiology.

Signs and symptoms:
- Vary greatly depending on infecting organism
- Classic clinical picture:
- Fever
- Sputum production
- Productive cough, dyspnea
- Tachycardia, pleuritic chest pain
- Additional findings may include:
- Hemoptysis, blood-tinged sputum, history of upper respiratory infection
- Weakness, general malaise, anorexia, recent weight loss
- Rales, decreased sounds, rhonchi and wheezing on auscultation
- Dullness to percussion, increased tactile fremitus
- Severe tachycardia, tachypnea, fever, and hypotension associated with pneumonia are ominous signs, and could herald respiratory failure or be suggestive of septicemia.

Lab values, diagnostics, and imaging studies:
- Leukopenia: suggestive for sepsis
- Leukocytosis with a left shift indicates bacterial infection
- Rapid antigen detection kits: can detect influenza, RSV, parainfluenza, and other viruses rapidly
- Chest radiograph:
- May reveal consolidation, pleural effusion, patchy interstitial or alveolar infiltrates, or peribronchial thickening
- Findings may be lobular, multilobular, unilateral, or bilateral.
- ABG:
  - May reveal hypoxemia in severe cases of pneumonia

- Summary of the laboratory results that influence the decision for hospitalization:
  - leukopenia less than 4000–5000 cells/mm^3
  - Leukocytosis greater than 30,000 cells/mm^3
  - PaO_2 less than 50 mmHg
  - Involvement of more than 50 percent of the lung.

e. Pneumothorax

A pneumothorax occurs when a hole in the lung, the chest wall, or both, penetrates the visceral or parietal pleura and transforms the intrapleural region from a potential space into an actual one. Without the subatmospheric (negative) pressure within the pleural cavity to hold the lung up to the inner chest wall, the lungs tendency to collapse is unopposed.

Spontaneous pneumothoracies are those that occur without a prior event or any other apparent cause. A spontaneous pneumothorax that occurs in an individual without any underlying lung disease is termed a primary spontaneous pneumothorax, and one that occurs in the presence of underlying disease is termed a secondary spontaneous pneumothorax. Traumatic pneumothorax results from direct or indirect trauma to the thorax and can be further delineated as iatrogenic or noniatrogenic.

Primary spontaneous pneumothorax results from the rupture of a subpleural emphysematous bleb, most often in the upper lobe. Secondary spontaneous pneumothorax occurs as a complication of lung disease, most often COPD.

Iatrogenic pneumothorax occurs secondary to transthoracic needle aspiration, needle thoracentesis, subclavicular catheterization attempts, bronchoscopy, pericardiocentesis, nasogastric tube placement into the bronchial tree, mechanical ventilation, and CPR. Utilizing the low tidal volume, minimal PEEP method of ventilation detailed in the ARDS section may prove helpful in preventing iatrogenic pneumothorax in patients with underlying lung disease.

Signs and symptoms of pneumothorax:
- Pleuritic chest pain
- Dyspnea
- Tachycardia
- Decreased or absent lung sounds
- Ipsilateral hyper-resonance and decreased chest wall motion with large pneumothoracies
  Signs and symptoms of developing tension pneumothorax in a mechanically ventilated patient:
- Acute onset of:
  - Decreased SaO_2
  - Hypotension
  - Tachycardia
  - Increases in airway pressure
  - PEA
  - Combativeness, restlessness, and "fighting the vent"

Lab, diagnostic, and imaging studies:
- Chest radiograph:
  - P/A upright film: thin pleural line, absence of lung marking between the pleural line and the chest wall
  - A/P supine film: wide and deep costophrenic angle (sulcus sign), enlarged ipsilateral hemithorax secondary to contralateral shift of the mediastinum
- ABG:
  - Not necessary for the diagnosis of pneumothorax
  - Hypocapnia secondary to an elevated respiratory rate and excess CO_2 elimination early on
  - Hypoxia and hypercapnia may be seen, as well as a respiratory acidosis in severe cases

4. Discuss how the following assessment parameters assist in determining the severity of a pulmonary emergency:

a. Inspection
p. 591

Begin the physical examination with a general global view of the patient. Is the patient conscious and alert? Does he seem aware of his surroundings? Is he agitated or combative? Does he have an altered mental status?

Look for obvious signs of respiratory distress. Is the patient posturing to help facilitate breathing? Inspect for accessory muscle use, nasal flaring, purse-lipped breathing, a gaping mouth, and head bobbing. Note the color of the patient's skin and observe for pallor or cyanosis. Evaluate the trachea, assuring that it is midline.

Expose and inspect the chest. Note the presence of accessory muscle use and intercostal, supraclavicular, or supersternal retractions. Assess for symmetry of the chest wall, and assess the rate and quality of respirations. Observe the amount of chest expansion. Note the duration of inspiration and expiration. Abnormal breathing patterns (Biot's, Cheyne-Stokes, Kussmaul's, and apneustic respirations) should be identified and corrected.

Assess the contour of the chest wall closely. The air trapping common in obstructive pulmonary disease often causes an increased AP diameter, commonly referred to as a "barrel chest." Other chest contour variations include funnel chest, pigeon breast, scoliosis, and kyphosis. Assess the chest for the presence of surgical scars and evidence of recent trauma. Observe closely for new or healing stab or gunshot wounds, abrasions, contusions, lacerations, hematomas, burns, or any other indicator of traumatic insult to the chest wall.

Some patients with critical pulmonary disorders or traumatic thoracic injuries may have a chest tube placed prior to transport. Chest tubes are inserted primarily to serve as a drainage system for the thoracic cavity. The chest tubes can remove air, fluid, or blood from the plural space, promote the normal re-expansion of a collapsed lung, prevent the reflux of drainage back into the chest, and allow the return of the negative intrapleural pressure needed for normal lung function.

Patients with chest tubes in place require additional ongoing inspection. Frequent assessment of the patient and drainage system should be performed by the critical care paramedic to include assessment for proper tube placement (not outward displaced, allowing the chest tube eyelets to exit the thorax); also check for an absence of any air leaks, dressing integrity around the chest tube insertion site, water seal integrity to include water level, and drainage. Also assess the insertion sites of the chest tube, or any central lines for that matter, for infection. Signs of an infection can be seen if the skin surrounding the insertion site displays swelling, redness, weeping, or purulent discharge from the insertion site. Note the presence of blood or fluid in a chest tube drainage chamber. Be sure to inquire if the system has been emptied, and assure that you are aware of the total amount of fluid drained.

b. Palpation p. 592

Palpation often occurs simultaneously with inspection, and both should include the anterior, lateral, and posterior chest walls. Attempt to identify pain, tenderness, masses, or the presence of subcutaneous emphysema. Palpate for chest wall symmetry with deep inspiration. Asymmetry can indicate the presence of trauma or unilateral ventilation issues. The trachea should be palpated from its origin inferior to the larynx to the supersternal notch for deviation from the midline. Conditions such as tension pneumothorax, pleural effusion, and hemothorax may result in deviation away from the affected side, while atelectasis, fibrosis, and phrenic nerve paralysis may result in deviation toward the affected side. Tracheal tugging, if it is observed, may be due to obstruction of bronchi.

Assess for tactile fremitus by placing the palmar or ulnar surface of one hand on the patient's chest wall. Palpable vibrations are transmitted from the bronchial tree through the chest wall when the patient speaks. Fremitus is best appreciated in thin, healthy males, and is more pronounced over the larger bronchi, dissipating toward the distal bronchial tree. The patient is asked to repeat the word "ninety-nine" as the examiner moves his hand over the patient's chest wall, palpating for disparity between bilateral regions. Tactile fremitus is increased over areas of lung consolidation, such as in pneumonia, and decreased over areas where the bronchi are obstructed, the lung is hyperinflated, or where the pleural space is occupied by air.

c. Percussion p. 592

The five types of sounds produced by percussion are resonant, hyper-resonant, flat, dull, and tympanic and should be described in terms of their pitch, intensity, and duration. Resonant sounds are the normal sounds associated with the lungs and are of low pitch, low intensity, long duration, and often described as "hollow" sounding.

Hyper-resonant sounds are abnormal sounds percussed over the lungs, and are suggestive of air building up in the thoracic cavity, as in emphysema. Hyper-resonant sounds are of low pitch, low intensity, and long duration, and are often described as a "booming" sound when compared to the "hollow" sound of resonant. Tympanic sounds occur secondary to significant free air buildup in the thoracic cavity, as in cases of pneumothorax, and are normally heard over hollow organs such as the empty stomach and bowel. They are of high pitch, loud intensity, and long duration. Dull sounds appear in the chest exam when there is air removed from the lung field, as in atelectasis or consolidation. Dull sounds are of high pitch, low intensity, and short duration. Flat sounds are normally percussed over solid organs such as the liver, and appear in the chest exam when the thorax is filled with blood, fluid, or a solid mass. Flat sounds are of higher pitch than dull sounds, low intensity, and very short duration.

d. Auscultation   p. 593

It is important to be familiar not only with adventitious lung sounds, but with normal lung sounds as well. Normal lung sounds are described as tracheal, bronchial, bronchovesicular, and vesicular. Tracheal breath sounds are loud, harsh sounds with an equal inspiratory and expiratory duration appreciated over the trachea. Bronchial sounds are loud and high-pitched with a longer expiratory phase normally heard over the manubrium. Bronchovesicular sounds are of medium pitch, have an almost equal inspiratory and expiratory phase, and are heard over the mainstem bronchi and larger divisions of the bronchial tree. Vesicular lung sounds are auscultated over the majority of the lung fields, and are the result of air being ventilated into and out of the bronchi and alveoli. They are described as soft, low-pitched sounds with a long inspiratory phase and a short expiratory phase.

Adventitious lung sounds include rales, rhonchi, wheezes, and friction rub. Rales, often referred to as crackles, can be described as fine, coarse, and audible. Fine crackles are often described as small "pops" or akin to the sound hair makes when rolled and rubbed together between one's fingers next to the ear. This sound is the result of deflated, slightly edematous alveoli reinflating during inspiration and is often appreciated at the end of inspiration. Coarse crackles are produced when the alveoli are more filled with fluid, pus, or blood, and are heard earlier in the inspiratory phase. They are present in pathologies such as pneumonia or pulmonary edema. They commonly have a moister, wet sound than do fine crackles. Audible crackles are appreciated when edema buildup is significant enough to include the larger bronchial airways, and are often associated with fulminating pulmonary edema.

Rhonchi are produced when mucus or secretions are present in the larger divisions of the bronchial tree. The sound is often described as a wet, sticky, deep and low-pitched noise akin to the sound of sucking a thick liquid out of the bottom of a cup through a straw. Because of the mucous in the larger airways, often asking the patient to cough forcibly will cause the mucous to shift and produce a change in the characteristics of the sound.

Wheezes are the result of airflow through a constricted or partially obstructed airway as occurs in asthma, emphysema, chronic bronchitis, pneumonia, and allergic reactions. Wheezes are often described as a musical, high-pitched sound that can occur late in the expiratory phase with slight constriction and obstruction and progress over the whole respiratory cycle in cases of severe constriction and obstruction.

Friction rub is a cracking, grating sound appreciated during both inspiration and expiration, caused by the inflamed visceral and parietal pleuras rubbing together. The presence of infection, pus, or fluid in the pleural space can also create the sound. Etiologies include pneumothorax, pleural effusion, and pleurisy.

To evaluate egophony, the patient is instructed to verbalize a long "E" (i.e., "eeeee"), while the stethoscope is on the thorax. If the long "E" sound that is spoken sounds like a flat "A" sound, then "E to A" egophony is said to be present. What this assessment finding infers is that there is consolidation of lung tissue beneath the stethoscope (i.e., pneumothorax, tumor, pulmonary edema, pleural effusion, hemothorax, and so on.). The denser tissue from the consolidation creates the "E to A" change. With the absence of egophony, there should be no discernable "flat A" sound auscultated.

Whispered pectoriloquy is the presence of a loud and clear sound auscultated while the patient is speaking in a whispered voice. Again, the finding indicates lung consolidation and the finding exists because sound vibration travels better through dense lung tissue rather than normally aerated lung tissue.

e. Arterial blood gases   p. 594

An ABG analysis provides information regarding a patient's ventilation and perfusion status, as well as data concerning the overall acid-base balance status. Information provided by an

ABG includes the SaO_2, PaO_2, $PaCO_2$, pH, and bicarbonate (HCO_3^-) level. Normal values for an ABG are as follows:

- SaO_2: 94–99 percent
- PaO_2: 80–100 mmHg
- $PaCO_2$: 35–45 mmHg
- pH: 7.35–7.45
- HCO_3^-: 22–26 mEq/L

ABGs are useful in both the evaluation of respiratory function in a patient, as well as determining the need for and efficacy of therapeutic interventions. ABG analysis can identify hypercapnia, hypoxemia, acidosis, alkalosis, and compensatory measures utilized to reverse these disturbances.

f. Pulse oximetry p. 594

It is known that when arterial oxygen saturations are above 70 percent, the oxygen saturation recorded by pulse oximetry varies from actual arterial saturation by only about 3 percent. This makes it an ideal tool for continuous monitoring and evaluation of therapeutic interventions. In addition, it is a valuable tool for identifying and recording hypoxemic episodes. Compared to ABG determination of arterial oxygenation, pulse oximetry is as accurate, is faster, is less invasive, has fewer complications, and is less expensive. In addition, pulse oximetry allows for continuous monitoring of arterial blood oxygenation, making it ideal for transport situations, especially in intubated patients. The following chart is a rough estimate that may be used when estimating PaO_2 from SpO_2:

Monitored SpO_2	Estimated PaO_2
90 percent	60 mmHg
80 percent	50 mmHg
70 percent	40 mmHg

Given this relationship, it is easy to understand why a pulse oximeter reading less than 90 percent is considered to be an "objective" sign of severe hypoxemia (as would a PaO_2 level of 60 mmHg or less). Normal SpO_2 is 98 percent to 99 percent, with an acceptable SpO_2 value being greater than 95 percent. SpO_2 readings between 90 percent and 95 percent are in that "gray" zone of not being too low, but not being "normal," requiring a thorough pulmonary assessment. A critical limitation of pulse oximetry is that while it does offer information regarding oxygenation, it does not offer information regarding ventilation. Thus, a patient can be oxygenated adequately and demonstrate an acceptable SpO_2 reading but could still have issues with pulmonary gas exchange, resulting in hypercapnia.

g. End-tidal capnography p. 595

The end-tidal carbon dioxide level ($ETCO_2$) is an approximation of $PaCO_2$ since both are a reflection of alveolar ventilation. Whereas a normal disparity between $PaCO_2$ and $ETCO_2$ may exist (end tidal is usually 1–2 mmHg lower than arterial carbon dioxide), the monitoring of exhaled carbon dioxide still allows gross interpretation as to the quality of alveolar ventilation in the spontaneously breathing or mechanically ventilated patient.

The exhaled carbon dioxide levels can be displayed via a waveform on the monitor, thus the capnogram is a continuous and graphic reading of exhaled carbon dioxide with each breath. As mentioned previously, exhaled carbon dioxide equates roughly with arterial carbon dioxide, and as such, any elevations or depressions in the $ETCO_2$ value can reflect a change in the patient's physiological status, mechanical change in ventilation, or both.

$ETCO_2$ monitoring does have its limitations; it does not detect mainstem intubations, it may be affected by high concentrations of oxygen (false-low readings), and it can be influenced by excessive water vapor (false-high readings). The use of end-tidal carbon dioxide monitoring (and even the use of pulse oximetry, for that matter), was never intended to be a sole diagnostic device and should never be used as such.

5. Discuss the basic management of the following specific pulmonary diseases:

a. Acute respiratory failure p. 588

As discussed in Objective 2, acute respiratory failure (ARF) can be defined as a state of inadequate gas exchange, and it occurs when the respiratory system is unable to absorb oxygen

©2007 Pearson Education, Inc.
Critical Care Paramedic

and/or excrete carbon dioxide. ARF occurs as a result of many etiologies and may be the patient's primary problem, or a secondary result of an existing disease process. As such, the management of ARF revolves around first securing the airway, assuring adequate oxygenation and ventilation and then managing the *cause* of the ARF, the etiology responsible for the state of inadequate gas exchange.

b. Asthma p. 601

The goal of the treatment of asthma is to reverse bronchoconstriction and airway inflammation and edema to increase ventilation, oxygenation, and CO_2 elimination. The medications utilized to achieve this goal include oxygen, β-agonists, anticholinergics, corticosteroids, theophylline, and magnesium. Patients who do not respond to pharmacological therapy and who are in impending respiratory arrest are candidates for intubation and mechanical ventilation.

β-agonists and anticholinergics are considered first-line medications in an asthma attack. While dramatic improvement can be expected in the early phase of an asthma exacerbation, these medications tend to result in limited improvement in patients experiencing late-phase asthma exacerbations.

β-agonists, preferably β-2 specific agonists, are beneficial in asthma for three reasons: they result in bronchial smooth muscle relaxation of the smaller airways, they inhibit mediator release, and they promote mucociliary clearance. Inhaled forms of β-agonists are preferred over the oral, intravenous, or subcutaneous routes. Aerosolization can be achieved via a nebulizer or metered-dose inhaler (MDI), provided that a properly fitted spacing device and proper technique are utilized. Parenteral routes can be considered in patients who are too dyspneic to take the adequate tidal volumes needed to deposit the medication on the bronchiole smooth muscle. Another consideration for the extremely dyspneic patient in extremis is elective endotracheal intubation; with this intervention, aerosolized β-agonists can be administered via the endotracheal tube.

Anticholinergic drugs act as a competitive antagonist to acetylcholine at the acetylcholine receptor. This action blocks vagal tone to the larger central airways, resulting in bronchodilation. Used in conjunction with a β-agonist, bronchoconstriction is thus addressed from both the sympathetic and parasympathetic influences. Aerosolized ipratropium bromide, a synthetic derivative of atropine sulfate, is the anticholinergic most often used , and it is administered in doses of 0.5 mg via a nebulizer every 15 to 20 minutes or continuously if needed. MDI preparations are also available.

Corticosteroids are highly effective in reducing the airway inflammation and edema characteristic of asthma, and are used in the management of both acute and chronic asthma. As the onset of action can be four to eight hours by both the intravenous and oral routes, the goal of the critical care paramedic should be to get corticosteroids administered as soon as possible. Common treatment regimes include oral prednisone 40–60 mg, or intravenous Solu-Medrol 60–125 mg every six hours for the first 24 hours.

The use of theophylline or IV aminophylline as a first-line treatment for asthma remains controversial. When used to treat acute exacerbation of asthma, oral theophylline, in combination with inhaled β-agonists, appears to increase the toxicity of treatment, but not the efficacy. When used to manage chronic asthma, oral theophylline contributes to a decrease in airway inflammation and swelling, but its overall bronchodilatory effects are limited. Theophylline toxicity occurs at plasma levels greater than 30 mcg/mL, with cardiac dysrhythmia and seizures a serious risk. The arguably meager benefits of theophylline or aminophylline must be weighed against the potentially undesirable side effects.

Intravenous magnesium sulfate relaxes bronchial smooth muscle via the blocking of calcium channels in muscle cells. In addition, it may inhibit mast cell degranulation, resulting in decreased airway inflammation and edema, and can improve respiratory muscle function in cases of serum magnesium deficiency. Magnesium seems to benefit those patients with severe exacerbations (FEV_1 greater than 25 percent predicted). The medication is usually administered 1 to 2 g in 50 mL of normal saline over 20 to 30 minutes.

Patients with severe asthma and hypercapnia who are unresponsive to pharmacological and supplemental oxygen therapy, are hemodynamically stable, and still possess an adequate respiratory drive may benefit from noninvasive positive-pressure ventilation (NPPV). This intervention works by providing a constant "backpressure" of air that the patient must exhale against. The backpressure helps keep the alveoli open, diminishes alveolar fluid accumulation, assists in keeping smaller bronchioles open (which allows more effective ventilation), and decreases the work of breathing during inhalation due to the positive pressure in the airway. There are two forms of NPPV, continuous positive airway pressure (CPAP), and bilevel positive airway pressure (BiPAP).

Any patient who experiences progressive lethargy, near exhaustion, somnolence, or apnea will require intubation. Nasotracheal intubation may be better tolerated in a conscious patient, but the orotracheal route permits the use of a larger diameter endotracheal tube (ETT), allowing for deep suctioning of the airway and the use of a bronchoscope, if necessary. In addition, a larger diameter ETT will lower the resistance in the airway circuit. Sedation may be necessary in a conscious patient, but the use of neuromuscular blocking agents should be avoided if at all possible. In addition, the use of opioids or barbiturates should be avoided, as they both encourage histamine release and can worsen bronchoconstriction.

There is significant potential for barotrauma in a patient who is receiving mechanical ventilation when severe airflow obstruction leads to air trapping and the "stacking" of respirations. Stacking can be avoided by administering ventilations at a rapid inspiratory flow rate with a frequency of 12 to 14 breaths per minute, then allowing for a prolonged respiratory phase. While this "relative hypoventilation" may not resolve an elevated $PaCO_2$, it is adequate for maintaining a PaO_2 above 90 mmHg. This methodology has been termed permissive hypoventilation.

c. Chronic obstructive pulmonary disease   p. 608

The goal in treatment of acute exacerbation of COPD is to improve oxygenation and CO_2 elimination, correct reversible bronchospasm, and begin (or continue) treatment of the underlying etiology of the exacerbation. The methods utilized to achieve this goal are similar to those used in the management of asthma and include oxygen, β-agonists, anticholinergics, corticosteroids, and theophylline. Patients who do not respond to pharmacological therapy and are in impending respiratory arrest are candidates for intubation and mechanical ventilation.

The patient should be provided high flow oxygen via the oxygenation adjunct most appropriate for the patient's minute ventilation. SpO_2 values above 95 percent are desired in the acute setting.

The use of aerosolized β-agonist and anticholinergic medications are considered first-line therapies in the management of acute exacerbation of COPD. See information on these medications presented in the asthma section.

While the use of corticosteroids in the treatment of acute exacerbation of COPD is fairly widespread, controversy remains as to whether or not they are truly beneficial. What is fairly certain is that they are not harmful if administered for a few days. The general consensus is that while there may be a benefit in mild exacerbation of COPD, their efficacy in moderate and severe exacerbation is unknown.

Likewise, the use of theophylline in acute exacerbation of COPD is also controversial. The current trend calls for their use when other pharmacological management has failed, or when plasma theophylline levels in a chronic user are subtherapeutic. As stated in the asthma section, the risk of significant side effects from theophylline is significant, its therapeutic index narrow, and its bronchodilatory effects limited.

Antibiotics should be administered in acute exacerbation of COPD when the clinical condition suggests infection. Mild to moderate exacerbations are usually treated with older, broad-spectrum antibiotics such as doxycycline, trimethoprim-sulfamethoxazole, and amoxicillin. Treatment with penicillins, fluoroquinolones, and third-generation cephalosporins or aminoglycosides is often used in patients with severe exacerbations.

The indications for NPPV and endotracheal intubation in the management of acute exacerbation of COPD mirror that of asthma. Despite hypercapnia, hyperventilation is to be avoided in the intubated COPD patient, who is chronically hypercapnic and has developed renal compensation to maintain normal acid-base balance. Hyperventilation will result in the excess elimination of CO_2, leaving the compensatory metabolic alkalosis that is present unchecked. In addition, as in asthma, hyperventilation can result in "air stacking," hyperinflation, and subsequent barotrauma.

d. Acute respiratory distress syndrome

p. 609

The primary goal of management for ARDS is to ensure oxygenation to a SpO_2 of greater than 90 percent. Early in the disease process, this may be accomplished by use of a nonrebreather mask, while late phases of the disease will require endotracheal intubation and the use of significant positive end-expiratory pressure (PEEP).

Whatever the delivery modality, the FiO_2 should be kept low, 50 percent or lower, in an effort to minimize the risk of oxygen toxicity. Lung parenchyma destruction can occur with the long-term administration of high concentrations of oxygen, a powerful oxidant. Endogenous pulmonary antioxidants in the lung usually protect against the destructive nature of oxygen, but are overwhelmed by the development of ARDS. If an FiO_2 of 50 percent is insufficient to achieve a SpO_2 of 90 percent, external PEEP should be provided incrementally to increase oxygenation at nontoxic levels.

The growing consensus is that intubated patients with ARDS should be ventilated at low-tidal volumes to prevent overpressure injuries to the lung. To prevent overinflation injury, an effort should be made to limit PIP to 35 cm H_2O by utilizing tidal volumes of 7–10 mL/kg. A suggested strategy is to initiate mechanical ventilation at 10 mL/kg. If the PIP is greater than 35 cm H_2O, the tidal volume is reduced in increments of 2 mL/kg until PIP is 35 cm H_2O or lower. If inflation pressures less than 6 cm H_2O result, PEEP should be utilized to prevent distal airway and alveolar collapse. PEEP should be added in increments of 2 cm H_2O until adequate ventilation is achieved. Late in ARDS, especially when there is significant interstitial edema and fibrosis, significant PEEP (>20 cm H_2O) may be needed to ensure airway patency and adequate ventilation.

One emerging trend with the mechanical ventilation of the ARDS patient is to decrease the delivered tidal volume in order to keep airway pressures low and avoid barotrauma. Doing this, though, has a tendency to allow the arterial levels of carbon dioxide to rise. This "permissive hypercapnia" is felt by some to be a reasonable trade-off in the attempt to avoid excessive airway pressures and barotrauma from mechanical ventilation.

Along with permissive hypercapnia, some pulmonary physicians will reverse the inspiratory/expiratory (I/E ratio) times on the ventilator so that the inhalation phase is longer than the exhalation phase. A longer inhalation time will typically lower peak airway pressures, promote a less turbulent gas flow, and provide more time for good tidal volume distribution through the damaged lung tissue.

In intubated patients who are resisting mechanical ventilation, sedation or neuromuscular blockade should be considered. "Fighting the vent" can result in poor oxygenation, high airway pressures and barotraumas, and episodes of hypotension secondary to the high intrathoracic pressures generated during combativeness.

e. Pneumonia

p. 613

The management of a patient with pneumonia will be mostly supportive, consisting primarily of oxygenation and ventilatory support. In cases of severe pneumonia, endotracheal intubation may be necessary.

Treatment with antibiotic therapy should be initiated within the first 8 hours, if possible, as the early administration of antibiotics has been shown to improve morbidity and mortality for those patients who are going to require hospitalization for their pneumonia. Typical treatment for unidentified etiologies includes a second or third-generation cephalosporin or penicillin, plus a beta-lactamase inhibitor. Patients may also receive a macrolide to address atypical agents. If the etiology has been determined, more specific antibiotic treatment can be initiated.

For those patients with wheezing audible upon auscultation, an inhaled agonist may be considered, but its benefit should be weighed against the potential for cardiac involvement of the drug.

f. Pneumothorax

p. 616

The management goals for pneumothorax include the removal of intrapleural air, ensuring proper oxygenation, and preventing recurrences.

Many small, primary pneumothoracies do not require treatment other than the administration of oxygen at 3 to 4 lpm and a serial chest radiograph to ensure that the injury is not expanding. Needle aspiration is also an option in a small, primary pneumothorax.

Chest tube thoracostomy is standard of care for almost all cases of secondary spontaneous pneumothorax, and is always required if mechanical ventilation is going to be utilized.

Other indications for tube thoracostomy include a pneumothorax greater that 40 percent, a pneumothorax that does not respond to aspiration, and ABG abnormalities.

The development of tension pneumothorax necessitates the need for immediate needle decompression of the affected side of the chest. A chest thoracostomy tube should not be used to treat a tension pneumothorax unless it can be performed more rapidly than needle decompression.

Case Study

As you pull into the ambulance spot at 0130 hours, there are only two other cars visible in the parking lot. This tiny emergency department is 50 miles from your facility, which is the next closest hospital, and has a reputation for generating some very sick patients. The physician assistant had your team called to transfer a patient to the tertiary care center where your program is based. She tells you that the patient, a 76-year-old male, is well known to her, and has a long history of COPD. The COPD has increased in severity over the past year, requiring several admissions and at least two intubations. He has an 80 pack-year smoking history and is normally oxygen dependent on 3 lpm at home. He also has a history of hypertension, for which he takes enalapril, and gout. He uses a Spiriva® HandiHaler® and has an albuterol metered-dose inhaler that he had been using every half-hour today without significant relief. He came to the emergency department this evening via EMS, complaining of a three-day history of productive cough and increasing shortness of breath. He arrived on a NRM with an SpO_2 of 88 percent. Since arrival, he has received three nebulized albuterol treatments, the first of which was mixed with ipratropium bromide, and 125 mg of methylprednisolone IV push, with minimal improvement in his respiratory status. He was also given levofloxacin 500 mg IV. Lab values are normal except for a slightly elevated white blood cell count without a "left shift" and the arterial blood gas. The ABG on arrival showed pH 7.31, $PaCO_2$ 57 mmHg, PaO_2 78 mmHg and HCO_3^- 35 mEq/L. Chest X-ray shows a barrel-shaped chest and hyperinflated lung fields with flattened diaphragms. Upon your arrival, the PA was trying to decide between intubating the patient and starting him on noninvasive positive pressure ventilation. Although she feels it would be better for the patient to avoid intubation, NPPV is new to this facility and she tells you that she is relatively inexperienced with it and would appreciate your input.

Your patient is sitting on the ED stretcher in high Fowler's position with oxygen being administered via a nonrebreather mask. With his hypertrophic accessory muscles, barrel chest, and purse-lipped expirations he is the textbook picture of a patient with emphysema. "Still," you think, "this guy is definitely working harder than normal to breathe." His head is bobbing with each respiratory cycle, and when you introduce yourself to him and discuss the transfer, he just nods his head in response. He can speak only one word at a time. His breath sounds are diminished and with expiratory wheezes, and adventitious sounds are auscultated in all fields. The nurse informs you that the patient's current vital signs are: temperature 37.5 degrees C, respirations 32 per minute and shallow, with purse-lipped exhalations and an SpO_2 of 90 percent, pulse 110 bpm and regular with the monitor showing a sinus tachycardia, and a blood pressure of 168/98.

After discussing the patient with the PA, you elect to give NPPV a try, and your partner sets it up while you explain the procedure to the patient. The NPPV is attached to the patient and he tolerates the therapy well, with only minor coaching. His respirations decrease slightly and his SpO_2 improves to 92 percent as you begin transport. Unfortunately, the patient's SpO_2 and mental status both decrease enroute requiring you to intubate him. Intubation significantly improves his status, however, and by the time you reach the ICU he is alert and following commands better than he was when you first met.

DISCUSSION QUESTIONS

1. What is acute respiratory failure?
2. What are the general treatment modalities available for the management of the following pulmonary emergencies?
   A. Asthma
   B. Exacerbation of chronic obstructive pulmonary disease
   C. Adult respiratory distress syndrome
   D. Pneumonia

Content Review

MULTIPLE CHOICE

_____ 1. The respiratory zone of the respiratory system extends from the:
   A. respiratory bronchioles to the alveoli.
   B. entrance of the nasal and oral cavities to the terminal bronchioles.
   C. glottic opening to the alveoli.
   D. entrance of the nasal and oral cavities to the glottic opening.

_____ 2. The combination of goblet cells and ciliated epithelium form the _____, which traps and removes foreign debris from the upper and lower airway.
   A. mucus apparatus   C. mucociliary escalator
   B. respiratory epithelium   D. trachea

_____ 3. The upper airway's primary function is to:
   A. ensure that food boluses are directed down the esophagus.
   B. warm, humidify, and filter inspired air.
   C. support the larynx.
   D. provide a conduit for air exchange with the lower airway.

_____ 4. The cartilaginous components of the larynx include the:
   A. thyroid cartilage, cricoid cartilage, and epiglottis.
   B. C-shaped cartilaginous rings, thyroid cartilage, and cricoid cartilage.
   C. corniculoid cartilage, arytenulate cartilage, and thyroid cartilage.
   D. none of the above.

_____ 5. The _____ ligament connects the thyroid and cricoid cartilages.
   A. extrinsic   C. intrinsic
   B. entrinsic   D. thyroid

_____ 6. The trachea bifurcates at the carina to form the right and left:
   A. primary bronchi.   C. secondary bronchi.
   B. lungs.   D. none of the above.

_____ 7. Cartilaginous support of the bronchi stops at the level of the :
   A. respiratory bronchi.   C. terminal bronchioles.
   B. tertiary bronchi.   D. terminal bronchi.

_____ 8. Smooth muscle control of the lower airway begins at the level of the:
   A. respiratory bronchi.   C. terminal bronchioles.
   B. tertiary bronchi.   D. terminal bronchi.

_____ 9. Gas exchange is first able to take place in the lower airway at the level of the:
   A. respiratory bronchi.   C. terminal bronchioles.
   B. tertiary bronchi.   D. terminal bronchi.

_____ 10. The alveolar capillary membrane is made up of _____ layers consisting of the:
   A. two, alveolar epithelial cell and capillary endothelial cell.
   B. three, alveolar epithelial cell, capillary endothelial cell, and fused basil lamina of each.
   C. three, alveolar epithelial cell, capillary endothelial cell, and the interstitial space.
   D. none of the above.

_____ 11. Factors that will decrease the efficacy of gas exchange between the respiratory and circulatory systems include all of the following except:
   A. increased width of the interstitial space.
   B. interruption of the alveolar epithelial membrane.
   C. lack of perfusion of the pulmonary capillaries.
   D. decreased PaO_2.

_____ 12. Pores of Kohn and canals of Lambert allow for:
  A. the easy migration of Type III alveolar cells within the lung parenchyma.
  B. better gas exchange across the alveolar-capillary membrane with only slight increases in airway resistance.
  C. collateral circulation between adjacent alveolar and bronchiolar structures without an increase in airway resistance.
  D. the "venting off" of areas of increased intralobular pressure, decreasing the risk of barotrauma.

_____ 13. Type II alveolar cells:
  A. produce pulmonary surfactant.
  B. allow gas exchange.
  C. roam the alveolar epithelium surface, engulfing foreign material.
  D. none of the above.

_____ 14. Pulmonary surfactant:
  A. consists of an assortment of phospholipid substances.
  B. decreases the surface tension of water.
  C. prevents alveolar collapse and atelectasis.
  D. all of the above.

_____ 15. The negative pressure between the visceral and parietal pleura of the thorax is created by:
  A. the hydrostatic attraction of water molecules in the pleural fluid.
  B. the normal elasticity of the lung parenchyma.
  C. both A and B.
  D. none of the above.

_____ 16. The production of angiotensin-converting enzyme takes place in the:
  A. pulmonary artery.   C. pulmonary capillaries.
  B. pulmonary arterioles.   D. pulmonary venules.

_____ 17. The _____ supply(ies) arterial blood to the tissue of the bronchial tree.
  A. aorta   C. pulmonary artery
  B. bronchial arteries   D. bronchiole arteries

_____ 18. Acute respiratory failure (ARF) can be described as:
  A. a state of inadequate respiratory gas exchange.
  B. apnea.
  C. a triad consisting of tachypnea, cyanosis, and acidosis.
  D. none of the above.

_____ 19. It is generally accepted that ARF exists when:
  A. $PaO_2 < 60$ mmHg, $PaCO_2 > 50$ mmHg, and pH > 7.30 on room air.
  B. $PaO_2 < 50$ mmHg, $PaCO_2 > 60$ mmHg, and pH < 7.30 on room air.
  C. $PaO_2 < 50$ mmHg, $PaCO_2 > 60$ mmHg, and pH > 7.30 on room air.
  D. $PaO_2 < 60$ mmHg, $PaCO_2 > 50$ mmHg, and pH < 7.30 on room air.

_____ 20. Which of the following is not recognized as a mechanism that can result in oxygenation failure?
  A. Cardiogenic shock   C. Hyperventilation
  B. Ventilation/perfusion mismatch   D. Low FiO_2

_____ 21. Oxygenation failure secondary to hypoventilation can occur as a result of all of the following except:
  A. multiple sclerosis.   C. sedation.
  B. pleural effusion.   D. pulmonary embolis.

©2007 Pearson Education, Inc.
Critical Care Paramedic

_____ 22. A ventilation/perfusion mismatch occurs when:
   A. the V/Q ratio falls below 1.0.
   B. either ventilation or perfusion to an area of the lung decreases.
   C. both ventilation and perfusion to the lungs decreases.
   D. none of the above.

_____ 23. A ventilation/perfusion mismatch can occur secondary to:
   A. poor lung compliance.   C. decreased pulmonary perfusion pressures.
   B. increased airway resistance.   D. all of the above.

_____ 24. A patient suffering from a large pulmonary embolus can be expected to have an A/Q ratio:
   A. = 0.8.   C. > 0.8.
   B. < 0.8.   D. none of the above.

_____ 25. A _____ is created in part by the introduction of deoxygenated blood into the pulmonary vein from the drainage of the coronary and bronchial veins.
   A. physiologic shunt   C. V/Q mismatch
   B. ventilation/perfusion mismatch   D. left-to-right shunt

_____ 26. Which of the following statements regarding a right-to-left shunt is false?
   A. It occurs when an area of the lung has normal perfusion but is not adequately ventilated.
   B. It will result in a V/Q ratio of > 0.8.
   C. PaO_2 can be expected to decrease.
   D. It results in blood returning to the right atrium with some degree of under oxygenation.

_____ 27. Normal oxygen transport to the peripheral tissues is about:
   A. 200 to 600 mL/min.   C. 400 to 1,600 mL/min.
   B. 600 to 1,000 mL/min.   D. 600 to 1,200 mL/min.

_____ 28. Which of the following does not directly contribute to a diffusion deficit resulting in decreased oxygenation?
   A. Decreased cardiac output   C. Plasma in the alveoli
   B. Interstitial edema   D. All of the above

_____ 29. Decreased oxygenation secondary to a low FiO_2 can occur secondary to:
   A. altitude.
   B. inadequate flow rate through a nonrebreather mask.
   C. containment in an enclosed, unventilated space.
   D. all of the above.

_____ 30. Ventilation failure resulting in hypercapnia is best measured by:
   A. pulse oximetry.   C. ABG analysis.
   B. capnometry.   D. venous blood gas analysis.

_____ 31. Which of the following statements regarding the relationship between dead air space and $PaCO_2$ is true?
   A. As dead air space decreases, $PaCO_2$ increases.
   B. As dead air space increases, $PaCO_2$ increases.
   C. As dead airspace increases, $PaCO_2$ decreases.
   D. As dead airspace decreases, $PaCO_2$ decreases.

_____ 32. One of the earliest signs of developing hypoxia is:
   A. a decreasing mental status.   C. altered level of consciousness.
   B. respiratory failure.   D. accessory muscle use.

_____ 33. Normal expiration is about _____ times as long as inspiration, and a prolonged expiratory phase could indicate _____.
   A. 1.5, the presence of hypoxia   C. 2, a developing pneumothorax
   B. 1.5, air trapping   D. 2, air trapping

_____ 34. The ratio of anteroposterior (AP) to lateral diameter of the thorax is:
A. 1:2.
B. 1:1.
C. 1:2.5.
D. 2:1.

_____ 35. Accessory muscles utilized to aid respiration include the:
A. scalenes.
B. sternocleidomastoid.
C. trapezius.
D. all of the above.

_____ 36. Which of the following is the most accurate indicator that a chest tube has been displaced outward from the thorax?
A. The patient experiences increased difficulty breathing.
B. Lung sounds are diminished on the affected side.
C. Chest tube fenestrations are visible outside the thorax.
D. An air leak exists at the chest tube/thorax interface.

_____ 37. Which of the following is not part of the normal assessment of a chest tube that has been placed prior to your arrival?
A. Check for the presence of air leaks.
B. Pull on the chest tube to ensure that it is adequately secured in place.
C. Assess for the presence of blood or fluid in the drainage chamber.
D. Inquire whether the system has been emptied prior to your arrival.

_____ 38. Tactile fremitus is best appreciated in:
A. emaciated elderly males.
B. obese, young females.
C. emaciated elderly females.
D. thin, healthy males.

_____ 39. A paramedic assessing tactile fremitus would expect an increase over an area of:
A. consolidation.
B. hyperinflation.
C. injury.
D. none of the above.

_____ 40. Types of sounds appreciated by performing percussion include:
A. flat.
B. dull.
C. resonant.
D. all of the above.

_____ 41. Vesicular lung sounds are best auscultated over the:
A. mainstem bronchi.
B. majority of the lung fields.
C. trachea.
D. manubrium.

_____ 42. Bronchovesicular lung sounds are best described as:
A. soft, low-pitched sounds with a long inspiratory phase and a short expiratory phase.
B. loud, high-pitched sounds with a longer expiratory phase.
C. of medium pitch with an almost equal inspiratory and expiratory phase.
D. loud, harsh sounds with an equal inspiratory and expiratory phase.

_____ 43. Course crackles are produced when:
A. deflated, slightly edematous alveoli reinflate during inspiration.
B. mucus or secretions are present in the bronchi and bronchioles.
C. air flows through a constricted airway.
D. pus, blood, or fluid fills the alveoli.

_____ 44. Which of the following is the best example of a normal arterial blood gas (ABG) from a healthy patient?
A. $SaO_2 = 96\%$, $PaO_2 = 84$ mmHg, $PaCO_2 = 37\%$, pH = 7.36, $HCO_3^- = 25$ mEq/L
B. $SaO_2 = 98\%$, $PaO_2 = 94$ mmHg, $PaCO_2 = 39\%$, pH = 7.4, $HCO_3^- = 28$ mEq/L
C. $SaO_2 = 99\%$, $PaO_2 = 100$ mmHg, $PaCO_2 = 40\%$, pH = 7.341, $HCO_3^- = 20$ mEq/L
D. $SaO_2 = 92\%$, $PaO_2 = 84$ mmHg, $PaCO_2 = 32\%$, pH = 7.34, $HCO_3^- = 28$ mEq/L

_____ 45. Which of the following cannot be determined with an ABG?
A. Hypercapnia
B. Hematocrit
C. Hypoxemia
D. Alkalosis

_____ 46. The affinity for oxygen on the heme subunits of the hemoglobin molecule _____ as the total number of heme sites occupied increases.
    A. increases
    B. decreases
    C. remains the same
    D. all of the above

_____ 47. The release of oxygen from hemoglobin is dependant of all of the following except:
    A. 2,3-DPG.
    B. blood pH.
    C. hemoglobin concentration.
    D. temperature.

_____ 48. A SpO_2 value of 90 percent correlates with a PaO_2 of about:
    A. 40 mmHg.
    B. 50 mmHg.
    C. 60 mmHg.
    D. 70 mmHg.

_____ 49. Pulse oximetry provides information on the effectiveness of ventilation and oxygenation.
    A. True
    B. False

_____ 50. $ETCO_2$ can be expected to be _____ compared to $PaCO_2$.
    A. 1–2 mmHg lower
    B. 10–20 mmHg lower
    C. 1–2 mmHg higher
    D. none of the above

_____ 51. The third phase, or plateau, of a capnographic waveform represents:
    A. the exhalation of CO_2 from the bronchi and bronchioles.
    B. the beginning of the expiratory phase.
    C. the exhalation of CO_2 from the terminal airways and alveoli.
    D. none of the above.

_____ 52. A patient suffering from an acute exacerbation of her asthma can be expected to have which characteristic waveform?
    A. Plateau
    B. "Shark fin appearance"
    C. Flattening of the shoulder of the waveform
    D. None of the above

_____ 53. All of the following could result in an increased, or continuously rising, $ETCO_2$ except:
    A. fever.
    B. decreased minute ventilation.
    C. rebreathing of CO_2 in the vent circuit.
    D. pulmonary embolis.

_____ 54. All of the following could result in an decreased, or continuously lowering, $ETCO_2$ except:
    A. cardiac arrest.
    B. hyperventilation.
    C. high levels of PEEP in a ventilated patient.
    D. displacement of an endotracheal tube.

_____ 55. Which of the following is not a limitation of $ETCO_2$ monitoring?
    A. False-high values can result from the presence of excessive water vapor.
    B. False-low values can result from high concentrations of oxygen.
    C. $ETCO_2$ does not detect right mainstem intubations.
    D. $ETCO_2$ cannot be used to titrate a respiratory rate in mechanically ventilated patients.

_____ 56. It is generally accepted that intubation is required when $PaO_2 < 60$ mmHg, $PaCO_2 > 50$ mmHg, and arterial pH is < 7.30 on room air.
    A. True
    B. False

_____ 57. Asthma can be best described as a:
   A. condition of lower airway hyper-responsiveness resulting in bronchospasm and decreased gas exchange.
   B. chronic condition of the lower airways characterized by airway hyper-responsiveness to various stimuli resulting in decreased gas exchange.
   C. chronic inflammatory disorder of the lower airways characterized by hyper-responsiveness, inflammation, edema, and increased mucus production.
   D. syndrome of allergic reaction, bronchoconstriction, decreased air exchange, and developing hypoxia.

_____ 58. The first phase of an acute exacerbation of chronic asthma is characterized by:
   A. significant inflammation, mucus production, and edema.
   B. submucosal cell damage, basement membrane thickening, hypertrophy of airway smooth muscle, and increased numbers of goblet cells.
   C. mast cell degranulation, mediator release, bronchoconstriction, developing submucosal edema, vascular congestion, mucus production, and impaired mucociliary clearance.
   D. none of the above.

_____ 59. The second phase of an acute exacerbation of chronic asthma is characterized by:
   A. significant inflammation, mucus production, and edema.
   B. submucosal cell damage, basement membrane thickening, hypertrophy of airway smooth muscle, and increased numbers of goblet cells.
   C. mast cell degranulation, mediator release, bronchoconstriction, developing submucosal edema, vascular congestion, mucus production, and impaired mucociliary clearance.
   D. none of the above.

_____ 60. Pulses paradoxus greater than 20 mmHg is considered indicative of serious asthma exacerbation.
   A. True
   B. False

_____ 61. All of the following are 12-lead ECG findings characteristic of asthma except:
   A. early R-wave progression.   C. right axis deviation.
   B. left ventricular strain.   D. sinus tachycardia.

_____ 62. The right ventricular strain that may accompany an exacerbation of asthma occurs secondary to:
   A. decreased pulmonary resistance secondary to damaged and fibrotic capillary endothelium.
   B. increased intrathoracic pressure secondary to air trapping.
   C. increased pulmonary resistance secondary to hyperinflation.
   D. none of the above.

_____ 63. Changes in PEFR and FEV1 often precede the clinical manifestations of acute exacerbations of asthma, providing warning of a worsening condition.
   A. True
   B. False

_____ 64. Radiograph findings associated with asthma include:
   A. a flattened diaphragm.   C. focal atelectasis.
   B. a normal radiograph.   D. all of the above.

_____ 65. ABG analysis is not indicated in mild exacerbations of chronic asthma.
   A. True
   B. False

_____ 66. During the early stages of an acute exacerbation of asthma, a tachypneic patient can be expected to have a $PaCO_2$ that is:
   A. slightly lowered.   C. slightly elevated.
   B. normal.   D. extremely elevated.

©2007 Pearson Education, Inc.
Critical Care Paramedic

_____ 67. _____ are considered first-line medications in an asthma attack.
   A. Magnesium sulfate and corticosteroids
   B. Anticholinergics and beta-agonists
   C. Oxygen and corticosteroids
   D. Theophylline and aminophylline

_____ 68. The airway inflammation and edema characteristic of phase II of an exacerbation of asthma is best treated with:
   A. anticholinergics and beta-agonists.
   B. magnesium sulfate.
   C. corticosteroids.
   D. theophylline.

_____ 69. The bronchoconstriction characteristic of phase I of an exacerbation of asthma is best treated with:
   A. anticholinergics and beta-agonists.
   B. magnesium sulfate.
   C. corticosteroids.
   D. theophylline.

_____ 70. All of the following are ways that noninvasive positive pressure ventilation (NPPV) assists the asthma patient except:
   A. the positive pressure keeps the lower airways open, allowing for better ventilation.
   B. the positive pressure decreases the work of breathing during inhalation.
   C. the positive pressure reduces the accumulation of fluid in the alveoli, increasing the efficacy of gas exchange.
   D. the positive pressure reduces airway edema and bronchoconstriction, allowing for better ventilation.

_____ 71. Advantages of using a larger endotracheal tube via the orotracheal route rather than performing nasotracheal intubation in an asthma patient who requires intubation include:
   A. the ability to suction more effectively.
   B. decreased air resistance in the vent circuit.
   C. the ability to utilize a bronchoscope.
   D. all of the above.

_____ 72. The use of sedative agents such as opiates and barbiturates are recommended for all asthma patients undergoing intubation.
   A. True
   B. False

_____ 73. The asthma patient who is being mechanically ventilated is at increased risk of barotrauma secondary to:
   A. air trapping and the "stacking" of ventilations.
   B. an increased inspiratory phase.
   C. a decreased expiratory phase.
   D. hypoxia.

_____ 74. The risk of barotrauma in the mechanically ventilated asthma patient can be lowered by:
   A. increasing oxygen concentration and allowing for a prolonged expiratory phase.
   B. decreasing respiratory rate, increasing inspiratory flow rate, and allowing for a prolonged expiratory phase.
   C. increasing respiratory rate and allowing for a prolonged expiratory phase.
   D. none of the above.

_____ 75. Asthma affects about _____ of the total population of the United States.
   A. 2–4 percent
   B. 4–5 percent
   C. 5–7 percent
   D. 6–10 percent

_____ 76. Chronic obstructive pulmonary disease (COPD) represents the _____ leading cause of death in the United States.
   A. third
   B. fourth
   C. fifth
   D. sixth

_____ 77. The pathological changes associated with COPD include all of the following except:
A. alveolar wall destruction and bleb formation.
B. goblet cell hypertrophy.
C. increased α_1-antitrypsin production.
D. thickening of pulmonary capillary endothelial walls.

_____ 78. Hypoxemia develops in COPD secondary to:
A. the destruction of the alveolar membrane and destruction of capillary walls.
B. the development of a right-to-left shunt.
C. the creation of a V/Q mismatch.
D. all of the above.

_____ 79. Patients with COPD exacerbation will often breathe through pursed lips to:
A. prolong expiration.
B. create a physiological positive end-expiratory pressure.
C. increase tidal volume.
D. increase minute ventilation.

_____ 80. All of the following are factors that can exacerbate existing COPD except:
A. increased FiO_2.   C. underlying respiratory infection.
B. cardiovascular deterioration.   D. increased bronchospasm.

_____ 81. Signs and symptoms of COPD exacerbation include:
A. tachypnea, rales, rhonchi, decreased SpO_2, and increased anteroposterior chest diameter.
B. tachypnea, wheezing, rhonchi, decreased SpO_2, and increased anteroposterior chest diameter.
C. tachypnea, silent chest, decreased SpO_2, JVD, and peripheral edema.
D. none of the above.

_____ 82. Stage III, or severe COPD, is defined according to the GOLD methodology as:
A. $FEV_1/FVC < 70\%$, $FEV_1 < 30$–50% of predicted, with chronic symptoms.
B. $FEV_1/FVC < 70\%$, $FEV_1 < 50$–80% of predicted, with or without chronic symptoms.
C. $FEV_1/FVC < 70\%$, $FEV_1 < 30$–50% of predicted, with or without chronic symptoms.
D. $FEV_1/FVC < 70\%$, $FEV_1 < 50\%$ of predicted, with chronic symptoms.

_____ 83. Chest radiographs are valuable tools in the initial diagnosis and determination of the severity of an acute exacerbation of COPD.
A. True
B. False

_____ 84. Which of the following can be a useful tool in monitoring a COPD patient's response to therapy?
A. SpO_2 C. Both of the above
B. Serial spirometry   D. None of the above

_____ 85. Respiratory failure in the COPD patient is suggested by which of the following ABG analysis findings?
A. $PaO_2 < 60$ mmHg, $SpO_2 < 90\%$ on room air
B. $pH > 7.40$, $PaO_2 < 80$ mmHg, $PaCO_2 > 45$ mmHg
C. $pH < 7.30$, $PaCO_2 > 70$ mmHg on room air
D. $pH < 7.40$, $PaCO_2 < 80$ mmHg, $PaCO_2 < 35$ mmHg

_____ 86. Ventilatory failure in the COPD patient is suggested by which of the following ABG analysis findings?
A. $PaO_2 < 60$ mmHg, $SpO_2 < 90\%$ on room air
B. $pH > 7.40$, $PaO_2 < 80$ mmHg, $PaCO_2 > 45$ mmHg
C. $pH < 7.30$, $PaCO_2 > 70$ mmHg on room air
D. $pH < 7.40$, $PaCO_2 < 80$ mmHg, $PaCO_2 < 35$ mmHg

_____ 87. SpO$_2$ readings may be artificially lower in the patient with COPD secondary to:
   A. air trapping.
   B. polycythemia.
   C. hypoxia.
   D. the administration of high-flow, 100% oxygen.

_____ 88. The administration of high-flow, 100 percent oxygen should be avoided in patients with COPD because of the risk of respiratory depression secondary to hypoxic drive.
   A. True
   B. False

_____ 89. Management of exacerbation of chronic COPD includes:
   A. anticholinergics and beta-agonists.   C. corticosteroids.
   B. antibiotics.   D. all of the above.

_____ 90. Antibiotics administered to treat mild-to-moderate exacerbations of COPD include:
   A. penicillins, fluoroquinolones, and third-generation cephalosporins or aminoglycosides.
   B. penicillins, fluoroquinolones, trimethoprim-sulfamethoxazole, and amoxicillin.
   C. doxycycline, trimethoprim-sulfamethoxazole, and amoxicillin.
   D. none of the above.

_____ 91. Antibiotics administered to treat mild-to-moderate exacerbations of COPD include:
   A. penicillins, fluoroquinolones, and third-generation cephalosporins or aminoglycosides.
   B. penicillins, fluoroquinolones, trimethoprim-sulfamethoxazole, and amoxicillin.
   C. doxycycline, trimethoprim-sulfamethoxazole, and amoxicillin.
   D. none of the above.

_____ 92. Hyperventilation is to be avoided in the patient with COPD because:
   A. air trapping can lead to barotrauma.
   B. excess ventilation will leave the normal compensatory alkalosis present in COPD exacerbation unchecked.
   C. both of the above.
   D. none of the above; hyperventilation is necessary in the treatment of COPD.

_____ 93. Acute respiratory distress syndrome (ARDS) is characterized by:
   A. chronic airflow limitation that is not fully reversible.
   B. hyper-responsiveness of the airways to various stimuli, inflammation and edema of the airways, and increased mucus production.
   C. infection of the gas-exchange units of the lungs leading to progressive hypoxemia secondary to bronchospasm, fluid and pus accumulation, and decreased lung compliance.
   D. impaired oxygenation, rapidly progressive hypoxemia, the presence of diffuse bilateral infiltrates on chest radiograph, and decreased lung compliance following a known predisposing insult.

_____ 94. Which of the following is not representative of the pathophysiology of ARDS?
   A. Activated neutrophils and macrophages adhere to the pulmonary capillary endothelium, where they release proteases, oxygen metabolites, and leukotrines.
   B. Inflammation and capillary permeability results in the accumulation of interstitial and alveolar edema.
   C. Submucosal cell damage results in basement membrane thickening and hypertrophy of airway smooth muscle.
   D. Lung compliance decreases, and blood flow to the lung is reduced.

_____ 95. All of the following are factors associated with ARDS except:
   A. pulmonary contusion, multi system trauma, and near–drowning.
   B. pneumonia, sepsis, and gastric aspiration.
   C. fat embolism and acute pancreatitis.
   D. diabetes, hypertension, and heart failure.

_____ 96. The same process that leads to ARDS can occur in any organ system in the body, resulting in multisystem organ dysfunction syndrome (MODS)
   A. True
   B. False

_____ 97. Signs and symptoms of ARDS include:
   A. rapidly worsening dyspnea and hypoxia, JVD, and S_3 heart sound.
   B. rapidly worsening dyspnea, tachypnea, hypoxia, and crackles upon auscultation.
   C. rapidly worsening tachypnea and hypoxia, wheezes and crackles upon auscultation, and signs of left ventricular overload.
   D. none of the above.

_____ 98. Diagnostic criteria for ARDS includes:
   A. bilateral infiltrates on chest radiograph, a $PaO_2 < 80$ mmHg, and no evidence of left heart failure.
   B. lack of bilateral infiltrates on chest radiograph, a $PaO_2 < 80$ mmHg on an FiO_2 of 100%, no evidence of left atrial hypertension in a patient with a defined risk factor for ARDS, and no history of pulmonary disease.
   C. lack of consolidation on chest radiograph, a $PaO_2 < 80$ mmHg on an FiO_2 of 100%, evidence of left atrial hypertension in a patient with a defined risk factor for ARDS, and no history of pulmonary disease.
   D. bilateral infiltrates on chest radiograph, a $PaO_2/FiO_2 < 100$, no evidence of left atrial hypertension in a patient with a defined risk factor for ARDS, and no severe chronic pulmonary disease.

_____ 99. Management of ARDS includes the administration of oxygen at an FiO_2 of:
   A. < 25%.   C. < 50%.
   B. 40–60%.   D. 50–75%.

_____ 100. In the treatment of ARDS, if an FiO_2 of 50 percent is insufficient to achieve a SpO_2 of 90%, _____ should be provided to increase oxygenation.
   A. positive end-expiratory pressure
   B. increases in FiO_2 up to 75%
   C. exogenous administration of pulmonary surfactant
   D. none of the above

_____ 101. Ventilation management of ARDS may include all of the following except:
   A. permissive hypercapnia.
   B. mechanical ventilation with low-tidal volumes.
   C. a reversed I/E ratio.
   D. allowing for a prolonged expiratory phase.

_____ 102. Pharmacological management of the patient with ARDS may include:
   A. corticosteroids.   C. dobutamine.
   B. loop diuretics.   D. dopamine.

_____ 103. Pneumonia is the _____ leading cause of death in the United States.
   A. third   C. seventh
   B. fifth   D. ninth

_____ 104. Atypical agents that can cause pneumonia include:
   A. _Mycoplasma._   C. _Legionella._
   B. _Streptococcus pneumoniae._ D. _Chlamydia._

©2007 Pearson Education, Inc.
Critical Care Paramedic

_____105. Normal defense mechanisms that protect against pneumonia include:
   A. filtration and humidification of inspired air as it passes through the upper airway.
   B. the cough reflex.
   C. cellular immunity and humoral immunity.
   D. all of the above.

_____106. Which of the following does not increase the risk of pneumonia?
   A. Increased circulating neutrophils
   B. Impaired mucociliary clearance
   C. Increased risk of aspiration
   D. Immunocompromization

_____107. Risk factors for nosocomial pneumonia include:
   A. an increased length of stay in the hospital.
   B. intubation and mechanical ventilation.
   C. the use of antacids and/or H-blockers.
   D. all of the above.

_____108. Commonly accepted clinical criteria for the identification of serious pneumonia includes:
   A. tachypnea greater than 20 breaths per minute, temperature greater than 101.9°F, hypotension, and a decreased level of consciousness.
   B. tachypnea greater than 30 breaths per minute, temperature greater than 100°F, hypoxia, and an altered mental status.
   C. tachypnea greater than 30 breaths per minute, temperature greater than 101°F, hypotension, and an altered mental status.
   D. tachypnea greater than 24 breaths per minute, temperature greater than 101°F, hypertension, hypoxia, and an altered mental status.

_____109. The absence of leukocytosis rules out the possibility of pneumonia.
   A. True
   B. False

_____110. Which of the following correctly lists the laboratory results that influence the decision for hospitalization of a patient with pneumonia?
   A. Leukopenia < 4000-5000 cells/mm^3, leukocytosis > 30,000 cells/mm^3, PaO_2 < 50 mmHg, and involvement of > 50% of the lung
   B. Leukopenia > 4000-5000 cells/mm^3, leukocytosis < 30,000 cells/mm^3, PaO_2 < 50 mmHg, and involvement of < 50% of the lung
   C. Leukopenia < 4000-5000 cells/mm^3, leukocytosis < 30,000 cells/mm^3, PaO_2 < 60 mmHg, and involvement of > 50% of the lung
   D. Leukopenia > 4000-5000 cells/mm^3, leukocytosis > 30,000 cells/mm^3, PaO_2 < 50 mmHg, and involvement of > 40% of the lung

_____111. ABG analysis is required in all cases of pneumonia, regardless of the level of severity.
   A. True
   B. False

_____112. Common chest radiograph findings consistent with pneumonia include all of the following except:
   A. peribronchial thickening.
   B. pleural effusion.
   C. patchy interstitial or alveolar infiltrates.
   D. flattening of the diaphragm.

_____113. The management of a patient with pneumonia consists primarily of:
   A. oxygenation, ventilatory support, and antibiotic and diuretic administration.
   B. endotracheal intubation and mechanical ventilation.
   C. oxygenation, ventilatory support, and antibiotic administration.
   D. oxygenation, ventilatory support, antibiotic administration, and inhaled beta-agonists.

_____114. Iatrogenic pneumothorax occurs:
   A. secondary to the rupture of a subpleural emphysematous bleb.
   B. secondary to a medical procedure.
   C. as a complication of lung disease.
   D. without a prior event or any other apparent cause.

_____ 115. The most dependable signs and symptoms of a pneumothorax can include all of the following except:
   A. decreased breath sounds on the affected side.
   B. decreased SpO_2.
   C. pleuritic chest pain.
   D. increased $ETCO_2$.

_____ 116. The transport environment is commonly noisy, making the completion of some parts of the physical exam difficult. The most reliable signs and symptoms of developing tension pneumothorax in the mechanically ventilated patient in a noisy, transport environment include:
   A. decreased breath sounds on the affected side, decreasing SpO_2, decreasing level of consciousness, and hypotension.
   B. absent breath sounds on the affected side, tracheal deviation, and increases in airway pressure.
   C. decreased SaO_2, hypotension, tachycardia, and increases in airway pressure.
   D. absent breath sounds on the affected side, decreased breath sounds on the unaffected side, and increases in airway pressure.

_____ 117. The "gold standard" chest radiograph for the diagnosis of pneumothorax is considered to be a:
   A. 6-foot upright posteroanterior view.   C. 4-foot supine anteroposterior view.
   B. 6-foot upright anteroposterior view.   D. 4-foot upright posteroanterior view.

_____ 118. Chest radiograph findings suggestive of pneumothorax include all of the following except:
   A. a deep suclus sign.
   B. a thin pleural line.
   C. an absence of lung marking between the pleural line and the chest wall.
   D. a widened mediastinum.

_____ 119. Immediate management of a tension pneumothorax may include:
   A. needle decompression.   C. BVM ventilation.
   B. chest thoracostomy.   D. both A and B.

_____ 120. Intrapleural air is reabsorbed at a rate of:
   A. 1.25% per hour.   C. 1.25% per day.
   B. 1.25% per kg/day.   D. 1–2% per kg/day.

_____ 121. Most small, primary pneumothoraces are treated with:
   A. oxygen 3–4 lpm, chest thoracostomy, serial chest radiographs, and observation.
   B. oxygen 3–4 lpm, serial chest radiographs, and observation.
   C. oxygen 3–4 lpm, chest thoracostomy, serial CT scans, and observation.
   D. none of the above.

_____ 122. Chest thoracostomy is:
   A. standard of care for almost all cases of secondary spontaneous pneumothorax.
   B. always required if mechanical ventilation is going to be utilized.
   C. required for pneumothoraces greater than 40%.
   D. all of the above.

Cardiovascular Emergencies

Review of Chapter Objectives

Upon completion of this chapter, the student should be able to:

1. **Understand and discuss the anatomy and physiology of the heart as it pertains to the critical care paramedic.** p. 623

   The heart is located in the mediastinal cavity just to the left of the sternum. The superior border of the heart rests at approximately the second intercostal space, and the inferior border at the level of the sixth rib. The heart is rotated slightly to the left, making the right ventricle the anterior surface.

   The heart is divided into four chambers, two atria and two ventricles. Valves ensure that no retrograde flow of blood occurs within the heart. The mitral and tricuspid valves, collectively termed the atrioventricular (AV) valves, are tethered by the *chordae tendoneae* and papillary muscles, which prevent them from prolapsing into the atria when the ventricles contract. The pulmonary and aortic valves, collectively termed the semilunar valves, prevent the retrograde flow of blood from the pulmonary and aorta arteries, respectively, back into the ventricles of the heart. The left and right sides of the heart are considered separate systems, with the left being a high-pressure system and the right, a low-pressure system.

   The myocardium must operate in a rhythmic fashion in order for there to be forward propulsion of blood. Two types of cells contribute to pumping blood: conduction cells and contractile cells. Conduction cells transmit the electrical signal initiated at the sinoatrial (SA) node throughout the entire myocardium in an organized fashion. The components of the myocardial conduction system are:

   - SA node
   - Intra-atrial pathways
   - AV node
   - Purkinje fibers

   Some locations within the electrical conduction system can act as a pacemaker site should the intrinsic heart rate fall below its set point. Specific sights and their intrinsic firing rates are:

   - SA node: 60–100 impulses per minute
   - AV node: 40–60 impulses per minute
   - Purkinje fibers: 20–40 impulses per minute
   - Ventricular myocardium: less than 20 impulses per minute

   The contractile force of the myocardium is generated from the second type of cardiac cell, the contractile cell, which makes up the vast majority of cells in the myocardium. In fact, when we use the term myocardium, we are, for all intents and purposes, referring to the contractile cells of the heart. The contractile cell is where the actual work of pumping the blood happens. As the electrical current generated from the conductive cells passes through a contractile cell, the contractile cell shortens in length, and blood is ejected from the heart as the chamber size decreases in response to this contraction. Myocardial cells have specific properties that make them unique from other cells in the body; they possess:

- Automaticity
- Conductivity
- Excitability
- Contractility

Myocardial blood supply is provided via the coronary arteries, which originate at the base of the aorta. Perfusion of coronary arteries occurs during diastole. The right coronary artery perfuses the:

- SA node
- AV node
- Right atrium
- Right ventricle
- Posterior myocardium
- Inferior wall of the left ventricle

The left coronary artery branches into the left anterior descending (LAD) and left circumflex arteries. They perfuse:

- LAD
  - Septal wall
  - Anterior left ventricle
- Circumflex
  - Lateral, posterior left ventricle

Cardiac auscultation is an important part of cardiac assessment at the critical care level. The proper equipment is required, as is a quiet environment, which admittedly may be difficult in some critical care situations. Specific heart sounds include:

- S_1
- S_2
- Split S_1
- Split S_2
- S_3
- S_4

S_1 and S_2 represent the basic "lub-dub" sound of the heart. S_1 is created by the closing of the AV valves during ventricular systole, and S_2 is created by the closing of the semilunar valves at the end of ventricular systole/beginning of ventricular diastole.

A split S_1 is caused by the closing of the louder aortic valve followed by the closing of the quieter pulmonic valve, and is referred to as "physiologic splitting." It is a result of increased venous return and negative intrathoracic pressure, and can be heard on inspiration. Increased intrathoracic pressure delays emptying of the right ventricle, which delays closing of the pulmonic valve, resulting is a "lub dubdub" being auscultated.

A split S_2 occurs when the closing of AV valves does not occur in unison, and is the sound of the louder mitral valve followed by the softer tricuspid. A split S_2 tends to be harder to auscultate than split S_1. An especially loud mitral closure may mask a split S_2.

An S_3, also known as a "ventricular gallop," occurs secondary to rapid filling of a noncompliant ventricle. The stiff ventricle cannot distend to accept blood, and the resultant turbulent blood flow results in vibration of valve and ventricle. It follows S_2, and may be confused with a split S_2.

An S_4, also known as an "atrial gallop," precedes S_1, and occurs late in the diastolic phase. It occurs secondary to vibration created as the atria contract and propel blood into a noncompliant ventricle, and is, therefore, similar to S_3 etiology.

A heart murmur is a sound created when:

- Blood flows through a stenosed valve
- Blood regurgitates through an improperly functioning valve

Heart murmurs are longer in duration than normal heart sounds. Systolic murmurs are the result of blood flowing retrograde through a faulty AV valve, and are appreciated between S_1 and S_2, during ventricular systole; the sound can be described as a crescendo-decrescendo. Diastolic murmurs that are the result of blood flowing retrograde through a faulty semilunar valve occur after S_2, during ventricular diastole. The sound typically decreases in intensity. Diastolic murmurs that are the result of AV stenosis occur a short time after, and can be described as a low-frequency, decrescendo-crescendo.

The Levin scale classifies murmurs by intensity as a grade of I–V, but this scale is extremely subjective.

2. **Understand the pathophysiology, clinical manifestation, diagnostics, and management guidelines of patients with the following disorders:**

   a. **Acute coronary syndrome**   p. 631
      Pathophysiology
      Coronary artery disease involves the development of atherosclerosis and atheromas. As the narrowing of the coronary arteries progresses, it leads to the clinical spectrum of myocardial ischemia, injury, and infarction known as acute coronary syndrome (ACS). Myocardial ischemia occurs as oxygen demand exceeds supply, leading to the injury of myocardial cells; if the oxygen deficit is not corrected, ischemia will lead to infarction and cell death. Impaired oxygen delivery to the myocardium can occur secondary to:
      - Coronary artery occlusion
        - Coronary artery spasm
        - Stenosis
        - Thrombus formation
      - Hypotension
      - Tachycardia

      Clinical exam findings
      The "classic" signs and symptoms, though present in only 50 percent of all ACS, are:
      - Chest pain, discomfort, pressure
        - Radiating to left arm or jaw
      - Dyspnea
        - Diaphoresis, tachycardia
      Atypical signs and symptoms of ACS include:
      - Dyspnea
      - Syncope
      - Fatigue
      - Nausea and vomiting
      - Sharp/pleuritic chest pain
      - Confusion, stroke-like symptoms

      Women have been shown to have different signs and symptoms than the "classic" presentation:
      - Indigestion/gas pain
      - Dizziness, nausea
      - Weakness, fatigue
      - Pain/discomfort between shoulder blades
      - Recurring chest discomfort
      - Feeling of impending doom

      Risk factors for ACS include:
      - Past history of coronary or vascular disease
      - Family cardiac history
      - Smoking
      - Hypertension
      - Hyperlipidemia
      - Diabetes mellitus

- Contraceptive use
- Artificial/early menopause

Diagnostic exam findings

An electrocardiogram (ECG) is useful to support the diagnosis of AMI and to screen patients with atypical presentations. It is important to remember that ECG will be nondiagnostic in > 50 percent of patients, so the lack of ECG evidence does not rule out AMI. Changes suggestive of AMI include:
- ST segment elevation > 0.1 mm in at least two continuous leads
- Reciprocal ST depression
- Presence of Q wave

AMI is now classified based on ECG findings; AMI without ST segment elevation on ECG is termed a non-ST elevation myocardial infarction (Non-STEMI), and AMI with ST segment elevation on ECG is termed an ST elevation myocardial infarction (STEMI).

Cardiac enzymes that can be diagnostic in AMI include creatine kinase and troponin. Creatine kinase, myocardial band (CK-MB) immunochemical testing is possible within several hours after onset of AMI. At 3 hours, sensitivity and specificity are greater than 90 percent, and at 10 to 12 hours there is almost 100 percent sensitivity. If the value of CK-MB is elevated and the ratio of CK-MB to total CK (relative index) is more than 2.5 to 3, it is likely that myocardium was damaged. A high CK with a relative index below this value suggests that skeletal muscle was damaged.

Troponin is a family of proteins found in skeletal and cardiac muscle, though the test used for AMI detects only the troponin released from damaged myocardium into the blood, troponin T. Troponin T is present in blood 3 to 4 hours post myocardial injury, and remains elevated for up to 14 days. Troponin T has a 98 percent diagnostic accuracy for AMI.

Management

Approach to ACS includes the following:
- Increase myocardial oxygen supply
  - Administration of supplemental oxygen
  - Nitrates
  - Calcium channel blockers
  - Fibrinolytic therapy
  - PTCA
  - Bypass surgery
- Decrease myocardial oxygen demand
  - Nitrates
  - Calcium channel blockers
  - Beta blockers
- Correct rhythm and rate disturbance
- Prevent reocclusion of coronary arteries
  - Aspirin
  - GP2b3a inhibitors
- Reduce pain and relieve stress
  - Goal for pain reduction is no pain
  - Achieved with:
    - Oxygen
    - Nitrates
    - Nitrous oxide
    - Morphine sulfate

b. Aortic aneurysm   p. 639
Pathophysiology

An aortic aneurysm is a localized dilation of the aorta secondary to a weakened vessel wall. All three layers, the tunica intima, media, and adventitia, are involved, and aneurysms most often evolve below the level of the renal arteries. There is no universal standard as to when localized dilatation is termed an aneurysm, but it is generally accepted that an infrarenal aortic diameter greater than 3 cm can be defined as an abdominal aortic aneurysm (AAA). Aortic aneurysm is different than aortic dissection; dissection involves separation of the intimal and media layers and typically originates in the thoracic aorta with 90 percent developing within 10 cm of the aortic valve.

An aortic aneurysm occurs when the loss of collagen and connective tissue leads to a weakening of the aortic wall, allowing the high pressure in the aorta to distend the weakened wall. Risk factors for aortic aneurysm include:
- Age
- Male gender
- Peripheral vascular disease
- Extremity arterial aneurysms
- Family history of AAA

Criteria for surgical intervention of an aortic aneurysm include:
- 5 cm diameter
- 1 cm growth in 12 months
- Symptomatic pain or hypertension

Clinical exam findings
Most abdominal aortic aneurysms are clinically silent until they rupture. However, clinical manifestations may include:
- Abdominal pulsations
- Back pain
  - Throbbing, colicky
- Oliguria
- Sensation of abdominal "fullness"
- Decreased femoral pulses, abdominal bruits
- Hypotension
  - Late sign
  - Indicates ruptured AAA

Diagnostic exam findings
Signs of AAA are seen on plain radiographs in two-thirds to three-fourths of cases. Either ultrasound or abdominal CT best determines the diagnosis of abdominal aortic aneurysm.

Management
Initial management of AAA revolves around the decision for emergency surgery versus medical intervention; hemodynamic status drives the decision making. Rupture requires immediate surgical intervention, while unruptured AAA may be treated medically. The sudden onset of hypotension with, or without, new onset of pain is suggestive of rupture, and should be treated aggressively. The patient should be transported to the nearest appropriate emergency department in a facility that has immediate surgical capabilities. Multiple large bore IVs or a central venous catheter should be placed. Crystalloid infusion is the most immediate supportive measure; however, avoid overaggressive fluid resuscitation to limit blood loss. Infusion of blood products may be necessary and, therefore, the patient should be immediately typed and cross-matched for 10 units of blood.

c. **Aortic dissection**   p. 641
Pathophysiology
An aortic dissection is the separation of the tunica intima and media layers of the aorta, which results in altered blood flow through the aorta. An intimal tear results in subintimal hematoma formation, and the expanding hematoma separates the intima and the media layers, creating a false lumen between the layers. The dissection can extend both distal and proximal from the site of the intimal tear. Distal extension can affect the aortic valve, and proximal extension can involve branching arteries such as the carotid and subclavian. Up to 90 percent of dissections occur within 10 cm of the aortic valve.

Known risk factors for aortic dissection are:
- Hypertension
- Marfan's disease
- Inflammatory disorders of the aorta
- Smoking
- Pregnancy

Categorization of aortic dissection can be accomplished using the DeBakey Classification system:
- DeBakey Type I
  - Intimal tear in the ascending aorta
  - Extends to involve the aortic arch and the descending aorta
- DeBakey Type II
  - Intimal tear confined to the ascending aorta
- DeBakey Type III
  - Intimal tear confined to the descending aorta, distal to the subclavian artery

Clinical exam findings

Clinical exam findings can vary with the type of dissection that occurs, and can include:
- Sharp, tearing pain
  - Chest pain radiating to the upper back
  - Arm or neck pain
- Hypertension
- Variable BPs between the left and right side of the body
- Unilateral/bilateral decrease in carotid pulse pressure
- Paraplegia, extremity paresthesias
- Pleural effusion, diastolic murmur
- Decreased bowel sounds, hematuria
- Dyspnea
- Loss of speech
- AMI, abdominal pain

Diagnostic exam findings

A patient with a dissected aorta may present with ECG changes consistent with AMI. Therefore, an ECG positive for AMI on a patient presenting with chest pain does not rule out aortic dissection. Further workup and clinical correlations need to be made in order to rule out the presence (or absence) of dissection. The ECG in this situation may show evidence of LVH and left axis deviation that reflects long-standing hypertension. Aortography, CT, and MRI are useful in diagnosis.

Management

All patients suspected of having an aortic dissection should have ongoing monitoring of the cardiac rhythm, blood pressure, and urine output. Therapy is geared at decreasing the forces that favor progression of the dissection. This is accomplished by maintaining systolic blood pressure between 100 and 120 mmHg and by reduction of cardiac contractility. For patients who present with hypertension, prompt reduction of blood pressure can be accomplished in a controlled manner with sodium nitroprusside infused at 0.5 to 3.0 mcg/kg/min. The rate is adjusted to maintain the blood pressure between 100 and 120 mmHg. A beta-adrenergic blocker should be used in conjunction with nitroprusside to decrease cardiac contractility and heart rate. Propranolol may be administered with a starting dose of 1 mg IV every five minutes with a target reduction of heart rate to 60 to 80 beats/min. Esmolol, a short-acting beta blocker administered by continuous infusion at 50 to 200 mcg/kg/min, may be preferable. Unlike AAA, nearly all aortic dissections must undergo surgical intervention.

In some instances, critical care transport may be utilized to transport postoperative patients recovering from aortic dissection. Care should be taken to maintain antihypertensive and anticoagulation medications as ordered by the physician. In addition, utilization of a "cough pillow" helps the patient minimize the increased thoracic pressure associated with coughing, which, in turn, decreases the likelihood of damaging the repaired structures. The critical care paramedic provider should be on the lookout for any signs or symptoms suggestive of a leaking or ruptured repair.

d. Cardiogenic shock   p. 643
Pathophysiology
Cardiogenic shock is defined as circulatory failure after the heart has suffered pump failure. It results in inadequate end-organ perfusion secondary to:
- Decreased preload
- Decreased contractile force
- Decreased ejection fraction
- Decreased stroke volume
- Increased afterload

Causes of cardiogenic shock include:
- MI
- Cardiomyopathy
- Myocarditis
- Myocardial contusion
- Valvular dysfunction
- Ventricular septal defect

Clinical exam findings
Clinical exam findings indicative of cardiogenic shock include:
- Cool, pale, diaphoretic skin
- Tachycardia, tachypnea
- Restlessness, anxiety, altered mental status
- Oliguria
- CHF
- JVD
- Peripheral edema

Diagnostic exam findings
Labs studies useful in the evaluation of cardiogenic shock include ABG, which may reveal hypoxemia and acidosis and the presence of cardiac markers such as troponin T and CK-MB. ECG findings consistent with cardiogenic shock include:
- AMI
- Cardiomyopathy
- Myocarditis
- Myocardial contusion

A Swan-Ganz catheter can be used to measure pulmonary capillary wedge pressure (PCWP) and central venous pressure (CVP). Cardiogenic shock may be indicated by a PCWP greater than 18 mmHg and a cardiac index of less than 1.8 $L/min/m^2$.

Management
After a controlled airway and adequate ventilation with 100 percent oxygen have been assured, pharmacological management can be considered. It includes:
- Inotropic agents
  - Increase cardiac contractility
- Vasodilators
  - Decrease afterload
- Vasoconstrictors
  - If hypotension develops
- Diuretics
  - If volume overload exists

Fluid volume administration should be considered if right ventricular infarction is present, and a PCWP can help in guiding fluid resuscitation in cases where left ventricular preload is hard to determine. An intra-aortic balloon pump can be used as a bridge to percutaneous coronary intervention (PCI) or coronary artery bypass graft (CABG) surgery to decrease myocardial workload and improve end-organ perfusion. Left-ventricular assist devices are used when more long-term maintenance is required.

e. Adult cardiomyopathies   **p. 647**
Pathophysiology
Cardiomyopathies are cardiac disorders whose dominant feature is pathologic change to the myocardium. Primary cardiomyopathies are those in which no underlying cause can be identified, while secondary cardiomyopathies have a demonstrable underlying cause. There are three major categories of cardiomyopathies:

- Dilated cardiomyopathies
- Hypertrophic cardiomyopathies
- Restrictive cardiomyopathies

In dilated cardiomyopathy, the chambers of the heart become enlarged or dilated. All four chambers can be involved. Decreased stroke volume (SV) and ejection fraction (EF) result in an increased end-systolic volume, increased end-systolic pressure and dilated chambers. Pulmonary hypertension and CHF can also result as a consequence of the backup of pressure. Dilated cardiomyopathy is often idiopathic, though toxic, metabolic, and infectious factors may be involved.

Hypertrophic cardiomyopathy (HCM) involves a nondilated, hypertrophic left ventricle of unknown etiology; it is thought to be genetic. Asymmetric thickening of septum and the ventricular wall results in asymmetric tension on papillary muscles which causes valvular regurgitation. The end result is:

- Decreased ventricular compliance
- Decreased ventricular end-diastolic volume
- Increased pressure gradient

Restrictive cardiomyopathy is characterized by ventricular stiffness that leads to diastolic dysfunction. This stiffness occurs secondary to endocardial and myocardial lesions, and results in progressive limitation of ventricular filling and eventual reduced cardiac output.

Clinical exam findings

Dilated Cardiomyopathy	*Hypertrophic Cardiomyopathy*	*Restrictive Cardiomyopathy*
Fatigue, weakness, progressive S/S of CHF, right and left side S_3 and S_4 summation gallop, mitral/tricuspid regurgitation murmurs	Patients often asymptomatic, systolic murmur, dyspnea, chest pain, angina, palpitations, fatigue, weakness, vertigo, syncope	Chest pain, dyspnea with exertion, exercise intolerance, evidence of right ventricular failure

Diagnostic exam findings
Diagnostic findings with dilated cardiomyopathy include:

- Radiograph
  - Cardiomegaly
  - Pulmonary edema
  - Pleural effusion
- Echocardiogram
  - Dilated ventricle
  - EF < 45 percent
- ECG
  - Often nonspecific
  - BBB, or intraventricular conduction delay

Diagnostic findings with hypertrophic cardiomyopathy include:

- Radiograph
  - Left ventricular hypertrophy
- Echocardiogram
  - Decreased left ventricular ejection fraction

- ECG
  - Nonspecific intraventricular conduction
  - Bundle branch block

Diagnostic findings with restrictive cardiomyopathy include:
- Radiograph
  - Pulmonary congestion
- ECG
  - Sinus tachycardia
  - Atrial fibrillation
  - Biventricular hypertrophy

Management

Management of dilated cardiomyopathy includes:
- Nitrates
  - Reduce preload and afterload
- Diuretics
  - Decrease blood volume
  - Decrease preload and afterload
- Anticoagulants
  - Prevent clot and emboli formation

Management of hypertrophic cardiomyopathy includes:
- Beta blockers
  - Propranolol
  - Reduce pressure gradient across outflow tract
  - Lengthen diastolic filling time
  - Decrease risk of dysrhythmia
- Calcium channel blockers
  - Verapamil

f. Cardiopulmonary arrest p. 649

Pathophysiology

Cardiopulmonary arrest is the absence of normal cardiac function resulting in inadequate cardiac output; blood flow ceases and systemic circulatory failure occurs. Irreversible ischemic brain damage develops after four to six minutes of cessation of blood flow. Etiologies of cardiopulmonary arrest include:
- CAD
- Ischemia
- Dysrhythmias
- Cardiomyopathies
- Valvular disease
- Respiratory failure
- Pulmonary embolus
- Trauma
- Shock
- Drug OD/toxic exposure
- Environmental factors

Clinical exam findings

Clinical exam findings consistent with cardiopulmonary arrest include:
- Pulselessness
- Apnea
- Unconsciousness
- Fixed, dilated pupils

Diagnostic exam findings

ECG may reveal the presence or absence of electrical activity. End-tidal CO_2 detection equipment will not register the presence of CO_2. A pulse oximeter will indicate no pulse and no oxygen saturation.

Management

Management of cardiopulmonary arrest is in accordance with AHA ACLS guidelines and includes determining the presence of, and treating, reversible causes, such as:

- Hypoxia
- Hypovolemia
- Hyper-hypokalemia
- Hypothermia
- Hydrogen ion (acidosis)
- Tamponade, cardiac
- Tension pneumothorax
- Tablets (ingestion)
- Thrombosis, coronary
- Thrombosis, pulmonary

g. **Congestive heart failure**   p. 651

Pathophysiology

Congestive heart failure (CHF is a pathophysiological state in which the left ventricle of the heart is unable to pump enough blood to meet the metabolic needs of the body. The most serious complication of CHF, pulmonary edema, occurs when increased pulmonary capillary pressure results in the leakage of fluid from the intravascular space into the interstitial space and alveoli of the lung. Right heart failure can also occur secondary to failure of the right ventricle, resulting in the backflow of blood into the vena cava. Left heart failure results in a reduced cardiac output secondary to a reduction in stroke volume (SV), heart rate (HR), or both. Failure of the body's normal compensatory mechanisms (increased HR, activation of renin-angiotension system, increased peripheral vascular resistance) results in hemodynamic instability. Etiologies of CHF include:

- CAD
- Myocardial disease
- Valvular disease
- Obstructive causes

Clinical exam findings

Clinical exam findings associated with left and right heart failure are as follows:

- Left heart failure
  - Shortness of breath
  - Orthopnea
  - Paroxysmal nocturnal dyspnea
  - Crackles
  - Apical pulse displaced
  - Split S_2, S_3 gallop
- Right heart failure
  - JVD
  - Peripheral edema
  - S_3, tricuspid regurgitation

Diagnostic exam findings

The following clinical exam data are suggestive for CHF:

- Radiograph
  - Cardiomegaly
  - Pulmonary congestion/edema
- ECG
  - Ischemia
  - Left ventricular hypertrophy
- Lab data
  - Cardiac enzymes may indicate AMI as cause of acute failure
  - ABG
    - May reveal hypoxemia, acidosis, V/Q mismatch, hypercapnia

- BNP: Beta natriuretic peptide
  - Can help differentiate CHF from other causes of dyspnea
- Invasive monitoring
  - Elevated PCWP
  - Elevated SVR
  - Decreased CO

Management

The general management of patients with congestive heart failure involves decreasing cardiac workload by reducing both preload and afterload, increasing SV, decreasing the work of breathing, and clearing the alveoli of fluid to increase the effectiveness of gas exchange. Common management strategies to achieve these goals include:

- Preload reduction
  - NTG
  - Morphine
  - Diuretics
- Afterload reduction
  - ACE inhibitors
  - Beta blockers
- Improve SV
  - Dobutamine
- Decrease work of breathing, clear alveolar fluid accumulation
  - CPAP/BiPAP
  - Diuretics

h. Hypertensive emergencies   p. 652

Pathophysiology

The most common category of hypertension is primary or essential hypertension. Essential hypertension is a hypertensive state in which no specific cause has been identified. Essential hypertension is chronic in nature; seldom do patients with essential hypertension progress to hypertensive emergencies.

Several theories exist with respect to the acute onset of hypertensive emergencies. One popular theory stems from the belief that chronic hypertensive disease eventually causes permanent changes in arterial wall smooth muscle, resulting in overreactive vasoconstriction. Other theories suggest that these emergencies stem from a loss of autoregulatory mechanisms in the central nervous system. A hypertensive emergency is defined as severe, accelerated hypertension, with a diastolic blood pressure greater than 140 mmHg and a constellation of findings representing end-organ damage.

Clinical exam findings

Hypertension in the face of an acute MI is likely to manifest with signs of left ventricular heart failure. Symptoms progress nearly identical to that of any acute MI, but with a greater likelihood of pulmonary edema. Specific signs and symptoms include:

- Shortness of breath
- Dyspnea on exertion (DOE)
- Chest pain
- Cyanosis
- Crackles
- Production of pink, frothy sputum, and hemoptysis
- JVD
- S_3 or S_4 gallop

Patients with intracranial hemorrhage and hypertensive encephalopathy may present initially with:

- Severe headaches
- Nausea and vomiting
- Drowsiness, confusion

- Decreased level of consciousness
- Seizures
- Blindness
- Neurological deficits, coma, and death

Aortic dissections associated with hypertension may present with:

- Severe onset of "tearing" back or chest pain
- Partial or full paralysis
- Syncope
- Cardiac tamponade
- Shortness of breath
- Varying blood pressures on the left side compared to the right

Hypertensive emergencies during pregnancy are considered to be an impending sign of eclampsia, and require rapid intervention. An increase of greater than 30 mmHg systolic or 15 mmHg diastolic is clinically significant for hypertension in gravid females. A blood pressure of 160/110 is considered representative of severe preeclampsia and impending seizures. Physical manifestations include:

- Swelling and edema of the face and distal extremities
- Visual changes
- Headache with nausea and vomiting
- Epigastric pain
- Seizures

Malignant hypertension results from end-organ damage secondary to both acute and chronic episodes of hypertension. Therefore, clinical signs and symptoms can vary with the organs involved. Changes in vision are significant indicators of changes within the retinal arteries. Exudates, cotton wool spots, or punctate hemorrhages may be present on funduscopic exam. Hematuria and oliguria are present with renal damage. Systemic signs and symptoms include headache with blurred vision, dyspnea, chest pain, and neurological changes. It is extremely difficult to differentiate malignant hypertension from other etiologies by exam alone.

Diagnostic exam findings

Diagnostic exam findings in hypertensive patients with AMI may include:

- ECG
  - Characteristic AMI findings on 12-lead ECG
  - Left ventricular hypertrophy from chronic hypertension
- Elevated cardiac enzymes
- Pulmonary congestion on chest X-ray
- Increased pulmonary wedge pressures and decreased cardiac output are indicative of left ventricular failure

Patients with intracranial hemorrhage or hypertensive encephalopathy:

- Serum chemistries to rule out any metabolic causes of altered mental status
- CT
  - Normal in encephalopathy
  - Diagnostic for intracranial hemorrhage

A high index of suspicion for aortic dissection should exist in hypertensive patients with chest pain. Ultrasonography may rapidly reveal a clinically significant aortic dissection. Additional tests that are useful include transesophageal ultrasound, CT or MRI, and aortography. These additional tests will make a more definitive case where the providers are uncertain of the diagnosis.

The American College of Obstetricians and Gynecologists define the following hypertensive categories:

- *Pregnancy-induced hypertension*—systolic BP > 140 or diastolic > 90 on more than one occasion
- *Mild preeclampsia*—systolic BP > 140 or diastolic BP > 90 on more than one occasion and proteinuria

©2007 Pearson Education, Inc.
Critical Care Paramedic

- *Severe preeclampsia*—systolic BP > 160 or diastolic BP > 110 on two occasions more than 6 hours apart with patient resting, OR 24-hour urine output < 400 mL OR proteinuria greater than 5 g/24 hr, OR visual disturbances, pulmonary edema, or cyanosis
- *Eclampsia*—seizures without underlying CNS lesion in a patient with preeclampsia

To make the diagnosis of malignant hypertension, patients must demonstrate evidence of end-organ damage in addition to elevated blood pressures.

- Blood chemistry
  - Elevated kidney function tests (BUN and creatinine), suggest kidney damage.
- Urinalysis
  - Hematuria and proteinuria, suggest kidney damage.
- ECG
  - Left ventricular hypertrophy with strain pattern.
- Radiograph
  - Cardiomegaly and pulmonary congestion on chest X-ray suggest end-organ damage to the heart.
- Blood smear
  - Red blood cell fragments and fibrin degradation products suggest microangiopathic hemolytic anemia.

Management

The overall goal is to judiciously lower MAP, aiming for a 20 to 25 percent decrease in MAP or a decrease in diastolic blood pressure to between 100 and 110 mmHg. Specific strategies are determined by etiology:

- AMI
  - Nitrate infusion
  - Diuretics
  - Beta blockers
- Intracranial hemorrhage/hypertensive encephalopathy
  - Nitroprusside infusion
  - Beta blockers
  - Calcium channel blockers
- Aortic dissection
  - Goal is systolic pressure between 100–120 mmHg
  - Nitroprusside infusion
  - Beta blockers
  - Surgical repair
- Pregnancy
  - Magnesium sulfate
  - Hydralazine
  - Labetalol
- Malignant hypertension
  - Nitroprusside
  - Labetalol
  - Diuretics
  - Ace inhibitors

i. **Pericarditis, pericardial effusion, and cardiac tamponade**　　　　　　　p. 656
Pathophysiology

Pericarditis is an inflammation, infection, or infiltration of the pericardium that results in the accumulation of pericardial fluid, which can lead to pericardial tamponade.

A pericardial effusion is an abnormal buildup of fluid in the pericardial sac, and can occur secondary to pericarditis or trauma. The fluid buildup places pressure on the heart, decreases diastolic filling pressures, and decreases cardiac output.

Cardiac tamponade is the accumulation of fluid in the pericardial sac, and is considered a life-threatening emergency as it results in decreased cardiac output. Tamponade can occur secondary to trauma, viral and bacterial infections, and drug therapy. The speed of accumulation determines hemodynamic effects; the faster the accumulation, the worse the hemodynamic effects. Detrimental hemodynamic effects can be seen with the rapid accumulation of as little as 150–200 mL of fluid. The developing, increased intrapericardial pressures result in decreased right ventricular filling pressures and decreased cardiac output.

Clinical exam findings

Clinical exam findings associated with pericarditis include:
- Substernal chest pain
  - Retrosternal
  - Sharp, pleuritic, may radiate to shoulder
- Pericardial friction rub
- Muffled heart sounds
- JVD

Clinical manifestations of pericardial effusion include:
- Beck's triad
  - Hypotension
  - JVD
  - Muffled heart sounds
- Pulsus paradoxus
- Tachycardia, tachypnea
- Pericardial friction rub

Clinical manifestations of cardiac tamponade include:
- Beck's triad
  - Hypotension
  - JVD
  - Muffled heart sounds
- Fatigue, malaise, weakness
- Dyspnea, othopnea
- Chest pain
- Oliguria
- Friction rub
- Pulsus paradoxus

Diagnostic exam findings

Lab and diagnostic exam findings typical of pericarditis include:
- WBC
- Elevated in infection
- ESR
  - Elevated in infection
- ECG
  - Diffuse ST segment changes
  - PR segment depression
  - "Lucid interval" as condition progresses
  - Inverted T waves

Studies useful in the diagnosis of pericardial effusion include:
- Radiograph
  - Enlarged cardiac silhouette
- CT
- ECG
- Pericardiocentesis

Diagnosis of cardiac tamponade should be made on clinical grounds, but the following may be useful:
- Chest radiograph
- Echocardiography
- 12-lead ECG findings suggestive for tamponade:

- Sinus tachycardia
- Low-voltage QRS
- Electrical alternans
- PR depression

Management

Treatment of pericarditis consists of:

- Nonsteroidal anti-inflammatory drugs (NSAIDs)
- Oral steroids
- Antiuremic or antibiotic therapies may be indicated

Treatment of cardiac tamponade includes:

- Aggressive fluid volume administration
  - Increase preload
- Pericardiocentesis
- Antibiotic therapy, anti-inflammatory drugs, surgery to treat cause

Treatment for pericardial effusion includes:

- Pericardiocentesis
- Supportive care

j. Valvular dysfunction p. 658

Valvular dysfunction can be categorized by its two basic presentations: valvular stenosis and valvular insufficiency. They result from myriad congenital and acquired causes and are further exacerbated by continuous immunologic or hemodynamic stressors. Each of the four valves of the heart may become involved in either category, though some are more serious than others. The following valvular heart diseases involving the aortic and mitral valves are among the more significant with respect to hemodynamic compromise. This is primarily due to the location of the aortic and mitral valves on the left side of the heart and their effect on cardiac output.

k. Disorders of the aortic valve p. 659

Pathophysiology: Aortic valve stenosis

Aortic valve stenosis is the most common isolated valvular lesion. Causes include:

- Congenitally acquired bicuspid aortic valve
- Calcific degeneration
- Rheumatic disease
- Infection
- Idiopathic calcification

A stenotic aortic valve obstructs forward blood flow into the aorta. To compensate, the left ventricle attempts to increase SV and CO, resulting in left ventricular hypertrophy. Cardiac output is usually maintained until the valve orifice is less than 1.0 cm or the pressure gradient across the valve greater than 50 mmHg.

Clinical exam findings: Aortic valve stenosis

Aortic valve stenosis may present with:

- Triad of:
  - Angina
  - Exertional syncope
  - Dyspnea on exertion
- Crescendo-decrescendo systolic murmur
- Pulsus parvus et tardus
- Narrowing pulse pressure
- Fixed A2-P2 split
- Ejection click

Diagnostic exam findings: Aortic valve stenosis

Diagnostic modalities useful in the evaluation of aortic valve disorders include:

- Radiograph
  - Left ventricular hypertrophy

- Pulmonary congestion
- Aortic calcification
- ECG
  - Findings consistent with left ventricular hypertrophy
  - Idioventricular conduction delay
  - Left axis deviation
  - Left atrial enlargement
- Echocardiography
  - Provides definitive diagnosis
  - Evaluates:
    - Aortic root size
    - Valvular anatomy
    - Left ventricle size
    - Aortic anatomy

Management: Aortic valve stenosis

Once symptomatic, surgery is the only definitive option for aortic valve disorders. Asymptomatic patients or symptomatic patients considered to be poor surgical candidates may receive medical therapy consisting of:
- Medical therapy
  - Digitalis
  - Diuretics
  - Nitrates
  - Inotrophic agents

If the patient is hemodynamically unstable, management may consist of:
- IABP as a bridging device
- Valve replacement

Pathophysiology: Aortic regurgitation

Aortic regurgitation occurs secondary to incomplete valve closure and results in retrograde flow of blood during diastole. Rising left ventricular pressures result in:
- Left ventricular dilation
- Left ventricular hypertrophy
- Left heart failure

Causes of aortic regurgitation include:
- Marfan's disease
- Rheumatic fever
- Endocarditis
- Aortic dissection
- Calcification

Clinical examination: Aortic regurgitation

Patients with aortic regurgitation may present with:
- Angina
- Signs or symptons of CHF
- Hypotension
- Decrescendo murmur
- Widened pulse pressure
- Corrigan's pulse

Diagnostic and lab findings: Aortic regurgitation

Diagnosis of aortic regurgitation is made with echocardiogram, multiple-gated acquisition scan (MUGA), or ventriculogram. Other diagnostic findings that are suggestive for aortic regurgitation include:
- Radiograph

- Acute disease:
  - Pulmonary congestion
  - Normal cardiac silhouette
- Chronic disease:
  - Enlarged left ventricle
  - Dilated aorta
- ECG
  - Normal early in disease
  - Left axis deviation, left ventricular hypertrophy in chronic disease

Management: Aortic regurgitation

As in aortic stenosis, aortic regurgitation is treated by surgical valve replacement.

I. Disorders of the mitral valve   p. 660

Pathophysiology: Mitral stenosis

Mitral stenosis (MS) is typified by a stenotic valve that obstructs forward blood flow from the left atrium into the left ventricle, which can result in elevated left atrial pressure, pulmonary hypertension, and right ventricular failure. Causes include:

- Rheumatic fever
  - Most common cause
- Neoplasms
- Rheumatologic disorders
- Congenital defects
- Calcification

Clinical exam findings: Mitral stenosis

Patients with mitral stenosis may present with:

- Exertional dyspnea, orthopnea
- Fatigue, malaise
- Hemoptysis
- S_1 snap, palpable diastolic thrill
- Diastolic murmur

Diagnostic exam findings: Mitral stenosis

An echocardiogram is used for the diagnosis of mitral stenosis. Other imaging modalities include:

- Radiograph
  - Increased vascular markings
  - Pulmonary edema
  - Left atrial enlargement
- ECG
  - Atrial fibrillation
  - Left atrial enlargement
  - Right ventricular hypertrophy

Management: Mitral stenosis

Management of mitral stenosis is directed at treating the symptoms of congestive heart failure and controlling the ventricular rate if atrial fibrillation is present; surgical intervention is an option when stenosis reaches an advanced stage.

- Treat symptoms of congestive heart failure
  - Diuretics
  - Nitrates
- Treat atrial fibrillation
  - Digitalis
  - Anticoagulation for new-onset atrial fibrillation
- Surgical intervention

Pathophysiology: Mitral regurgitation

Mitral regurgitation occurs when incomplete closure of the mitral valve results in retrograde blood flow during systole. The left ventricle compensates by increasing SV and CO, and left atrial enlargement and atrial fibrillation may develop. Causes of mitral regurgitation include:

- Rheumatic fever
- Mitral valve prolapse
- Infection
- Trauma
- Cardiomyopathies
- AMI

Clinical exam findings: Mitral regurgitation

Presentation of MR is often insidious, and patients may remain asymptomatic throughout their lifetimes.

- Acute presentation
  - Signs or symptoms of CHF
  - Crescendo-decrescendo murmur
  - S_3, S_4 heart sounds
- Chronic presentation
  - Fatigue
  - Dyspnea
  - Palpitations
  - Palpable thrill at apex
  - Holosystolic murmur best heard at apex
  - S_1 decreased or obscured, S_2 widely split

Diagnostic exam findings: Mitral regurgitation

Diagnosis of mitral regurgitation is made via echocardiogram. Other diagnostic modalities of use and their findings include:

- ECG
  - Atrial fibrillation
  - AMI, if cause of mitral regurgitation
  - Left ventricular hypertrophy
- Radiograph
  - Right atrial enlargement

Management: Mitral regurgitation

The management of mitral regurgitation is the same as for mitral stenosis.

3. **Be familiar with those procedures with which competency is expected in the critical care transport environment including:**

a. **Ventricular assist device**   p. 645

The left ventricular assist device (LVAD) allows an injured myocardium to rest by diverting blood from the natural ventricle to an artificial pump that maintains the circulation. LVADs are indicated when profound cardiogenic shock develops despite maximal conventional therapy. There are typically three groups of patients that can benefit from the use of a ventricular assist device: (1) patients in cardiogenic shock secondary to acute myocardial infarction, (2) patients with postcardiotomy left ventricular failure who cannot be weaned from cardiopulmonary bypass, and (3) candidates for cardiac transplantation whose condition deteriorates before a donor can be found.

Transport of patients in cardiogenic shock requiring the use of either the IABP or LVAD requires organizing a smooth and safe transition from the critical care area to the receiving facility. This requires a team effort to ensure that the hemodynamic stability of the patient is not adversely affected. All equipment must be properly secured prior to transport. During transport, whether by ground or air, the transport team must be able to adequately visualize the patient, monitors, and medication pumps. Adequate supplies of oxygen, medical air if needed to power devices, and electrical power must be readily available to complete the transport safely.

b. Arterial line placement   p. 662

Indications:
- Hemodynamic monitoring for:
  - Hypotension
  - Arterial hypertension requiring vasodilator therapy
- Unstable ischemic heart disease
- Postcardiac surgery
- Inotropic therapy
- Frequent blood gas sampling
- Intra-aortic balloon pump use

Precautions:
   Allen test to ensure adequate collateral circulation

Technique:
1. Equipment
   a. 20-gauge, non-tapered, 1.5- or 2-inch over-the-needle catheter
   b. Fluid-filled noncompliant tubing with stopcocks
   c. A constant flush device
   d. 4–0 suture material
   e. 1 percent lidocaine
2. Perform the Allen's test and/or Doppler examination of the wrists to ensure collateral circulation.
3. Utilize appropriate body substance isolation precautions.
4. Place the hand in 30 to 45 degrees of dorsiflexion.
   a. Roll of gauze and armband as aid
5. Prepare and drape the volar aspect of the wrist.
6. Infiltrate 0.5 mL of lidocaine on both sides of the artery using a 25-gauge needle.
7. Puncture the skin approximately 5 cm proximal to the wrist crease at an angle of 30 to 60 degrees.
8. Advance until blood is noted in the syringe hub.
9. Advance the needle into the lumen of the artery.
10. Attach the catheter to the Luer-Lock three-way stopcock, which in turn is attached to:
    a. Pressure-infused heparin solution
    b. Maintain continuous infusion of 1–3 mL per hour
    c. Intraflow device
    d. Arterial pressure monitor
11. Suture the catheter in place, and apply antibiotic ointment and sterile dressing.
12. Zero the transducer and observe the waveform.
    a. Correlate the invasive blood pressure with the noninvasive reading.

Complications:
- Pain at insertion site
- Exsanguinating hemorrhage
- Thrombosis
- Hematoma formation
- Limb ischemia
- Infection
- Air embolism

c. Central venous access   p. 664
Subclavian vein cannulation

Indications:
- Emergency intravenous route in seriously ill or injured patients
- Central venous pressure monitoring
- Insertion of transvenous pacemaker
- Intravenous access in patients without peripheral veins

- Infusion of hypertonic or irritant solutions

Precautions
- Significant increase in serious complications when performed on uncooperative or agitated patients
- Rates of complication directly influenced by operator experience
- Maintain control of the J-wire at all times when using the Seldinger technique.
- This procedure is contraindicated in patients with:
  - Deformity of the chest wall
  - Previous surgery or trauma in insertion area
  - Fibrotic changes in insertion area
  - Anatomy distortion in insertion area

Technique:
1. Equipment
   Double- or triple-lumen, J-wire-guided subclavian kit
   Saline or heparin flush
2. Utilize appropriate body substance isolation.
3. Prepare equipment.
   a. If using a triple-lumen catheter, flush the two accessory ports with heparin.
4. Place the patient in 10 to 20 degrees Trendelenburg.
5. Prep and drape the area appropriately.
6. Locate the appropriate landmarks.
7. If the patient is conscious and his condition warrants anesthesia:
   a. A skin wheal of 1 percent lidocaine is raised at the proposed vena puncture site
   b. 2 cm lateral to the medial and middle thirds of the clavicle
8. Attach the 18-gauge introducer needle to a syringe.
   a. Line up the bevel of the needle with the markings on the syringe.
9. Insert the needle through the skin at the vena puncture site.
10. Advance the needle into the side of the clavicle.
11. Place the index finger of your left hand in the sternoclavicular notch.
12. Apply a downward pressure on the needle with the thumb of your left hand until the needle goes under the clavicle.
13. Keeping the angle of the needle shallow, advance the needle forward, directed toward the target landmark, just above the sternoclavicular notch.
    a. Too deep an angle increases the likelihood of puncturing the lung and causing a pneumothorax.
14. Continue to advance the catheter, maintaining negative pressure on the syringe, until blood is noted to flow freely into the syringe.
15. Rotate the syringe 90 degrees so that the markings on the syringe are pointed toward the patient's feet.
16. Place the J-wire through the side port and advance the wire, then remove the catheter over the wire.
    a. Make sure to always maintain control of the wire.
17. Make a small incision through the skin at the site of the wire, large enough to easily advance the dilator catheter through the skin.
18. Place the dilator over the wire, and advance the dilator to the hub.
19. While maintaining stability of the wire, remove the dilator.
20. Place the triple-lumen catheter over the wire and advance so that the catheter is in the proximal aspect of the superior vena cava.
21. Remove the wire and assure that there is free flow of blood into the syringe.
22. Attach intravenous tubing to the catheter and ensure that the line is flowing properly.
23. Apply antibiotic ointment and suture the catheter in place.
24. Apply a sterile gauze dressing.
25. Confirm proper placement with chest radiograph.

Complications:
- Pneumothorax
- Venous thrombosis

- Thrombophlebitis
- Hematoma formation
- Infection

Femoral vein cannulation   p. 666
Indications:
- Emergency intravenous route when unable to find access elsewhere
- When rapid placement of a large-bore central venous catheter is necessary
- Need for hemodynamic monitoring or medications that require administration through a central venous catheter

Precautions:
- Operator inexperience may increase the number of attempts required and rate of complications.
- As with all central venous catheterizations, caution must be exercised to prevent air embolis.
- A common error is to direct the needle tip medially, toward the umbilicus.
- All central lines should be flushed prior to insertion.
- Application of a knee immobilizer will limit movement of the cannulated extremity.
- The femoral vein should not be used if there is infection or lesions at the site, or if there is known thrombosis of the vessel.

Technique:
1. Utilize appropriate body substance isolation.
2. Locate the vein by palpating the femoral artery pulse.
   a. Located 1 cm medial to the artery
   b. Extend an imaginary line between the symphysis pubis and the anterior superior iliac spine.
   c. Vein is located midway between the two structures.
3. Anesthetize the area with 1 percent lidocaine if the patient is conscious.
4. Position the catheter approximately 2 cm distal to the inguinal ligament and medial to the artery.
5. Direct the needle cephalad at a 45-degree angle with the skin.
6. Advance the catheter, maintaining negative pressure on the syringe, until a flash of blood is noted in the hub.
7. Advance the catheter while removing the needle.
8. Attach intravenous tubing to the catheter and ensure that the line is flowing properly.
9. Apply antibiotic ointment and secure the catheter and tubing in place.
10. Apply a sterile gauze dressing to insertion site.

Complications:
- Venous thrombosis
- Thrombophlebitis
- Hematoma formation
- Infection
- Septic arthritis of the hip
- Femoral nerve damage

Internal jugular vein cannulation   p. 667
Indications:
- Emergency intravenous route in seriously ill or injured patients
- Central venous pressure monitoring
- Insertion of transvenous pacemaker
- Intravenous access in patients without peripheral veins
- Infusion of hypertonic or irritant solutions

Precautions:
- Significant increase in serious complications when performed on uncooperative or agitated patients.
- Use with caution in patients with known coagulopathies.

Technique:
1. Equipment
   a. Double- or triple-lumen, J-wire-guided subclavian kit
2. Utilize appropriate body substance isolation.
3. Prepare equipment.
   a. If using a double- or triple-lumen catheter, flush the accessory ports with heparin.
4. Place the patient in 10 to 20 degrees Trendelenburg position.
5. Turn the patient's head to the contralateral side.
6. Prep and drape the area appropriately.
7. Locate the appropriate landmarks.
8. Anterior approach:
   a. Locate the triangle formed by the sternal and clavicular heads of the sternocleidomastoid muscle and the clavicle inferiorly.
   b. Point of insertion is at the apex of the triangle.
   c. Direct the needle inferiorly and laterally toward the ipsilateral nipple.
9. Posterior approach:
   a. Site of insertion is along the posterior border of the sternocleidomastoid muscle just cephalad to where the external jugular vein crosses that border.
   b. Advance the needle under the sternocleidomastoid, aiming at the midpoint of the suprasternal notch.
10. If the patient is conscious and his condition warrants anesthesia, a skin wheal of 1 percent lidocaine is raised at the proposed vena puncture site.
11. Attach the 18-gauge introducer needle to a syringe.
    a. Line up the bevel of the needle with the markings on the syringe.
12. Insert the needle through the skin at the vena puncture site described above.
13. Advance the catheter, maintaining negative pressure on the syringe, until blood is noted to flow freely into the syringe.
14. Rotate the syringe 90 degrees so that the markings on the syringe are pointed toward the patient's feet.
15. Place the J-wire through the side port and advance the wire, then remove the catheter over the wire.
    a. Make sure to always maintain control of the wire.
16. Make a small incision through the skin at the site of the wire, large enough to easily advance the dilator catheter through the skin.
17. Place the dilator over the wire.
18. Advance the dilator to the hub.
19. Remove the dilator.
20. Place the triple-lumen catheter over the wire and advance so that the catheter is in the proximal aspect of the superior vena cava.
21. Remove the wire and check to assure that there is free flow of blood into the syringe.
22. Attach intravenous tubing to the catheter and ensure that the line is flowing properly.
23. Apply antibiotic ointment and suture the catheter in place.
24. Apply a sterile gauze dressing.
25. Confirm proper placement with chest radiograph.

Complications:
- Pneumothorax
- Venous thrombosis
- Thrombophlebitis
- Hematoma formation
- Infection
- Arterial catheterization

d. Intra-aortic balloon pump   p. 671

Indications for IABP:
- Cardiogenic/septic shock
- Unstable angina/myocardial infarction
- Weaning from cardiopulmonary bypass

- Preoperative and postoperative myocardial dysfunction
- Bridge to transplantation
- Percutaneous coronary angioplasty

Precautions:
- CCT team members will not be responsible for the insertion of intra-aortic balloon pumps but will be responsible for maintaining both triggering and timing during interfacility transfers.
- Keep a 60-cc syringe present in order to exercise the balloon in the event of pump failure.
- Consider placing the patient's leg (with the IABP insertion site) in a knee immobilizer to prevent movement.
- Do not allow the patient to sit up greater than 30 degrees.
- Maintain access to cannulation site and monitor leads.
- Determine the patient's ability to tolerate brief periods without counterpulsation prior to departing the sending facility.
- Most triggering problems are due to an ECG with an R wave of low amplitude.
- Timing should be rechecked every one to two hours and whenever there is a greater than 20 percent change in heart rate, change in cardiac output, development of an arrhythmia, or change in triggering mode.
- Do not use the central lumen of the intra-aortic balloon catheter for blood sampling.
- Ensure that the patient does not have a history of AAA or AV insufficiency.

Transport technique:
- Equipment:
  - Intra-aortic balloon pump
  - IABP equipment kit:
    - 60-cc slip-tip syringe
    - Appropriate IAB/IABP adapters
    - Scissors
    - Kelly clamp
    - ECG patches
    - Extra helium tank
    - ECG cable and arterial pressure cable
    - IABP flow sheet
    - IABP operator's manual
- Review the patient condition and current triggering and timing of the IABP with the referring physician.
- Review the postinsertion X-ray to confirm proper placement.
  - Second to third intercostal space, below left subclavian
- Verify clean ECG and arterial pulse (AP) transducer signals on the monitor.
- Check the IABP battery for sufficient charge.
- Verify that an adequate amount of helium is available to complete transport safely.
- If the patient can tolerate the reduction in counterpulsation, set the assist ratio to 1:2 and confirm timing.
- Return to a 1:1 ratio after confirming proper timing.
- Secure the IABP in the ambulance.
- Constantly monitor the console and make adjustments for timing errors as needed during transport.
- Timing is evaluated by utilizing timing markers on the arterial pressure waveform, ensuring that inflation and deflation correspond with appropriate stages of diastole.
- Blood in the connecting tubing is a hallmark of balloon rupture and requires immediate cessation of counterpulsation to prevent cerebral gas embolization.
- Alarms indicated on the console are accompanied by an indicated corrective action.

Complications:
- Aortic wall dissection, rupture, or local vascular injury
- Balloon rupture with helium embolus or catheter entrapment
- Limb ischemia or compartment syndrome
- Infection
- Thrombocytopenia

- Hemorrhage
- Obstruction of the left subclavian artery, carotid arteries, renal arteries, or mesenteric arteries

e. Pericardiocentesis   p. 672
Indication:
- Suspected cardiac tamponade

Precautions:
- Temporizing measure only
  - Not a definitive therapeutic procedure

Technique:
1. Equipment
   a. Iodinated prep solution
   b. Sterile towels
   c. 10 cc and 50 cc syringes
   d. 3-inch 18-gauge spinal needle
2. Prep the skin in the substernal area with Betadine solution and drape the area.
3. Attach the limb leads of the ECG to the patient.
4. Place the patient with the upper torso elevated at 30 degrees.
5. Attach an 18-gauge spinal needle to a syringe via a three-way stopcock.
6. Attach one end of an alligator clip to the base of the spinal needle and the other end to the chest lead of an electrocardiograph.
7. Place the four limb leads normally on the extremities.
8. Introduce the spinal needle into the left costal arch and direct the tip toward the right shoulder or directly cephalad.
   a. The needle may be aimed at the tip of the left shoulder.
9. Pass the needle through the diaphragm while maintaining negative pressure on the syringe.
10. Entrance into the pericardial sac is indicated by the loss of negative pressure in the syringe, and/or introduction of blood or fluid into the syringe barrel.
11. Carefully monitor the V lead of the ECG for the appearance of a myocardial injury pattern.
    If an injury pattern is noted, the needle is in contact with the epicardium,
    Withdraw the needle 1–2 mm until the normal ECG complex returns.
12. With the needle tip in the pericardial sac, perform aspiration of fluid.
13. Withdraw the catheter and apply a sterile dressing.
14. Repeated aspirations may be necessary as the patient's condition warrants.

Complications:
- Myocardial injury
- Coronary artery injury
- Arrhythmias
- Pneumothorax

4. Understand the general considerations for interfacility critical care transport   p. 673

General considerations for interfacility transport include:

- Perform independent patient evaluation.
- Review:
  - Lab tests
  - Imaging tests
  - Patient history
- Recommend other transport options if your unit cannot provide the necessary care.
- Secure all equipment prior to transport.
- Report to receiving facility.

5. Understand the special considerations related to air critical care transport.

a. Preparation for flight   p. 674
Flight and ground times should be determined to ensure that adequate oxygen is available, as well as an adequate power supply; plug adaptors in the aircraft and battery life will determine power limitations.

b. Alterations in cardiovascular physiology at altitude   p. 674

Physiological changes occur as barometric pressure at altitude decreases, causing a reduction in the alveolar pressure of oxygen. A reduction in alveolar pressure leads to a reduction in the amount of oxygen that perfuses into the blood, which, in turn, decreases the amount of oxygen available to the tissues. The body attempts to compensate for the decreased oxygen supply by increasing the respiratory rate, heart rate, and cardiac output; patients with cardiovascular disease may not be able to support a response to compensate for the decreased oxygen supply. Patients with CAD who are unable to compensate for the increased workload imposed on the heart by decreased oxygen tension of high altitude may experience chest pain, congestive heart failure, pulmonary edema, cardiac dysrhythmias, or cardiac arrest. As such, all patients with cardiovascular disease should receive supplemental oxygen while in flight. The American College of Chest Physicians has recommended altitude limits for patients with known cardiovascular disease when supplemental oxygen is not available. Limiting the cabin altitude pressure to a maximum of 6,000 feet has been shown to eliminate problems for people with cardiovascular disease.

c. Handling in-flight cardiopulmonary arrest   p. 674

The flight team must be aware of the patient's Do Not Resuscitate order or code status prior to leaving the referring facility. In addition, before transport, the patient and family members accompanying the patient on flight should be made aware of the risks of air medical transport and the potential for diversions should the patient's condition deteriorate.

The flight critical care paramedic must address the issues of a full cardiopulmonary arrest during transport. The flight medic must consider:

1. Code status of the patient
2. Company policies and procedures for in-flight arrests
3. The decision to return, divert, or proceed to the destination
4. Availability of resuscitation equipment
5. Time frames and endurance of the air medical personnel

If a patient's code status is "full resuscitation" or "full code" and the patient suffers a cardiopulmonary arrest, then the company's policies and procedures must be followed and must take into consideration the legal aspects of interstate transport and state laws. The program's policies and procedures should clearly delineate what should be done if a patient arrests in flight. The flight team must weigh both state and interstate laws. The team may need to weigh distance and time factors to decide the appropriate destination. This may require returning to the sending facility, diverting to the closest facility, or continuing to the receiving facility. The flight team may need to consider terminating resuscitative efforts based on the amount of resuscitative medications available, the time anticipated to get the patient to an appropriate facility, and the endurance capabilities of the medical personnel onboard. Usually consultation with medical direction to determine cessation of resuscitation is recommended.

Preparation for in-flight cardiac arrest includes ensuring that resuscitative equipment is easily accessible. Oxygen should be readily available and ACLS drugs must be labeled and within easy reach. The flight team must establish well-defined roles and responsibilities in order to effectively respond in the event of a cardiac arrest. There must be access to the patient's head so that endotracheal intubation can be performed. A cardiac defibrillator must be readily available. Studies have shown that defibrillation with current equipment can be safely administered. Standard defibrillation precautions should be followed. If the patient is at high risk for cardiopulmonary arrest, defibrillation pads should be placed on the patient's chest and equipment readied prior to transport.

Case Study

Your aeromedical critical care transport team has been called to a Park Service health center about 100 miles from the nearest hospital for a patient complaining of chest pain. This particular health center is staffed by an advanced practice paramedic who lives on site to assist in the medical needs of the Park Service staff. Your patient is a maintenance worker who came to the health center complaining of "indigestion." On presentation to the health center, the patient reported an aching sensation in his epigastric area that started approximately four hours ago, after he drank a cup of hot cocoa. The pain was constant and radiated intermittently to his right shoulder. He rated the pain as a "6" on a 0 to 10 scale. He denied any nausea, shortness of breath, diaphoresis, or palpitations. A 12-lead ECG showed a sinus rhythm with a deep Q-wave in lead III with 2 mm ST segment elevations in leads II, III and aVF. The patient was started on oxygen, given 324 mg of aspirin, and IV access was obtained. The patient's pain decreased to "2" on 0 to 10 after the oxygen and aspirin. He was then given 0.4 mg sublingual nitroglycerin with complete resolution of his pain.

After introducing yourself to the patient, he tells you that he remains pain free and feels completely normal. He has the following vital signs: temperature 37° C, respirations 18 breaths per minute with an SpO_2 of 98 percent, pulse 88 bpm and regular with the monitor showing a normal sinus rhythm, and a blood pressure of 146/78. A repeat 12-lead ECG shows no changes. Breath sounds are clear to auscultation and heart sounds are normal. While your partner establishes another IV, you question the patient and determine that he has no contraindications to the use of fibrinolytic therapy. You discuss the patient with your medical control physician and it is decided that, since the patient remains pain free and onset was over 4 hours ago, fibrinolytics will be withheld in favor of primary percutaneous coronary intervention (PCI). Your partner gives a 4,000 unit bolus of heparin and then starts a continuous infusion at 1,000 units/hour while you hang a nitroglycerin infusion at 5 mcg/min. Both IVs are administered through a three-channel infusion pump. The patient remains stable during the 45-minute flight and arrives without change. The patient is taken directly into the catheterization lab where two stents are placed in the right coronary artery, resulting in complete reperfusion.

DISCUSSION QUESTIONS

1. What is the definition of acute coronary syndrome?
2. What diagnostics can be used to help confirm the diagnosis of acute coronary syndrome?
3. What pharmacological agents may be used in the management of acute coronary syndrome?

Content Review

MULTIPLE CHOICE

_____ 1. The _____ is/are open during ventricular systole.
   A. semilunar valves
   B. AV valves
   C. mitral valve
   D. tricuspid valve

_____ 2. The _____ is/are conductive fibers that carry impulses to the contractile cells of the ventricular myocardium to promote uniform contraction of the ventricles.
   A. internodal pathways
   B. AV junction
   C. Purkinje fibers
   D. Bundle of His

_____ 3. The right coronary artery perfuses the:
   A. SA node, AV node, right atrium, and right ventricle.
   B. septal and anterior walls of the left ventricle.
   C. lateral and posterior wall of the left ventricle.
   D. posterior wall of the right ventricle, internodal pathways, and inferior wall of the left ventricle.

_____ 4. To best auscultate the tricuspid valve, a stethoscope should be placed at the:
   A. fifth ICS to the left of the sternum.
   B. second ICS to the right of the sternum.
   C. second ICS to the left of the sternum.
   D. fifth ICS on the midclavicular line.

_____ 5. The basic "lub-dub" sound of the heart can be described as:
A. S_1.
B. S_2.
C. split S_2.
D. S_1 and S_2.

_____ 6. The S_1 heart sound is produced by the:
A. closing of the semilunar valves.
B. closing of the aortic valve.
C. closing of the AV valves.
D. none of the above.

_____ 7. The S_2 heart sound is produced by the:
A. closing of the semilunar valves.
B. closing of the aortic valve.
C. closing of the AV valves.
D. closing of the pulmonic valve.

_____ 8. The first "normal" heart tone heard on auscultation is:
A. S_1.
B. S_2.
C. S_3.
D. S_4.

_____ 9. A _____ occurs as a result of increased venous return and negative intrathoracic pressure which delays emptying of the right ventricle and closing of the pulmonic valve.
A. split S_1
B. split S_2
C. ventricular gallop
D. murmur

_____ 10. An S_3 can form when:
A. increased venous return and negative intrathoracic pressure delays closing of the pulmonic valve.
B. the atrial wall vibrates as blood is forced into a noncompliant ventricle.
C. a stiff ventricle cannot distend to accept blood, resulting in turbulent blood flow and vibration of the AV valve and ventricle.
D. a stiff atria cannot effectively pump blood into the ventricle, resulting in delayed closing of the AV valves.

_____ 11. An S_4 heart sound is also known as a(an):
A. ventricular gallop.
B. heart murmur.
C. lub dub-dub.
D. atrial gallop.

_____ 12. Which heart sound is best auscultated at the apex ausculatory point?
A. S_1
B. S_2
C. S_3
D. S_4

_____ 13. Which heart sound is best auscultated at the lower left sternal border with the patient turned to the left?
A. S_1
B. S_2
C. S_3
D. S_4

_____ 14. A systolic murmur occurs:
A. between AV valve closure and semilunar valve opening.
B. between semilunar valve closure and AV valve opening.
C. during ventricular systole.
D. during atrial systole.

_____ 15. Systolic regurgitation murmurs result from:
A. high atrial pressure.
B. faulty AV valves.
C. faulty semilunar valves.
D. faulty aortic or semilunar valves.

_____ 16. A diastolic murmur occurs:
A. after S_2 and before the next S_1.
B. after S_1 and before S_2.
C. during S_1.
D. during S_2.

_____ 17. A diastolic semilunar murmur can occur secondary to:
A. high atrial pressure.
B. faulty AV valves.
C. stenotic AV valves.
D. faulty aortic or pulmonary valves.

_____ 18. An AV valve murmur can be described as a:
   A. decreasing in intensity.
   B. high-frequency, crescendo-decrescendo.
   C. low-frequency, decrescendo-crescendo.
   D. none of the above.

_____ 19. According to the Levin scale, a heart murmur that can be heard when the stethoscope is off the chest wall would be considered a:
   A. Grade I.   C. Grade VI.
   B. Grade V.   D. Grade VII.

_____ 20. Acute coronary syndrome can be best described as:
   A. the presence of chest pain, diaphoresis, nausea, and ST segment changes on 12-lead ECG.
   B. a spectrum of coronary artery disease (CAD) processes from myocardial ischemia and myocardial injury to myocardial infarction.
   C. a situation in which myocardial infarction is occurring.
   D. the presence of chest pain, diaphoresis, and nausea.

_____ 21. Unstable angina is defined as angina that:
   A. occurs at rest and lasts longer than 20 minutes.
   B. is new in onset.
   C. is crescendoing in nature.
   D. all of the above.

_____ 22. Coronary artery disease involves:
   A. atherosclerosis.   C. decreased myocardial blood flow.
   B. atheroma formation.   D. all of the above.

_____ 23. Thrombus formation associated with coronary artery disease most often occurs secondary to:
   A. coagulopathy.   C. disruption of an atherosclerotic plaque.
   B. atrial fibrillation.   D. genetic factors.

_____ 24. Risk factors associated with coronary artery disease include all of the following except:
   A. renal disease, liver disease, and stress.
   B. family history of coronary or vascular disease.
   C. smoking, hypertension, hypercholesterolemia, and diabetes mellitus.
   D. artificial or early menopause and the use of contraceptives.

_____ 25. The pain associated with myocardial infarction is most likely to be described as:
   A. gradual onset, left-sided pain radiating to the right arm and jaw.
   B. acute onset, substernal pain or heaviness radiating to the left arm or jaw.
   C. acute onset, sharp, and reproducible with palpation.
   D. gradual onset, dull, and radiating between the shoulder blades.

_____ 26. Females, compared to males, may have atypical complaints associated with acute coronary syndrome, including:
   A. gradual onset, and retrosternal pain radiating to the left arm and jaw.
   B. tachycardia, tachypnea, and diaphoresis.
   C. indigestion, weakness, dizziness, and nausea.
   D. none of the above.

_____ 27. A Q wave on a 12-lead ECG can be used to estimate the size and age of a myocardial infarction.
   A. True
   B. False

_____ 28. The ECG finding most indicative of evolving acute myocardial infarction (AMI) is:
  A. reciprocal ST segment depression.
  B. presence of a Q wave.
  C. presence of a bundle branch block.
  D. ST segment elevation of > 0.1 mm in at least two continuous leads.

_____ 29. Which leads on a 12-lead ECG correspond with the lateral left ventricular wall?
  A. II, III, and aVF   C. V3 and V4
  B. I, aVL, V5, and V6   D. V1, V2, and V3

_____ 30. The specific serum cardiac markers utilized to diagnose myocardial infarction include:
  A. CK-T and troponin I.   C. CK-MB and troponin T.
  B. CK and troponin I.   D. CK-MB and troponin.

_____ 31. The management of acute coronary syndrome includes all of the following except:
  A. increasing myocardial oxygen supply.
  B. reducing pain and relieving stress.
  C. increasing preload and afterload.
  D. preventing reocclusion of coronary arteries.

_____ 32. ST segment elevation in leads II, III, and aVF indicates acute _____ myocardial infarction.
  A. right ventricular   C. septal wall
  B. left ventricular   D. inferior wall

_____ 33. In patients with right ventricular infarct, the CCP should consider:
  A. prompt administration of vasodilators to decrease afterload.
  B. the early administration of vasopressors such as dopamine to correct hypotension.
  C. withholding the administration of fluid to prevent fluid overload.
  D. administration of a fluid bolus prior to the administration of a vasodilator to prevent hypotension.

_____ 34. Analgesics are useful in the treatment of acute coronary syndrome because they:
  A. decrease myocardial oxygen demand.   C. both A and B.
  B. decrease pain.   D. none of the above.

_____ 35. Which of the following statements about aspirin is false?
  A. Aspirin works by inhibiting platelet formation during the thrombotic response to ruptured coronary artery plaque.
  B. Standard doses range from 160 to 324 mg given orally.
  C. Aspirin has a significant synergistic effect with heparin in reducing AMI and death.
  D. Aspirin accelerates the action of antithrombin III and activated Factors IX, X, and XI.

_____ 36. Medications used to decrease myocardial oxygen demand during AMI include all of the following except:
  A. beta blockers.   C. calcium channel blockers.
  B. anticoagulants.   D. analgesics.

_____ 37. The therapeutic goals of lysing clots and preventing further clot propagation can be achieved with the administration of:
  A. fibrinolytics.   C. antiplatelets.
  B. anticoagulants.   D. all of the above.

_____ 38. The biggest risk associated with the administration of fibrinolytics and anticoagulants is:
  A. hemorrhage.   C. thrombosis.
  B. allergic reaction.   D. hyperkalemia.

_____ 39. The most commonly used mechanical reperfusion technique is:
  A. PTCA.   C. LVAD.
  B. IABP.   D. CABG.

_____ 40. Candidates for mechanical reperfusion include those patients with:
  A. postinfarct or postreperfusion ischemia.
  B. contraindications to fibrinolytic therapy.
  C. persistent hemodynamic instability.
  D. all of the above.

_____ 41. A localized dilation of the aorta involving all three layers of the arterial wall is called a/an:
  A. aortic dissection.   C. aortic aneurysm.
  B. aortic transection.   D. none of the above.

_____ 42. Aortic dissections most commonly originate in which area?
  A. abdominal aorta   C. pelvic aorta
  B. thoracic aorta   D. descending aorta

_____ 43. Criteria for surgical intervention of an AAA includes:
  A. dilatation greater than 6 cm in diameter.
  B. dilation greater than 1 cm growth in 24 months.
  C. symptomatic pain or hypotension.
  D. all of the above.

_____ 44. Which of the following imaging modalities is best for the diagnosis of abdominal aneurysm?
  A. CT   C. MRI
  B. radiograph   D. doppler ultrasonography

_____ 45. The sudden onset of hemodynamic instability in a patient with an AAA is suggestive for:
  A. rupture.   C. transection.
  B. dissection.   D. AMI.

_____ 46. Profound hypotension associated with AAA rupture is best treated with:
  A. crystalloid solution.   C. colloid solution.
  B. vasopressors.   D. whole blood or blood products.

_____ 47. An aortic dissection in which the intimal tear is confined to the descending aorta distal to the left subclavian artery is classified a Debakey Type:
  A. I.   C. III.
  B. II.   D. IV.

_____ 48. Pain associated with an aortic dissection is most commonly described as:
  A. throbbing or colicky back pain.
  B. sharp and tearing, radiating to upper back.
  C. sharp pain between the shoulder blades.
  D. throbbing, pulsating abdominal pain.

_____ 49. Cardiogenic shock can occur secondary to:
  A. increased preload.   C. increased afterload.
  B. increased stroke volume.   D. all of the above.

_____ 50. Left ventricular preload can be indirectly evaluated by measuring:
  A. pulmonary capillary wedge pressure (PCWP).
  B. systolic blood pressure (SBP).
  C. central venous pressure (CVP).
  D. mean arterial pressure (MAP).

_____ 51. Pharmacological agents used in the treatment of cardiogenic shock include:
  A. nitroprusside.   C. furosemide.
  B. norepinephrine.   D. all of the above.

_____ 52. An intra-aortic balloon pump:
  A. can augment cardiac output by 10 to 20 percent.
  B. is inflated during systole.
  C. is percutaneously inserted into the iliac artery.
  D. creates a rapid drop in afterload during inflation.

53. Patients who are candidates for a left ventricular assist device include those:
  A. in cardiogenic shock secondary to acute myocardial infarction.
  B. with postcardiotomy left ventricular failure that cannot be weaned from cardiopulmonary bypass.
  C. who are candidates for cardiac transplantation but whose condition deteriorates before a donor can be found.
  D. all of the above.

54. During air medical transport of a patient on an IABP, repriming may be required:
  A. during ascent.
  B. at cruising altitude.
  C. during descent.
  D. all of the above.

55. Categories of cardiomyopathy include:
  A. dilated cardiomyopathy.
  B. hypotrophic cardiomyopathy.
  C. constrictive cardiomyopathy.
  D. all of the above.

56. The most reliable diagnostic finding for the diagnosis of cardiac arrest is:
  A. lack of end-tidal CO_2 detection.
  B. ventricular rhythm on the ECG monitor.
  C. lack of a palpable pulse.
  D. lack of a reading on a pulse oximeter.

57. Which of the following is most likely to occur if a patient arrests at a sending facility prior to aeromedical transport?
  A. Aeromedical transport to the receiving facility will be initiated immediately.
  B. Resuscitation will be attempted in the facility and transport considered if the resuscitation is successful.
  C. Resuscitation will be attempted in the facility and transport initiated after intubation, IV access, and one round of ACLS medications have been administered.
  D. Ground transport will be initiated.

58. Which of the following is least likely to contribute to congestive heart failure in the adult patient?
  A. thyrotoxicosis
  B. pulmonary embolism
  C. alcohol/drug abuse
  D. congenital heart defect

59. Right heart failure most often occurs secondary to:
  A. hypertension.
  B. valvular disease.
  C. left heart failure.
  D. AMI.

60. Chest radiograph findings suggestive for congestive heart failure include:
  A. cardiomegaly and pulmonary congestion.
  B. pulmonary edema and widened mediastinum.
  C. air trapping and atelectasis.
  D. none of the above.

61. Diagnostic findings associated with congestive heart failure may include:
  A. elevated PCWP.
  B. elevated SVR.
  C. decreased cardiac output.
  D. all of the above.

62. All of the following medications are used to reduce preload in patients with CHF except:
  A. morphine.
  B. ACE inhibitors.
  C. nitrates.
  D. furosemide.

63. An adult patient is considered to have severe hypertension if they present with:
  A. a systolic BP of 140 mmHg, renal failure, and AMI.
  B. a BP of 142/108 mmHg and a headache.
  C. a diastolic BP of 140 mmHg, papilledema, and acute renal failure.
  D. a BP of 156/108 mmHg, acute renal failure, and CHF.

_____ 64. Clinical exam findings that suggest severe preeclampsia include all of the following except:
  A. systolic BP > 160 or diastolic BP > 110 on two occasions more than six hours apart with patient resting.
  B. 24-hour urine output > 400 mL.
  C. proteinuria greater than 5 g/24 hours.
  D. visual disturbances, pulmonary edema, or cyanosis.

_____ 65. Which of the following suggests the presence of malignant hypertension in a hypertensive patient?
  A. increased BUN and creatinine
  B. hematuria and proteinuria
  C. pulmonary congestion on radiograph
  D. all of the above

_____ 66. When treating hypertension, treatment should be directed at producing:
  A. a 20 to 25 percent decrease in MAP.
  B. a diastolic BP of 100 to 110 mmHg.
  C. both A and B.
  D. none of the above.

_____ 67. Pharmacological treatment of a pregnant patient with a hypertensive emergency may include all of the following except:
  A. captopril.
  B. labetalol.
  C. hydralazine.
  D. magnesium sulfate.

_____ 68. Which of the following medications is least desirable for the treatment of a patient with a malignant hypertension?
  A. nifedipine
  B. labetalol
  C. nitroprusside
  D. furosemide

_____ 69. Which of the following classes of medication is least likely to be used in the treatment of pericarditis?
  A. NSAIDs
  B. steroids
  C. antibiotics
  D. beta blockers

_____ 70. The immediate treatment for hemodynamically significant pericardial effusion is:
  A. steroids.
  B. pericardiocentesis.
  C. antibiotics.
  D. beta blockers.

_____ 71. The progression of pericardial effusion to tamponade is manifested by all of the following except:
  A. hypotension.
  B. widening pulse pressure.
  C. muffled heart sounds.
  D. JVD.

_____ 72. A (an) _____ is performed prior to the insertion of an arterial line into the radial artery in the wrist to ensure adequate arterial flow distal to the insertion site.
  A. arteriogram
  B. pulse check
  C. neurological exam
  D. Allen's test

_____ 73. If a hematoma forms over an arterial line insertion site during transport, the CCP should immediately:
  A. provide direct pressure to control bleeding for 5 to 10 minutes.
  B. remove the arterial line and apply a constrictive bandage.
  C. administer a 250 mL fluid bolus.
  D. check the arterial line waveform on the monitor.

_____ 74. Common sites for arterial line insertion include all of the following arteries except the:
  A. radial.
  B. dorsalis pedis.
  C. carotid.
  D. brachial.

_____ 75. You are preparing to transport a patient with an IABP. Which of the following findings would indicate a potential serious complication?
  A. presence of a headache
  B. absence of a left radial pulse
  C. redness around the catheter insertion site
  D. a postinsertion radiograph that shows the balloon tip in the aorta at the level of the third intercostal space

_____ 76. Blood in the IABP connecting tube indicates:
  A. thrombis formation.
  B. increased intrathoracic pressure.
  C. balloon rupture.
  D. the need for a saline flush.

Review of Chapter Objectives

Upon completion of this chapter, the student should be able to:

1. Develop and enhance neurologic assessment skills.   p. 688

A detailed neurological assessment is an important diagnostic tool for all clinicians, including the CCP. The approach to a patient with a possible neurological insult should be systematic and comprehensive. Recommendations for evaluation of the conscious patient are as follows:

- Assess patient's ability to open his eyes.
  - Ability to acknowledge examiner and track movement
- Assess extraocular movement in all extremes of the visual field.
  - Note abnormal findings such as nystagmus, gaze restriction
- Assess for visual field deficit.
- Ask the patient about the presence of visual changes.
  - Blurred vision
  - Diplopia
  - Perception of "floaters," spots of light
  - Loss of vision, transient or ongoing
- Assess facial symmetry.
- Ask the patient to stick out his tongue and say "ah."
  - Tongue deviation
  - Bilateral rise of the soft palate
- Determine orientation.
  - Patients may be able to successfully answer orientation questions but still be confused.
  - Be alert to strange behavior, affect, repetitive questioning, or other indications of confusion.
- Assess speech for clarity.
- Assess for presence of aphasia.
  - Forms of aphasia
    - Expressive: patient unable to speak or formulate words clearly
    - Receptive: patient unable to understand speech
    - Global: both receptive and expressive
    - Conductive: speech fluent but dysphasic with inappropriate words, yet good comprehension
- Assess for motor weakness and a pronator drift.
- Assess for cerebellar ataxia.
- Assess motor strength.
  - Hand grasps are a subjective indicator of motor strength.
  - Assess motor strength in the legs by asking the patient to lift them against resistance.
- Ask the patient about parasthesias or other sensory abnormalities.

Recommendations for evaluation of the unresponsive patient are as follows:

- If the patient is not responsive, determine if they have been chemically paralyzed.
  - MBAs greatly reduce the efficacy of your neurological exam.
  - Cranial nerves are affected.
- If the patient is not sedated or chemically paralyzed, assess for spontaneous respirations.
- If the patient does not open his eyes, note the presence of a gaze preference, disconjugate gaze, or strange eye movement.
  - Repetitive or "roving" eye movements may be indicative of seizure activity.
- Assess presence of blink reflex.
- Assess for presence of overt seizure activity.
- Assess for motor response with a brisk sternal rub.
  - If no response, consider applying nailbed pressure to each extremity
- Assess the Babinski reflex.
- Assess for clonus.
  - Presence of clonus may indicate a seizure state or other abnormal tone.
- Assess for presence of blink reflex.
- Assess for the presence of a gag reflex.
  - Insert a rigid tonsil tip suction catheter into the patient's oropharnyx
- Assess cough reflex.
  - Patient coughs on his endotracheal tube.
  - Responds to deep tracheal suctioning
- Assess for CSF drainage from the ears, nose, or from a surgically placed drain.

2. **Identify common neurologic emergencies that may result in the need for critical care intervention.** p. 691

Cerebrovascular disorders
Cerebrovascular disorders, discussed in detail in Objective 4, include ischemic stroke, hemorrhagic stroke, and intracerebral hemorrhage.

Infectious processes
Infectious processes that can affect the brain include meningitis, encephalitis, and brain abscesses, and are discussed in detail in Objective 6.

CNS tumors
CNS tumors are not uncommon, and their severity can vary from benign to malignant. Brain tumors can be primary or metastatic lesions, and benign or malignant. Factors determining a tumor's malignancy include its histological origin, speed of growth, and degree of cellular differentiation.

Tumors within the brain can arise anywhere within the brain and supporting structures, are pathological space-occupying lesions, and are capable of causing mass effect, vasogenic edema, hydrocephalus, and increased intracranial pressure.

Diagnostic modalitites used to identify CNS tumors include MRI, CT, and lumbar puncture, and treatment is based on the type and location of the tumor.

Gliomas are tumors of the neuroglia, the supportive cells within the brain. These include astrocytomas, oligodendrogliomas, and ependymomas. Treatment typically includes surgical debulking and radiation therapy.

A meningioma is a tumor of the meninges, and does not include brain parenchyma. It is usually benign, can be subclinical, and the most effective treatment is surgical excision. Other types of intracranial tumors include those that originate from neurons, vascular structures, nerve sheaths, and epithelial cells.

Encephalopathy
Encephalopathy is a progressive, neuronal degeneration and dysfunction resulting from pathological changes that occur outside the CNS, the etiologies of which include hypoxia, hypercapnia, blood glucose extremes, metabolic disorders, organ failure, toxins, and alcoholism.

The progression of encephalopathy is variable, and are dependent on the causative agent. Gradual onset encephalopathy typically follows a predictable progression of findings: subtle changes in behavior, memory, and movement are followed by worsening disorders of thought and movement, then frank dementia, coma, and death.

Specific forms of encephalopathy are AIDS encephalopathy, Wernicke's encephalopathy, hepatic encephalopathy, and toxin-induced encephalopathy.

HIV encephalopathy occurs in patients infected with HIV. HIV-infected CD4 cells travel to the brain and infect neural and glial cells, resulting in progressive degeneration and destruction. Treatment is mainly supportive in nature, and antiretroviral therapy may slow the disease progression.

Wernicke's encephalopathy occurs secondary to Vitamin B_1 (thiamine) deficiency that is typically seen with chronic alcoholism, poor nutrition, and impaired absorption and storage of thiamine.

Signs and symptoms of Wernicke's encephalopathy include:

- Korsakoff's psychosis
  - Progressive retrograde and anterograde amnesia
  - Flattening of affect
  - Intellectual slowing
- Nystagmus
- Impaired extraocular movement
- Cerebellar ataxia with gait disturbance

Treatment consists of supportive care and thiamine administration.

Hepatic encephalopathy occurs as a result of a buildup of toxic by-products of metabolism secondary to liver disease. Normally, protein metabolism results in the formation of ammonia, which is converted in the liver to urea and then excreted by the kidneys. Hepatic insufficiency results in an increase of serum ammonia, which has an intoxicating effect on the CNS. Signs and symptoms associated with hepatic encephalopathy include:

- Impaired cortical function
- Cerebellar ataxia
- Asterixis
- Altered level of consciousness
- Coma
- Death

Hepatic encephalopathy can be acute or chronic, and acute encephalopathic changes can be triggered by infection, GI bleeding, and metabolic derangements.

Treatment is supportive in nature, and centers around reversal of the precipitating cause. Removal of serum ammonia can be accomplished with the administration of Lactulose, and patients with known hepatic insufficiency may be placed on a low protein diet in order to decrease ammonia production.

Toxin-induced encephalopathy may occur in abusers of volatile solvents (butane "huffing" and glue sniffing), IV drug abusers, and patients in contact with industrial chemicals, heavy metals, or organophosphates.

Seizure disorders
Seizures are the result of paroxysmal and abnormal electrical activity within the brain and can occur secondary to hypoxia, hypoglycemia, metabolic derangement, or unknown etiologies.

The presentation of a seizure can vary; not all seizures present as grand mal. Seizures that originate from an epileptic focus in the cerebral cortex commonly begin with focal symptoms that may progress to generalized seizure activity. Seizures that originate from ectopic foci in deeper structures of the brain tend to immediately present with generalized seizure activity. Signs and symptoms of seizure include:

- Behavioral changes, inattentiveness
- Sensory complaints such as:

- Tinnitus
- Parasthesias
- Gustatory, auditory, or visual abnormalities
- Repetitive actions such as:
  - Lip smacking
  - Finger activity
- Eye rolling, roving
- Tonic/clonic movement
  - May be subclinical, requiring EEG
- Todd's paralysis
  - Appreciated in postictal phase of seizure
  - Signs/symptoms consistent with ischemic stroke
    - Hemiparesis
    - Facial droop
    - Other focal symptoms
- Tachycardia, hypertension
  - May be the only signs in a patient who has received NMBAs

Status epilepticus is seizure activity with little or no recovery between episodes, and is considered a potential life-threatening event because of the myriad complications that may occur, including apnea, hypoxia, acidosis (metabolic and respiratory), renal compromise secondary to rhabdomyolysis, cardiovascular insufficiency, hyperthermia, hypertension, elevated ICP, and neuronal destruction.

Treatment of seizures centers around airway control, oxygenation, ventilation, and cessation of seizure activity.

- ABCs
- Cessation of seizure activity
  - Reversal of underlying cause
    - Hypoglycemia
    - Hypoxia
  - Benzodiazepenes
  - Antiepileptics
    - Phenytoin
- Cool patient, if hyperthermic

Alzheimer's disease
Alzheimer's disease is a primary dementia that occurs secondary to cortical and hippocampal degeneration and the formation of neurofibrillary tangles and senile plaques; neurotransmitter deficiency and viral infection appear to be two major causes of Alzheimer's. Signs and symptoms include:

- Short-term memory loss, forgetfulness, difficulty in retaining newly learned information
- Motor function effects, behavioral impairment
- Mental and physical debilitation

Treatment is primarily supportive, but several therapeutic agents designed to slow the progression of disease are commonly administered.

Parkinson's disease
Parkinson's disease is a degenerative brain disorder that occurs secondary to loss of dopamine-secreting neurons, and dopamine deficiency in the extrapyramidal nuclei. Signs and symptoms include:

- Tremors
  - Begin in upper extremities, spread to lower extremities as disease progresses
- Muscular rigidity
- Bradykinesia

Treatment involves the administration of anticholinergic agents and exogenous dopamine precursors.

Multiple sclerosis (MS)

MS is an autoimmune disease characterized by the inflammation, demyelination, and scarring of CNS tissue; subsequently, nerve impulses are slowed through unmyelinated nerve. The course of the disease can be relapsing, remitting, or progressive.

Signs and symptoms of MS include:

- Vague sensory alterations, fatigue, diminished visual acuity
- Cerebellar ataxia, loss of sphincter control
- Motor disturbances
  - Spasticity, weakness, paraplegia
- Cognitive dysfunction or behavioral changes

Treatment for MS centers around supportive care and the administration of corticosteroids.

Amyotrophic lateral sclerosis (ALS)

ALS, also known as Lou Gehrig's disease, is a degenerative muscular disease characterized by progressive degeneration of upper and lower motor neurons resulting in progressive muscle weakness and atrophy. The critical stage of disease is reached when atrophy of respiratory muscles occurs, resulting in inefficient ventilation, when cranial nerve involvement results in the inability to protect the airway, increasing the risk of aspiration pneumonia. Treatment is supportive only.

Guillain-Barré syndrome

Guillain-Barré syndrome is an autoimmune disorder characterized by the inflammatory destruction of the myelin sheaths surrounding spinal cord nerve roots. Inflammation can extend into the anterior horn of the spinal cord and the motor nuclei of cranial nerves. Nerve impulse conduction is impaired, resulting in muscle weakness. Impairment begins distally and inferiorly, and ascends up the limbs and trunk. The disease may be self-limiting. Treatment consists of:

- Supportive care
  - Cardiopulmonary
  - Respiratory
  - Plasmapheresis
- Administration of IV immunoglobulin
- Administration of beta blockers for autonomic instability

Myasthenia gravis

Myasthenia gravis is an autoimmune disorder characterized by the destruction of acetycholine receptors at the neuromuscular junction, resulting in impaired nerve impulse transmission to skeletal muscle and subsequent muscular weakness. Involvement of the diaphragm and intercostal muscles can lead to respiratory compromise, known as a "gravid," or "myasthenic" crisis. Treatment consists of:

- Supportive care
  - Respiratory
- Administration of ACE inhibitors
- Thymectomy
- Plasmapheresis

Neuroleptic malignant syndrome (NMS)

NMS is a profound reaction to neuroleptic agent use; specific neuroleptic medications include haloperidol, prochlorperazine, promethazine, risperidone, and metoclopramide.

Idiopathic blockade of dopamine-2 receptors in the hypothalamus can cause severe hyperthermia and muscular rigidity, leading to increased heat generation, decreased heat dissipation, acid–base disturbances, and a risk of rhabdomyolisis. A cascade response of the sympathetic autonomic nervous system also occurs, with life-threatening tachycardia and hypertension possible. Signs and symptoms of NMS include:

- Muscular rigidity
- Hyperthermia

- Tachycardia, hypertension
- Development of rhabdomyolysis

Treatment consists of:

- Supportive care
- Administration of muscle relaxants
- Administration of dopamine receptor (D-2) agonists
- Active cooling

Malignant hypertension syndrome (MHS)
Malignant hypertension syndrome occurs as a result of a genetic abnormality. Administration of succinylcholine or anesthesia creates profound hyperthermia secondary to increased calcium release from the sarcoplasmic reticulum of skeletal muscle, resulting in abnormal, sustained muscular contractions. Signs and symptoms of malignant hypertension syndrome include:

- Muscular rigidity
- Hyperthermia

Treatment involves supportive care and dantrolene administration; active cooling may also be necessary.

Creutzfeldt-Jakob disease (CJD) and Bovine spongiform encephalopathy (BSE)
CJD and BSE are two transmissible degenerative diseases caused by prion deposition in the brain that cause widespread glial and neuronal destruction with eventual and inevitable death. The transmission of these disorders depends on their etiology. CJD can follow a familial pattern of genetic transmission, while variants of this disease use animal vectors to infect humans. Of those that utilize an animal vector, BSE is the most widely recognized thanks to the widespread media attention that it has enjoyed in the past decade. All prion disorders are fatal, often within a period of several months. The mechanism whereby they cause CNS tissue destruction is not readily apparent; however, patients will present with progressive encephalopathic changes until coma ensues and death occurs.

Myelomeningocele (spina bifida)
Spina bifida is a congenital disorder (thought to be the result of maternal folate deficiency) that results in the improper formation of the neural tube during embryonic development; the neural tube is the precursor to the central nervous system. Incomplete formation of the spinal column allows the exposure of meningeal and CNS tissue to the outside environment with the obvious risk of infection and damage. In the more severe forms, the meninges and spinal cord tissue protrude from a defect in the patient's back. Such defects are typically located at the level of the lumbar spine. The disease is associated with varying degrees of paralysis, and neurological deficit. Surgical correction is possible.

3. **Recognize the potential for secondary injury and understand treatment options to minimize its effects.** p. 690

The central nervous system reacts to hypoperfusion and hypoxia the same way in the neuromedical patient as it does in the trauma patient. As such, regardless of the mechanism, the patterns of histopathologic secondary brain injury are the same. Infarcted tissue will become edematous and swell just as contused tissue will. Bleeds that are atraumatic in origin, such as from a ruptured aneurysm, are just as dangerous and have the same sequelae as bleeds that are caused by trauma; in some cases, bleeds of an atraumatic origin can be more dangerous.

The trauma principles of the prevention of secondary injury, ICP monitoring and treatment, and maintenance of cerebral perfusion pressure (CPP) apply to the neuromedical patient. Some neurologic emergencies have greater predisposition to certain types of secondary injuries than others, and some have other complications of their own above and beyond those seen in the trauma population.

©2007 Pearson Education, Inc.
Critical Care Paramedic

4. Become familiar with the pathophysiology of thromboembolic and hemorrhagic cerebrovascular accidents as well as the treatment for both.   **p. 691**

A cerebrovascular accident, or stroke, is characterized by the acute loss of perfusion to an area of the brain and resultant loss of neurological function. Strokes are classified as ischemic or hemorrhagic, and ischemic stroke can occur secondary to thrombosis or embolism. Ischemic stroke accounts for about 85 percent of all strokes. Risk factors for acute thromboembolic ischemic stroke include:

- Hypertension
- Hyperlipidemia, diabetes mellitus
- Smoking, obesity
- Genetic predisposition
- Elevated hematocrit
  - Polycythemia vera
- Hypercoaguable states, oral contraceptive use
- Prolonged airplane or car trips
- Valvular dysfunction, chronic atrial fibrillation, persistent patent foramen ovale

Blockage of a cerebral artery results in cerebral tissue ischemia and a transition to anaerobic metabolism. Anaerobic glycolysis occurs, but insufficient adenosine triphosphate (ATP) production results in Na^+/K^+ transmembrane pump insufficiency, and intracellular accumulation of sodium follows. Extracellular water moves into the cell along the created osmotic gradient, resulting in cellular edema and death. In any area of infarction, there are two clinically significant regions, the zone of infarction and the penumbra. The zone of infarction is comprised of brain tissue that will become necrotic in the absence of perfusion. The penumbra surrounds the zone of infarction, and consists of brain tissue threatened with cellular death, though death can be prevented with reperfusion.

As with all neurologic disorders, the signs and symptoms, as well as the prognosis, depend on the area of brain tissue affected by hypoperfusion and secondary changes. Signs and symptoms of middle cerebral artery (MCA) occlusion include:

- Global aphasia (if on the dominant side)
- Contralateral upper motor neuron facial weakness
- Ipsilateral gaze preference
  - Eyes look toward the lesion
  - Homonymous hemianopsia in the visual fields contralateral to the side of the lesion
- Damage to the motor function governing a patient's oral motor mechanics
  - High risk for aspiration

MCA infarction can result in significant edema and secondary injury. The degree of deficit resulting from infarct depends on the amount of tissue involved and directly correlates to the proximity of the lesion to the circle of Willis; infarction of more distal aspects of the vessel will result in similar, but less severe or incomplete, deficits.

The anterior cerebral artery (ACA) perfuses the medial aspects of the temporal and parietal lobes and the majority of the frontal lobes. Signs and symptoms of ACA occlusion include:

- Contralateral lower extremity weakness
- Intellectual and behavioral changes
  - Secondary to frontal lobe involvement

Signs and symptoms of posterior cerebral artery (PCA) occlusion include:

- Visual acuity loss
- Total vision loss
- Cortical blindness
- Contralateral hemisensory loss
  - With occlusion affecting the thalamus
- Contralateral hemiplegia
  - With involvement of pyramidal motor tracts

Vertebral and basilar artery occlusion can be catastrophic, with varying degrees of motor and sensory loss. Signs and symptoms of cerebellar artery occlusion include:

- Contralateral and ipsilateral patterns of:
  - Ataxia
  - Motor weakness
  - Sensory deficit
  - Vertigo
- Edema resulting in hernia and death

Lacunar infarction syndromes are symptoms caused by patterns of small infarctions and areas of neuronal necrosis within the deep white matter structures of the brain that tend not to be as severe as infarcts of larger vessels. Lacunar infarction syndromes present with similar symptoms to classic stroke:

- TIAs
- Motor, sensory, and movement disorders
  - Dysarthria/clumsy hand syndrome
- Facial muscle paresis
- Unilateral ataxia

Watershed infarctions are numerous small areas of infarcted tissue at the periphery of the cerebral arteries. Peripheral tissue is particularly vulnerable to hypoperfusion because of lack of collateral circulation.

Numerous stroke scales exist to aid in the evaluation of stroke, and include the National Institute of Health (NIH) stroke scale, the Cincinnati Stroke Scale, and the Los Angeles (LA) Stroke Scale. The NIH Stroke Scale is an objective evaluation based on the level of consciousness, motor and sensory function, and the degree of cognitive impairment. Because of its complexity, it is an impractical assessment to render in the prehospital setting.

The Cincinnati Stroke Scale is an effective and more succinct means of determining the presence of neurological deficit. Any abnormal finding is considered to be evidence of intracerebral pathology. The scale evaluates for the presence or absence of facial droop, arm weakness, and clarity of speech.

The treatment for thrombotic stroke is fibrinolytic or antiplatelet therapy, discussed in Objective 5.

Hemorrhagic stroke occurs secondary to an intracranial hemorrhage, and, in fact, the two terms are interchangeable. Intracranial hemorrhage accounts for about 15 percent of all strokes and is associated with a higher mortality than ischemic stroke. Cerebral aneurysm or arteriovenous malformation rupture can cause injury to brain tissue in three primary ways; through the mass effect of accumulated blood (dependent on the size and location of the bleed), hypoperfusion, and cerebral vasospasm.

Subarachnoid hemorrhage (SAH), the severity of which can be graded on the Hunt and Hess or Fisher scales, results when intracerebral bleeding occurs into the subarachnoid space. Blood in subarachnoid space overwhelms the arachnoid villi's ability to reabsorb CSF, secondary to the fluid (CSF + blood) volume increase and mechanical obstruction from clotting. This results in rapidly developing hydrocephalus, which must be corrected via the insertion of an extraventricular drain (EVD). Signs and symptoms of SAH include:

- Headache
- Decreased level of consciousness, loss of consciousness, seizures
- Focal motor weakness
- Neck pain/stiffness
- Photophobia
- Nausea
- Findings consistent with AMI
  - ECG changes
  - Elevated troponin
  - Decreased CO
  - Ventricular wall dysfunction

- Hypertension
- Increased ICP
- Positive CT
  - Differentiates hemorrhagic from ischemic stroke

During the course of a developing SAH, blood in the brain parenchyma may irritate arterial vessels, resulting in vasospasm and decreased blood flow distal to vasospasm; cerebral hypoperfusion and subsequent infarction are possible secondary injuries. Large areas of infarction can cause cytoxic cerebral edema, resulting in increased ICP, decreased CPP, hypoperfusion, and wider zones of infarction.

The Lindegaard ratio, the ratio of the velocity of blood traveling through the MCA to that traveling through the vertebral artery, can be determined with transcranial Doppler study. Typical onset of SAH varies from three to 21 days post injury, with a peak between days eight and 12. Management of cerebral vasospasm includes:

- ICP monitoring
- Venous and arterial pressure monitoring
- Calcium channel blockers
  - Nimodipine
- "Triple-H" therapy: forces blood into areas not adequately perfused
  - Hypertense
  - Hypervolumize
  - Hemodilute

An intracerebral hemorrhage (ICH) occurs when blood vessels located in the brain bleed directly into the brain parenchyma. Hematoma formation occurs, and can extend into the subarachnoid space and/or ventricles. There is risk of secondary injury as a result of mass effect, which can produce herniation and hydrocephalus. Intracerebral hemorrhages generally occur as a result of chronic hypertension or hypertensive crises.

Amyloid angiopathy, a vascular disorder, is a possible etiology for ICH in those patients not suffering from hypertension. Amyloid deposits in the walls of cerebral vessels weaken the vessel walls, resulting in the formation of microaneurysms. Bleeds from amyloid angiopathy tend to be superficial compared to those secondary to hypertension, and have a high incidence of recurrence. Management of intracerebral hemorrhage involves the control of mean arterial pressure, and the surgical repair and evacuation of the injury and accumulated blood.

5. Identify patients who are candidates for fibrinolytic therapy.   p. 695

The primary purpose of fibrinolytic therapy is the lyses of thromboembolic clots. The intent of fibrinolytic therapy is to minimize or eliminate the necrosis of hypoperfused tissue, thereby preserving the function of that tissue; we are aiming for preservation of neurons and improvement in functional outcome. As "time equals brain tissue," it is imperative that fibrinolytic therapy is initiated within a very narrow time frame after the onset of symptoms. As such, all members of the critical care transport team should be familiar with the inclusion and exclusion criteria for fibrinolytic therapy.

Inclusion criteria for fibrinolytic therapy is as follows:

- The patient must:
  - Be between 18 and 75 years of age.
  - Have a clinical diagnosis of stroke with significant neurological compromise to warrant the risk of fibrinolytic therapy.
  - Have symptoms with a definite onset of less than three hours prior to the initiation of thrombolysis.
  - Have a CT scan that demonstrates the absence of any sort of intracranial hemorrhage.

Exclusion criteria for fibrinolytic therapy is as follows:

- The patient must not:
  - Have deficits that are improving without treatment.
  - Have a CT that demonstrates any suggestion of ICH.

- Have a history of ICH or known aneurysm.
- Have had a seizure when symptoms began.
- Have had a stroke or serious head injury within the prior 3 months.
- Have a history of IV drug abuse.
- Be under the influence of cocaine.
- Have undergone major surgery or sustained major trauma within the prior 2 weeks.
- Have suffered gastrointestinal or genitourinary hemorrhage within the prior 3 weeks.
- Require ongoing aggressive treatment to lower blood pressure.
- Have sustained an arterial puncture at a noncompressible site or lumber puncture within 1 week.
- Have undergone heparin therapy within 48 hours.
- Have evidence of pericarditis.
- Have a known bleeding diathesis.
- Be pregnant or breast-feeding.

Recommended exclusion vital signs:

- Systolic BP greater than 185 mmHg
- Diastolic BP greater than 110 mmHg

Recommended exclusion laboratory values:

- Serum glucose < 50mg/dL or >400mg/dL
- Platelet count greater than 100,000/uL
- Patients currently on anticoagulant therapy with prothrombin time (PT) more than 15 seconds or International Normalized Ratio (INR) greater than 1.7

Firbrinolysis is accomplished with the administration of tissue plasminogen activator (tPA) at a dose of 0.9 mg/kg IV, with 10 percent of the total dose as bolus, and the remaining 90 percent infused over 60 minutes. Maximum dose is 90 mg total.

Antiplatelet therapy is an option for those patients excluded from fibrinolytic therapy, and includes the use of aspirin and clopidogrel (Plavix).

6. **Identify infectious processes found in the central nervous system and their effects.** p. 701

Infectious processes that can affect the brain include meningitis, encephalitis, and brain abscesses. Meningitis is an infection of the meninges of the brain and spinal cord. Common etiologies include viruses and bacteria, specifically:

- Viruses
  - Mumps
  - Herpes
  - Epstein-Barr virus
- Bacterial
  - *Neisseria meningitides*
  - *Streptococcus pneumoniae*
  - *Haemophilus influenzae*
  - *Klebsiella pneumoniae*
- Other
  - Syphilis
  - Lyme disease
  - *Leptospira interrogans*
  - Toxoplasmosis
  - Malaria

Morbidity and mortality of meningitis is dependant on etiology, secondary complications, speed of onset, and speed of treatment, as the CNS has a poor capacity to respond to infection. Patients particularly at risk include those with open infection pathways secondary to skull fractures, CSF leaks, or ventricular drains, and patients with a recent history of viral or bacterial illness, such as HIV or tuberculosis.

Signs and symptoms of meningitis:

- High fever, headache, neck/back pain
- N/V, photophobia, seizures
- Purpuric or petechial rash with meningococcal meningitis

Complications of meningitis include hydrocephalus secondary to mechanical obstruction of CSF flow, infarction or secondary infection from vascular inflammation, and cranial nerve involvement.

Evaluation for meningitis includes CT scan, lumbar puncture, and blood cultures, with treatment centering around antimicrobial therapy.

Encephalitis is an infection of the brain parenchyma, distinct from meningitis, etiologies of which include the herpes simplex virus, cytomegalovirus, *Toxoplasma gondii,* mumps virus, Epstein-Barr virus, and the Eastern Equine and West Nile viruses.

Encephalitis results in elevated ICP, diffuse cerebral edema, and hydrocephalus. Treatment is supportive in nature; the antiviral azithromycin is used to treat encephalitis secondary to herpes infection.

Bacterial infections of the brain tend to occur as localized abscesses, and can occur anywhere within the cranial vault. They can arise from skull fractures or surgical incision, and can spread in the blood to form local infection elsewhere in the body. Abscesses act as space-occupying lesions, and can result in elevated ICP, mass effect, and herniation. Treatment options include surgical intervention and antibiotic therapy.

Immunocompromised individuals are more susceptible to CNS infection from bacteria, viral, and fungal sources. Specific microbes include *Toxoplasma gondii,* cytomegalovirus, and cryptococcal encephalitis.

Case Study

Your critical care ground transport team has been called to a small, rural hospital for an inpatient transfer to University Medical Center, approximately 75 miles away. The nurse on the floor advises you and your partner that your patient is a 73-year-old female who was admitted with back pain and lower extremity weakness. She had been admitted to the same facility approximately 6 weeks ago for overnight observation and IV hydration secondary to a diarrheal illness. The diarrhea later proved to be caused by a *Campylobacter* infection and resolved with antibiotic treatment.

Since her admission, the patient's back pain has resolved but the weakness has been increasing in severity over the past 24 hours. The patient's weakness has been ascending, and in the past 12 hours, she has lost the use of her arms and is no longer able to raise her head off the pillow. You are told the patient has been diagnosed with Guillain-Barré syndrome and is being transferred for plasmapheresis. The nurse finishes her report as the three of you walk into the patient's room. As she starts to introduce you to the patient, she stops in midsentence. "Catherine!" she says in alarm to the patient. Looking up at you she says, "She's gotten so much worse in the past half hour!" The patient does look very ill. Her skin is pale and ashen. Although her eyes look at you and her lips are moving softly, she is unable to respond verbally. Her airway has soft audible rhonchi and she is showing weak respiratory effort, with shallow diaphragmatic breaths. "She needs to be ventilated," you say to the nurse. "Would you please let her physician know?" She turns and quickly leaves the room. Fortunately, you always bring your assessment/airway bag in on transfers, so all necessary equipment is close at hand. While you explain the procedure to the patient and work out a system of yes/no for eyelid blinking, your partner readies the intubation equipment. The nurse returns and tells you that the patient's physician has left for the day, but that she spoke to him on the phone and he said to tell you to "do whatever you need to do." Using etomidate for induction and avoiding the use of neuromuscular blocking agents, your partner quickly and easily passes the endotracheal tube into the trachea. Tube placement is confirmed with auscultation and EtCO$_2$, which is initially elevated but begins to normalize after the first dozen ventilations. After intubation, the patient's heart rate is 112, sinus tachycardia on the monitor, and she has a blood pressure of 158/92. The patient's color has improved and her SpO$_2$ is 95 percent with 100 percent oxygen administered via BVM.

The patient is moved into the ambulance and switched over to the transport ventilator without any incident. During the transport, you make a conscious effort to ensure that the patient's extremities are secured and protected from injury and to keep the patient informed and reassured. The patient remains stable throughout transport and she is transferred into a bed in University's ICU without any further deterioration. You later learn that the patient failed to regain sufficient muscle strength to breathe off the ventilator. She was subsequently transferred by one of your colleagues to a long-term ventilator care facility.

DISCUSSION QUESTION

1. What is the importance of managing airway, breathing, and circulation in preventing secondary injury in the neurologic patient?

Content Review

MULTIPLE CHOICE

_____ 1. The cerebrum is divided laterally into left and right hemispheres in the midline by the:
A. sulci.
B. gyri.
C. longitudinal fissure.
D. frontal fissure.

_____ 2. The white matter of the brain contains:
A. neuronal axons.
B. neuronal cell bodies and supporting structures.
C. the functional units of the brain.
D. the cortex.

_____ 3. Which of the following statements regarding the cerebellum is true?
A. It is responsible for the coordination and stabilization of fine and complex movements.
B. It is responsible for proprioception.
C. It connects to the brainstem via the cerebellar peduncles.
D. All of the above.

_____ 4. The _____ controls the autonomic nervous system, helps to regulate sleep-wake cycles, and regulates body temperature.
A. thalamus
B. midbrain
C. hypothalamus
D. epithalamus

_____ 5. The brainstem consists of the:
A. cerebrum, cerebellum, and midbrain.
B. midbrain, pons, and medulla.
C. thalamus, hypothalamus, and epithalamus.
D. none of the above.

_____ 6. The primary structures of the ventricular system are the:
A. paired lateral ventricles, superior ventricle, and inferior ventricle.
B. paired lateral ventricles, third ventricle, and fourth ventricle.
C. first ventricle, second ventricle, third ventricle, and fourth ventricle.
D. lateral ventricle, middle ventricle, superior ventricle, and inferior ventricle.

_____ 7. Which layer of the meninges is continuous with the periosteum?
A. pia mater
B. arachnoid membrane
C. subarachnoid space
D. dura mater

CRITICAL CARE PARAMEDIC

8. The anatomical structures that divide the spinal cord into two lateral halves are the:
   A. anterior median fissure and posterior median sulcus.
   B. posterior and lateral funiculus.
   C. anterior and lateral funiculus.
   D. none of the above.

9. Which of the following statements regarding the spinal cord is true?
   A. The spinal cord's vascular supply runs cephalocaudally along the lateral aspects of the cord.
   B. The ventral root of the spinal nerve carries efferent motor impulses from the cell bodies in the posterior horns of the white matter to the skeletal muscles.
   C. The dorsal root of the spinal nerve carries afferent sensory information from the body's periphery through the dorsal root ganglion and into the spinal cord to the brain.
   D. All of the above are true.

10. The white matter of the spinal cord contains several nerve tracts that carry:
    A. afferent impulses.   C. both afferent and efferent impulses.
    B. efferent impulses.   D. neither afferent or efferent impulses.

11. Which of the following, if no compensation occurs, would directly lead to an increase in cerebral perfusion pressure?
    A. an increase in ICP
    B. an increase in MAP
    C. a decrease in MAP
    D. an equal increase in MAP and decrease in ICP

12. All blood supply to the brain originates from the:
    A. vertebral arteries.   C. spinal arteries.
    B. carotid arteries.   D. aorta.

13. The circle of Willis is composed, in part, by all of the following arteries except the:
    A. basilar.   C. anterior cerebral.
    B. posterior cerebral.   D. posterior communicating.

14. Examples of the venous sinuses that help collect blood returning to the circulation from the brain include all of the following except the:
    A. cavernous sinus.   C. central sinuses.
    B. sagittal sinus.   D. transverse sinuses.

15. The frontal lobe is separated from the parietal lobe by a structure known as the:
    A. precentral gyrus.   C. pyramidal sulcus.
    B. central sulcus.   D. pyramidal gyrus.

16. The premotor cortex:
    A. has control over the intent and higher thought surrounding voluntary movement, as well as learned patterns of complex voluntary motor repetition.
    B. is responsible for the initiation of, and physical formation of, speech.
    C. controls fine motor movement, coordination, and balance.
    D. none of the above.

17. Patients exhibiting expressive aphasia most likely have damage to which of the following areas of the brain?
    A. Broca's area   C. the cerebral peduncles
    B. the internal capsule   D. the corticobulbar tract

18. Upper motor neuron lesions affect:
    A. the ipsilateral side of the body.
    B. the contralateral side of the body.
    C. both sides of the body equally.
    D. the central nervous system only, with no observable manifestations.

_____ 19. The extrapyramidal motor system:
   A. receives and interprets information concerning light touch, pain, pressure, stretching, and temperature.
   B. allows for voluntary muscle control.
   C. provides involuntary control of musculature.
   D. none of the above.

_____ 20. The "extrapyramidal effects" of certain medications, particularly antipsychotic medications such as thorazine derivatives, includes:
   A. athetosis, tardive dyskinesia, tremors, or other abnormal disorders of movement.
   B. paralysis, paresthesia, and decreased range of motion.
   C. increased pain, pressure, and light sensitivity, and decreased temperature tolerance.
   D. altered mental status, loss of consciousness, coma, and death.

_____ 21. Partial decussation of the optic nerve occurs at the:
   A. circle of Willis.   C. basal ganglia.
   B. somatosensory association area.   D. optic chiasma.

_____ 22. The cortical areas involved with the processes of smell and taste are located in the:
   A. frontal lobe.   C. parietal lobe.
   B. temporal lobe.   D. occipital lobe.

_____ 23. The cortical areas involved with the processes of hearing are located in the:
   A. frontal lobe.   C. parietal lobe.
   B. temporal lobe.   D. occipital lobe.

_____ 24. Primary control of the autonomic nervous system is governed by the:
   A. pituitary gland.   C. endocrine system.
   B. thalamus.   D. hypothalamus.

_____ 25. The preganglionic fibers of the sympathetic nervous system are mediated by the neurotransmitter _____, while the postganglionic fibers secrete the neurotransmitter _____.
   A. norepinephrine, acetylcholine   C. acetylcholine, norepinephrine
   B. dopamine, acetylcholine   D. epinephrine, norepinephrine

_____ 26. Which of the following statements regarding the parasympathetic nervous system is true?
   A. The parasympathetic autonomic nervous system's preganglionic fibers tend to be much shorter than those of the sympathetic.
   B. The parasympathetic nerve fibers originate from the brainstem and the sacral region of the spine, from S2 through S4.
   C. Both the presynaptic and postsynaptic ganglia secrete the neurotransmitter norepinephrine.
   D. The vagus nerve alone is responsible for a very limited amount of parasympathetic control over the body.

_____ 27. The area of the brain that responds to a variety of physiological and sensory input to define the brain's response to emotion and contributes heavily to the formation and integration of memory is the:
   A. limbic system.   C. somatosensory association area.
   B. lentiform system.   D. spinocerebellar tracts.

_____ 28. A patient is said to have global aphasia when the patient:
   A. is unable to speak or formulate words clearly.
   B. is unable to understand speech.
   C. is unable to speak or formulate words clearly and is unable to understand speech.
   D. has good comprehension, and speech that is fluent but dysphasic with inappropriate words.

©2007 Pearson Education, Inc.
Critical Care Paramedic

_____ 29. Assessing a patient for pronator drift is an assessment of which area of the brain?
   A. cerebrum
   B. brainstem
   C. occipital lobe
   D. cerebellum

_____ 30. Which of the following neurological assessment techniques is appropriate to use on a conscious patient?
   A. Flick your hand toward the patient's face to elicit a reflexive blink.
   B. Attempt to elicit a motor response with a brisk sternal rub.
   C. Insert a rigid tonsil tip suction catheter into the patient's oropharynx and assess both sides for the presence of a gag reflex.
   D. None of the above.

_____ 31. The most widely utilized imaging modality for CNS tissue is:
   A. transcranial doppler ultrasound.
   B. CT.
   C. MRI.
   D. cerebral angiography.

_____ 32. Which of the following are risk factors for stroke?
   A. hypertension and diabetes mellitus
   B. genetic predisposition and hyperlipidemia
   C. smoking and obesity
   D. all of the above

_____ 33. During acute stroke, the area known as the penumbra:
   A. consists of brain tissue that is threatened with cellular death from hypoperfusion, but that may be spared with timely treatment.
   B. is the area surrounding the infarct, that experiences increased blood flow and perfusion.
   C. is the center of the infarction, and is comprised of brain tissue that will become necrotic in the absence of perfusion.
   D. results in a feeling of altered sensorium.

_____ 34. What percentage of strokes is the result of ischemic, rather than hemorrhagic, insult?
   A. 15 percent
   B. 20 percent
   C. 80 percent
   D. 85 percent

_____ 35. The anterior cerebral artery perfuses the:
   A. medial aspects of the temporal and parietal lobes of the brain, near the midline, and much of the frontal lobes.
   B. the lateral aspects of the frontal, temporal, and parietal lobes.
   C. the anterior aspects of the frontal, temporal, and parietal lobes, and the entire occipital lobe.
   D. the brainstem.

_____ 36. A watershed infarction involves:
   A. patterns of small infarctions and areas of neuronal necrosis within the deep white matter structures of the brain.
   B. complete, total-body loss of motor control with the exception of minimal extraocular movement and aphasia.
   C. numerous small areas of infarcted tissue at the periphery of the smallest extensions of the cerebral arteries.
   D. infarct of the visual processing cortex.

_____ 37. Thromboembolic strokes may be differentiated from hemorrhagic strokes with:
   A. a good neurologic exam.
   B. CT scan.
   C. transcranial Doppler ultrasound.
   D. all of the above.

_____ 38. Normal cerebral blood flow is about:
   A. 10–15 mL/100g/min.
   B. 30–35 mL/100g/min.
   C. 50–55 mL/100g/min.
   D. 100 mL/100g/min.

_____ 39. Which of the following would exclude a patient as a candidate for fibrinolytic therapy to treat acute ischemic stroke?
A. a blood pressure of 180/110
B. a platelet count of 10,000/uL
C. a patient currently with a prothrombin time (PT) of 12 seconds and an International Normalized Ratio (INR) of 1.2
D. history of a stroke three years ago

_____ 40. Which of the following best represents the initial loading dose of tPA for a 100 kg patient?
A. 0.9 mg IV
B. 9 mg IV
C. 90 mg IV
D. 900 mg IV

_____ 41. Patients with acute ischemic stroke who do not receive fibrinolysis should receive:
A. antiplatelet therapy.
B. clopidogrel.
C. aspirin.
D. all of the above.

_____ 42. Special considerations for patients who have been administered tPA include all of the following except:
A. administration of heparin IV.
B. strict monitoring of MAP.
C. withholding of invasive procedures unless absolutely necessary.
D. frequent assessment for internal and external hemorrhage.

_____ 43. Which of the following stroke etiologies might be treated with fibrinolytic therapy, providing no exclusion, and all inclusion, criteria are met?
A. thromboembolism
B. subarachnoid hemorrhage
C. intracranial hemorrhage
D. intracerebral hemorrhage

_____ 44. A CT scan showing a diffuse layer of subarachnoid blood would be considered a Fisher grade _____.
A. I
B. II
C. III
D. IV

_____ 45. A patient with acute stroke presenting with confusion, lethargy, and focal motor deficit would receive a Hunt and Hess grade _____.
A. II
B. III
C. IV
D. V

_____ 46. Patients with intracranial hemorrhage are at high risk for:
A. cerebral arterial vasospasm.
B. AMI.
C. increased ICP.
D. all of the above.

_____ 47. A Lindegaard ratio of 5 indicates what degree of cerebral artery vasospasm?
A. none
B. mild
C. moderate
D. severe

_____ 48. The goal during the treatment of hemorrhagic stroke is to maintain:
A. a MAP of 65–75 mmHg.
B. a CPP of at least 80–90 mmHg.
C. a ICP of 20–30 mmHg.
D. all of the above.

_____ 49. The common goal in the treatment of hemorrhagic and ischemic stroke is to:
A. achieve maximum perfusion of brain parenchyma.
B. lyse the blood clot causing brain ischemia.
C. surgically repair the defect causing the brain ischemia.
D. decrease MAP and CPP to prevent secondary injury to the brain.

_____ 50. The management of a patient with an intracerebral hemorrhage and cerebral artery vasospasm may include all of the following except:
A. ICP, central venous, and arterial pressure monitoring.
B. calcium channel blockers.
C. beta blockers.
D. "Triple-H" therapy: hypertense, hypervolumize, and hemodilute.

©2007 Pearson Education, Inc.
Critical Care Paramedic

_____ 51. Patients at high risk for meningitis include those with:
   A. HIV.
   B. tuberculosis.
   C. open skull fractures.
   D. all of the above.

_____ 52. Which of the following is the least useful in the evaluation of a patient with meningitis?
   A. CT scan
   B. skull radiograph
   C. lumbar puncture
   D. blood cultures

_____ 53. _____ is an infection of the brain parenchyma.
   A. Encephalitis
   B. Meningitis
   C. Gliomatitis
   D. Cytomegalovirus

_____ 54. Encephalitis may result in:
   A. decreased ICP.
   B. localized cerebral edema.
   C. hydrocephalus.
   D. all of the above.

_____ 55. Immunocompromised individuals are more susceptible to CNS infection from _____ sources.
   A. bacterial
   B. viral
   C. fungal
   D. all of the above

_____ 56. Bacterial infections within the brain tend to result in:
   A. diffuse encephalitis.
   B. localized abscesses.
   C. meningitis.
   D. encephalitis.

_____ 57. Factors determining a brain tumor's malignancy include:
   A. histological origin.
   B. speed of growth.
   C. degree of cellular differentiation.
   D. all of the above.

_____ 58. A developing brain tumor may contribute to an increase in ICP secondary to:
   A. mass effect.
   B. vasogenic edema.
   C. hydrocephalus.
   D. all of the above.

_____ 59. Which of the following is not a diagnostic modality used to identify CNS tumors?
   A. MRI
   B. CT
   C. transcranial doppler ultrasound
   D. lumbar puncture

_____ 60. Which of the following statements regarding meningioma is true?
   A. It is a tumor of the meninges.
   B. It typically involves the brain parenchyma.
   C. It is usually malignant.
   D. All of the above.

_____ 61. Which of the following statements regarding gliomas is false?
   A. They are tumors of the neuroglia.
   B. They affect astrocytomas, oligodendrogliomas, and ependymomas.
   C. Treatment typically includes chemotherapy.
   D. None of the above.

_____ 62. Encephalopathy is a (an):
   A. infection of the meninges of the brain and spinal cord.
   B. progressive neuronal degeneration and dysfunction resulting from pathological changes that occur outside the brain.
   C. infection of the brain parenchyma.
   D. none of the above.

_____ 63. Etiologies of encephalopathy include:
   A. blood glucose extremes.
   B. metabolic disorders and organ failure.
   C. toxins and alcoholism.
   D. all of the above.

_____ 64. Gradual onset encephalopathy typically follows a predictable progression of findings that include all of the following except:
   A. subtle changes in behavior, memory, and movement.
   B. paralysis and paresthesia.
   C. worsening disorders of thought and movement.
   D. coma.

_____ 65. Specific forms of encephalopathy include all of the following except:
   A. AIDS encephalopathy.
   B. Wernicke's encephalopathy.
   C. myocardial encephalopathy.
   D. hepatic encephalopathy.

_____ 66. Korsakoff's psychosis, nystagmus, impaired extraocular movement, and cerebellar ataxia with gait disturbance are signs of:
   A. AIDS encephalopathy.
   B. Wernicke's encephalopathy.
   C. myocardial encephalopathy.
   D. hepatic encephalopathy.

_____ 67. The management of hepatic encephalopathy may include all of the following except:
   A. reversal of the precipitating cause.
   B. the administration of Lactulose.
   C. high-protein diet.
   D. airway management and mechanical ventilation.

_____ 68. Toxin-induced encephalopathy may occur secondary to all of the following except:
   A. metabolic derangement.
   B. IV drug abuse.
   C. contact with industrial chemicals.
   D. contact with organophosphates.

_____ 69. Seizures that present immediately with generalized seizure activity commonly originate from an epileptic focus in the:
   A. occipital region.
   B. cerebellar region.
   C. cerebral cortex.
   D. deep structures of the brain.

_____ 70. Seizures may occur secondary to:
   A. hypoxia.
   B. hypoglycemia or other metabolic derangement.
   C. unknown etiologies.
   D. all of the above.

_____ 71. A patient who is actively seizing should immediately receive _____ in an attempt to stop their seizure activity:
   A. phenytoin IV
   B. diazepam IV
   C. magnesium sulfate IV
   D. phenobarbitol IV

_____ 72. Parkinson's disease is a (an):
   A. degenerative muscular disease characterized by progressive degeneration of upper and lower motor neurons.
   B. autoimmune disease characterized by the inflammation, demyelination, and scarring of CNS tissue.
   C. degenerative brain disorder that occurs secondary to loss of dopamine-secreting neurons and dopamine deficiency in the extrapyramidal nuclei.
   D. autoimmune disorder characterized by the inflammatory destruction of the myelin sheaths surrounding spinal cord nerve roots.

_____ 73. Myasthenia gravis is a (an):
   A. autoimmune disorder characterized by the destruction of acetycholine receptors at the neuromuscular junction.
   B. autoimmune disorder characterized by the inflammatory destruction of the myelin sheaths surrounding spinal cord nerve roots.
   C. profound reaction to neuroleptic agent use.
   D. congenital disorder (thought to be the result of maternal folate deficiency) that results in the improper formation of the neural tube during embryonic development.

_____ 74. A patient experiencing chronic mental and physical debilitation, short-term memory loss, forgetfulness, and difficulty retaining newly learned information is most likely suffering from:
   A. Parkinson's disease.
   B. Guillain-Barré syndrome.
   C. Alzheimer's disease.
   D. delirium.

_____ 75. Treatment of Guillain-Barré syndrome includes all of the following except:
   A. plasmapheresis.
   B. administration of IV immunoglobulin.
   C. administration of beta blockers.
   D. thymectomy.

_____ 76. Medications that may result in the onset of neuroleptic malignant syndrome include all of the following except:
   A. haloperidol.
   B. lorazepam.
   C. prochlorperazine.
   D. risperidone.

_____ 77. The management of malignant hypertension syndrome includes:
   A. administration of muscle relaxants.
   B. administration of dopamine receptor (D-2) agonists.
   C. administration of dantrolene.
   D. all of the above.

_____ 78. _____ is thought to occur secondary to folic acid deficiency.
   A. Myelomeningocele
   B. Creutzfeldt-Jakob disease
   C. Myasthenia gravis
   D. None of the above

24 Gastrointestinal Emergencies

Review of Chapter Objectives

Upon completion of this chapter, the student should be able to:

1. Describe basic gastrointestinal anatomy and physiology.   p. 720

The digestive tract is an approximately 9-meter muscular tube consisting of the oral cavity, pharynx, esophagus, stomach, small intestine (duodenum, jejunum, and ileum), large intestine (colon), and rectum.

Accessory organs to the digestive tract include the salivary glands, the liver, and the pancreas. These structures secrete various enzymes, buffers, and other digestive aids to increase the effectiveness of the breakdown and absorption of nutrients.

The wall of the digestive tract can be divided into four distinct layers: the mucosa, the submucosa, the muscularis externa, and the serosa. The mucosa is made up of a layer of simple or stratified epithelium, depending on the location, and is moistened by the secretions of mucus glands. The mucosa is arranged into distinct circular and longitudinal smooth muscle layers called plicae, which contract to create peristalsis.

The loose connective tissue of the lamina propria contains small blood vessels, smooth muscle, lymphatic tissue, and lymphatic vessels. In addition to its role as part of the immune system, the lymphatic vessels absorb long-chain fatty acids from the intestinal lumen as chylomicrons, depositing them in the venous blood via the thoracic duct.

The submucosa is a layer of dense connective tissue surrounding the mucosal and muscularis layers. It contains exocrine glands, larger blood vessels, lymphatic tissue, and collections of nerve fibers called Meissner plexus. The muscularis externa contains muscle layers arranged in an inner, circular layer covered by an outer, longitudinal layer, as in the muscularis mucosae. Stimulation of the parasympathetic nervous system stimulates peristaltic motion, while sympathetic stimulation attenuates peristaltic motion. The serosa is a serous membrane that is continuous with the mesentery and covers the muscularis externa of all parts of the intestinal tract located in the peritoneal cavity.

Mechanical digestion of food begins in the oral cavity and occurs secondary to chewing food. Chemical digestion of carbohydrate begins with the release of the enzyme, amylase, in the saliva. Lingual lipase, secreted by glands on the tongue, also adds to saliva in the oral cavity and initiates the digestion of triglycerides. Saliva also serves to lubricate ingested material, facilitating passage through the esophagus, and it is produced and secreted from the parotid, sublingual, and submandibular salivary glands. This process of mechanical digestion, chemical digestion, and lubrication is termed mastication.

The tongue helps form the masticated food debris into a bolus, which is then directed to first, the oropharynx, and then, the laryngopharynx. Pharyngeal muscles contract to push the bolus further along into the esophagus, the superior portion of which is located at the level of C6. Involuntary muscle contractions of the esophagus produce the peristaltic esophageal wall motion that delivers the bolus the length of the esophagus to the stomach. The esophagus receives a rich arterial blood supply, with the superior portion located in the neck supplied by the external carotid and thyrocervical arteries, the mediastinal portion supplied by branches of the bronchial and the esophageal arteries, and the inferior portion supplied by the gastric artery. Venous blood from the esophagus drains into the esophageal, azygos, and gastric veins. Veins draining the inferior esophagus, as well as the cardia of the stomach, communicate with the hepatic portal vein.

The majority of the stomach lies in the upper left quadrant of the abdomen, immediately inferior to the diaphragm, between the level of vertebrae T7 and L3. The exact size and extension can be variable among individuals and meals. The stomach receives food from the upper GI tract via the esophagus and empties through the pyloric sphincter into the duodenum. It is divided into four regions: the cardia, fundus, body, and pylorus. The cardia is so named due to its proximity to the heart located just across the diaphragm. The fundus lies superior to the gastroesophageal junction and comes into contact with the abdominal surface of the diaphragm. The body, the largest of the four regions, extends from the fundus to the pylorus. The pylorus connects to the duodenum via the pyloric sphincter.

The stomach has a rich vascular supply consisting of the left gastric artery and branches of the splenic and common hepatic arteries. These arteries together comprise the three branches of the celiac artery, which itself branches off the abdominal aorta. The digestive functions of the stomach are carried out by chemical and mechanical means. Chyme exits the stomach through the pyloric sphincter and enters the small intestine, where further digestion and up to 90 percent of nutrient absorption will take place.

The small intestine is located in every abdominal quadrant and takes up the majority of space in the peritoneal cavity. It is suspended in place by the mesentery and protected by the greater omentum. Its divisions are the duodenum, jejunum, and ileum.

The duodenum is the shortest segment of the small intestine, and its majority is located in the retroperitoneal cavity. It reenters the peritoneal cavity just before its transition with the jejunum. In addition to chyme from the stomach, it receives digestive secretions from the pancreas and gallbladder, which aids in digestion and lowers the pH of the chyme. The jejunum is the site of the bulk of digestion and absorption within the small intestine. The most distal segment of the small intestine is the ileum. The ileocecal valve, at its terminus, regulates the flow of material into the first segment of the large intestine, the cecum. The large intestine takes a horseshoe-shaped route around the small intestine to its terminus at the anus. It is responsible for the resorption of water, electrolytes, and some vitamins from the intestinal contents and its divisions are the cecum, colon (consisting of the ascending, transverse, and descending colons), and rectum.

The cecum is a small, expandable pouch that receives material from the ileum and begins the process of fecal collection. The ascending colon, considered a retroperitoneal structure, ascends the right posterolateral wall of the abdominal cavity, turns at the hepatic flexure below the liver, and transitions into the transverse colon. The transverse colon is suspended in place by the mesentery, and curves anteriorly to reenter the peritoneal cavity before transitioning into the descending colon at the splenic flexure. The descending colon travels inferiorly along the left posterolateral wall of the abdominal cavity until its transition to the sigmoid colon, which takes place at the level of the iliac fossa with the sigmoid flexure before ending at the rectum. The rectum, the last six inches of the digestive tract, serves as a storage area for fecal material prior to defecation.

The abdominal cavity divided into three spaces, the peritoneal space, the retroperitoneal space, and the pelvic space. Organs located in each of the spaces are as follows:

- Peritoneal space
  - Stomach
  - Proximal duodenum
  - Ascending colon
  - Transverse colon
  - Sigmoid colon
  - Liver
  - Gallbladder
  - Spleen

- Retroperitoneal space
  - Kidneys
  - Ureters
  - Distal duodenum
  - Descending colon
  - Pancreas
- Pelvic space
  - Urinary bladder
  - Rectum
  - In the female, the ovaries and the fallopian tubes are also located in the pelvic cavity.

The visceral peritoneum, parietal peritoneum, and mesentery form a large, continuous sheet of serous membrane that lines the peritoneal space, and also serves to cover (and suspend) the peritoneal organs. The mesentery is a double layer of serous membrane connected by loose connective tissue that extends inferiorly from the posterior wall of the abdominal cavity and acts as a supportive structure for the digestive tract, preventing the movement and entanglement of the intestines. The space between the double layer serves as a conduit for the vast vascular network, nerves, and lymphatic structures to and from the large and small intestines.

The greater and lesser omentum are similar double-layer membranes hanging from the greater and lesser curvatures of the stomach, respectively. The greater omentum lies over and conforms to the abdominal viscera; its adipose tissue provides padding, protection, and insulation to the underlying structures. The lesser omentum lies in the space between the liver and stomach and provides an access route for blood vessels entering the liver and support for the stomach.

Accessory organs of the digestive tract include the liver, gallbladder, and pancreas. The liver is located in upper right quadrant of the abdomen within the peritoneal cavity, and is afforded some bony protection from the inferior rib cage. The falciform ligament bisects the liver, dividing it into the left and right lobes while anchoring it to the posterior and anterior abdominal walls. The inferior margin of the falciform ligament thickens to form the ligamentum teres, the remnant of the fetal umbilical vein. The hepatic artery provides the liver's blood supply. Venous return is via the hepatic vein, which deposits blood into the inferior vena cava. In addition to a rich arterial supply, the liver receives all venous blood exiting the digestive system through the hepatic portal vein. The hepatic portal vein, hepatic artery, nerves, lymphatic structures, and the hepatic bile ducts pass through the hilus. The liver is encapsulated in a tough, fibrous layer that is itself covered with a layer of visceral peritoneum. Liver function can be divided into three categories: metabolic regulation, hematologic regulation, and bile synthesis and secretion. With regard to metabolic regulation, the liver monitors circulating levels of carbohydrates, fats, and amino acids. Hematologic regulation is accomplished by the removal of old or damaged red blood cells from circulation and the synthesis of plasma proteins. Bile is produced in the liver, stored in the gallbladder, and excreted into the duodenum where it aids in the digestion of fats.

The gallbladder is located on the posterior surface of the liver and stores and concentrates bile produced in the liver prior to secretion into the duodenum. A system of ducts and sphincters connect the liver, gallbladder, and duodenum; these structures include the cystic duct, common hepatic duct, common bile duct, and the hepatopancreatic sphincter.

While bile production is continuous, secretion into the duodenum only occurs when acidic chyme in the duodenum increases serum cholecystokinin (CCK) levels. In response to rising CCK, muscular contractions of the gallbladder wall propel bile into the small intestine. Rising CCK levels result in the relaxation of the pancreohepatic sphincter, allowing the secretion of bile; chyme rich in lipids results in a greater release of bile. The pancreatic duct shares this terminus, and the hepatopancreatic sphincter controls the secretion of bile and pancreatic juice into the duodenal ampulla, which empties into the duodenum via the duodenal papilla.

The pancreas is a retroperitoneal structure whose exocrine functions include the secretion of digestive enzymes, buffers, and pancreatic juice into the duodenum. Pancreatic juice is a mixture of water, sodium bicarbonate, and digestive enzymes including lipase and amylase. Endocrine functions include the secretion of insulin, glucagon, and somatostatin. Arterial blood supply to the pancreas is via the pancreatic and pancreaticoduodenal arteries, and venous blood is drained via the splenic vein.

2. Discuss and differentiate the pathology of common gastrointestinal diseases and complications.

p. 728

Gastrointestinal (GI) bleeding

GI bleeding is divided into upper GI bleeds (UGIBs) and lower GI bleeds (LGIBs). Causes of UGIBs include peptic ulcer disease, gastritis, esophageal and gastric varices, and Mallory-Weiss syndrome. The most common cause of LGIBs is diverticular disease.

UGIBs are hemorrhages that occur proximal to the ligament of Treitz. Etiologies, in order of decreasing frequency of occurrence, include peptic ulcer disease, gastritis and esophagitis, esophageal and gastric varices, and Mallory-Weiss tears.

Peptic ulcer disease (PUD) is the formation of an ulcer that results secondary to the destruction and sloughing off of the mucosa of the digestive tract, allowing the hydrochloric acid and pepsin present in gastric juice to destroy underlying tissue. Peptic ulcers tend to appear in areas of the digestive tract that are exposed to these contents. Common sites of ulcer formation are the esophagus, pylorus, stomach, and duodenum.

PUD involving the stomach and duodenum accounts for the vast majority of cases, up to 50 percent, of all UGIB. Bleeding results secondary to arterial erosion within the ulcer, and hemorrhage from vessels greater than 1.5 mm in diameter is associated with an increased mortality rate. Large vessels capable of resulting in exsanguinating hemorrhage are usually located deep in the duodenal and gastric submucosa and serosa, and, as such, require significant ulcer progression for inclusion and subsequent rupture. Bleeding secondary to a peptic ulcer will resolve spontaneously in about 80 percent of cases, and rebleeding is associated with a higher mortality; gastric ulcers are more likely to rebleed than are duodenal ulcers. Risk factors for PUD include *Helicobacter pylori* infection (recognized as the leading etiology of PUD), history of NSAID use (second most common etiology) alcohol abuse, stress, and chronic renal failure.

Stress ulcers can occur in the stomach and duodenum of critically ill patients secondary to stress from trauma, burns (Curling's ulcer), sepsis, hypotension, cranial or CNS disease (Cushing's ulcer), and long-term ventilatory support.

Long-term ventilatory support and coagulopathy have been identified as the two main risk factors for stress-related erosive syndrome (SRES). Occult bleeding secondary to SRES occurs in over 25 percent of critically ill patients, and about 10 percent experience overt hemorrhage. Normal defensive mechanisms include an intact mucosal lining, the secretion of alkaline buffers, gastric epithelial migration to areas of mucosal disruption, and the production of mucosal prostaglandin. These factors are significantly impaired in critically ill patients.

Gastritis is the superficial erosion and chronic inflammation of the gastric mucosa, and can be thought of as a precursor to an ulcer. Cells of the immune system infiltrate the gastric tissue, resulting in edema irritation. Chronic episodes of gastritis commonly lead to peptic ulcers, perforation, and hemorrhage. *H. pylori* infection occurs in 30 to 50 percent of cases, resulting in localized edema, irritation, and disruption of the mucosal barrier, allowing further irritation and erosion by stomach acids. Autoimmune gastritis occurs when circulating antibodies mistake the cells of the gastric mucosa for foreign antigens, resulting in destruction of the gastric mucosa layer. The resulting chronic inflammation can result in pernicious anemia secondary to decreased vitamin B_{12} absorption. Chemical gastritis occurs secondary to the reflux of pancreatic enzymes and bile into the stomach, and to the chronic use of NSAIDs, salicylates, alcohol, and coffee. Compared to other gastritis etiologies, the inflammation associated with chemical gastritis is minimal. Radiation gastritis can occur at relatively small doses of radiation (<1,500 RAD). Mucosal damage is reversible and isolated to the epithelial cells and lamina propria, while higher doses of radiation can result in irreversible changes including mucosal erosion, blood vessel compromise, and mucosal ischemia.

Esophageal and gastric varices are most often the result of alcoholic and viral cirrhosis of the liver; about 60 percent of patients with chronic liver disease will develop varices, and 25 to 30 percent of those who develop varices will experience hemorrhaging. In chronic cirrhotic liver failure, hepatocyte destruction and resultant fibrosis result in increased resistance to blood flow. The portal vein supplies approximately 1,500 mL/min of blood to the liver, and any resistance to blood flow will result in an increase of portal venous pressure. Blood in the splenic system is diverted to the superior and inferior vena cava via collateral circulation through veins in the submucosa of the esophagus, stomach, and anterior abdominal wall. The absence of valves in the portal vasculature aids in the retrograde flow of blood. Normal venous pressure in the portal system is 5 to 10 mmHg, and pressures in excess of 10 mmHg will result in variceal formation.

Mallory-Weiss syndrome is an UGIB secondary to a longitudinal tear in the cardio-esophageal region, and it occurs secondary to a rise in intragastric pressure such as by retching, vomiting, or forceful coughing. It is also associated with long-term NSAID, salicylate, or alcohol use.

LGIBs are hemorrhages that occur distal to the ligament of Treitz. The most frequent etiology of LGIB is diverticular disease. A diverticula is an outpouching of the colonic mucosa. An exact mechanism of diverticular formation is not well understood, though it is thought that areas of increased intraluminal pressure within the colon cause defects in the colon wall. Another hypothesis holds that colonic muscle abnormalities or connective tissue disorders weaken the colon wall and contribute to diverticula formation. Whichever the cause, the acute complications of diverticular disease include inflammation and bleeding. Bleeding (diverticulosis) can occur secondary to perforation of a blood vessel by a developing diverticula. The pain of diverticular disease is sometimes characterized as a "left-sided appendicitis."

Clinical signs and symptoms associated with GI hemorrhage include:

- History of weakness, dizziness, near syncope or syncope, and angina, particularly with exertion
- Hypotension, tachycardia, diaphoresis
- Coffee-ground emesis and hematemesis
- Hematochezia and melena

A history of retching and vomiting followed by hematemesis is suggestive for a Mallory-Weiss tear. Hematochezia and melena is generally suggestive of a LGIB, but can also occur secondary to an UGIB. A bleed producing at least 200 mL of blood is generally needed for the formation of melena, but a tarry stool may be passed with as little as 60 mL of blood in the GI tract.

Laboratory data useful in the evaluation of GI bleeding includes:

- Hemoglobin and hematocrit
  - Normal—early
  - Decreased—late
- Serum glucose
  - Decreased
- WBC count
  - Decreased
- Coagulation studies
  - Normal—early
  - May be decreased late
- Electrolytes
  - Vary
- BUN
  - Increased
- Creatinine
  - Normal
- Ammonia
  - Increased

In acute blood loss, H&H values remain unchanged from baseline for any type of hemorrhage, GI or otherwise. Hematocrit may fall secondary to crystalloid infusion and re-equilibration of extracellular fluid into the intravascular space. In less acute hemorrhagic situations, the hematocrit and hemoglobin values would be expected to be lowered. The serum blood glucose and white blood cell count may be elevated secondary to stress. Coagulation studies are useful for determining liver function, especially in those patients with hepatic disease and those on anticoagulant therapy. Prolonged prothrombin (PT) and partial thromboplastin (PTT) times are not necessarily suggestive for GI hemorrhage, but do suggest that the patient is at high risk for one. In a patient with normal liver function, a prolonged bleed can result in consumption of coagulation factors, resulting in prolonged times. It is not abnormal for a healthy individual to have a normal PT and PTT with a GI bleed, especially early in its course. Electrolyte abnormalities can include hypokalemia, hypocalcemia, and in cases of severe bleeding from any source, elevated lactate. The BUN can increase secondary to decreased hepatic perfusion and the digestion of blood and subsequent absorption of hemoglobin. In patients with a suspected GI bleed, a BUN greater than 40 with a normal creatinine is suggestive for a substantial hemorrhage. The BUN can be expected to return to normal about 12 hours after the cessation of bleeding. Ammonia can be expected to rise as blood in the GI tract is digested and its metabolites absorbed.

Diagnostic and imaging studies used in the assessment of GI hemorrhage are discussed in Objective 3 and include:

- Endoscopy/colonoscopy
- Scintigraphy
- Angiography
- Radiograph
  - No use in the acute patient
  - Very limited use in the chronic patient

Pancreatitis

The exact physiological mechanism of pancreatitis remains unidentified. It is postulated that premature activation of pancreatic enzymes that are still within the acinar cells of the pancreas results in the autodigestion of pancreatic tissue. Activation of these digestive enzymes results in edema, vascular damage, interparenchymal hemorrhage, coagulation, and tissue necrosis. This damage results in a local inflammatory reaction that further increases vascular permeability and edema. Poor pancreatic blood flow can cause the ischemic pancreas to release myocardial depressant factor (MDF). MDF decreases heart contractility and cardiac output leading to multiorgan dysfunction. The clinical course of pancreatitis can range from mild to severe and includes multiple organ failure, sepsis, and death.

Etiologies of pancreatitis include obstructive, traumatic, toxin-induced, metabolic, infectious, vascular, and idiopathic causes. Signs and symptoms of pancreatitis include:

- Midepigastric or upper left quadrant abdominal pain
  - Constant, boring pain
  - Radiates to the back and flanks
  - Acute onset after the ingestion of a meal
- Nausea and vomiting
- Low-grade fever
- Tachycardia
- Abdominal guarding and rigidity
- Abdominal swelling or distension
- Abdominal pain with palpation
- Hyperactive or absent bowel sounds in the case of paralytic ilius
- Grey Turner's sign or Cullen's sign in severe cases
- Shock and multisystem organ failure in severe cases

Laboratory data commonly utilized in the identification of pancreatits include:

- Amylase
  - Elevated early
- Lipase
  - Elevated
- ABG

Serial ABGs are useful in tracking the progression of severe pancreatitis, as pulmonary involvement is a common extrapancreatic sequelae in such cases. While serum amylase and lipase are the two most commonly utilized serum markers for pancreatitis, both lack the sensitivity and specificity to be used as the sole indicators of disease and should be used in conjunction with the entire clinical picture. Amalyase is elevated early and returns to normal within 3 to 4 days, even in instances of continued inflammation. Lipase remains elevated for several days after serum amylase returns to normal.

Other lab studies that may be helpful in determining the extent of cases other than mild pancreatitis include:

- Serum calcium
- Hematocrit
- Base deficit
- BUN
- White blood cell count
- Glucose
- Lactate dehydrogenase
- Asparate aminotransferase

Imaging studies useful in the assessment of pancreatitis include CT scanning, MRI, and ultrasound. CT is the imaging study of choice, as it provides unsurpassed anatomical detail, allowing not only the diagnosis of pancreatitis, but also the grading of the severity of the disease. However, CT is not useful in ruling out pancreatitis, as it is insensitive to mild and early disease. MRI is as effective as CT in identifying and grading pancreatitis. Ultrasound is useful in the evaluation of pancreatitis secondary to biliary obstruction or dilation, but it has limited value in the evaluation of nonbiliary etiologies and practically no value in determining the extent of pancreatic injury. Abdominal radiographs have no use in the evaluation of the pancreas, but can be used to exclude conditions that may mimic pancreatitis, such as bowel infarction.

Liver failure

Liver failure often occurs secondary to hepatitis, which along with cirrhosis is responsible for the vast majority of liver failure cases in the United States. Hepatitis is an inflammation of the liver parenchyma including the Kupffer's cells, bile ducts, and blood vessels. Inflammation leads to disruption of the hepatic structures, leading to an interrupted blood supply, ischemia, and eventual necrosis. Dead liver cells are removed via the immune system, and some regeneration takes place, which allows for the recovery of some degree of liver function. Chronic active hepatitis, along with alcoholic liver disease and diseases causing biliary obstruction, can lead to cirrhosis of the liver. Fulminant liver failure is acute liver failure associated with hepatic encephalopathy. Signs and symptoms of liver disease can be vague, but include:

- Nausea, vomiting, abdominal discomfort, anorexia
- Dark urine, clay-colored stools
- Enlarged liver, pain with palpation
- Jaundice

Signs and symptoms of cirrhosis include:

- Enlarged or firm liver upon palpation
- Ascites
- Esophageal and gastric bleeding secondary to varices

Severe liver failure may present with:

- Altered mental status
- Decreased LOC
- Coma

Laboratory data useful in identifying liver dysfunction:

- Alanine transferase (ALT or AGOT)
  - Elevated
  - May be normal in liver failure
- Aspartate aminotransferase (AST or SGPT)
  - Elevated
  - May be normal in liver failure
- Alkaline phosphatase
  - Elevated

- PT
  - Prolonged
- Albumin
  - Decreased
- Bilirubin
  - Elevated
- Serum ammonia
  - Elevated

3. **Discuss diagnostic studies available to aid in the diagnosis of gastrointestinal disease and complications.** p. 734

Endoscopy/colonoscopy

Both are useful diagnostic, as well as therapeutic, modalities. Endoscopy is utilized to identify and treat UGIBs, and is a more proven intervention than colonoscopy. Colonoscopy is utilized to treat LGIBs.

Scintigraphy

Also known as technetium-labeled red blood cell scan, is an effective diagnostic test in cases of brisk GI bleeding of 0.5 to 2.0 mL/min or greater. Extravasation of blood is identified on radiograph by the presence of radiolabeled blood found in the GI tract.

Angiography

Particularly useful in the identification of LGIBs, angiography requires a relatively brisk bleeding rate of 0.5 to 2.0 mL/min or greater to be effective. Identification of radio-opaque dye in the GI tract via fluoroscopy is diagnostic for hemorrhage.

Radiograph

Routine abdominal radiographs are of little diagnostic value in the diagnosis of GI bleeding, but have a role in the diagnosis of pancreatitis. Barium studies for GI hemorrhage have the disadvantage of contaminating and obscuring the GI tract wall, making the subsequent use of colonoscopy or endoscopy less effective.

CT

CT is the imaging study of choice for pancreatitis and liver disease, as it provides unsurpassed anatomical detail. It allows for, not only, the diagnosis of pancreatitis, but also, the grading of the severity of the disease. It is not useful in ruling out pancreatitis, as it is insensitive to mild and early disease process.

MRI

MRI is as effective as CT in identifying and grading pancreatitis and liver disease.

Ultrasound

Ultrasound is useful in the evaluation of pancreatitis secondary to biliary obstruction or dilation, with a 67 percent sensitivity and 100 percent specificity. It has limited value in the evaluation of nonbiliary etiologies and practically no value in determining the extent of pancreatic injury. It is also useful in the evaluation of liver disease and for evaluation of the hepatic blood supply.

4. **Discuss the management of specific gastrointestinal diseases and complications.** p. 735

GI hemorrhage

The management of GI hemorrhage begins with addressing the ABCs. The administration of volume-expanding agents may be necessary to correct hypotension; crystalloid solutions are often utilized. For severe hemorrhages, the need for blood products administration should be determined based on clinical findings suggestive of severe volume depletion. Bleeding control can be achieved in the traditional method, direct pressure, with a Sengstaken-Blakemore tube. Otherwise, ligation or sclerotherapy, the administration of vasopressin, somatostatin, or octreotide, or the placement of a transjugular intrahepatic portosystemic shunt (TIPS) is required to control bleeding.

All patients with significant GI bleeding should have a NG tube placed, and contrary to popular belief, it will not result in bleeding in patients with varices. The tube should be placed and the stomach evacuated of any contents, and a gentle gastric lavage performed if blood is aspirated from the stomach. Acid-reducing therapy with an IV proton pump inhibitor (PPI) is the standard of care. In addition, histamine receptor antagonists (H_2RAs), sucralfate, and antacids are commonly used.

Pancreatitis

Management of the patient with pancreatitis includes keeping the patient NPO to "rest the pancreas"; no chyme in the duodenum means no release of pancreatic juice. Of course, no food via the enteral route requires TPN. NG tube insertion can be used to clear the stomach of acidic contents to further decrease the release of pancreatic enzymes as well as to decompress the stomach. IV hydration with crystalloid solution should be titrated to a urine output of 100 mL/hr, as with a Foley catheter. Analgesics should be used to control pain and provide physical comfort.

Liver failure

Management of liver failure is supportive, as the definitive treatment is liver transplant. Obviously, the airway, breathing, and circulation status will demand the attention of the critical care transport team. A patient with hepatic encephalopathy can lose the ability to control his airway and may develop breathing irregularities, and as such, will require an advanced airway and ventilatory support. Hypoalbuminemia can result in changes in oncotic pressure and subsequent fluid shift out of the vascular space, requiring volume support. Alteration in coagulation may require the administration of coagulation factors.

5. **Understand how to manage various types of gastric management tubes that may be encountered during transport.** p. 739

Nasogastric (NG) tube

A NG tube is a large bore (14 to 16 French) tube that may be inserted for a number of reasons including:

- Decompression of gastric air during artificial ventilation
- Removal of gastric contents in cases of obstruction
- Ileus
- Drug overdose
- Removal of gastric acids in cases of ulcerative disease
- Control of bleeding in cases of variceal bleeding
- Diagnostic purposes
  - evaluation of gastric pH
  - determine the presence of blood in the stomach

Types of NG tubes include the Salem sump tube and Levine tube. Prior to transport, a team member should confirm tube placement, confirm tube patency, evaluate tube drainage, and secure the tube adequately.

Nasointestinal tubes

Nasointestinal tubes are commonly referred to as feeding tubes, and the most common is the Dobhoff tube. It is a small bore (8 to 10 French) tube inserted into the small intestine to support nutrition, and can be kept in place for two to three weeks. Nasointestinal tubes are placed in the same manner as NG tubes, though advanced further along the digestive tract past the pyloric sphincter and into the duodenum or ileum. Prior to transport, a team member should confirm placement, confirm patency, secure adequately, and slow or stop flow rate during transport.

Nasointestinal tubes are sometimes used to clear obstructions of the small bowel in patients who are considered high-risk surgical candidates; common tubes are the Miller-Abbott, Anderson, and Cantor tubes. They are long (up to 10 feet), wide diameter tubes with a weighted distal end that is pulled along the intestinal tract by peristalsis. Low continuous suction is applied to aid in the removal of impacted fecal material, and irrigation can be utilized to facilitate breakup and removal of impacted material. Transport considerations are the same as for NG and nasointestinal tubes.

Transabdominal feeding tubes

Three types of transabdominal feeding tube procedures often utilized are gastrostomy, jejunostomy, and gastrojejunostomy. Feeding tube placement can be via open surgical technique by a surgeon, under endoscopy by a gastroenterologist, or percutaneously by an interventional radiologist. Prior to transport, a team member should confirm placement, confirm patency, secure adequately, slow or stop flow rate during transport, and assess for complications of the procedure. Potential complications include perforated bowel, stomach or liver, tube-site infections, leakage at the tube site, catheter occlusion, and catheter dislodgement.

T-tube

A T-tube derives its name from its shape, and is used to collect bile from the gallbladder after liver transplant, cholecystectomy, or other surgery of the common bile duct. T-tubes are frequently left in for up to 6 weeks, and secured with a suture.

Esophageal tube

Esophageal tubes are used to control bleeding from esophageal and gastric varices; specific types include the Sengstaken-Blakemore and Minnesota tubes. The Sengstaken-Blakemore tube is inserted through a nare, down the esophagus, and into the stomach, where a gastric balloon is inflated to apply pressure at the cardioesophageal junction; inflation of the esophageal balloon compresses esophageal varices and controls bleeding. Traction is applied at the proximal end of the tube to hold the tube in place and can be maintained with a pulley system or by taping the tube to a helmet placed on the patient's head. Gastric contents, including blood, can be aspirated via the gastric port by gastric lavage or low pressure intermittent suction. Swallowing is inhibited with the gastric balloon inflated, and secretions will accumulate above the balloon; suction can be provided via insertion of a Salem sump or Levine tube and the application of low pressure intermittent suction.

The Minnesota tube is similar to the Sengstaken-Blakemore, but has an esophageal aspiration lumen that allows for the suctioning of collected esophageal secretions and does not require the additional placement of an NG tube. Prior to transport, a team member should evaluate airway patency and formulate a maintenance plan, ensure continued traction to the proximal end of the tube, and consider that changes in atmospheric pressure may alter the pressure within the balloon or cuff.

Ostomy collection bags

An ostomy is the attaching of the proximal bowel to the surface of the abdomen after an intestinal resection. Normal defecation is not preserved, and must take place through this opening. The opening is termed an ileostomy when the ileum is involved and a colostomy when the colon is involved. As defecation through an ostomy is uncontrollable, the use of a collection bag is required. Prior to transport, a team member should empty the bag, ensure adequate seal to the skin, and ensure that the collection bag can be vented, if necessary, during transport.

Rectal tubes

Rectal tubes are employed as temporary measures to control and collect liquid stool. They are usually 25 to 35 cm long, 18–30 French in diameter, and may or may not have a distal balloon to keep them in place. If a distal balloon is used, care must be taken to prevent pressure necrosis of the rectal mucosa. Prior to transport, a team member should assure patency and adequate securing, determine the need for periodic deflation of the cuff to prevent pressure necrosis, and assess for signs of rectal perforation and hemorrhaging.

Surgical wound drainage systems

Commonly used surgical wound drainage systems include the Penrose drain, Jackson-Pratt drainage system, the Hemovac drainage system, and sump tubes. A Penrose drain is a flat, 0.5 to 1.0 inch diameter, single-lumen tube inserted into a surgical site to promote drainage of large amounts of fluid. It is a passive drainage method, relying on gravity to move fluid into a collection container, and is usually held in place with layers of absorbent dressings. A Jackson-Pratt drainage system is a hand-grenade-sized bulb that is compressed and then attached to the proximal end of the drainage tube, creating a closed, low-pressure system; it is an active drainage system. The Hemovac drainage system has a rigid plastic housing with internal springs. Compressing the device, attaching the proximal end of the drainage tube, and plugging a vent hole creates a closed, low-pressure system. Both the Jackson-Pratt and Hemovac devices have graduations on the collection

©2007 Pearson Education, Inc.
Critical Care Paramedic

chamber, making accurate measurement of drainage volume possible, and are often held in place with absorbent dressings only. Sump tubes are Penrose tubes with a double-lumen sump tube inserted inside, resulting in a triple-lumen drainage tube. It is often inserted into the abdominal compartment, and is useful in draining large abscesses and large amounts of fluid and debris. One port is connected to low continuous suction, another to air to prevent the buildup of large suction pressures and subsequent tissue damage, and the third port connected to slow, continuous irrigation if needed. For all of these systems, prior to transport, a team member should ensure patency, empty collection chambers prior to transport, and ensure that tubes will not be dislodged during transport. If a collection chamber must be emptied during transport, first, clamp drainage tube, remove, empty, and then reattach the drainage chamber, then remove the clamp to continue suction. Record the amount of discarded drainage.

Peritoneal dialysis catheters
The Tenckhoff catheter is the most commonly used peritoneal dialysis catheter. It is a flexible, siliconized rubber catheter surgically placed into the abdominal cavity to facilitate the administration and removal of dialysate solutions. A cuff is placed into the subcutaneous layer of the skin, and scarring around the cuff firmly anchors it in place. Prior to transport, a team member should assess a newly placed catheter for external and intraabdominal bleeding, assure proper securing, and assure that the catheter is capped when not in use.

Tube checklist
Regardless of the type of tube encountered by the critical care transport crew, the following checklist can be utilized to ensure that all pertinent considerations are addressed prior to transport:

- What is the tube's purpose?
- Has proper placement been confirmed?
- Is it patent?
- Is it properly secured?
- What amount and type of drainage can be expected?
- How, and with what frequency, should the tube and equipment be assessed?
- What are the potential complications?
- What are the instructions for the care and maintenance of the tube during transport?
- What information needs to be documented?

Case Study

Your patient is a 22-year-old male who was eating at a local restaurant when he began to choke. Although his airway was never completely obstructed, he had a severe retching episode and is now complaining of severe substernal chest pain and is unable to swallow due to the pain. The patient was brought to the emergency department via EMS who, on orders of medical control, administered glucagon IV to relax the esophageal musculature in case the patient's symptoms were caused by an impacted food bolus. The glucagon had no apparent effect, other than making the patient nauseous. The attending MD tells your crew that the patient presented complaining of severe pain, dysphagia, and mild dyspnea. The patient refuses to swallow due to the pain, and intermittently spits saliva. He is nauseous, but has had no further retching episodes while in the department. The chest X-ray clearly showed peritoneal free air under both diaphragmatic leaflets, and the patient was diagnosed with a Boerhaave's syndrome.

The MD explains that although most esophageal ruptures are iatrogenic in nature, caused by endoscopy, 10 to 15 percent are caused by events that cause transient increases in intraesophageal pressure, such as retching or vomiting. Distal perforations have a mortality rate of between 20 and 50 percent. The mortality increases the longer surgical repair is delayed because esophageal contents including undigested food, digestive enzymes, stomach acid, and bacteria are dumped into the mediastinum and peritoneal cavity. You are told this can induce immediate shock or overwhelming sepsis. Therefore, it is important that the patient is expeditiously transported to a center with a cardiothoracic surgery service that can manage this type of injury.

A nasogastric tube was placed to drain the stomach and limit further contamination of the peritoneum and mediastinum by gastric contents, and the patient was instructed not to swallow his saliva. IV analgesia and broad spectrum antibiotics were administered prior to your arrival. The physician introduces you to your patient and you explain how the transfer works and begin your assessment. His breath sounds are clear, but as you listen to his heart, you look up at the physician in surprise since you are hearing a short burst of crackles with each heart beat. He smiles and says, "That's a Hamman's crunch. It is caused by mediastinal air being moved by the beating heart." Moving on in your assessment, you find that the patient's abdomen is rigid and very tender to light palpation. His vital signs are: respirations 22 and regular, pulse 112, sinus tachycardia on the monitor, and blood pressure 132/74. The patient is packaged for transport and moved into the ambulance.

During the transport you apply intermittent suction to the patient's NG tube by switching the on board unit on for a few seconds every couple of minutes and maintain an IV infusion of normal saline at 250 mL/hr. The patient remains pain free with stable vital signs enroute and arrives at St. Mary's Medical Center without change.

DISCUSSION QUESTIONS

1. What diagnostic studies are available to assist in the diagnosis of gastrointestinal disease?
2. During the management of patients with gastrointestinal disease, what types of tubes and catheters may be encountered and how are they managed?

Content Review

MULTIPLE CHOICE

_____ 1. The four layers of the digestive tract wall are the:
   A. serosa, mucosa, submucosa, and epithelium.
   B. mucosa, submucosa, muscularis externa, and serosa.
   C. duodenum, jejunum, ileum, and large intestine.
   D. mucosa, submucosa, basement membrane, and epithelium.

_____ 2. The process of mechanical digestion, chemical digestion, and lubrication is termed:
   A. mastication.   C. digestion.
   B. chewing.   D. ingestion.

_____ 3. Veins draining the inferior esophagus as well as the cardia of the stomach communicate directly with the:
   A. inferior vena cava.   C. great hepatic vein.
   B. superior vena cava.   D. hepatic portal vein.

_____ 4. The esophagus enters the stomach at the:
   A. body.   C. cardia.
   B. pylorus.   D. fundus.

_____ 5. The duodenum receives digestive secretions from the _____ to aid in the digestion of chyme from the stomach.
   A. pancreas.   C. pancreas and gallbladder.
   B. gallbladder.   D. liver.

_____ 6. Food enters the stomach from the esophagus through the _____ and exits the stomach into the duodenum through the_____.
   A. cardiac sphincter, pyloric sphincter   C. esophagus, small intestine
   B. pyloric sphincter, cardiac sphincter   D. esophagus, cardiac sphincter

_____ 7. The bulk of digestion and absorption in the small intestine takes place in the:
     A. duodenum.   **C.** ileum.
     B. jejunum.   **D.** none of the above.

_____ 8. The large intestine is responsible for the absorption of:
     A. water.   **C.** vitamins.
     B. electrolytes.   **D.** all of the above.

_____ 9. The vermiform appendix is usually attached to the:
     A. retroperitoneal aspect of the ascending colon.
     B. anteromedial aspect of the cecum.
     C. posteromedial aspect of the cecum.
     D. posteriolateral aspect of the colon.

_____ 10. Which one of the following organs is not retroperitoneal?
     A. transverse colon   **C.** pancreas
     B. ureters   **D.** distal duodenum

_____ 11. The abdominal cavity can be divided into three spaces, the:
     A. pelvic space, abdominal space, and retroperitoneal space.
     B. pelvic space, peritoneal space, and retroperitoneal space.
     C. peritoneal space, retroperitoneal space, and subperitoneal space.
     D. none of the above.

_____ 12. Organs and structures located within the peritoneal space include the:
     A. proximal duodenum.   **C.** liver and spleen.
     B. ascending colon.   **D.** all of the above.

_____ 13. Functions of the liver include:
     A. detoxification, red blood cell production, and glycogen storage.
     B. glucose storage, bile synthesis and secretion, and hormone synthesis and secretion.
     C. metabolic regulation, hematologic regulation, and bile synthesis and secretion.
     D. none of the above.

_____ 14. The gallbladder releases bile into the duodenum when:
     A. chyme enters the duodenum.   **C.** both A and B.
     B. serum CCK levels increase.   **D.** none of the above.

_____ 15. Pancreatic juice contains:
     A. insulin, glucagon, and pancreatic polypeptide.
     B. water, digestive enzymes, and insulin.
     C. water, sodium bicarbonate, digestive enzymes, and insulin.
     D. water, sodium bicarbonate, carbohydrases, lipases, proteinases, peptidases, and nucleases.

_____ 16. The functional unit of the exocrine pancreas are the:
     A. pancreatic acini.   **C.** F-cells.
     B. islets of Langerhans.   **D.** alpha cells.

_____ 17. An upper GI hemorrhage is a bleed that occurs in the:
     A. esophagus, stomach, or duodenum.
     B. esophagus, stomach, duodenum, or jejunum.
     C. esophagus, stomach, duodenum, jejunum, or ileum.
     D. esophagus, stomach, duodenum, jejunum, ileum, or cecum.

_____ 18. The most common cause of lower GI bleeding is:
     A. angiodysplasia.   **C.** diverticular disease.
     B. neoplasia.   **D.** colitis.

_____ 19. _____ is recognized as the leading cause of peptic ulcer disease.
   A. The use of NSAIDs and salicylate drugs
   B. *H. pylori* infection
   C. Alcoholism
   D. Stress, both physical and emotional,

_____ 20. In the majority of cases, bleeding secondary to a peptic ulcer will resolve spontaneously.
   A. True
   B. False

_____ 21. Increased mortality secondary to upper GI bleeds is associated with:
   A. age over 60 years and coexistent organ disease.
   B. blood transfusions in excess of 5 units, persistent hypotension, and the need for surgery.
   C. stress including surgery, sepsis, ventilatory support, and trauma.
   D. all of the above.

_____ 22. The formation of stress ulcers in the stomach and duodenum of critically ill patients secondary to stress from trauma or illness is termed:
   A. stress-related ulcer formation (SRUF).
   B. syndrome of stress-related ulcers (SSRU).
   C. stress-related erosive syndrome (SRES).
   D. serious recurring erosive syndrome (SRES).

_____ 23. Which of the following is not a normal defensive mechanism in the GI tract?
   A. intact mucosal lining
   B. inhibition of mucosal prostaglandin production
   C. secretion of alkaline buffers
   D. gastric epithelial migration to areas of mucosal disruption

_____ 24. A _____ is a superficial erosion and chronic inflammation of the gastric mucosa.
   A. peptic ulcer   C. gastritis
   B. Mallory-Weiss injury   D. varix

_____ 25. Subcategories of gastritis include:
   A. chemical gastritis.   C. radiation gastritis.
   B. autoimmune gastritis.   D. all of the above.

_____ 26. In the United States, esophageal and gastric varices are most often the result of:
   A. alcoholic and viral cirrhosis of the liver.
   B. hepatitis.
   C. human immunodeficiency virus.
   D. hepatic cancer.

_____ 27. Esophageal and gastric varices form secondary to:
   A. decreased hepatic portal pressure and the diversion of blood into the splenic system.
   B. increased hepatic portal pressure and the diversion of blood into the splenic system.
   C. increased hepatic portal pressure and the diversion of blood into the vena cava through veins in the submucosa of the esophagus and stomach.
   D. increased resistance to blood flow in the hepatic vein, leading to the retrograde flow of blood into the veins in the submucosa of the esophagus and stomach.

_____ 28. _____ is a UGIB secondary to a longitudinal tear in the cardioesophageal region.
   A. Mallory-Weiss tear   C. Esophageal varix
   B. Peptic ulcer disease   D. Mallory-Weiss syndrome

_____ 29. _____ are outpouchings of the colonic mucosa, and _____ can occur secondary to perforation of a blood vessel by such an outpouching.
   A. Diverticulosis, diverticula   C. Varices, hemorrhage
   B. Diverticula, diverticulosis   D. None of the above

_____ 30. Which of the following is not a sign or symptom normally associated with gastrointestinal hemorrhage?
A. hypertension
B. history of weakness, dizziness, near syncope
C. nausea, "coffee-grounds" emesis, and hematemesis
D. hematochezia

_____ 31. A patient with GI hemorrhage may present with signs and symptoms of compensated shock.
A. True
B. False

_____ 32. Which of the following statements regarding laboratory data in the assessment of GI hemorrhage is true?
A. Serum glucose and the white blood cell (WBC) count will be lowered.
B. Electrolyte studies will show acute changes in serum calcium, potassium, and sodium.
C. Hemoglobin and hematocrit values will be lowered in non-acute cases.
D. Prolonged prothrombin (PT) and partial thromboplastin (PTT) times are suggestive for GI hemorrhage.

_____ 33. In cases of GI hemorrhage, the BUN can _____ secondary to _____
A. increase, the digestion of blood and subsequent absorption of hemoglobin.
B. increase, increased hepatic perfusion.
C. decrease, increased hepatic perfusion.
D. decrease, the decreased hepatic perfusion and the digestion of blood and subsequent absorption of hemoglobin.

_____ 34. In patients with a suspected GI bleed, a BUN _____ with a _____ creatinine is suggestive of a substantial hemorrhage
A. < 40, elevated   C. > 60, lowered
B. > 40, normal   D. < 20, normal

_____ 35. _____ are useful diagnostic as well as therapeutic modalities in cases of GI hemorrhage.
A. MRI and CT scan   C. Endoscopy and colonoscopy
B. Scintigraphy and endoscopy   D. None of the above

_____ 36. In _____, radio-opaque dye is injected into the gut vasculature, which is then inspected under a fluoroscope.
A. endoscopy   C. angiography
B. colonoscopy   D. scintigraphy

_____ 37. Hematocrit levels are a reliable indicator for the need for volume replacement in patients with GI hemorrhage.
A. True
B. False

_____ 38. A nasogastric (NG) tube should not be used in patients with esophageal or gastric varices, as it may instigate or worsen hemorrhage.
A. True
B. False

_____ 39. All of the following are treatments to control the bleeding of esophageal and gastric varices except:
A. band ligation or sclerotherapy.
B. balloon tamponade with a Sengstaken-Blakemore tube.
C. TIPS procedure.
D. administration of oxytocin.

_____ 40. Acid-reducing therapies for patients with, or at risk for, peptic ulcer formation may include:
  A. histamine receptor agonists (H₂RAs).
  B. proton pump agonists.
  C. sucralfate and antacids.
  D. all of the above.

_____ 41. _____ is/are considered standard of care for the treatment or prevention of peptic ulcers.
  A. Proton pump inhibitors (PPIs)
  B. Proton pump antagonists
  C. Sucralfate
  D. Antacids

_____ 42. The etiologies of acute pancreatitis can be categorized as:
  A. traumatic, obstructive, autoimmune, vascular, toxin-induced, metabolic, and idiopathic.
  B. infectious, autoimmune, obstructive, traumatic, toxin-induced, catabolic, and idiopathic.
  C. obstructive, infectious, vascular, traumatic, toxin-induced, metabolic, and idiopathic.
  D. obstructive, infectious, autoimmune, traumatic, metabolite-induced, catabolic, and idiopathic.

_____ 43. Changes in pulmonary function that may occur secondary to pancreatitis include:
  A. arterial hypozemia.
  B. atelectasis and pleural effusions.
  C. acute respiratory failure (ARF) and acute respiratory distress syndrome (ARDS).
  D. all of the above.

_____ 44. The release of _____ during pancreatitis can lead to decreased myocardial contractility and cardiac output.
  A. pancreatic enzymes
  B. myocardial depressant factor
  C. trypsin
  D. lipase and phospholipase A

_____ 45. The most common complaint associated with acute pancreatitis is:
  A. midepigastric or upper left quadrant abdominal pain.
  B. lower left quadrant abdominal pain.
  C. nausea and vomiting.
  D. low-grade fever and tachycardia.

_____ 46. Severe cases of pancreatitis may present with:
  A. Grey Turner's sign.
  B. Cullen's sign.
  C. multisystem organ failure.
  D. all of the above.

_____ 47. The "gold standard" diagnostic study in the diagnosis of pancreatitis is:
  A. CT scan.
  B. ultrasound.
  C. pathologic examination of the pancreas.
  D. MRI.

_____ 48. Serum amylase and lipase are the two most commonly utilized serum markers for pancreatitis, but lack the sensitivity and specificity to be used as the sole indicators of disease.
  A. True
  B. False

_____ 49. Which of the following is the imaging study that best allows for the diagnosis and grading of pancreatitis?
  A. MRI
  B. ultrasound
  C. radiograph
  D. CT

_____ 50. Which of the following is not considered part of the normal treatment of pancreatitis?
  A. keeping the patient NPO
  B. insertion of an NG tube and gastric lavage
  C. IV volume replacement therapy
  D. IV imipenem or a quinolone in combination with metronidazole

_____ 51. _____ is an inflammation of the liver parenchyma including the Kupffer cells, bile ducts, and blood vessels.
A. Cirrhosis
B. Liver failure
C. Hepatitis
D. Fulminant hepatic failure

_____ 52. _____ causes the generation of fibrotic tissue which causes severe changes in the structure and function of hepatic cells.
A. Cirrhosis
B. Liver failure
C. Hepatitis
D. Fulminant hepatic failure

_____ 53. _____ is a medical emergency that is described as acute liver failure associated with hepatic encephalopathy.
A. Cirrhosis
B. Liver failure
C. Hepatitis
D. Fulminant hepatic failure

_____ 54. Clinical exam findings suggestive of liver failure include all of the following except:
A. nausea, vomiting, abdominal discomfort, and anorexia.
B. production of dark urine and clay-colored stools.
C. jaundice and ascites.
D. JVD and hypertension.

_____ 55. Hepatic encephalopathy may result in:
A. altered mental status.
B. decreased level of consciousness.
C. coma.
D. all of the above.

_____ 56. Liver failure can result in significant fluid shifts out of the _____ secondary to _____.
A. vascular space, hypoalbuminemia
B. vascular space, increased diuresis
C. intracellular space, hyperalbuminemia
D. interstitial space, hyperalbuminemia

_____ 57. Which of the following serum markers of heptic function would be expected to be lowered in cases of liver dysfunction?
A. bilirubin
B. ammonia
C. alkaline phosphatase
D. potassium

_____ 58. A _____ prothrombin time (PT) and a _____ albumin suggest decreased or diminishing hepatic function.
A. normal, decreased
B. prolonged, decreased
C. shortened, increased
D. prolonged, increased

_____ 59. The treatment of liver failure is least likely to include:
A. airway support and ventilation.
B. administration of coagulation factors.
C. administration of diuretics.
D. intravascular volume support.

25

Renal and Acid-Base Emergencies

Review of Chapter Objectives

Upon completion of this chapter, the student should be able to:

1. Describe the anatomical structures of the renal system. p. 751

The kidneys are located in retroperitoneal space at the level of the costovertebral angle, between vertebrae T12 and L3. The left kidney lies slightly superior to the right kidney. The renal arteries, which originate from the abdominal aorta at about the same level as the superior mesenteric artery, supply blood to the kidneys, which receive about 25 percent of cardiac output, equivalent to about 1,200 mL of blood/min. The renal veins return blood to the inferior vena cava. The renal artery and vein enter the kidney at the hilum, as do the renal nerves and ureter.

A layer of collagen fibers termed the renal capsule covers the outer surface of each kidney, providing protection. The renal capsule also lines the renal sinus, an internal cavity within the kidney, where it serves as an anchoring point for the ureter and renal blood vessels and nerves. The interior of the kidney can be divided into the superficial renal cortex and the deeper renal medulla. The functional unit of the kidney, the nephron, is mostly located in the renal cortex, though part does extend into the medulla. The renal medulla is divided into distinct triangular structures called the renal pyramids. The renal pelvis is a large, funnel-shaped chamber that collects urine produced in the nephron and funnels it into the ureter, which drains the kidney.

The nephron, working with the renal cortex and medulla, is responsible for the filtration, reabsorption, and secretion of fluids, electrolytes, and waste products through the formation of urine. Each nephron consists of a renal corpuscle and renal tubule, which together contain the Bowman's capsule, glomerulus (glomerular capillaries and podocytes), proximal tubule, loop of Henle, distal tubule, and collecting duct.

Each renal corpuscle contains a Bowman's capsule and a glomerulus. The Bowman's capsule houses the glomerulus, which consists of a capillary network that allows for the filtration of blood. Pores in the glomerular capillaries allow fluid and small molecules to pass into the capsule. In addition, podocytes, specialized cells with comblike projections (pedicels), wrap around the glomerular capillaries, aiding in the filtration of blood. Filtrate then enters the renal tubule. Three critical functions occur in the renal tubule: the reabsorption of water, the reabsorption of desirable nutrients in the filtrate, and the secretion of unwanted waste products into the tubule for elimination in the urine.

The renal tubule has three parts, the proximal convoluted tubule, the loop of Henle, and the distal convoluted tubule. The loop of Henle partially extends into the medulla. The filtrate, now considered tubular fluid, changes in composition as it travels the length of the tubule; water, glucose, ions, small proteins, and amino acids are reabsorbed, and waste products, ions, and water are excreted as needed. The processes of filtration, reabsorption, and secretion are discussed in greater detail in Objective 2. After traveling the length of the tubule, the tubular fluid, now considered urine, enters the collecting duct. Urine then travels through the papillary duct, minor calyx, major calyx, and renal pelvis before entering the ureter.

2. Understand the basic physiology of the renal system. p. 752

To successfully fulfill their contribution to homeostasis, the kidneys must perform three functions: filtration, reabsorption, and secretion.

About 20 percent of CO passes through, and is filtered by, the glomerulus (the "missing" 5 percent perfuses the renal parenchyma). Filtrate is composed of water, ions, glucose, amino acids, and small proteins (albumin).

Filtration across the glomerulus is driven by hydrostatic pressure gradient between the glomerulus and Bowman's capsule, across the glomerulur capillaries. Higher pressure within the glomerulus is required for filtration. Fenestrations in the capillaries and small, fingerlike projections from structures called podocytes, allow the passage of small molecules only. As such, the molecular size of any given substance determines if it will be filtered or not. Plasma concentration of solute can affect the *amount* of solute filtration, the higher the plasma concentration, the greater the amount of filtration of that substance.

Glomerular filtration rate (GFR) is the amount of filtrate the kidney produces each minute, and is equal to about 125 mL/min; at this rate, the circulating blood volume is filtered around 20 to 25 times per day.

After filtrate leaves Bowman's capsule, reabsorption takes place along the length of the nephron. Substances reabsorbed include water, glucose proteins (albumin), amino acids, and ions such as sodium, calcium, potassium, hydrogen, and bicarbonate.

Reabsorption methods in the kidney include osmosis, facilitated transport, cotransport, and passive reabsorption. Osmosis occurs secondary to the osmotic gradient created by the increased solute concentrations within the renal cortex and medulla compared to the filtrate in the tubule. Water then moves from an area of low solute concentration (tubule) to an area of high solute concentration (renal parenchyma). Facilitated transport occurs via specialized transport (carrier) proteins, termed transporters, located on the tubule walls. This transport occurs along a concentration gradient (high to low), and no energy is expended. In cotransport, two substances share a carrier protein. This action always follows the concentration gradient of at least one of the transported substances. Two forms of passive reabsorption include "solvent drag" and diffusion. In solvent drag, solute is caught up in the osmotic flow of water, while in passive diffusion, substances move from an area of high concentration to low concentration. An overwhelming number of transporters can occur when increased glomerular filtration of solute overrides the reabsorption mechanisms; solute that is unabsorbed spills over into urine; an example would be glucosuria accompanying hyperglycemia.

Filtrate that is not reabsorbed by the kidney travels the length of the tubule (proximal convoluted tubule, loop of Henle, distal convoluted tubule) to the collecting duct, enters the collecting system, and is secreted as urine. Normal urine is about 95 percent water and 5 percent solute, but the kidney can concentrate urine based on physiological requirements. Normal urine output is greater than 500 mL/day, and less than 500 mL/day is considered oliguria.

3. Identify three major causes of acute renal failure. p. 755

Renal failure can be classified according to the origin of the insult with regard to anatomy. The classifications are prerenal renal failure, intrarenal renal failure, and postrenal renal failure.

Prerenal renal failure occurs secondary to decreased renal perfusion which results in decreased GFR and decreased urine output. In other words, the cause of prerenal renal failure is somewhere outside the kidney. Specific causes of prerenal renal failure include hypovolemia (hemorrhage, dehydration) and cardiac failure (decreased CO).

The accumulation of metabolic waste products in blood results in increased BUN and creatinine levels. Treatment of prerenal renal failure involves correcting the underlying cause of the hypoperfusion, for example:

- Hypovolemia
  - Control active hemorrhaging
  - IV crystalloids, blood, and blood products

- Cardiac failure
  - Diuretics
- Nitrates
- Inotropic agents
- Vasopressors

Intrarenal renal failure results from damage to the renal parenchyma. Specifically, insult to the glomerulus, tubule, interstitial tissue, and renal microvasculature can result in failure. In addition to trauma, some of the more common specific etiologies include glomerulonephritis, ischemic acute tubular necrosis, rhabdomyolysis, massive hemolysis, and nephrotoxins such as radio contrast die and aminoglycosides. Damage to the renal interstitium can occur secondary to acute interstitial nephritis (drug reactions), infectious agents, or autoimmune disease, and damage to the renal vasculature can occur secondary to hypertension.

As in prerenal renal failure, management is directed at treating the underlying cause.

Postrenal renal failure occurs secondary to an obstruction of urine flow; urine backs up into the kidney, and filtration at the glomerulus can't occur. Causes of obstruction include prostatic hypertrophy, renal calculi, neoplasms, and urinary tract infections.

Treatment of postrenal renal failure includes:

- Correction of obstruction
- Urine clearance
  - Foley catheter
  - Suprapubic urinary catheter

4. Describe emergent treatment of renal failure. p. 756

While all of the different etiologies of acute renal failure have specific management priorities (which is beyond the scope of this text), a common management modality among them all, and with chronic renal failure as well, is dialysis. Dialysis is a method of removing toxins from blood when the kidneys are not able to do so. It is utilized in patients with kidney failure or those who have suffered acute poisoning from toxins or drugs. Blood is circulated through a dialyzer, which contains filters made up of semipermeable membranes. The blood is pushed through the dialyzer in one direction, and dialysate is pushed through in the opposite direction, creating a countercurrent flow. The semipermeable membrane (filter) separates the blood and dialysate, and solutes move across the membrane along their chemical gradients. The dialysate can be tailored to a patient's specific blood chemistry, assuring that a patient's specific dialysis needs are met. Regular angiocatheters are not sufficient to provide the blood flow needed for dialysis, so dialysis catheters are required. Permanent vascular access via arteriovenous fistula or arteriovenous graft is used in patients with CRF, and temporary or tunneled catheters can be utilized in patients with ARF who do not have permanent access. In patients with CRF, a typical dialysis schedule is three times per week, 3 to 4 hours each. Noncompliance can lead to fluid volume overload, electrolyte imbalance, and cardiopulmonary compromise.

The most significant life threat from renal failure or noncompliance with dialysis is hyperkalemia, treatment of which centers around three goals. First, the myocardial membrane must be stabilized to discourage the formation of lethal dysrhythmia. Second, potassium must be pushed into the intracellular space, removing it from the intravascular space, where it can harm the myocardium. Third, potassium levels must be lowered by promoting its excretion in the urine, stool, or by dialysis. Specifically, these goals are accomplished in the following manner:

- Stabilize the myocardial membrane
  - Calcium gluconate or chloride
- Promote an intracellular shift of potassium
  - Insulin/glucose
  - Albuterol
  - Sodium bicarbonate
- Excretion of potassium
  - Diuretics: if patient is producing urine
  - Potassium-binding resins
  - Dialysis

5. Describe the kidney's role in acid-base physiology. p. 758

The human body is able to adjust for fluctuations in pH; this is a good thing, as life would be incompatible with the metabolic derangements that would occur otherwise. A combination of the buffer, respiratory, and renal systems maintain pH within the normal 7.35–7.45 range.

The buffering systems are used for short-term pH control; they tie up hydrogen ions. Four types of buffering systems are at work in the human body: the protein buffering system, the hemoglobin buffering system, the carbonic acid-bicarbonate buffering system, and the phosphate buffering system.

The respiratory and renal systems are used for long-term acid-base balance, and achieve this end by removing H^+ from body and by manipulating pH with CO_2, HCO_3^-, and H^+ secretion and/or retention. Increased $PaCO_2$ results in increased H^+ concentration (in accordance with the carbonic acid equation) decreasing pH. Central and peripheral chemoreceptors detect changes in CSF CO_2 and $PaCO_2$, respectively. Stimulation of chemoreceptors results in an increase of the respiratory rate, resulting in the CO_2 "blowing off" of CO_2 in the lungs. $PaCO_2$ drops, and H^+ concentration follows (again, in accordance with the carbonic acid equation). With the drop in $PaCO_2$, chemoreceptor stimulation decreases, and respiratory activity decreases.

The renal system is the slowest of three systems, and may take 24 to 48 hours to react to pH changes. There are three methods of buffering within the kidney: the carbonic acid-buffering system, ammonia buffering system, and the phosphate buffering system. The carbonic acid-bicarbonate buffer system regulates pH balance through the selective excretion/reabsorption of HCO_3^- and H^+. The ammonia buffer system combines H^+ with NH_3 in tubular lumen to form NH_4, which is then excreted in the urine. The phosphate buffer system combines HPO_4^{2-} with H^+ in tubular lumen to form HPO_4^-, which is then excreted in urine.

All of these methods result in the excretion of hydrogen ions, effectively increasing pH (lowering acidity). In addition, the carbonic acid-bicarbonate buffer system can address alkalosis by excreting bicarbonate when needed.

6. Discuss the varying etiologies of acid-base disturbances. p. 760

Metabolic alkalosis (pH > 7.45) can result from increased HCO_3^- intake or increased H^+ loss. Specific etiologies include excessive bicarbonate ingestion, blood transfusion, vomiting, nasogastric suctioning, and drug therapy or abuse.

Metabolic acidosis (pH < 7.35) can result from increased H^+ reabsorption, decreased HCO_3^- production, decreased HCO_3^- intake, or impaired HCO_3^- reabsorption. Specific etiologies include drug therapy or abuse, toxic ingestion (paraldehyde, methanol, ethylene glycol, salicylates), metabolic disturbances such as lactic acidosis or DKA, hypermetabolic state, anaerobic metabolism, infection, acute or chronic renal, hepatic, and pancreatic failure, and diarrhea.

Respiratory acidosis (pH < 7.35) can result from decreased ventilation or decreased CO_2 exchange across the alveolar-capillary membrane. Specific etiologies include apnea, bradypnea, COPD, neuromuscular disease, CNS-depressing drugs, and obesity hypoventilation syndrome.

Respiratory alkalosis (pH > 7.45) results from hyperventilation, and specific etiologies include pain, anxiety, fever, infectious disease, dehydration, sepsis, tumors, psychosis, hypoxemia, drugs (nicotine, catecholamines, salicylates, methylxanthines, progesterone), pregnancy, and mechanical ventilation.

7. Define the MUDPILES mnemonic and its effect on acid-base balance. p. 761

The MUDPILES mnemonic is a useful tool to help recall some of the most common causes of metabolic acidosis.

- M: Methanol
- U: Uremia
- D: Diabetic Ketoacidosis (DKA)
- P: Paraldehyde
- I: Infection
- L: Lactic acidosis
- E: Ethylene Glycol
- S: Salicylates

©2007 Pearson Education, Inc.
Critical Care Paramedic

Case Study

Case #1

Your ground transport team is called as an ALS intercept to a BLS ambulance for a patient with vomiting. The patient is a 72-year-old female with chronic renal failure who uses home peritoneal dialysis. She states that she has not been feeling well for a couple of days and has not performed her scheduled dialysis. She was awakened from sleep this morning with abdominal pain and vomiting. Her vital signs are: temperature 39 degrees C, respiratory rate 24 and shallow, heart rate 128 and irregular, and blood pressure 92/60. She is guarding her abdomen, which is very tender to palpation.

Case #2

The patient is a 19-year-old male who was found semiconscious and brought to the emergency department by friends. They reported that he had the "flu" for three or four days. He has the following vital signs: respirations 30, deep but nonlabored, pulse 122, blood pressure of 92/50, and a temperature of 38.7 degrees C. His ABG showed: pH 7.27, pCO_2 25 mm/Hg, pO_2 112 mm/Hg, HCO_3^- 12 mmol/L. His CBC shows an elevated white blood cell count. His basic metabolic panel showed the following abnormalities: sodium—150, potassium—5.9, CO_2—10, BUN—66 and glucose—615 mg/dL. His urine was positive for ketones.

Case #3

A 57-year-old female needs to be transferred for admission to the ICU. She was brought to the emergency department via EMS for increasing shortness of breath and productive cough. She has a 70-pack-year smoking history. She has the following vital signs: respirations 26 and shallow, heart rate 110, and blood pressure 166/98. Her SpO_2 is 90 percent on 4 lpm nasal cannula. Her arterial blood gas shows: pH 7.29, pCO_2 76 mm/Hg, pO_2 70 mm/HG, and HCO_3^- 36 mmol/L.

DISCUSSION QUESTIONS

1. For each of the scenarios above:
   a. Determine the most likely cause for the patient's problem or acid-base disturbance.
   b. Briefly outline an appropriate management plan for the correction of that disturbance.

Content Review

MULTIPLE CHOICE

_____ 1. The _____ is the functional unit of the kidney.
   A. nephron
   B. loop of Henle
   C. cortex
   D. tubule

_____ 2. The nephron is composed of all of the following except the:
   A. glomerulus.
   B. loop of Henle.
   C. distal convoluted tubule.
   D. cortex.

_____ 3. Functions of the kidney include:
   A. the reabsorption of water.
   B. the reabsorption of ions.
   C. the secretion of ions.
   D. all of the above.

_____ 4. The bulk of the nephron is located in the:
   A. renal medulla.
   B. renal cortex.
   C. renal pyramid.
   D. none of the above.

_____ 5. Which of the following is not considered part of the renal tubule?
A. proximal convoluted tubule
B. distal convoluted tubule
C. loop of Henle
D. glomerulus

_____ 6. Filtration of blood occurs in the:
A. renal corpuscle.
B. renal tubule.
C. collecting duct.
D. proximal convoluted tubule.

_____ 7. The secretion of antidiuretic hormone (ADH) results in the production of:
A. small volumes of dilute urine.
B. small volumes of highly concentrated urine.
C. large volumes of dilute urine.
D. large volumes of highly concentrated urine.

_____ 8. Reabsorption of substrate (water, ions, glucose, etc.) occurs in all of the following structures except:
A. Bowman's capsule.
B. loop of Henle.
C. distal convoluted tubule.
D. collecting duct.

_____ 9. A patient who produces 300 mL of urine over a 24-hour period is considered:
A. normouric.
B. hypouric.
C. anuric.
D. oliguric.

_____ 10. Acute renal failure occurring secondary to glomerulonephritis is considered:
A. prerenal renal failure
B. intrarenal renal failure.
C. postrenal renal failure.
D. none of the above.

_____ 11. Acute renal failure occurring secondary to hypovolemia is considered:
A. prerenal renal failure.
B. intrarenal renal failure.
C. postrenal renal failure.
D. none of the above.

_____ 12. Acute renal failure occurring secondary to an occluded urethra is considered:
A. prerenal renal failure.
B. intrarenal renal failure.
C. postrenal renal failure.
D. none of the above.

_____ 13. A connection created between an artery and a vein using blood vessels using a synthetic bridge is called a (an):
A. arteriovenous fistula.
B. arteriovenous bridge.
C. arteriovenous conduit.
D. arteriovenous graft.

_____ 14. A patient in the CCU with acute renal failure requires immediate hemodialysis but is considered too unstable to make the transport to a dialysis unit across the hospital grounds. Which of the following treatments would be most beneficial to this patient?
A. peritoneal dialysis
B. continuous veno-venous hemofiltration (CVVH)
C. administration of calcium chloride, bicarbonate, and lasix
D. hemodialysis in the dialysis unit after the patient is stable

_____ 15. Complications associated with chronic renal failure include all of the following except:
A. anemia.
B. pericarditis.
C. peripheral neuropathy.
D. hypokalemia.

_____ 16. The management of hyperkalemia in a patient with CRF who is not producing urine includes the administration of all of the following except:
A. calcium chloride.
B. insulin.
C. albuterol.
D. furosemide.

_____ 17. An intracellular shift of potassium can be promoted by the administration of all of the following except:
A. insulin and glucose.
B. albuterol.
C. potassium exchange resin.
D. sodium bicarbonate.

©2007 Pearson Education, Inc.
Critical Care Paramedic

_____ 18. Which of the following set of lab values is consistent with a diagnosis of renal failure?
   A. BUN: 30 mg/dL
      Creatinine: 6 mg/dL
      Potassium: 12.3 mEq/L
      pH: 7.30
   B. BUN: 3 mg/dL
      Creatinine: 2.3 mg/dL
      Potassium: 4.7 mEq/L
      pH: 7.35
   C. BUN: 3.1 mg/dL
      Creatinine: 0.2 mg/dL
      Potassium: 1.8 mEq/L
      pH: 7.4
   D. BUN: 20 mg/dL
      Creatinine: 1.5 mg/dL
      Potassium: 12 mEq/L
      pH: 7.41

_____ 19. Which of the following correctly expresses the carbonic acid equation?
   A. $CO + H_2O \Leftrightarrow H_2CO_2 \Leftrightarrow H^+ + HCO_2^-$
   B. $H^+ + HCO_3^- \Leftrightarrow H_2CO_3 \Leftrightarrow CO_2 + H_2O$
   C. $CO_2 + H^+ \Leftrightarrow H_2CO_3 \Leftrightarrow H_2O + HCO_3^-$
   D. $CO + H_2O \Leftrightarrow H_2CO_3 \Leftrightarrow H^+ + HCO_3^-$

_____ 20. The most common extracellular buffer is _____, and the most common intracellular buffer is _____.
   A. bicarbonate ion, phosphate
   B. phosphate, bicarbonate ion
   C. bicarbonate ion, hydrogen ion
   D. carbonic acid, bicarbonate ion

_____ 21. As $PaCO_2$ rises, the production of carbonic acid _____, and the production of hydrogen ions _____.
   A. decreases, decreases
   B. decreases, increases
   C. increases, decreases
   D. increases, increases

_____ 22. An overproduction of bicarbonate ions creates a (an):
   A. actual acidosis
   B. actual alkalosis
   C. relative acidosis
   D. relative alkalosis

_____ 23. An overelimination of hydrogen ions creates a (an):
   A. actual acidosis
   B. actual alkalosis
   C. relative acidosis
   D. relative alkalosis

_____ 24. Continuous nasogastric suctioning may most likely result in:
   A. metabolic acidosis.
   B. metabolic alkalosis.
   C. respiratory acidosis.
   D. respiratory alkalosis.

_____ 25. The development of ketoacidosis may most likely result in:
   A. metabolic acidosis.
   B. metabolic alkalosis.
   C. respiratory acidosis.
   D. respiratory alkalosis.

_____ 26. Which of the following represents the ABG findings consistent with a metabolic acidosis with respiratory compensation?
   A. pH: 7.32
      HCO_3^-: 30
      PCO_2: 42
   B. pH: 7.40
      HCO_3^-: 24
      PCO_2: 35
   C. pH: 7.30
      HCO_3^-: 18
      PCO_2: 26
   D. pH: 7.48
      HCO_3^-: 30
      PCO_2: 62

_____ 27. Which of the following represents the ABG findings consistent with a respiratory alkalosis with renal compensation?
   A. pH: 7.40
      HCO_3^-: 24
      PCO_2: 35
   B. pH: 7.31
      HCO_3^-: 32
      PCO_2: 44
   C. pH: 7.50
      HCO_3^-: 18
      PCO_2: 26
   D. pH: 7.47
      HCO_3^-: 28
      PCO_2: 58

_____ 28. A 19-year-old female presents with a 3-day history of fever, vomiting, and diarrhea. Her ABG comes back with the following values: $PaO_2 = 110$, $PaCO_2 = 40$, $HCO_3^- = 23$, pH = 7.41. Based on the history and ABG analysis, which of the following acid-base disturbances does the patient most likely have?
   A. metabolic acidosis
   B. metabolic acidosis with respiratory compensation
   C. metabolic acidosis with a respiratory alkalosis
   D. no acid base disturbance is indicated

_____ 29. Causes of metabolic acidosis include all of the following except:
   A. salicylate toxicity.
   B. methanol toxicity.
   C. sepsis.
   D. diuretic use.

_____ 30. Management of methanol toxicity may include the administration of all of the following except:
   A. ethanol.
   B. activated charcoal.
   C. bicarbonate.
   D. fomepizole.

_____ 31. The accumulation of urea and other nitrogen-containing waste products in the blood is called:
   A. uremia.
   B. oliguria.
   C. anuria.
   D. none of the above.

_____ 32. A patient presents with a blood glucose of 460 mg/dL, a bicarbonate of 11 mEq/L, a pH of 7.33, and ketone bodies in the urine and blood. Which of the following is the most accurate diagnosis?
   A. Hyperglycemia
   B. Ketoacidosis
   C. Metabolic alkalosis
   D. Metabolic alkalosis with renal compensation

_____ 33. A patient presents to the ED complaining of a 3-day history of fever and vomiting, and ringing in his ears that started this morning. PE reveals tachycardia and tachypnea. Lab studies reveal a PT of 18 seconds, a platelet count of 175,000, $PaO_2 = 100$, $PaCO_2 = 22$, $HCO_3^- = 18$, and pH = 7.31. Based on the history, you would most likely expect _____ toxicity.
   A. methanol
   B. ethanol
   C. salicylate
   D. paraldehyde

Infectious Disease Emergencies

Review of Chapter Objectives

Upon completion of this chapter, the student should be able to:

1. **Discuss the importance of infectious disease knowledge and prevention in the critical care setting.** **p. 774**

   Health care workers have a professional responsibility to prevent the spread of infectious and communicable diseases. This includes stopping (or minimizing) the spread of infection to and from patients, coworkers, themselves, and their families and friends. To fulfill this obligation, it is incumbent on every health care professional to be knowledgeable about the principles of infection control and the recognition and treatment of those infectious diseases that they may reasonably expect to encounter in their work.

2. **Describe the basic types of disease-causing organisms including the following:**

   a. **Bacteria** **p. 774**

   Bacteria are prokaryotic, unicellular microorganisms that come in a variety of cell morphologies including coccus (round), bacillus (rod-shaped), coccobacillus (oval), spirillum (spiral), and vibrio (curved bacillus). They live in soil, water, organic matter, or in the bodies of plants and animals, and, as such, are capable of reproducing outside of a living host organism. The human body is host to trillions of bacteria, and, in fact, we have a symbiotic relationship to many species, such as *e. coli*, which assists humans with digestion in the gut. Bacteria have a remarkable ability to survive in extreme conditions, surviving in temperatures well below freezing and far above the boiling point of water. Different species of bacteria "eat" everything from sugar to sunlight (via photosynthesis), and sulfur to hydrogen gas to iron. Bacteria are also the cause of animal and human disease, and antibiotics are effective against most bacterial infections.

   Aerobic bacteria survive only in the presence of oxygen and are the causative agent of diseases such as streptococcal throat diseases (Group A Streptococci), syphilis (*Treponema pallidum*), tuberculosis (*Mycobacterium tuberculosis*), food poisoning (*Salmonella*), meningococcal diseases (*Neisseria meningitidis*), plague (*Yersinia pestis*), pertussis (*Bordetella pertussis*), diphtheria (*Corynebacterium diphtheriae*), and cholera (*Vibrio cholerae*).

   Anaerobic bacteria survive in the absence of free oxygen and can cause infections such as colitis (*clostridium difficile*), tetanus (*clostridium tetani*), and abdominal infections (*bacteroides fragilis*).

   b. **Viruses** **p. 774**

   A virus is one of the smallest microorganisms, and it is also one of the simplest; they are commonly described as DNA housed in a protein coat and come in various shapes including helical, polyhedral, enveloped, or complex. They are neither prokaryotes or eukaryotes; rather, viruses walk a fine line between living and nonliving; they remain inert while free in the environment, but once in contact with a suitable living organism (plant, animal, or human) a virus will take over the host's reproductive apparatus to create its own progeny, often destroying the cell they have invaded in the process. As a result of this nature, viruses are often referred to as obligate intracellular parasites. Viruses do not require nutrients to live, in other words, they do not "eat." Viruses cause a variety of diseases including AIDS, hepatitis, measles, and rubella, smallpox and poliomyelitis, herpes, influenza and the common cold, rabies, and viral and equine encephalitis.

They are not generally susceptible to antibiotics although some antiviral drugs have been developed. Vaccines have been developed, or are under development, to prevent some of the more important viral infections.

c. Rickettsia p. 775

Rickettsia are prokaryotic organisms extremely similar to bacteria, and, in fact, are considered protobacteria, but are unable (with the exception of one species) to survive for long outside of their hosts because they are deficient in many metabolic activities and obtain needed metabolites from their hosts. Therefore, like viruses, rickettsia are obligate intracellular parasites. Since they do not survive long outside their host, rickettsia require a vector, most often an arthopod such as ticks, fleas, or lice. Rickettsia can be rod-shaped, coccoid, or diplococcus, and can cause a number of serious diseases including typhus, rickettsialpox, Rocky Mountain spotted fever, scrub typhus, and Q fever. Most rickettsia are responsive to antibiotic therapy.

d. Fungi p. 775

A fungus is a eukaryotic, saprophytic, parasitic, spore-producing organism that lacks chlorophyll. Fungi absorb nutrients through their cell wall from living or dead organic matter, and can live in water, soil, and on, and in, the human body (though they are not as pathogenic as bacteria and viruses). Three main groups of fungi are recognized: molds, mushrooms, and yeasts.

Those that are capable of producing disease in humans include actinomycetes (rat bite fever), dermatomycosis (ringworm), aspergillosis (infections of the external ear, pulmonary, sinus, and subcutaneous tissue), blastomycosis (abscesses of skin and subcutaneous tissue), candidiasis, and thrush.

Numerous antifungal agents have been developed for many of these infections.

e. Protozoa p. 775

Protozoa are eukaryotic unicellular organisms of considerable size when compared to bacteria and viruses. Protozoa are found in many habitats including water, soil, and animal and human bodies. Most obtain nutrients via phagocytosis, or engulfing material in their environment, and are quite mobile and able to "catch" their food. Specific protozoa that can infect humans include *Endamoeba histolytica* (amebiasis), trypanosoma (malaria, or sleeping sickness), leishmania (leishmaniasis), trichomonas (trichomoniasis), and toxoplasma (toxoplasmosis). Antimicrobial agents are available for the treatment of protozoa disease.

f. Metazoa-helminths p. 775

Helminths are parasitic worms, including tapeworms, liver flukes, roundworms, and pinworms. Antihelmintics are available to treat many of these infections.

g. Prions p. 775

A prion (short for proteinaceous infectious particle) is an abnormally structured protein that is able to enter cells and convert normal cellular proteins into abnormally structured proteins just like themselves. These proteins disrupt normal cellular processes and are the cause of various infectious diseases of the nervous system, classified as transmissible spongiform encephalopathies (TSEs) such as scrapie, Creutzfeldt-Jakob disease, and bovine spongiform encephalopathy (BSE). These diseases are all untreatable and fatal.

3. Discuss the cycle of infectious disease transmission. p. 775

Different pathogens have different modes of transmission, which are usually related to the areas of the body that the organism inhabits. For example, gastrointestinal organisms are usually transmitted via food or water contaminated with feces, and respiratory organisms spread via airborne transmission.

Sources of infection include persons with acute illnesses, those in the incubation period of a disease, and persons who are carriers of pathogenic microorganisms but are asymptomatic. Other sources of infection include one's own endogenous flora and objects that have become contaminated such as equipment, linens, and work surfaces.

Hosts are persons who may become infected with pathogenic microorganisms. A susceptible host is anyone who is capable of becoming infected with the disease being transmitted. Whether a person is susceptible to a particular pathogen is dependent on several factors including, but not limited to, their general health and hygiene, their immune status for various microorganisms, their age, the presence of any immunosuppressive diseases or therapies, and any break in the first lines of defense.

Microorganisms are passed from a source to a susceptible host through one of five routes of transmission; contact (direct and indirect), droplet, vehicle, vector-borne, and airborne.

Some pathogens (e.g., chickenpox) are capable of being transmitted through more than one route. Also, with some diseases, the infectious agent may make use of multiple transmission routes. Furthermore, in some cases, diseases have been shown to mutate and "change" how they move, both on an interspecies and on an intraspecies basis.

Direct contact is the ability of a pathogen to be transmitted from one person to another through direct personal contact, such as touching or kissing. Indirect contact occurs when a susceptible host becomes infected after contact with an object contaminated by the source organism, such as a contaminated needle or soiled dressings.

Droplet transmission occurs when an infected individual sprays moist droplets into the air during coughing, sneezing, or speaking, or during medical procedures such as suctioning or bronchoscopy. In fact, nothing is quite better at producing the proper droplet size for infection in humans than sneezes and coughs. Organisms capable of being transmitted by droplet spread infect a susceptible host when the droplet comes into contact with the mucous membrane of the host's mouth, nose, or eyes. It is possible for a host to facilitate the transmission by receiving the droplets on their hands and then immediately putting their hands to his eyes or mouth. Organisms transmitted on droplets are propelled for about two to three feet and will only remain in the air for a brief period of time before falling to the ground or other surface. The droplets will dry up quickly and the organism is no longer considered a source of infection.

Diseases that are spread by vehicles are transmitted through mediums such as food, water, blood, drugs, and occasionally contaminated instruments or equipment. Examples of diseases that are transmitted through vehicles include typhoid fever, hepatitis A, and giardia Lamblia.

Vector-borne diseases are transmitted through an intermediate host such as a fly, mosquito, or tick. These vectors can transmit the disease through simple mechanical means whereby an organism from an infectious source will stick to the legs or body of the vector and is then deposited on the susceptible host or medium, or through biological transmission in which the infecting organism enters the intermediate host and will go through some form of life cycle change before being passed on to a susceptible host. This mechanism usually requires the intermediate host to bite or sting the susceptible host and inject the microorganism. Examples of diseases transmitted by vectors include Rocky Mountain spotted fever, bubonic plague, hantavirus, and malaria.

Airborne diseases are infections caused by microorganisms capable of being transmitted through the air as droplet nuclei or on dust particles. These organisms are very small and are capable of surviving in the air for a longer period of time and may be dispersed through air currents. Diseases that are spread through the airborne route include tuberculosis, chickenpox, and measles.

4. Detail the role of the critical care paramedic in infectious disease prevention. p. 776

Preventing the transmission of infectious agents requires practicing good infection control measures including general precautions and transmission-specific isolation precautions. Critical care providers should be knowledgeable in a variety of techniques and isolation precautions because they will encounter infectious diseases through their work with different health care institutions.

5. Describe Universal Precautions and Body Substance Isolation Precautions as they pertain to critical care transport. p. 776

Standard Precautions combine the salient features of both Universal Precautions and Body Substance Isolation (BSI) Precautions and apply them to all patients. Universal Precautions were designed to reduce the risk of transmission of blood borne pathogens and were to be used specifically to prevent contact with blood and/or body fluids that may contain blood. Universal Precautions, however, provide neither protection against diseases transmitted via body secretions or excretions not involving blood, nor against any diseases transmitted via droplet or airborne routes.

Body Substance Isolation (BSI) Precautions were designed to reduce the risk of transmission of diseases via moist body substances. Gloves are to be worn before any contact with mucous membranes, nonintact skin, or moist body substances. Various parties have been critical of BSI Precautions in that they do not contain adequate provisions for diseases transmitted via droplet transmission, direct or indirect transmission from dry skin or environmental surfaces, or true airborne transmission of infections over long distances by floating droplet nuclei. In addition, BSI Precautions do not require that caregivers wash their hands after removing gloves.

The combination of Universal Precautions and BSI Precautions into Standard Precautions has resulted in precautions being applied to blood, all body fluids, secretions and excretions (except sweat), nonintact skin, and mucous membranes. Standard Precautions cover a variety of diseases previously addressed by the Centers for Disease Control and Prevention (CDC) guidelines under category or disease-specific isolation precautions. In addition, Standard Precautions eliminate the need for the previous CDC categories of isolation precautions (strict isolation, contact isolation, respiratory isolation, tuberculosis isolation, enteric isolation), the drainage/secretion precautions, and the old disease-specific precautions, replacing these with the three Transmission-Based Precautions: airborne, droplet, and contact.

Standard Precautions include the following:

- Hand washing
  - After touching blood, body fluids, secretions, excretions, and
  - Contaminated items whether gloves are worn or not
  - After removing gloves
  - Between patient contacts
  - Between procedures on the same patient
  - When otherwise indicated to prevent transmission of organisms
  - A plain (nonantimicrobial) soap should be used for routine hand washing.
  - Use an antimicrobial agent under specific circumstances.
- Gloves
  - Wear approved gloves when touching blood, body fluids, secretions, excretions, or contaminated items.
- Mask, eye protection, face shield
  - Wear during procedures that are likely to generate splashes or sprays of blood, body fluids, secretions, or excretions.
- Gown or outerwear protection
  - Wear during procedures likely to generate sprays or splashes of blood, body fluids, secretions, or excretions
- Patient care equipment
  - Handle all patient care equipment so as to prevent contamination of hands or other equipment.
  - Ensure that single-use equipment is appropriately disposed of.
- Environmental control
  - Ensure that adequate cleaning and disinfecting procedures are in place.
- Linen
  - Handle soiled or contaminated linens so as to prevent cross-contamination to other patients or environment.
- Occupational health and blood borne pathogens
  - Always use caution to prevent injuries when using sharps.
  - Use safer medical devices, such as sharps with engineered, sharps-injury protection and needleless systems

- Work practice controls such as never recapping needles, proper disposal of sharps in puncture-resistant containers, and use of mouthpieces and resuscitation bags as an alternative to mouth-to-mouth resuscitation

Airborne Precautions should be followed when caring for a patient with a known or suspected infectious disease that can be transmitted by airborne droplet nuclei that remain suspended in the air and can be widely dispersed. These precautions include:

- Transport
  - There should be a minimum of 6 to 12 air exchanges in transporting ambulance per hour.
  - Vent to the outdoors or high-efficiency filtration of recirculated air.
  - There should be separate air circulation between cab and patient compartment.
  - Keep door/window closed between cab and patient compartment
  - Air out vehicle after transport
- Respiratory protection
  - Use N95 respirators when entering room or location of patient with known or suspected infectious pulmonary tuberculosis
  - Susceptible persons should not enter the room of patients known or suspected to have measles or varicella if other caregivers are available.
- Patient transport
  - Limit movement to essential purposes only.
  - Have patient wear surgical mask if possible and tolerated.

Droplet Precautions are used when caring for a patient who carries or is infected with pathogens capable of being spread by droplets that can be generated when sneezing, coughing, and talking, or while performing procedures such as suctioning or bronchoscopy. These precautions include:

- Positioning
  - Placement of patient not within three feet of other persons
- Mask
  - Used when working within three feet of patient
- Patient transport
  - Limit transport to essential purposes only.
  - Place a surgical mask on patient, if possible and tolerated.

Contact Precautions are used with patients who are infected or colonized with epidemiologically important pathogenic organisms capable of being transmitted by contact including direct contact with the patient's dry skin or indirect contact with inanimate objects in the patient's environment or that have been contaminated by contact with the patient. These precautions include:

- Gloves and hand washing
  - Wear gloves when entering the patient's room.
  - Change gloves when grossly contaminated or between procedures to prevent cross-contamination.
  - Wash hands with an antimicrobial agent or waterless antiseptic agent immediately upon removal of gloves and whenever hands touch a potentially contaminated surface.
- Gown or outerwear
  - Worn when entering the patient's room if substantial contact with patient or potentially contaminated surfaces or objects in the room is anticipated
  - Properly dispose of, or decontaminate, gown or outerwear.
- Patient care equipment
  - Dispose of nonreusable equipment appropriately.
  - Nondisposable equipment must be cleaned and disinfected prior to being placed back in service.

Additional precautions are indicated for patients infected with vancomycin-resistant organisms.

6. Detail the recommendations for vaccination of health care workers. pp. 785, 786

Table 26-1   CDC Immunization Recommendations for Health Care Workers

Disease	Route of Transmission	Vaccine	Vaccine Schedule	Indications
Hepatitis B (HBV)	Percutaneous of permucosal exposure to blood or body fluids containing blood	Hepatitis B recombinant vaccine	Two doses IM 4 weeks apart; third dose 5 months after second; booster doses not necessary	HCWs at risk for exposure to blood or body fluids
		Hepatitis B immune globulin (HBIG)	0.06 mL/kg IM ASAP after exposure but no later than 7 days. A second dose should be administered 1 month later if the HB series has not been started	Postexposure for persons exposed to blood or body fluids containing HbsAg and who are not immune to HBV infection
Influenza	Airborne	Annual vaccination with current vaccine	IM per vaccine schedule	HCWs who have contact with patients at high risk for influenza or its complications; HCWs who work in chronic care facilities; HCWs with high-risk medical conditions or who are aged $\geq$ 65 years
Measles (rubeola)	Airborne	Measles live-virus vaccine. Measles-mumps-rubella (MMR) vaccine of choice if recipients likely to be susceptible to mumps or rubella as well as measles	One dose SC; second dose at least 1 month later	HCWs born during or after 1957 who do not have documentation of having received 2 doses of live vaccine on or after the first birthday or a history of physician-diagnosed measles or serologic evidence of immunity. Vaccination should be considered for all HCWs who lack proof of immunity, including those born before 1957
Mumps	Droplet and direct contact with saliva	Mumps live-virus vaccine. MMR vaccine of choice if recipients likely to be susceptible to measles or rubella as well as mumps	One dose SC; no booster	HCWs believed to be susceptible can be vaccinated. Adults born before 1957 can be considered immune

Rubella, German measles, three-day measles	Droplet and direct contact with naso-pharyngeal secretions	Rubella live-virus vaccine. MMR vaccine of choice if recipients likely to be susceptible to measles or mumps as well as rubella	One dose SC; no booster	Indicated for HCWs who do not have documentation of having received live vaccine on or after their first birthday or laboratory evidence of immunity. Adults born after 1957, except women who can become pregnant, can be considered immune
Pneumococcal disease	Droplet spread, direct oral contact or indirectly through contact with items soiled with respiratory secretions	Pneumococcal polysaccharide vaccine (23 valent)	One 0.5 mL dose, IM or SC; revaccination recommended for those at highest risk ≥ 5 years after the first dose.	Adults who are at increased risk of pneumococcal disease and its complications because of underlying health conditions; older adults, especially those age ≥ 65 who are healthy
Tetanus and diphtheria	Tetanus spores introduced into the body through contaminated puncture wounds. Contact with diphtheria patient or carrier or rarely contact with items soiled with discharges from lesions of infected persons	Tetanus and diphtheria (toxoids) Td	Two IM doses 4 weeks apart; third dose 6–12 months after second dose; booster every 10 years	All adults
Varicella, chickenpox or herpes zoster (shingles)	Direct contact, droplet, or airborne spread, indirect contact with items contaminated with discharges from vesicles or respiratory tract	Varicella zoster live-virus vaccine Varicella-zoster immune globulin (VZIG)	Two 0.5 mL doses SC 4–8 weeks apart if ≥ 13 years of age Persons < 50 kg: 125 units/10 kg IM; persons > 50 kg: 625 units	HCWs who do not have either a reliable history of varicella or serologic evidence of immunity

Source: Adapted from CDC "Immunization of Health-Care Workers: Recommendations of the Advisory Committee on Immunization Practices (ACIP) and the Hospital Infection Control Practices Advisory Committee (HICPAC)." MMWR (December 26, 1997): 46, RR-18.

7. **Discuss the etiology, transmission, pathophysiology, signs and symptoms, and treatment of the following epidemiologically important infectious diseases:**

a. **HIV/AIDS** p. 786

Etiology

AIDS is caused by the HIV virus. There are two identified types of HIV, Type 1: HIV-1, which is predominant worldwide, and Type 2: HIV-2 which is concentrated in West Africa.

Transmission

HIV transmission is via the blood borne route, and can occur secondary to sexual contact, the sharing of syringes and needles, accidental needle sticks (risk of infection 0.5 percent after stick), childbirth, and exposure to other potentially infectious materials (OPIM) such as semen, vaginal fluid, peritoneal fluid, pleural fluid, other fluid with visible blood, and breast milk.

Pathophysiology

HIV is a retrovirus with a high affinity for CD4-T lymphocytes and monocytes. The virus binds to and enters the cell, generates a copy of its DNA via reverse transcriptase, and replicates. Viral DNA combines with host DNA enabling further replication. The host cell is destroyed as viral progeny leave the cell and infect additional cells.

Signs and symptoms
- Fever, fatigue, chronic diarrhea
- Loss of appetite, weight loss
- Lymphadenopathy
- Pneumonia, cytomegalovirus infections, candidiasis, herpes
- HIV dementia, Kaposi's sarcoma

Treatment
- Directed at treating opportunistic infections, cancers
- Antiretroviral therapy
- No cure, no vaccine

b. **Viral hepatitis** p. 787

Etiology
- Hepatitis A: caused by hepatitis A virus (HAV)
- Hepatitis B: caused by hepatitis B virus (HBV)
- Hepatitis C: caused by hepatitis C virus (HCV)
- Hepatitis D: caused by hepatitis D virus (HDV)
- Hepatitis E: caused by hepatitis E virus (HEV)

Transmission

Hepatitis A and E are spread via the fecal-oral route. Hepatitis B, C, and D are spread by exposure to blood and body fluids including semen, vaginal fluid, and saliva. Specific methods of transmission include sexual intercourse, childbirth, and the sharing of syringes and needles.

Pathophysiology

Hepatitis, regardless of the strain, is an acute and chronic inflammatory process involving the liver. The hepatitis virus infects hepatocytes and uses their DNA replication machinery to reproduce.

Signs and symptoms
- Hepatitis A
  - Anorexia, N/V, fatigue, malaise, low-grade fever
  - Bilirubinemia
  - Jaundice, pruritus, scleral icterus
  - Abdominal pain
  - Hepatomegaly

©2007 Pearson Education, Inc.
Critical Care Paramedic

- Hepatitis B
  - Loss of appetite, fatigue, malaise, myalgia
  - N/V, abdominal pain, jaundice
  - Low-grade fever, rash
  - Abdominal pain
  - Hepatomegaly, spider angioma, palmer erythema
- Hepatitis C
  - Loss of appetite, fatigue, N/V
  - Abdominal pain
  - Jaundice, scleral icterus, palmer erythema
  - Bilirubinemia
  - Gynecomastia, ascites, caput medusae
- Hepatitis D
  - N/V, fever
  - Abdominal pain
  - Bilirubinemia
  - Jaundice, scleral icterus
- Hepatitis E
  - Similar to other hepatitis infections

Treatment

Hepatitis A
- Supportive

Hepatitis B
- Supportive care
  - Liver failure
  - Dehydration
- Medications
  - Antiviral agents
    - Alpha interferon
    - Lamivudine

Hepatitis C
- Supportive
- Pharmacologic intervention
  - Antiviral agents
    - Interferon
    - Ribavirin

Hepatitis D
- Supportive
- Pharmacological treatment
  - Antiviral agents
    - Interferons

Hepatitis E
- Supportive

c. **Respiratory infections**   p. 789

Etiology
Viruses, bacteria, and fungi can all contribute to respiratory infections.

Transmission
Transmission typically via airborne and droplet mechanisms

Pathophysiology
Upper and lower respiratory parenchyma is invaded and/or colonized by the pathogenic organism.

Signs and symptoms
Vary according to the pathogenic organism

Treatment
Specific to the pathogenic organism

d. Epiglottitis

Etiology
Epiglottitis occurs most often secondary to *Haemophilus influenza* Type B, though other causative agents include *S. pneumoniae, Pneumococcus, S. aureus,* and *H. parainfluenzae.*

Transmission
Transmission occurs via the airborne route and through direct contact with respiratory droplets.

Pathophysiology
Infection leads to inflammation and edema of the epiglottis and surrounding tissues. Glottic and airway edema can result in airway obstruction.

Signs and symptoms
- Fever, sore throat, dysphagia
- Tachycardia, tachypnea, retractions
- Horse or muffled voice, stridor
- Positioning, drooling
  - Leaning forward

Treatment
- Keep patient calm.
- Position effectively.
- 100 percent, high-flow oxygen via appropriate delivery method
- Airway control
  - Endotracheal intubation only if airway obstruction imminent
- Antibiotics:
  - Cefotaxime
  - Ceftriaxone
  - Ampicillin
  - Sulbactam

e. Influenza
p. 790

Etiology
Influenza results from infection with one of the three basic virus subtypes (A, B,C) classified within the Orthomyxoviridae family.

Transmission
Transmission occurs via the airborne route and through direct contact with respiratory droplets.

Pathophysiology
Infection occurs in the upper and lower respiratory tract when the virus enters respiratory epithelial cells in the trachea and bronchi. Viral replication results in the destruction of the host cell, and the virus is shed in respiratory secretions for five to ten days.

Signs and symptoms
- Headache, myalgia
- Sore throat, dry cough, chills
- Fever
- Rhinorrhea
- Wheezing, rhonchi

Treatment
- Vaccine

346 CRITICAL CARE PARAMEDIC

©2007 Pearson Education, Inc.
Critical Care Paramedic

- Supportive care
  - Respiratory
- Pharmacological treatment
  - Antiviral agents
    - Oseltamivir
    - Zanamivir
    - Rimantadine
    - Amantadine

f. Pneumonia   p. 790

Etiology

Pneumonia has various etiologies including viral, bacterial, and fungal organisms. Pneumonia is commonly classified as community-acquired versus hospital-acquired pneumonia and as typical infection versus atypical infection. Typical organisms include *S. pneumoniae*, Haemophilus, and Staphylococcus. Atypical organisms include *Legionella*, Chlamydia, and Mycoplasma.

Transmission

Transmission occurs via the airborne route and through direct contact with respiratory droplets.

Pathophysiology

Nosocomial infection commonly occurs secondary to aspiration of normal upper respiratory flora during sleep, and depends on factors such as the strength of host defenses and the number and virulence of the organisms reaching the lower respiratory tract.

Typical pneumonia commonly occurs secondary to the aerosolization of *S. pneumoniae* from the upper respiratory tract and deposition of the organism in the alveoli. The organism then infects alveolar type II epithelial cells and the surrounding epithelium. Pneumococci are able to spread among neighboring alveoli through the pores of Kohn, producing infection within whole lobar compartments. A strong association exists between pneumonia and viral infection, such as influenza, which increases pneumoccocal adherence to receptors on activated respiratory epithelial cells.

The organisms responsible for atypical pneumonia attach to respiratory epithelial cells by a variety of methods, causing injury to the cells and their cilia. Host defense is mounted via humoral and cell-mediated immune activity, and the majority of damage caused during the course of infection occurs secondary to the actions of the immune system, not the pathogenic organism.

Signs and symptoms

Clinical exam findings vary according to the pathogenic organism, severity of infection, and presence of comorbidities, but tend to include:
- Fever, malaise
- Adventitious lung sounds
  - Crackles, rhonchi over affected areas
  - Tactile fremitus
  - Sputum production
    - Blood-tinged
    - Purulent

Treatment

- Respiratory support
  - Supplemental oxygen
  - Airway control and mechanical ventilation, if necessary
- Antimicrobial therapy
  - For bacterial infections:
    - Directed at causative agent
      - Penicillin G or V
      - Amoxicillin
      - Cephalosporins

- Macrolides (azithromycin)
- Quinolones (levofloxacin)
- Gatifloxacin
- Moxifloxacin

g. Tuberculosis   p. 791

Etiology

Tuberculosis is a bacterial infection caused by *Mycobacterium tuberculosis*.

Transmission

Transmission occurs via the airborne route and through direct contact with respiratory droplets.

Pathophysiology

After being inhaled, *M. tuberculosis* bacilli are deposited in alveoli where they are ingested by macrophages. Macrophages then deliver the bacilli to lymph nodes where the bacilli may be destroyed, multiply and cause primary TB, become dormant, or enter a latent period before activation and multiplication. When the bacteria multiply, pulmonary disease ensues, and extrapulmonary infections are also possible and may include the lymph nodes, kidneys, pericardium, meninges, bones, joints, and skin.

Signs and symptoms

Signs and symptoms of pulmonary TB include:
- Fever, chills, chest pain
- Loss of appetite, weight loss, fatigue
- Productive cough, hemoptysis

Signs and symptoms of extrapulmonary TB include:
- Signs/symptoms related to organs or systems infected

Treatment
- Antimicrobial therapy
  - Isoniazid (INH)
  - Rifampin
  - Pyrazinamide
  - Ethambutol
  - Streptomycin
- Administered over a period of six to nine months

h. Severe acute respiratory syndrome (SARS)   p. 792

Etiology

SARS-associated coronavirus (SARS-CoV).

Transmission

Transmission occurs via the airborne route and through direct contact with respiratory droplets.

Pathophysiology

The pathophysiology of SARS is similar to that of pneumonia. There is an incubation period of two to seven days, and carriers are contagious as long as they have symptoms.

Signs and symptoms
- Sore throat, rhinorrhea, headache, diarrhea
- Chills, rigors, myalgia
- Productive cough, respiratory distress, respiratory failure

Treatment
- No medical protocol currently exists
- Supplemental oxygen
  - Respiratory support
- Mechanical ventilation, if necessary

- Bronchodilators
- Rehydration
- Antiviral medications have no proven efficacy

i. Meningitis

p. 794

Etiology

There are various etiologies of meningitis including, viral, fungal, bacterial (associated with the highest mortality), parasitic, and from medications.

Transmission

Transmission may occur via the droplet, contact, or airborne routes.

Pathophysiology

Meningitis is an inflammation of the meninges and underlying CSF. Depending on the onset of symptoms, meningitis can be classified as acute or chronic. Acute meningitis, usually bacterial in origin, evolves over hours to days. Chronic meningitis has an onset of weeks to months.

A number of factors influence the development of meningitis, including host defenses and virulence of the pathogen. Initially, an organism establishes a local infection within a host in an area such as the GI tract, skin, upper respiratory system, or GU tract. From the original site, the organism infiltrates the CNS via the blood stream, retrograde neuronal pathways, or direct spread through a created or sustained defect (otitis media, trauma, congenital malformations). Once in the CSF, the lack of a formidable defense allows proliferation of the offending organism. Organism exudates and cellular debris spread throughout the CSF, resulting in damage to cranial nerves, the induction of thrombophlebitis and vasculitis, and the clogging of CSF pathways. As brain edema progresses and ICP raises, CNS autoregulatory processes fail, resulting in hemodynamic instability and eventual death.

Signs and symptoms

- Fever, stiff neck, N/V
- Photophobia, headache
- AMS

Treatment

- Supportive
- Antimicrobial therapy if appropriate

j. Meningococcal infections

p. 794

Etiology

Meningococcal infections are caused by the gram-negative diplococcus *Neisseria meningitides* and can result in meningococcemia and meningococcal meningitis.

Transmission

Transmission may occur via the droplet, contact, or airborne routes.

Pathophysiology

The human nasopharynx serves as the only identified reservoir for *N. meningitides*, typically colonizing the mucosal surface without producing symptoms. In a worst-case scenario, the organism can invade the bloodstream and cause one of three possible outcomes: uncomplicated bacteremia, meningitis, or systemic infection, sepsis, and DIC.

The characteristic pathology of meningococcemia includes widespread vascular injury with epithelial necrosis, intravascular thrombosis, and perivascular hemorrhage.

Signs and symptoms

- Meningitis
  - Stiff neck, photophobia, headache, AMS
- Meningococcemia
  - Fever, petechiae, purpuric eruption

Treatment
- Antibiotic therapy
  - Penicillin G
  - Ceftriaxone
  - Chloramphenicol
  - Cefuroxime
- Supportive care

8. **Discuss the etiology, transmission, pathophysiology, signs and symptoms, and treatment of the following childhood diseases:**

a. Measles (rubeola) p. 795

Etiology
The measles virus is an enveloped, RNA virus of the Paramyxoviridae family.

Transmission
Transmission may occur via the droplet, contact, or airborne routes.

Pathophysiology
After initial introduction, the initial infection and viral replication occurs in bronchial and tracheal epithelial tissue. In two to four days, the virus spreads to and infects local lymphatic tissue, where further replication and amplification occurs.

A generalized immunosupression that follows a measles infection will render a patient more susceptible to bacterial infections such as bronchopneumonia and otitis media. Viremia ensues, and infection of endothelial and epithelial cells results in the formation of enanthems (Koplik spots) on the buccal mucosa and the characteristic maculopapular rash, respectively.

Signs and symptoms
- Cough
- Fever
- Conjunctivitis
- Coryza
- Malaise
- Anorexia
- Maculopapular rash, Koplik spots

Treatment
- Supportive
- Vitamin A supplements
  - in malnourished children
- Antibiotics
  - if evidence of bacterial pneumonia or otitis media

b. Mumps p. 795

Etiology
The mumps virus is a single-stranded RNA virus of the Paramyxoviridae family.

Transmission
Transmission may occur via the droplet or contact routes.

Pathophysiology
After initial introduction into the oropharynx, the virus invades the parotid and salivary glands and surrounding nervous tissue. Viral replication produces viremia that can spread the virus to the pancreas, testes, and ovaries. The virus can be isolated in blood, urine, saliva, and CSF.

Signs and symptoms
- Fever
- Swelling, tenderness to lymph nodes, parotid glands
- Tinnitus, ataxia, vomiting followed by loss of hearing

Treatment
- Supportive

c. **Rubella (German measles)**   p. 795

Etiology
The rubella virus is an RNA virus of the Togaviridae family.

Transmission
Transmission may occur via the droplet, contact, or airborne routes.

Pathophysiology
After initial colonization of the nasopharynx, the rubella virus invades the respiratory epithelium before producing viremia, which allows spread to the lympathatic system prior to invasion of, and replication in, the reticuloendothelial system tissue. A second viremia occurs about one to three weeks after initial infection, allowing for viral spread to the urine, CSF, breast milk, synovial fluid, and lungs. Viremia resolves soon after the appearance of a cutaneous rash.

Signs and symptoms
- Fever, chills, nausea
- Myalgia, sore throat
- Maculopapular rash
- Adults
  - May also develop URI, headache

Treatment
- Supportive

d. **Chickenpox (varicella)**   p. 796

Etiology
The varicella-zoster virus (VZV) is a double-stranded DNA virus of the Alphaherpesvirinae subfamily.

Transmission
Transmission may occur via the droplet, contact, or airborne routes.

Pathophysiology
After initial infection of the conjunctivae or upper respiratory tract mucosa, viral replication occurs in the regional lymph nodes within two to four days, and a viremia on about days four to six. Viral replication then occurs again, this time in internal organs such as the liver and spleen followed by a second viremia at 12 to 14 days postinfection. Invasion of capillary endothelial cells and the epidermis occurs during the second viremia, resulting in the characteristic varicella cutaneous vesicle. Exposure to VZV induces production of antibodies, including IgG, which persist for the life of the patient and provide immunity.

Signs and symptoms
- Slight fever, macropapular rash
  - Vescicular, eventually pustular

Treatment
- Supportive

9. **Discuss the transmission, signs and symptoms, and treatment of gastroenteritis.**   p. 796

Etiology
Etiologies of gastroenteritis include bacterial, viral, or parasitic infection.

Transmission
Transmission may occur via the droplet or fecal-oral routes.

Pathophysiology
Gastroenteritis is a nonspecific term used to describe the clinical syndrome of diarrhea, nausea and vomiting, malabsorption of electrolytes and carbohydrates, and stimulation of cAMP in the gut mucosa. The invading organism causes diarrhea by adherence, mucosal invasion, enterotoxin production, and/or cytotoxin production.

Signs and symptoms
- Diarrhea, N/V, abdominal pain
- Fever, myalgia, loss of appetite

Treatment
- Rehydration is a priority.
  - Electrolyte replacement
- Supportive care

10. **Discuss the prevention and treatment of tetanus.**   p. 796

Etiology
Tetanus is caused by the gram-positive, spore-forming, anaerobic bacilli, *Clostridium tetani.*

Transmission
Contact route is via puncture wounds.

Pathophysiology
The tetanus bacillus is found in soil, feces (human and animal), skin, and the human and animal GI tract. The spores require live tissue with the proper metabolic conditions (anaerobic) to germinate, and necrotic wound tissue serves as the perfect petrie dish. The bacillus does not require the classic "step on a rusty nail" for successful inoculation; a wound as unimpressive as a splinter will serve its purpose adequately. Upon germination, the bacteria produce two toxins, one of which produces the clinical manifestations of the disease. The toxin is transported through motor neurons at the spinal cord, where it binds to inhibitory neurons, resulting in uncontrolled release of acetylcholine and uncontrolled muscle contraction, the characteristic clinical finding of the disease. The word tetanus comes from the Greek *tetanos,* itself derived from the term *teinein,* meaning "to stretch."

Prevention
The disease can be prevented with a tetanus immunization.

Signs and symptoms
- Muscle stiffness
  - Facial; risus sardonicus ("sardonic smile")
  - Neck
  - Trunk
  - Extremities
- Hyperautonomic state

Treatment
- Human tetanus immunoglobin (TIG)

- Ventilatory support
  - Mechanical ventilation
  - Muscle relaxants
  - NMBAs
  - Sedation
- Beta blockers for autonomic dysfunction

11. Detail the pathophysiology and treatment of septicemia and toxic shock syndrome.   p. 797

Etiology
Various organisms may cause septicemia including bacteria, viruses, and fungi.

Pathophysiology
Prior to a discussion on septicemia and toxic shock syndrome, a quick review of terms associated with sepsis is necessary. Systemic inflammatory response syndrome (SIRS) is a clinical term used to describe the invasion of microorganisms into the bloodstream and the body's response to the invasion (tachycardia, fever, tachypnea, elevated white blood cell count). SIRS results in a symptomatic bacteremia.

Sepsis, derived from a Greek word meaning "putrid," is defined as SIRS with an identifiable infection and may or may not include the beginnings of organ dysfunction. Septicemia, or severe sepsis, exists when bacteria are actively multiplying in the bloodstream, resulting in an overwhelming infection and the beginning of organ dysfunction and development of hypotension. Septicemia also requires the presence of at least one of the following perfusion abnormalities: altered mental status, hypoxemia, oliguria, or lactic acidosis. Septic shock is defined as sepsis-induced hypotension despite aggressive fluid management in the presence of perfusion abnormalities such as altered mental status, hypoxemia, oliguria, or lactic acidosis. Multiple organ dysfunction syndrome (MODS) is the parallel or sequential dysfunction of at least two organs, and homeostasis cannot be maintained without medical intervention. Toxic shock syndrome occurs as result of *Staphylococcus aureus* or *Streptococcus pyogenes* infection. It is an inflammatory response syndrome characterized by fever, rash, multiorgan dysfunction, hypotension, and death. TSS is typically associated with tampon use in healthy women, though the disease also exists in men, neonates, and nonmenstruating women.

Treatment
- Shock management
  - Fluid volume replacement
  - Albumin
  - Vasopressors
- Identification and treatment of infection source
- Antibiotic therapy
  - Clindamycin
  - Vancomycin
  - Penicillin
- Supportive care

12. Discuss the causes, symptoms, and treatment guidelines for necrotizing fasciitis.   p. 798

Etiology
Necrotizing fasciitis is most commonly caused by infection with Group A beta-hemolytic streptococci, but can also occur secondary to *Haemophilus aprophilus* or *Staphylococcus aureus* infection.

Pathophysiology
Necrotizing fasciitis is a progressive, rapidly spreading infection of the deep fascia that spreads along superficial and deep fascial planes. The infection is initially insidious, but becomes overwhelming and results in tissue necrosis. The mortality is as high as 25 percent, and increases to 70 percent when associated with sepsis or renal failure.

Signs and symptoms
- Infection, initially unremarkable, if noticed
- Fever, chills
- Pain progressing to anesthesia
- Erythemia, progressing to supralesional vesiculation, ulcers, blistering necrosis
- Hypotension, altered level of consciousness

Treatment
- Antibiotic therapy
- Hyperbaric oxygen
- Intravenous immunoglobulin
- Surgical debridement

13. Discuss the importance of and precautions involved in treating infections by antibiotic-resistant organisms and multidrug-resistant organisms.   p. 798

Several antibiotic-resistant strains of pathogenic microorganisms have developed during the past several years including methicillin-resistant *Staphylococcus aureus* (MRSA) and vancomycin-resistant enterococcus (VRE). Infection or colonization with antibiotic-resistant organisms (AROs) has become a challenge for both the patient whose treatment is dependent on eradication of an infectious pathogen and for the health care institutions that must manage these patients within their organizations. Many health care professionals are uninformed or misinformed about AROs and believe these organisms to be more virulent. Antibiotic-resistant organisms are of special concern because they are multidrug resistant and, therefore, have limited treatment options. Patients who are colonized or infected with an ARO will often be managed with Standard Precautions and Contact Precautions. All health care organizations should have an infection control plan with policies and procedures in place for managing persons, including patients and employees, colonized or infected with AROs.

14. Describe the rising threat of bioterrorism.   p. 799

Shortly after September 11, 2001 the United States faced another terrorist attack on its citizens, but this time a biological weapon, anthrax, was used. Several letters laden with anthrax spores were mailed to various governmental offices and media companies. While the exact numbers of infected persons is not known at this time, at least 22 people became ill with cutaneous or inhalation anthrax including a 10-month-old baby, and at least six persons died of inhalation anthrax. The CDC, in their bioterrorism guidance materials for health care providers and public health officials, have identified the following biological agents as having the most concern from a public health standpoint:

- *Bacillus anthracis* (anthrax)
- *Yersinia pestis* (plague)
- Variola major (smallpox)
- *Clostridium botulinum* toxin (botulism)
- *Francisella tularensis* (tularemia)
- Filovirus (Ebola hemorrhagic fever, Marburg hemorrhagic fever)
- Arenaviruses (Lassa fever), Junin (Argentine hemorrhagic fever), and related viruses

The National Emergency Response and Rescue Training Center includes the following biological agents (in addition to those listed with the CDC guidance) in their training programs:

- *Vibrio cholerae* (cholera)
- *Coxiella burnetii* (Q fever)
- Venezuelan equine encephalitis
- Ricin
- Saxitoxin

- Staphylococcal enterotoxin B
- Brucellosis
- *Burkholderia mallei* (glanders)
- *Burkholderia pseudomallei* (melioidosis)
- *Salmonella typhi* (typhoid fever)
- *Rickettsia typhi* (typhus)
- Chikungunya virus
- Congo-Crimean hemorrhagic fever virus
- Dengue fever
- Rift Valley fever virus
- Yellow fever

15. **Discuss the etiology, transmission, pathophysiology, signs and symptoms, and treatment of the following bioterrorism agents:**

   a. **Anthrax**   p. 800

   ### Etiology
   Bacillus anthracis

   ### Transmission
   Cutaneous anthrax is transmitted by contact with the tissues, skin/hide, or hair of infected animals or by biting insects that have fed on infected animals. Inhalation anthrax is spread via the airborne route by the inhalation of spores. Intestinal anthrax is transmitted via the ingestion of contaminated food, especially meat.

   ### Pathophysiology
   Humans are fairly resistant to cutaneous invasion of anthrax, which requires a break in the skin for entry into the body. An ulcer forms, producing an area of coagulation necrosis, which leads to eschar formation and edema around the lesion. As anthrax multiplies, it may enter the bloodstream and travel to other organs.

   Inhalation anthrax occurs after spores are inhaled and deposited in the alveoli, where they are ingested by alveolar macrophages and carried to the lymph nodes. Infection spreads, resulting in pulmonary edema and hemorrhagic mediastinitis.

   Intestinal anthrax results in local lesions, similar to cutaneous form, predominately in the cecum.

   ### Signs and symptoms
   - Cutaneous anthrax
     - Itching, rash formation
     - Formation of black eschar
     - Septicemia, if infection spreads to blood
   - Inhalational anthrax
     - Fever
     - Respiratory distress, cyanosis
     - Shock
     - Widened mediastinum on chest radiograph
   - Intestinal anthrax
     - Abdominal pain. N/V, diarrhea
     - Loss of appetite
     - Fever, dehydration

   ### Treatment
   - Antibiotic therapy
   - Respiratory support

b. Smallpox p. 801

Etiology
Variola virus of the Orthpoxvirus genus.

Transmission
Transmission occurs via the contact and airborne routes.

Pathophysiology
After inhalation and deposition on the respiratory mucosa, the virus enters respiratory epithelial cells and multiplies. Asymptomatic viremia follows, resulting in infection of the brain, intestines, kidneys, liver, and skin. Viral multiplication in the skin results in a rash that turns into the characteristic pustule when the cell-mediated response kicks in. These pustules leave behind significant scars that stay with afflicted patients for the rest of their lives. A historical example of this is the pockmarked mummy of King Ramses V, Egypt.

Signs and symptoms
- Fever, chills, myalgia, headache, vomiting
- Initial papular, progressing to vesicular rash
- Lesions then become pustular prior to drying and scabbing

Treatment
- Supportive
- Vaccine if administered early in incubation period

c. Plague p. 801

Etiology
Caused by the anaerobic, intracellular, gram-negative bacillus *Yersinia pestis*.

Transmission
Plague is spread by the bites of arthropods (mainly fleas), the inhalation of airborne respiratory droplets, and contact with buboe fluid.

Pathophysiology
There are three forms of plague: bubonic, pulmonary, and septicemic.

In bubonic plague, the bite of a vector (flea) deposits the bacillis in the skin, and the lymph tissue is invaded. A bubo (inflamed, hemorrhagic, necrotic lymph node) is formed, and the infection spreads through the lymphatic system to the thoracic duct, where the bacillis enters the bloodstream. Bronchopneumonia, bacteremia, and septicemia ensue, and the bacillis can travel in the bloodstream to infect every organ. Pulmonic plague occurs when the inhaled bacillis is deposited in alveoli. Severe and rapid bronchopneumonia and septicemia ensues, and the infection may spread in the blood to all organs.

Septicemic plague occurs when bacilli are deposited directly into the vasculature, not the lymphatics. Sepsis occurs without the characteristic bubo.

Signs and symptoms
- Bubonic plague
  - Fever, chills, headache
  - Malaise, myalgia, swollen and painful lymph nodes
- Pneumonic plague
  - Productive cough
  - Hemoptysis
  - Respiratory distress, failure
- Septicemic plague
  - Abdominal pain
  - Shock, coma

Treatment
- Antibiotic therapy
  - Doxycycline
  - Ciprofloxacin
- Supportive care
  - Respiratory

d. Botulism   p. 802

Etiology
Botulism is caused by the gram-positive, spore-forming anaerobe bacteria *Clostridium botulinum*.

Transmission
Food botulism is spread when preformed toxins are ingested with food. Infant botulism occurs when toxins are spread by organisms colonizing the infant. Wound botulism occurs when toxins are spread by organisms infecting a wound.

Pathophysiology
Clostridium botulinum consists of seven different strains of organism (A–G), three of which are capable of disease in humans (A, B, and E). Regardless of the mode of entry into humans, once the toxin enters the bloodstream, it acts in a similar manner to produce the characteristic signs and symptoms. Botulism toxin binds to receptors on the presynaptic membranes of cholinergic synapses, is taken up into the terminal, and then interferes with neurotransmitter release from the terminal, creating paralysis.

Neurotransmitter blockade is permanent until the axon grows a new terminal to replace the damaged one. The toxin affects peripheral cholinergic nerve terminals, including those at neuromuscular junctions, postganglionic parasympathetic nerve endings, and peripheral ganglia. A characteristic bilateral descending paralysis of the muscles innervated by cranial, spinal, and cholinergic autonomic nerves results, but no impairment of adrenergic or sensory nerves occurs.

Signs and symptoms
- Blurred/double vision
- Descending weakness/paralysis
- Dysphagia, dry mouth
- Constipation, diarrhea, vomiting

Treatment
- Antitoxoin
- Antibiotic therapy
- Supportive care
  - Respiratory
  - Wound debridement

e. Tularemia   p. 802

Etiology
Tularemia is caused by the gram-negative, pleomorphic bacterium, *Francisella tularensis*.

Transmission
Transmission can occur via a tick bite, contact with open wounds, by ingesting contaminated food or water, or by inhalation of the bacteria.

Pathophysiology
Bacillus is introduced into the host via inhalation, ingestion, or intradermal injection, and the clinical progression reflects the mode of transmission. Inoculation via tick vector is the most common mode of transmission. Following an incubation period of one to 14 days, papulae formation and ulceration occur, followed by fever and swelling of the lymph nodes. The bacteria then become trapped in the reticuloendothelial system, where they can survive for a long period of time. Bacteremia develops. Inhalation of the bacillus can result in pulmonic tularemia.

Signs and symptoms
- Ulcer at infection site
- Swollen, painful lymph nodes
- N/V, abdominal pain, diarrhea
- Painful purulent conjunctivitis
- Signs or symptoms of septicemia, pneumonia

Treatment
- Antibiotic therapy
- Supportive care

f. and g. Filoviruses (hemorrhagic fevers: Ebola, Marburg; Arenavirus (Lassa fever).   p. 803

Etiology
Viral hemorrhagic fever (VHF) is caused by an RNA virus from several different viral families, Arenaviridae, Bunyaviridae, Filoviridae, and Flaviviridae.

Transmission
Transmission occurs via contact with infected blood and body fluids.

Pathophysiology
The primary effect of infection with any of the viruses that result in VHS is increased vascular permeability. Early signs of flushing, petechial hemorrhage, and conjuctival hemorrhage preceed the more dramatic frank hemorrhaging from the mucus membranes and subsequent hypotension, shock, multiple organ failure, and death.

Signs and symptoms
- Fever, malaise, myalgia, headache
- Vomiting, diarrhea
- Maculopapular rash
- Bleeding from gums, mucous membranes
- Shock, organ failure

Treatment
Supportive

h. Hantavirus   p. 803

Etiology
Hantaviruses are RNA zoonotic viruses that are members of the family Bunyaviridae.

Transmission
Inhalation via the aerosolization of rodent excrement is the route of transmission.

Pathophysiology
After infection via the inhalation of aerosolized virus, respiratory endothelial cells are the preferential target. Viral antigens produced by the host's immune response penetrate the respiratory epithelium. Increased pulmonary vasculature permeability results in pulmonary edema, and cardiac depression via an unknown mechanism ensues.

Signs and symptoms
- Fever, GI symptoms, myalgia
- Respiratory distress, respiratory failure, cardiogenic shock

Treatment
- Supportive care
  - Respiratory
  - Circulatory

©2007 Pearson Education, Inc.
Critical Care Paramedic

i. Cholera

p. 803

Etiology
Vibrio cholerae, a gram-negative aerobic bacillus.

Transmission
Transmission occurs via the ingestion of contaminated food or water.

Pathophysiology
Vibrio cholerae produces enterotoxin that promotes secretion of fluid and electrolytes into the small intestine and promotes an increase in cAMP activity, which blocks the absorption of sodium and chloride and increases secretion of chloride. The large volume of fluid entering the colon overwhelms the colon's ability to reabsorb water, and severe diarrhea results.

Signs and symptoms
- Acute onset of uncontrollable diarrhea

Treatment
- Fluid, electrolyte replacement
- Antibiotic therapy
  - Tetracycline
  - Erythromycin

j. Q fever

p. 804

Etiology
Q fever is a rickettsial disease caused by *C. burnetii.*

Transmission
Transmission of the rickettsia occurs via the airborne route.

Pathophysiology
The inhalation of a single organism can result in the disease, affecting the pulmonary system. The incubation period is 9 to 40 days.

Signs and symptoms
- Fever, chills, headache, myalgia, malaise, weakness
- Dry cough, dyspnea
- N/V, abdominal pain, maculopapular rash

Treatment
- Supportive care
- Antibiotic therapy

k. Brucellosis

p. 804

Etiology
Brucellosis is caused by members of the bacterial genus *Brucellae*, a gram-negative, non-spore-forming, aerobic organism.

Transmission
Transmission occurs via the airborne and contact routes.

Pathophysiology
Inhaled bacteria are deposited in the alveoli, where they are ingested by macrophages and delivered to the lymph nodes. The bacteria multiply in lymph nodes, then spread to cause local and systemic infections in the liver, kidney, spleen, and joints. The bacteria may also enter through breaks in the skin, and the mucus membranes with same result.

Signs and symptoms
- Weakness, lethargy, anorexia, weight loss, myalgias
- Diaphoresis, depression
- Abdominal pain, arthralgia, headache

Treatment
- Supportive care
- Antimicrobial therapy
  - Rifampin
  - Doxycycline
  - Streptomycin
  - Gentamycin
  - Trimethoprim-sulfamethaoxazole

16. **Discuss the effects and prevention of various toxins—both naturally occurring and weaponized:**

   a. **Ricin**   p. 804
      Ricin is a cytotoxin produced during processing of castor beans that inhibits protein synthesis and results in cell death.

   b. **Saxitoxin**   p. 805
      Saxitoxin is a neurotoxin produced by blue-green algae, crabs, and the blue-ringed octopus. It blocks the movement of sodium ions through voltage-dependent sodium channels in nerve and muscle membranes.

   c. **SEB**   p. 805
      SEB is an exotoxin produced by *Staphylococcus aureus*, with pathological characteristics similar to toxic shock syndrome.

   d. **Mycotoxins**   p. 805
      Mycotoxins are produced by fungi, and inhibit intracellular protein synthesis resulting in a breakdown in DNA and chromosomal abnormalities.

Case Study

Your critical care ground transport team has been called to a rural community hospital for a patient with a fever and cough. The attending physician tells you that the patient is a 42-year-old male who needs to be transferred to the tertiary center where your program is based for an infectious disease consult. The patient was recently relocated to the area after being displaced from a major metropolitan area by a natural disaster. The patient was homeless in his city of origin, but for the past two weeks has been living in a local shelter for displaced persons. Staff on the night shift at the shelter noted that he had a severe cough with a low-grade temperature, and sent the patient to the emergency department for evaluation. He was brought to the emergency department by EMS who gave him one nebulized, albuterol treatment en route. On arrival, he complained only of cough, which he felt had improved after the breathing treatment. He denies any medical history. He admits to a history of IV drug abuse, but says that he has been "clean" for a year. He has been homeless, living intermittently on the street or in shelters, since losing his job due to substance abuse problems. Laboratory data was significant only for a slightly elevated white blood cell count. Chest X-ray shows a right lower lobe infiltrate with hilar adenopathy. The patient was diagnosed with right lower lobe pneumonia and is being transferred to rule out tuberculosis. After donning gloves, gown, and an N95 respirator, you enter the patient's room and introduce yourself. He is alert, sitting up on the stretcher in no apparent distress, and receiving oxygen at 2 lpm via nasal prongs. As you begin your assessment, you discuss the details of the transfer with the patient, as well as the need to limit any unnecessary exposures to his respiratory secretions. He tells you that he understands and agrees to wear a mask in public areas and to be very careful about containing any coughs or sneezes. As you finish your assessment, your partner, who has also donned personal protective equipment, enters the room and tells you that the ambulance is ready. While you were assessing the patient, he shut the walk-through door between the cab and patient compartment, turned on the patient compartment vent and air conditioning, and set the cab ventilation to create a positive pressure environment. Giving the patient a mask to wear, you move to the ambulance. After loading the patient into the ambulance, your partner removes his PPE and moves to the cab. Throughout the transport you leave your PPE in place. You contact the receiving facility early in the transport to be sure they are aware of the need for an isolation room upon your arrival. The transfer is uneventful, and on arrival at the destination, the patient replaces his mask and your partner again applies PPE for the move into the facility. The patient is moved to a stretcher in a reverse airflow room in the emergency department and a report is given to the staff. After properly disposing of your PPE, you thoroughly wash your hands before writing your run report. In the meantime, your partner cleans and disinfects the ambulance.

DISCUSSION QUESTIONS

1. What is the importance of having a working knowledge of the infectious diseases commonly encountered in the critical care setting?
2. Define and explain the role of Standard, Airborne, Contact, and Droplet Precautions in preventing transmission of infectious disease.

Content Review

MULTIPLE CHOICE

_____ 1. Which of the following statements regarding infectious disease (ID) is false?
  A. ID is caused by the invasion and multiplication of pathogenic microorganisms in the body.
  B. Etiologies of ID include bacteria, viruses, fungi, and protozoa.
  C. In a healthy human, the body's natural defenses are capable of stopping all infectious pathogens from invading the body and causing disease.
  D. All of the above.

_____ 2. *Neisseria meningitides*, *Mycobacterium tuberculosis*, and *Clostridium tetani* are all examples of:
  A. bacteria.　　　　　　　　　　C. fungi.
  B. viruses.　　　　　　　　　　　D. rickettsia.

_____ 3. Hepatitis, measles, and rubella are examples of _____ diseases.
  A. viral.　　　　　　　　　　　　C. fungal.
  B. bacterial.　　　　　　　　　　D. protozoal.

_____ 4. Rocky Mountain spotted fever, scrub typhus, and Q fever are examples of _____ diseases.
  A. rickettsial　　　　　　　　　C. bacterial
  B. viral　　　　　　　　　　　　D. protozoal

_____ 5. _____ are abnormal proteins that enter CNS tissue and induce a change in the morphology of intracellular proteins, resulting in disease.
  A. Viruses　　　　　　　　　　　C. Helminthes
  B. Prions　　　　　　　　　　　　D. Metazoa

_____ 6. Tapeworms, roundworms, liver flukes, and pinworms are examples of:
  A. protozoa.　　　　　　　　　　C. helminths.
  B. prions.　　　　　　　　　　　D. rickettsia.

_____ 7. Persons or animals that become infected with pathogenic organisms are known as
_____ of the organism or infection.
   A. hosts   C. sources
   B. carriers   D. all of the above

_____ 8. A _____ is a living organism that transfers a pathogen to a host.
   A. vehicle   C. fromite
   B. vector   D. all of the above

_____ 9. A paramedic acquires MRSA from handling soiled bed linen after an interfacility
transport while not wearing gloves. The mode of transmission, in this case, is termed:
   A. direct contact.   C. vector.
   B. indirect contact.   D. none of the above.

_____ 10. Which of the following is an example of vehicle transmission of an infectious organism?
   A. transmission via a contaminated syringe
   B. inhalation of spores
   C. transmission via an arthropod bite
   D. contact with sputum located on the bench seat of an ambulance

_____ 11. BSI Precautions require that caregivers wash their hands after removing gloves.
   A. True
   B. False

_____ 12. Adherence to Universal Precautions provides protection against droplet and airborne
disease transmission.
   A. True
   B. False

_____ 13. Which of the following statements regarding Standard Precautions is true?
   A. Standard Precautions combine the salient features of Universal Precautions and Body
      Substance Isolation procedures.
   B. Standard Precautions protect against blood, all body fluids, secretions and excretions
      (except sweat), nonintact skin, and mucous membranes.
   C. Standard Precautions include specific recommendations to protect against the
      airborne, contact, and droplet routes of transmission.
   D. All of the above.

_____ 14. According to Standard Precaution guidelines, a patient diagnosed with tuberculosis
would require which of the following precautions?
   A. droplet precautions   C. contact precautions
   B. airborne precautions   D. all of the above

_____ 15. Immunizations are available for all of the following infectious diseases except:
   A. hepatitis B.   C. tuberculosis.
   B. mumps.   D. pneumococcal disease.

_____ 16. Unvaccinated healthcare workers, and those who fail to maintain their immunity, pose a
risk to:
   A. themselves.   C. friends.
   B. family.   D. all of the above.

_____ 17. Which of the following is the least likely clinical or lab finding expected to be found in a
patient with hepatitis?
   A. jaundice
   B. increased serum alanine aminotransferase (ALT) and aspartate
      aminotransferase (AST)
   C. dark urine and bilirubinemia
   D. hepatic atrophy

_____ 18. The organism most often associated with epiglottitis in children is:
A. *Haemophilus influenzae* type B.
B. *Streptococcus pneumoniae.*
C. *Pneumococcus.*
D. *Haemophilus parainfluenzae.*

_____ 19. The treatment of epiglottitis is least likely to include:
A. steroids.
B. antibiotics.
C. bronchodilators.
D. oxygen.

_____ 20. Influenza occurs secondary to a _____ infection.
A. bacterial
B. viral
C. fungal
D. rickettsial

_____ 21. The *M. tuberculosis* bacillis is transmitted primarily through which of the following routes?
A. airborne
B. contact
C. vector
D. vehicle

_____ 22. Infection with *M. tuberculosis* is most likely to result in which of the following clinical findings?
A. nonproductive cough, fever, diaphoresis
B. pleuritic chest pain, swollen lymph nodes, productive cough
C. chest pain, hemoptysis, weight loss, fatigue
D. anorexia, altered mental status, pulmonary edema

_____ 23. The critical care paramedic can protect himself from infection by *M. tuberculosis* during transport by:
A. placing a surgical mask on the patient.
B. using a N95 respirator.
C. opening the windows in the patient compartment of the ambulance.
D. all of the above.

_____ 24. Medications used to treat active TB include all of the following except:
A. rifampin.
B. isoniazid.
C. erythromysin.
D. ethambutol.

_____ 25. The pathogen responsible for severe acute respiratory syndrome (SARS) is a:
A. bacteria.
B. coronavirus.
C. adenovirus.
D. rotavirus.

_____ 26. Individuals infected with SARS are considered to be contagious:
A. for ten to 14 days.
B. as long as they have symptoms.
C. for up to ten days after fever has abated.
D. only during the incubation period.

_____ 27. The management of SARS is least likely to include which of the following?
A. administration of oxygen
B. administration of intravenous fluids
C. ABG analysis
D. administration of antibiotics

_____ 28. Which of the following best describes meningitis?
A. Meningitis is an infection of the meninges of the brain resulting from viral infection.
B. Meningitis is a life-threatening infection of the central nervous system tissue.
C. Meningitis is a potentially life-threatening viral or bacterial infection of the meninges and cerebral spinal fluid.
D. Meningitis is a potential life-threatening illness, resulting from bacterial invasion of the central nervous system.

_____ 29. Which of the following diagnostic exams is the least useful in the evaluation of meningitis?
A. radiograph
B. rapid antigen panels
C. lumbar puncture and CSF examination
D. CT scan

_____ 30. Symptoms associated with meningitis include:
   A. photophobia, anorexia, listlessness, and negative Babinski reflex.
   B. fever, headache, photophobia, mental status changes, and altered mental status.
   C. sunken fontanels, positive Babinski reflex, tachycardia, and listlessness.
   D. URI symptoms, petechial rash, fever, and altered level of consciousness.

_____ 31. Meningococcal infections are caused by the invasion of the blood stream by the organism:
   A. *Streptococcus pneumoniae.*   C. meningoencephalitis.
   B. *Haemophilus meningococcus.*   D. *Neisseria meningitides.*

_____ 32. Signs and symptoms associated with meningococcal infection include:
   A. fever, conjunctivitis, coryza, malaise, and anorexia.
   B. photophobia, anorexia, listlessness, and a negative Babinski reflex.
   C. URI symptoms, petechial rash, fever, and altered level of consciousness.
   D. fever, headache, photophobia, mental status changes, and altered mental status.

_____ 33. Patients with meningococcal infection are considered noninfectious:
   A. 24 hours after the beginning of effective antibiotic therapy.
   B. after all signs and symptoms have abated.
   C. when serum white blood cell counts return to normal.
   D. after antibody titers return to normal levels.

_____ 34. Management of meningococcal infection is least likely to involve which of the following?
   A. administration of antiviral medications
   B. providing the patient with a quiet, darkened environment
   C. administration of dopamine
   D. administration of penicillin G

_____ 35. Which of the following complications is least likely to occur with meningococcal infection?
   A. bacteremia   C. hepatitis
   B. meningitis   D. dehydration and electrolyte imbalance

_____ 36. There is no vaccine available to prevent meningococcal infection.
   A. True
   B. False

_____ 37. The measles virus can be transmitted via:
   A. droplet contact.   C. direct contact.
   B. indirect contact.   D. all of the above.

_____ 38. Which of the following infectious diseases does not typically present with a macropapular rash?
   A. measles   C. mumps
   B. chickenpox varicella D. measles

_____ 39. A vaccine is available for which of the following infectious diseases?
   A. mumps   C. measles
   B. rubella   D. all of the above

_____ 40. A patient with chicken pox is considered infectious until:
   A. after the 21st day from exposure.   C. either A or B.
   B. all lesions are dry.   D. none of the above.

_____ 41. Which of the following classes of medications is least likely to be used in the treatment of gastroenteritis?
   A. diuretics   C. antibiotics
   B. antivirals   D. antiemetics

42. Complications associated with gastroenteritis include:
   A. hypotension, necrotizing enteritis, pulmonary edema, and cardiogenic shock.
   B. hypotension, hypovolemic shock, kidney failure, and DIC.
   C. hypovolemic shock, liver failure, MSOD, and increased ICP.
   D. necrotic bowel, electrolyte abnormalities, hypertension, and shock.

43. *Clostridium tetani* requires a deep puncture wound for transmission to occur and infection to develop.
   A. True
   B. False

44. If allowed to progress, tetanus will lead to:
   A. contraction of the respiratory muscles, respiratory failure, and death.
   B. cardiac tetany, heart failure, and death.
   C. hepatic failure, encephalopathy, and coma.
   D. none of the above.

45. Treatment of tetanus may include all of the following except:
   A. use of NMBAs.
   B. administration of TIG.
   C. tetanus antitoxin.
   D. antiviral agents.

46. Uncontrolled muscular contractions starting at the neck and progressing to the trunk are characteristic for which of the following infections?
   A. *Clostridium tetani*
   B. *Staphylococcus aureus*
   C. *Haemophilus aphrophilus*
   D. none of the above

47. Septicemia can develop secondary to the introduction of a pathogenic organism into the bloodstream via:
   A. rupture of organs.
   B. surgical or diagnostic procedures.
   C. intravenous catheters.
   D. all of the above.

48. Treatment of septicemia is least likely to include the administration of which of the following?
   A. antibiotics
   B. vasopressors
   C. nitrates
   D. fluid

49. _____ is a potentially life- and/or limb-threatening soft tissue infection characterized by widespread fascial necrosis.
   A. Toxic shock syndrome
   B. Necrotizing fasciitis
   C. Septicemia
   D. Gastroenteritis

50. Treatment for necrotizing fasciitis is likely to include all of the following except:
   A. administration of immunoglobulin.
   B. surgical debridement.
   C. hyperbaric oxygen.
   D. administration of steroids.

51. Which of the following is an example of an antibiotic-resistant strain of bacteria?
   A. methicillin-resistant *Streptococcus aureus*
   B. vancomycin-resistant *Haemophilus*
   C. penicillin-resistant enterococcus
   D. methicillin-resistant *Staphylococcus aureus*

52. The three categories of anthrax infection are:
   A. pulmonary, lymphatic, and gastrointestinal.
   B. inhalation, cutaneous, and intestinal.
   C. inhalation, lymphatic, and cutaneous.
   D. pulmonary, extrapulmonary, and cutaneous.

53. Which of the following is the preferred antimicrobial for the treatment of anthrax?
   A. penicillin
   B. ciprofloxacin
   C. anthrax antibody A1
   D. viromicinase

_____ 54. Which of the following diseases is caused by the variola virus?
   A. chickenpox
   B. measles
   C. smallpox
   D. botulism

_____ 55. A vaccine exists for the virus that causes smallpox.
   A. True
   B. False

_____ 56. A patient with smallpox is considered infectious until:
   A. 12 to 14 days after the abatement of signs and symptoms.
   B. he has a negative antibody titer.
   C. seven days after the abatement of fever.
   D. all lesions have dried and fallen off.

_____ 57. The treatment for a patient with smallpox who is noted to have flulike complaints and numerous postural lesions consists of:
   A. the administration of smallpox vaccine.
   B. the administration of steroids, diuretics, and analgesics.
   C. supportive measures only.
   D. none of the above.

_____ 58. Infection with the microorganism _Yersinia pestis_ results in which of the following diseases?
   A. smallpox
   B. plague
   C. botulism
   D. tularemia

_____ 59. The term "bubonic plague" describes:
   A. the characteristic "buboes" that appear on the chest radiograph of a patient with the disease.
   B. the painful abdominal masses that accompany the septicemic manifestation of the disease.
   C. the characteristic swollen, painful, and necrotic lymph nodes that accompany the disease.
   D. none of the above.

_____ 60. Patients with septicemic or pneumonic plague who do not receive treatment:
   A. will absolutely die.
   B. will probably die.
   C. have about a 50 percent chance of survival.
   D. almost always live.

_____ 61. A vaccine exists for the virus that causes the plague.
   A. True
   B. False

_____ 62. Postexposure prophylaxis for pneumonic plague includes:
   A. tetracycline and chloramphenicol.
   B. streptomycin or gentamycin.
   C. doxycycline or tetracycline.
   D. doxycycline or ciprofloxacin.

_____ 63. Treatment for a patient with pneumonic plague would most likely include supportive care along with the administration of:
   A. antibiotics and diuretics.
   B. NMBAs, sedatives, and diuretics.
   C. antibiotics.
   D. antiviral agents.

_____ 64. Which of the toxin types from the organism _Clostridium botulinum_ are most likely to cause disease in humans?
   A. C, D, F, and G
   B. A, B, and E
   C. A, B, C, D, and E
   D. none of the above

_____ 65. Which of the following is the definitive pharmacological treatment for botulism?
   A. antivirals
   B. antibiotics
   C. antitoxins
   D. antigens

_____ 66. Botulism is spread via the _____ transmission route.
   A. vehicle   C. airborne
   B. droplet   D. direct contact

_____ 67. Smallpox is spread via the _____ transmission route.
   A. airborne   C. indirect contact
   B. direct contact   D. all of the above

_____ 68. Anthrax is spread via the _____ transmission route.
   A. airborne   C. vehicle
   B. contact   D. all of the above

_____ 69. The pathogen *Francisella tularensis* is spread via the _____ transmission route.
   A. contact   C. vector
   B. vehicle   D. all of the above

_____ 70. Which of the following diseases is not considered a hemorrhagic fever?
   A. Lassa fever   C. Ebola
   B. Q fever   D. Marburg fever

_____ 71. Infection with which of the following pathogens may produce sudden onset of fever, headache, vomiting, diarrhea, maculopapular rash, and bleeding from gums and mucous membranes?
   A. arenavirus   C. *Francisella tularensis*
   B. hantavirus   D. variola virus

_____ 72. Which of the following statements regarding *Vibrio cholerae* is false?
   A. It is a bacteria.
   B. It produces an enterotoxin resulting in explosive diarrhea.
   C. The organism is transmitted by ingesting food or water contaminated with the feces or vomitus of infected persons.
   D. Most cases of *Vibrio cholerae* infection in the United States result from the ingestion of contaminated honey.

_____ 73. Antibiotic administration would be expected to have the least effect on which of the following organisms?
   A. *Coxiella burnetii*   C. *Brucella*
   B. *Vibrio cholerae*   D. staphylococcus enterotoxin

_____ 74. _____ is a neurotoxin produced by marine organisms such as the blue-ringed octopus and crabs.
   A. Saxitoxin   C. Rickettsia
   B. Mycotoxins   D. Ricin

_____ 75. Which of the following toxins has an existing vaccine?
   A. ricin   C. saxitoxin
   B. SEB   D. none of the above

_____ 76. Which of the following toxins has an existing antidote?
   A. ricin   C. saxitoxin
   B. mycotoxin   D. none of the above

27 Pediatric Medical Emergencies

Review of Chapter Objectives

Upon completion of this chapter, the student should be able to:

1. **Discuss why the critical care paramedic must remain aware of the special concerns surrounding the assessment and management of the pediatric patient.**   p. 812

Evaluation of the infant, child, or adolescent must be comprehensive and includes both physical and psychological factors. The need to understand the pediatric patient population and its pathophysiology is great, because more than 20,000 pediatric deaths occur each year in the United States. In addition, an increasing number of ill and injured pediatric patients require the services of the critical care transport team. As such, the critical care paramedic must have the ability to properly assess and manage the critical pediatric patient, and this cannot be overstated. Providing optimum care to these young patients can only be achieved by obtaining an appropriate clinical history and then coupling it with an effective physical exam. In fact, the critical care transport team must be capable of providing care to the pediatric patient in essentially the same manner that care would be delivered in a pediatric intensive care unit (PICU). When transporting pediatric patients, the critical care transport should be treated as an extension of the PICU.

2. **Understand the physiological differences between the adult and the pediatric patient.**   p. 813

Pediatric patients have significant physiological differences compared to an adult, differences that affect assessment, management, and transport decisions. Specific areas of concern are metabolism and thermoregulation, glucose requirements, airway, and the pulmonary and cardio systems.

Thermoregulation in the pediatric patient is affected by the increased surface area-to-volume ratio, which is four times that of an adult. With heat production only one and one-half times as high as that of an adult, there is a greater risk of hypothermia for a pediatric patient. Heat loss can occur as a result of convection, radiation, evaporation, or conduction.

Infants also have underdeveloped muscular innervation, which excludes shivering as a method of thermogenesis. An infant's higher basal metabolic rate (BMR) will result in the production of more heat, but also creates an increase in oxygen consumption (almost two times more than that of an adult), and a relatively faster onset of hypoxemia and hypercapnia during instances of inadequate oxygenation and ventilation.

Infants are at greater risk for developing hypoglycemia secondary to decreased glycogen stores, immature hepatic development resulting in decreased glycogenolysis, increased metabolic rate resulting in increased glucose requirements, or preexisting diabetes.

Pediatric patients have unique airway anatomy and physiology compared to adults that greatly affect their response to disease and trauma, as well as your approach to airway control. Specific differences in pediatric airway anatomy include:

- Larger tongue in relation to oropharynx
- Nares proportionally smaller

- Trachea more narrow and pliable
- Epiglottis is larger, less supported, and omega-shaped
- Larynx more superior, anterior
- Narrowest part of pediatric airway is at the level of the cricoid ring

A larger tongue in comparison to the oropharynx results in less room for airway swelling and a greater risk of airway occlusion. The smaller external nares may occlude easier from edema, mucus or blood accumulation, or tissue hypertrophy. The narrower and more pliable pediatric trachea is subject to occlusion from hyperextension/hyperflexion, and from occlusion secondary to swelling, mucus and blood accumulation, and neoplasm. The pediatric epiglottis may be difficult to identify and/or control during intubation. The pediatric larynx is located at the level of the first or second cervical vertebrae, compared to the adult level of fourth or fifth cervical vertebrae; it is superior and anterior compared to the adult. The narrow pediatric cricoid ring acts as a physiological cuff when an endotracheal tube is in place, and can also be the site of occlusion secondary to foreign body aspiration.

The pediatric rib cage, because it is incompletely calcified, is more flexible than that of an adult and unable to support the lungs during times of the great negative intrathoracic pressure that is typical of large volume ventilation attempts. In such instances, accessory muscles are recruited to aid in ventilation. However, because the ribs are more horizontally positioned, the leverage achieved during intercostal muscle contraction in an infant is less than that of an adult, which results in less rib lift during inspiration. In addition, the accessory muscles of infants are less developed, the younger the patient, the less developed the muscles. This, combined with decreased rigidity of the chest wall, contributes to diaphragmatic breathing in the infant. During inspiration, the infant experiences less increase in anterior/posterior chest diameter, less increase in intrathoracic volume, and a smaller tidal volume. Infants have a lower pulmonary reserve capacity than adults as the relatively large heart decreases available room for lung expansion. In addition, a small abdominal cavity filled with relatively large abdominal organs tends to impede diaphragmatic movement; decompressing the stomach can increase diaphragm motility.

The pediatric heart is able to increase heart rate, yet unable to increase contractility during efforts to improve cardiac output. As such, bradycardia is suggestive of drastically reduced cardiac output. Peripheral vascular resistance can be altered significantly through arterial vasoconstriction in an attempt to maintain systolic blood pressure. While the ability to maintain hemodynamically adequate systolic blood pressures is desirable, it is done at the expense of end-organ perfusion in the pediatric patient. A high index of suspicion is required to treat diminished end-organ perfusion before it is clinically evident.

3. **Recognize how the pediatric patient suffering from common medical emergencies may present with differing symptomatology as compared to the adult.** p. 816

Due to a decreased airway diameter, pediatric patients will develop stridor, or other adventitious sounds indicative of decreased airway diameter, such as wheezing, faster than an adult. The lower pulmonary reserve capacity of neonates and infants contributes to a more rapid development of hypoxia and hypercapnia and their associated signs and symptoms compared to an adult. In addition, infants will also "belly breath" in an attempt to increase intrathoracic area and alveolar ventilation, a sign not typically witnessed in adults with respiratory distress.

The pediatric myocardium can only increase the heart rate in an attempt to improve cardiac output and not the stroke volume (as can an adult); the pediatric heart has low compliance as it relates to volume and therefore cannot compensate by increasing stroke volume. Consequently, heart rate should be viewed as a significant clinical marker when monitoring cardiac output in the pediatric patient. Tachycardia is a sign of compensation of hemodynamic demise. When the pediatric patient becomes bradycardic, you should assume that the patient's cardiac output has been drastically reduced.

The second distinction that should be made pertains to the ability of the child to alter peripheral vascular resistance. Since the degree of arterial tone is the other determinant of perfusion pressure (systemic perfusion = cardiac output $\times$ systemic vascular resistance), the critical care paramedic should remember that this age group has the ability to promote vigorous arterial vasoconstriction. The end result is the maintenance of "acceptable" systolic blood pressure in the face of diminished end-organ perfusion. The critical care team should remember that blood pressure is a relatively nondescriptive variable in assessing the quality of peripheral perfusion. By the time there is a recognizable drop in systolic perfusion pressure, there will have already been a significant change in organ perfusion. The key is to maintain a high index of suspicion for conditions that may alter peripheral perfusion, and treat these conditions aggressively with fluids, medications, and the like in an attempt to thwart any diminishment of end-organ perfusion *before* it becomes clinically evident or physiologically significant.

4. Understand the importance of maintaining proficiency in supporting the pediatric patient's airway, breathing, and circulatory function. p. 818

It is important to remember at all times with neonatal, infant, and pediatric patients that the leading cause of cardiopulmonary arrest is airway and breathing insufficiency. If the airway and ventilatory systems are not carefully monitored and managed appropriately when compromises arise, the pediatric patient will degrade rapidly into cardiopulmonary failure and arrest, which carries with it even more abysmal rates for successful resuscitation than seen in the adult population. If early identification and treatment for a failed body system were ever to be stressed, it would involve the ability to maintain airway and ventilations in pediatrics. Support the airway and oxygenate and ventilate, and the cardiovascular system will follow.

That is not to say that cardiovascular support is not an important part of pediatric emergency management. While pediatric patients are capable of compensating for lost intravascular volume for long periods of time, when they decompensate, they decompensate rapidly. Early replacement of intravascular volume is necessary to prevent refractory shock or cardiopulmonary arrest and to reduce the risk of postshock end-organ dysfunction.

5. Be able to discuss the pathophysiology of respiratory complications in the pediatric patient. p. 821

Croup

Epidemiology
Croup is a viral infection that is most common in children after recent upper respiratory infection. There are 50 new cases per 1,000 children during second year of life, and the incidence decreases substantially after the sixth year. Infections typically occur in the fall and winter, with a recurrence rate of about 5 percent.

Pathophysiology
Croup is a viral infection of the subglottic airway. Swelling and edema of the airway results in the development of a barking cough and stridor. The distal airways may be affected by fluid accumulation, edema, and bronchospasm.

Signs and symptoms

- History of illness over past one to three days
- Fever, malaise
- Respiratory distress
- Barking cough

Treatment

- Goal is to prevent airway obstruction
- Maintain calm, quiet environment
- High-flow, high-concentration humidified oxygen as tolerated
  - Moisture aids in reducing airway edema
- Racemic epinephrine via nebulizer
- Steroids
  - Used in conjunction with racemic epinephrine to prevent rebound swelling of airways after epinephrine has worn off
  - Use as a primary means of swelling reduction is controversial
    - Dexamethasone
    - Budesonide

- Endotracheal intubation
  - Only when all other options have been exhausted

Epiglottitis

Epidemiology
There has been a progressive reduction of cases of epiglottitis since the mid 1980s as a result of the Hib vaccine. While it has been traditionally an illness seen in children aged two to seven years, epiglottitis is now being identified in more young adults than in children.

Pathophysiology
Epiglottitis typically results secondary to a bacterial infection, and is characterized by a rapid onset of fever and glottic edema, and upper airway obstruction from edema is possible.

Signs and symptoms
- Rapid onset of fever
- Sore throat, refusal to eat or drink
- Positioning, drooling
- Stridor, respiratory distress

Treatment
- Goal is to prevent upper airway obstruction
- Maintain calm, quiet environment
- High-flow, high-concentration humidified oxygen as tolerated
- BVM ventilations
  - Slow ventilation sequence
- Endotracheal intubation
  - Warranted only in cases of impending airway obstruction
- Needle, surgical cricothyrotomy if needed
- Antibiotic therapy
  - Wide-spectrum antibiotics prior to culture results

Asthma

Epidemiology
There were 14 million persons in the United States with asthma in 2000. Adverse outcomes and deaths from asthma tripled between 1983 and 1996.

Pathophysiology
Asthma may have intrinsic or extrinsic causes, and is a disease of airway edema, mucus production, and bronchoconstriction resulting in the narrowing of the lower airways.

Signs and symptoms
- Respiratory distress
- Wheezing
- Tachycardia
- Prolonged expiratory phase

Treatment
- Goal is to treat airway inflammation, reverse bronchospasm, and correct hypoxia
- High-flow, high-concentration oxygen
- Pharmacology
  - Beta-agonists
    - Often used in conjunction with anticholinergics
    - Albuterol (Proventil, Ventolin)
    - Levalbuterol (Xopenex)
    - Metaproterenol (Alupent)
    - Terbutaline (Breathine)

- Epinephrine
- Isoproterenol (Isuprel)
- Anticholinergics
  - Ipratropium (Atrovent)
  - Atropine
- Corticosteroids:
  - Methylprednisolone (Solu-Medrol)
  - Dexamethasone (Decadron)
  - Hydrocortisone sodium
- Methylxanthines:
  - Aminophylline
- BVM ventilations/endotracheal intubation
  - Allow for prolonged expiratory phase
  - Air trapping

Bronchiolitis

Epidemiology
Bronchiolitis is a viral infection that typically develops in children aged two to 24 months of age. The annual incidence is 11.4 percent in children younger than one year and 6 percent in children aged one to two years. The disease is responsible for about 4,500 deaths and 90,000 hospitalizations each year.

Pathophysiology
Bronchiolitis is most often caused by RSV infection of the lower airways, resulting in inflammation of the bronchial tissue. Infectious by-products accumulate in lower airways and interfere with gas exchange, as well as encourage bronchoconstriction.

Signs and symptoms
- Slow onset of symptoms
- Tachycardia, tachypnea
- Fever, mucus production
- Wheezing, coughing
- Chest tightness

Treatment
- Goal is to reverse bronchospasm, reduce airway inflammation, correct hypoxia, and identify and eradicate offending pathogen
- High flow, high-concentration oxygen
- Beta-agonists
  - Use is controversial
  - Drugs and dosages same as for asthma
- Ribavirin
  - For patients who are confirmed or at high risk for RSV infection
- Endotracheal intubation
  - If necessary, conservative approach recommended

Foreign Body Airway Obstruction (FBAO)

Epidemiology
In 1998, 3,200 deaths (1.2 per 100,000 people) from airway obstruction were reported in the United States. Children under four years of age had the highest mortality at 0.7 per 100,000 people.

Pathophysiology
When a foreign body lodges in the airway (supraglottic, glottic, or subglottic airway), a full or partial airway obstruction occurs, resulting in limited or no ventilation. The development of hypoxemia and hypercapnia, and death may occur if a totally occluded airway is left uncorrected.

Signs and symptoms
- Partial airway obstruction
  - Difficulty breathing
  - Stridor
  - Drooling, coughing
- Complete airway obstruction
  - Inability to:
    - Breathe
    - Talk
    - Cough

Treatment
- Basic airway maneuvers
  - Infants:
    - Back blows
    - Chest thrusts
  - Children
    - Heimlich maneuver
  - Finger sweep, if object visible
- Advanced airway maneuvers
  - Direct laryngoscopy
  - Magill forceps
  - Pushing object into right mainstem with endotracheal tube
  - Needle or surgical cricothyrotomy

6. Understand the pathophysiology of congenital heart disease that is common to the pediatric patient. p. 832

Many types of congenital anomalies exist. These may affect a single organ or structure or may affect many organs or structures. Congenital anomalies are the leading cause of death in infants—causing approximately one-quarter of infant deaths. Several recognized patterns, called *syndromes*, occur. Congenital heart defects (CHDs) are among the most common congenital anomalies encountered, though the cause of CHDs is largely unknown. CHDs are often classified by whether or not they increase pulmonary blood flow, decrease pulmonary blood flow, or obstruct blood flow.

Epidemiology
Congenital anomalies are the number one cause of death in infants over one year old, and the incidence of congenital heart disease (CHD) is about two to ten per 1,000 live births.

Pathophysiology
CHDs are often classified by pathophysiology and include defects that increase pulmonary blood flow, defects that decrease pulmonary blood flow, and defects that obstruct blood flow. Defects that increase pulmonary blood flow include patent ductus arteriosis (PDA), in which the ductus arteriosis fails to close, atrial septal defect, in which a passage between atria allows for mixing of blood, and ventricular septal defect, characterized by the existence of a passage between ventricles that allows for the mixing of blood between them.

Defects that decrease pulmonary blood flow include tetralogy of Fallot and transposition of the great vessels. Tetralogy of Fallot is a combination of four congenital defects: ventricular septal defect, pulmonary valve stenosis, hypertrophic right ventricle, and the positioning of the aorta over the ventricular septal defect. Transposition of the great vessels is a condition in which the positions of the pulmonary and aorta arteries are reversed.

Defects that result in obstruction of blood flow include coarctation of the aorta (the lumen of the aortic arc is narrowed and blood flow obstructed), aortic stenosis/atresia, mitral stenosis/atresia, and pulmonary stenosis/atresia.

7. **Discuss the steps of the initial assessment when caring for a pediatric patient.** p. 834

The following steps and principles should be considered for all pediatric patients, regardless of pathophysiology:

Airway
- Secure and maintain airway as soon as is required and possible.
- Consider RSI in the transport environment.
- Continued use of sedatives and paralytics during transport is helpful.
- Be cautious of, and vigilant for, accidental intubation.
- Use lateral restraints to:
  - Minimize lateral mobility.
  - Minimize likelihood of accidental extubation.

Breathing
- Avoid excessive tidal volume and airway pressures.
  - Risk of barotrauma
- Gastric decompression to reduce diaphragmatic impediment

Vascular access
- Can be difficult even for skilled/experienced providers
- Multiple vascular access options preferable
  - Venous routes
  - Intraosseous routes

Temperature regulation
- Prevent heat loss
- Aggressive warming, if necessary

Hypoglycemia
- Manage hypoglycemia with 25 percent dextrose
  - $D_{50}W$ contraindicated in pediatric population
- Correct hypoglycemia prior to transport

8. **Discuss the pathophysiology of hypoglycemia in the pediatric patient.** p. 836

Infants are at greater risk for developing hypoglycemia secondary to decreased glycogen stores, immature hepatic development, increased metabolic rate, and preexisting TI diabetes.

9. **Summarize the common denominator present in the majority of pediatric arrest situations.** p. 837

The common denominator for deaths seen in the pediatric population is hypoxia secondary to airway and breathing deficits.

Case Studies

Case #1

Your ground critical care transport team has been called to transport an infant to the pediatric intensive care unit (PICU) where your program is based. The patient is an eight-month-old female with respiratory failure. She was seen two days ago by her pediatrician for a 24-hour history of fever, runny nose, and cough. At that time, she was diagnosed with a viral upper respiratory infection (URI) and prescribed acetaminophen and increased fluids by mouth. Early the next morning, the parents brought the patient to the emergency department for respiratory distress. On presentation she had a temperature of 101.8 degrees F, and a weak, moist cough and wheezing.

Case #2

Your team has been called to provide an ALS intercept to a BLS ambulance for an infant with difficulty breathing. The patient is an 18-month-old male who was recently adopted from an orphanage in a socioeconomically depressed country and is behind in normal immunizations. He has had a 12-hour history of high fever and refuses to eat. He presents leaning forward and drooling.

Case #3

The small emergency department where the transfer originates is approximately 75 miles from the tertiary center where your program is based. The patient is a nine-week-old male with a fever and vomiting. The parents brought the baby to the ED because he is irritable and will not eat. The patient has poor muscle tone and his skin is cool and dusky with delayed capillary refill. You note a reddish, nonblanching, purple rash on his chest, arms, and shins. His respirations are rapid, but not labored. His heart rate is 166 beats per minute.

DISCUSSION QUESTIONS

1. For each of the scenarios above:
   a. Determine the most likely cause of the patient's medical emergency.
   b. Briefly outline an appropriate management plan for the patient.

Content Review

MULTIPLE CHOICE

_____ 1. All of the following are characteristic differences in the anatomy of the pediatric airway compared to the adult except:
   A. the trachea is narrower and less pliable.
   B. the tongue is larger in relation to the oropharynx.
   C. the epiglottis is larger and not as well supported.
   D. the larynx is funnel-shaped.

_____ 2. The pediatric larynx sits at about the level of the:
   A. first or second cervical vertebrae.
   B. third or fourth cervical vertebrae.
   C. fourth or fifth cervical vertebrae.
   D. fifth or sixth cervical vertebrae.

_____ 3. Which of the following statements regarding pediatric pulmonary A&P is true?
   A. Pediatric patients are able to recruit significant accessory muscle mass to assist ventilation during periods of respiratory compromise.
   B. The stiff, noncompliant pediatric rib cage allows for considerable increases in anteroposterior chest diameter.
   C. Reduced pulmonary reserve capacity is created in part by a relatively large heart taking up space in the thoracic cavity.
   D. Hypoxemia and hypercapnia take longer to develop in the pediatric patient than in an adult.

©2007 Pearson Education, Inc.
Critical Care Paramedic

_____ 4. The pediatric cardiovascular system will compensate for a decrease in cardiac output by:
A. increasing heart rate.
B. increasing heart rate and stroke volume.
C. increasing stroke volume.
D. none of the above.

_____ 5. The leading cause of cardiac arrest in children is:
A. sepsis.
B. trauma.
C. hypoglycemia.
D. respiratory arrest.

_____ 6. Clinical exam findings consistent with respiratory failure include all of the following except:
A. altered mental status.
B. pallor and cyanosis.
C. bradycardia.
D. inspiratory retractions.

_____ 7. _____ is an acute viral infection characterized by a "barking cough," stridor, and low-grade fever.
A. Epiglottitis
B. Croup
C. Bronchiolitis
D. Pneumonia

_____ 8. _____ is an acute infectious process of the lower respiratory tract common in children under 24 months of age, most often attributed to respiratory syncytial virus or Mycoplasma pneumoniae.
A. Epiglottitis
B. Croup
C. Bronchiolitis
D. Pneumonia

_____ 9. A six-year-old child presenting with rapid onset of a fever, sore throat, and unwillingness to eat or drink is most likely suffering from:
A. epiglottitis.
B. croup.
C. bronchiolitis.
D. asthma.

_____ 10. The management of croup is likely to involve all of the following except:
A. dexamethasone.
B. racemic epinephrine via nebulizer.
C. high flow, high-concentration humidified oxygen.
D. antibacterial agents.

_____ 11. Management of epiglottitis may include all of the following except:
A. racemic epinephrine via nebulizer.
B. antibiotic administration.
C. high flow, high-concentration humidified oxygen.
D. needle or surgical cricothyrotomy.

_____ 12. A conscious and alert five-year-old patient with a history of asthma presenting with acute onset respiratory distress, a SaO_2 of 93 percent, a PCO_2 of 38, pale skin, with moderate intercostal retractions and the ability to speak in partial sentences would be considered to be having a _____ exacerbation of her asthma.
A. mild
B. moderate
C. significant
D. severe

_____ 13. Pharmacological treatment of asthma is least likely to include which of the following?
A. metaproterenol
B. atropine
C. racemic epinephrine
D. aminophylline

_____ 14. _____ is a highly contagious subgroup of myxoviruses that are the predominant causative agent for bronchial infections in children.
A. Hepatitis B
B. HIV
C. Rotavirus
D. RSV

_____ 15. _____ is an acute infection of the lower respiratory tract, most often occurring in children aged two to 24 months.
   A. Epiglottitis
   B. Croup
   C. Bronchiolitis
   D. Asthma

_____ 16. Which of the following treatments for bronchiolitis is considered to have questionable efficacy?
   A. oxygen administration via nonrebreather mask
   B. nebulized beta-agonist administration
   C. administration of nebulized anticholinergics
   D. administration of Ribavirin

_____ 17. Findings consistent with complete FBAO include all of the following except:
   A. stridor.
   B. apnea.
   C. inability to speak.
   D. inability to cough.

_____ 18. Methods utilized to correct FBAO include all of the following except:
   A. use of Magill forceps.
   B. endotracheal intubation.
   C. BVM ventilation.
   D. cricothyroidotomy.

_____ 19. The onset of sepsis in the pediatric patient tends to be obvious and easily identifiable from noninfectious pathology.
   A. True
   B. False

_____ 20. Treatment of sepsis may include:
   A. antiviral therapy.
   B. antibiotic therapy.
   C. antibacterial therapy.
   D. all of the above.

_____ 21. Death secondary to asphyxia occurring within 24 hours of submersion is termed:
   A. drowning.
   B. near-drowning.
   C. wet drowning.
   D. none of the above.

_____ 22. The congenital heart defect in which mixing of atrial blood occurs through a hole between the atria is called a:
   A. ventricular septal defect.
   B. patent ductus arteriosis.
   C. atrial septal defect.
   D. tetralogy of Fallot.

_____ 23. A congenital heart defect that results in increased pulmonary blood flow is:
   A. tetralogy of Fallot.
   B. ventricular septal defect.
   C. coarctation of the aorta.
   D. aortic stenosis.

_____ 24. Congenital heart defects that result in a decrease of blood flow include all of the following except:
   A. mitral stenosis.
   B. patent ductus arteriosus.
   C. coarctation of the aorta.
   D. hypoplastic left heart syndrome.

_____ 25. Congenital heart defects that allow the mixing of oxygenated and deoxygenated blood include all of the following except:
   A. tetralogy of Fallot.
   B. hypoplastic left heart.
   C. tricuspid atresia.
   D. transposition of the great vessels.

_____ 26. The condition in which a defect in the diaphragm that allows some of the abdominal contents to enter the chest is called:
   A. diaphragmatic atresia.
   B. intestinal hernia.
   C. diaphragmatic hernia.
   D. hypoplastic diaphragm.

_____ 27. The management of hypoglycemia in the pediatric patient includes the administration of:
   A. $D_{25}W$ 0.5–1.0 g/kg IV.
   B. $D_{50}W$ 0.5–1.0 g/kg IV.
   C. $D_{10}W$ 0.5 g/kg IV.
   D. $D_{50}W$ 25 g IV.

_____ 28. Infants and small children are at a greater risk for the development of acute hypoglycemia because of:
   A. decreased glycogen stores.
   B. the ability to stimulate the release of stored glycogen from an immature liver.
   C. a decreased metabolic rate.
   D. all of the above.

_____ 29. Pediatric patients have lower basal metabolic rates than do adults.
   A. True
   B. False

_____ 30. Exposure of a pediatric patient to a cool environment or excessive airflow can result in hypothermia secondary to _____ heat loss.
   A. conductive
   B. convective
   C. evaporative
   D. radiative

28 High-Risk Obstetrical/ Gynecological Emergencies

Review of Chapter Objectives

Upon completion of this chapter, the student should be able to:

1. **Describe the anatomy and physiology of the organs and structures of the female reproductive system and fetal gestation.** p. 843

The female reproductive system consists of two ovaries and the female reproductive tract: the paired fallopian tubes, the uterus, and the vagina. This system functions to produce and secrete sex hormones, viable gametes, and also supports, protects, and delivers a developing fetus. After birth, the female reproductive system will provide nourishment to the newborn infant.

Gestation is the time from fertilization of an oocyte until birth, and in a human averages 266 days. A gestation of less than 37 weeks is considered premature, and a gestation of greater than 42 weeks is considered postmature. The gestational period is usually broken down into three trimesters, each three months in duration.

The first trimester is characterized by rapid cell division, implantation of the zygote in the uterine wall, completion of placental development, and development of the foundations of all the major organ systems.

Ovulation occurs at day 14 of the ovarian cycle in response to a surge in luteinizing hormone released from the anterior pituitary. During ovulation, an oocyte (egg) is released from an ovarian follicle located within an ovary. The ovarian follicle then atrophies into a structure called the corpus luteum, which secretes progesterone for a few days to prevent the onset of a new ovarian cycle. The released oocyte is guided into the lumen of the fallopian tube by the fimbriae of the fallopian tube. A combination of ciliary movement and peristaltic contractions propel the oocyte along the length of the isthmus of the fallopian tube. Fertilization, if it occurs, usually takes place in the first one-third of the fallopian tube. After fertilization, the zygote (fertilized egg) immediately divides and continues its travel down the length of the fallopian tube to the uterus.

About four days after fertilization, the zygote reaches the uterine cavity, and, over the next two to three days will continue to divide, forming a hollow sphere of cells called the blastocyst. The blastocyst adheres to the endometrium of the uterus and erodes a path through the epithelial cells and into the functional zone, where all fetal development will take place. During the first few days of implantation, human chorionic gonadotropin (HCG) is produced and this stimulates the corpus luteum to continue the release of progesterone, which prepares the uterus for pregnancy and prevents the start of new ovarian and menstrual cycles during pregnancy.

By day nine, the blastocyst, now termed a syncytial trophoblast, has spread into the surrounding endometrium, eroding endometrial capillaries. Maternal blood leaking from the eroded capillaries flows through channels called lacunae in the syncytial trophoblast. From days nine through 21, fingerlike projections called chorionic villi form on the trophoblast and extend into the endometrium. Embryonic blood vessels develop within the villi, and circulation in these vessels begins. As larger endometrial blood vessels become involved, maternal blood flow through the lacunae increases, and the first exchange between fetal and maternal blood takes place; a primitive placenta has been formed.

During this time period, the entire blastocyst is surrounded by the developing chorionic villi, which expand within the endometrium. As the chorion continues to enlarge, it pushes the endometrium into the lumen of the uterus. Within the chorion, the fetus and amniotic sac float in the fluid-filled chorionic chamber. As the fetus grows, it and the amnion will fill up the chorionic chamber, and amniotic fluid will accumulate in the amniotic sac.

By the end of week four, the embryo is about 5 mm long, weighs about 0.02 g, and has a heartbeat. The trachea, lungs, intestinal tract, liver, pancreas, eyes, and ears have begun to develop. By the end of week eight of gestation, the diaphragm, intestinal subdivisions, kidneys, axial and appendicular cartilage, and axial musculature have started to develop. It is at this point, the end of week eight, that the embryo is termed a fetus.

By the end of the first trimester (week 28), the gallbladder, gonads, brain, spinal cord, and appendicular musculature start to develop, and the fetus in about 80 mm in length and weighs about 25 g. The placenta has fully developed; its primary functions are to facilitate the exchange of nutrients and wastes between the mother and fetus and to produce hormones necessary for the maintenance of pregnancy and fetal development. Blood flows between the fetus and placenta via the umbilical cord, which contains the paired umbilical arteries and a single umbilical vein. The developing fetus represents a significant demand to the mother; a significant amount of maternal blood flow is redirected to the placenta. During the second and third trimesters, the placenta acts as an endocrine organ and will take over progesterone-releasing duties from the corpus luteum. In addition, the placenta produces the hormones HCG, estrogen, human placental lactogen, and relaxin.

The development of organ systems nears completion during the second trimester, and the developing fetus grows faster than the surrounding chorion. As a result, the outer surface of the amnion, which surrounds the fetus, comes into contact and fuses with the inner surface of the chorion, forming a single amniochorionic membrane. The fetus begins to move by the end of week 16, and by the end of the second trimester, the developing fetus has taken on distinctive human characteristics.

Early in the third trimester, the majority of organ systems have matured and become fully functional. In addition, the third trimester is characterized by rapid growth of the fetus, which at week 24 was approximately 230 mm in length and 0.65 kg in weight, grows to a length of about 345 mm and weighs about 3.2 kg at full gestation.

2. Describe the physiological changes that occur in the pregnant female. p. 847

The developing fetus is dependent on the maternal organ systems for nourishment and oxygen and the removal of metabolic waste. This places a significant strain on the mother, especially in the third trimester, and compensatory changes take place in maternal physiology. Systems affected in pregnancy include the cardiovascular, the respiratory, the reproductive, the gastrointestinal, and the urinary system.

Changes in the cardiovascular and respiratory system occur because the mother is, for all practical purposes, pumping blood and breathing for two. Blood flow to the placenta and uterus greatly reduces the volume available for systemic maternal circulation. In addition, fetal metabolism results in a decrease in the maternal PO_2 and an increase in PCO_2. As a result, rennin and erythropoietin production increases, resulting in an increased blood volume and red blood cell production. Volume increase is more pronounced than red blood cell increase, resulting in the dilutional edema common in pregnancy. Toward the end of gestation, maternal blood volume has increased by 45 to 50 percent, resulting in an increased resting heart rate, increased cardiac output, and flow murmurs may be appreciated on auscultation. In addition, slight decreases in peripheral vascular resistance result in a slight decrease in blood pressure during the first and second trimesters. Blood pressure rises to prepregnancy levels during the third trimester. In addition, intravascular fluid shifts into the intracellular space in dependent areas, especially the limbs, resulting in edema.

Although not a true physiologic change, a transient decrease in venous return to the heart and subsequent hypotension can occur when the gravid uterus compresses the inferior vena cava (IVC), most often when the pregnant female is laid supine. This condition, supine hypotensive syndrome, can be avoided by placing the pregnant female in a left lateral recumbent position during transport, allowing the gravid uterus to displace to the left and away from the IVC located to the right of the spinal column.

Changes in blood chemistry also occur in the gravid female. Pregnancy results in a hypercoagulable state, secondary to an increase of clotting factors and a decrease in fibrinolytic activity, and an increase in platelet activation and venous stasis. As such, pregnant women have two components of Virchow's triad: hypercoagulability and venous stasis. As a result, a pregnant female has an increased risk of DVT formation and a five times increase in the risk of developing venous thromboembolism, which is the most common cause of maternal mortality in the United States. Trauma to a pregnant female provides the third component of Virchow's triad, vascular injury, further increasing the risk of thromboembolism. Other changes to blood chemistry include a decrease in hematocrit and an increase in white blood cell (WBC) count.

A number of changes in the maternal respiratory system meet the increased needs for oxygen delivery and CO_2 removal. Maternal O_2 demand increases during pregnancy, and a 10 to 20 percent increase in O_2 consumption is typical. To help meet this demand, progesterone secretion results in the weakening of costal cartilage, allowing greater movement of the ribcage and a 35 to 40 percent increase in tidal volume. In addition, a mild increase in respiratory rate occurs; this, together with the increase in tidal volume, results in an increased minute volume. As a result, a mild compensated respiratory alkalosis is often present, creating a greater CO_2 gradient between fetal and maternal circulation and greater diffusion of CO_2 between the two.

The most obvious and significant change in the reproductive system for the critical care paramedic occurs in the uterus. For the first 14 weeks of pregnancy, estrogen and progesterone influence uterine enlargement. After this time the developing fetus stretches and enlarges the uterus to its full-gestational size of about 30 cm in length, 1,000 g in weight, and 5 L in volume. Considering that the nongravid uterus has a length of about 7.5 cm, a weight of about 60 g, and volume of 10 mL, this represents an enormous increase in both size and volume. By the end of gestation, the uterus receives about 15 percent of the maternal blood volume. Obviously, any insult to the uterus can result in significant, if not fatal, maternal blood loss.

The increased size of the uterus compresses and displaces the abdominal organs, making the assessment of the abdomen challenging. In addition, peristalsis is slowed, delaying gastric emptying and making bloating and constipation common. Maternal nutritional requirements increase 10 to 30 percent during pregnancy as a result of fetal metabolic demands.

As a result of the increase in maternal blood volume and renal blood flow, glomerular filtration rate (GFR) increases by about 50 percent, accelerating the renal excretion of fetal metabolic waste. As a result of increased GFR, glucose may not be sufficiently reabsorbed in the proximal tubule and subsequently excreted in the urine. The resulting glucosuria may be normal and not indicative of the development of gestational diabetes. Urine glucose is a poor indicator of serum glucose levels in a pregnant patient, and blood glucose levels should be obtained for a better appreciation of glucose control. Another consequence of increased GFR is a slight reduction in serum creatinine and BUN. Increased GFR, along with uterine compression of the bladder, results in increased urinary frequency in the gravid female.

3. List the components of a general assessment of the obstetric patient. p. 848

Determining the age of an obstetrical patient is important, as is determining the entire past medical history including chronic disease, recent illnesses, past trauma, and obstetric history. Medications and allergies to medications should be identified and recorded. Past medical history is of specific concern, as chronic disease concerns can be exacerbated by or complicate pregnancy. Specific diseases of concern include: diabetes, seizure disorders, heart disease, hypertension, and neuromuscular disorders.

Specific obstetric history concerns include:

- Gravida/para (G/P) status
- Number of living children
- Complications with previous pregnancies or deliveries

- History of preterm delivery
  - Gestational age
  - Outcome
- History of elective or spontaneous abortion
  - Was a D&C performed?
- Have all previous births been vaginal, or has a cesarean section been performed in the past?
- Has the patient delivered vaginally after a cesarean section?
- When was, and what was, the length of her last labor?
- With regard to the current pregnancy, what is the estimated date of confinement (EDC)?
- Has the patient received adequate, limited (defined as three or fewer visits), or no prenatal care?
- Has any problem with this pregnancy been identified and, if so, what?
- Have diagnostic tests such as ultrasound been performed?
  - If so, what were the results?
- Is the patient taking any medications for obstetric or nonobstetric reasons?
  - If so, what medications, in what doses, and has she been compliant?
- Is drug or alcohol abuse suspected and, if so, what substances, with what frequency, and when was the last use?
- Does the patient smoke?
- Has she experienced a normal weight gain with the pregnancy, or does she appear malnourished or obese?
- Is the patient presently having contractions and, if so, when did they begin and what are their frequency and duration?
- Is there an urge to defecate?
- Has the patient's amniotic sac ruptured, at what time, and was it a trickle or a gush of fluid?
- Was meconium present in the fluid or did it have a foul odor?
- Has the patient experienced any vaginal bleeding and, if so, is it painless or is there pain?
- If there is pain, is it associated with contractions or is it constant?
- Has the patient or transporting facility used sanitary napkins or other absorbent devices to soak up blood?
  - If so, how much?

With regard to the physical exam, the abdominal exam of a pregnant patient is basically identical to that of a nonpregnant patient, though displacement and compression of abdominal organs by the gravid uterus will make identification of familiar abdominal landmarks challenging. Palpate for pain, tenderness, guarding, masses, and uterine contractions. During uterine contractions, the fundus should be palpated for strength, frequency, and duration of contractions. A tocodynamometer can be a useful tool, as it records the strength, duration, and time between contractions. Information can be recorded and printed out continuously while the patient is hooked up to the monitor.

Fundal height (FH) of the uterus should be measured in centimeters from the symphysis pubis to the most superior portion of the fundus; each centimeter of FH corresponds roughly to the gestational age in weeks. The position of the fetus can be determined by palpating the uterus for the head and buttocks, and the fetal spine can often be palpated as well.

External genitalia should be examined for discharge, blood, mucus, a prolapsed cord, or crowning. Crowning should be evaluated for during a contraction. Internal vaginal exams are not normally within the scope of practice of the critical care paramedic and should not be performed. A physician's examination of the patient's cervix prior to transport may be warranted and requested as needed.

Vital signs should be assessed every 15 minutes or as frequently as the situation warrants. Important vital signs to note include: pulse, blood pressure, respiratory rate, temperature, and SpO_2.

Assessment of fetal heart tones (FHT) and monitoring should occur throughout transport. Electronic fetal monitoring is evaluating and monitoring uterine contractions and fetal heart rate with electronic methods, and is easily utilized in the transport environment.

4. Describe the evaluation assessment of fetal heart rate (FHR) patterns.   p. 851

The parameters of importance to the critical care paramedic, when evaluating and monitoring FHRs, are the baseline FHR, FHR variability, periodic changes in FHR, and the change in trends of FHR patterns over time.

Baseline FHR is the average FHR during a ten-minute period rounded off to the nearest five beats per minute. For baseline FHR to be established, there must be at least two minutes out of the ten-minute period in which there are no instances of episodic changes, periods of significant FHR variability, or segments of the baseline with differences greater than 25 beats per minute. Normal baseline FHR is 110 to 160 bpm.

Bradycardia exists when the FHR is less than 110 bpm for more than ten minutes; it is not uncommon for a term or postmature fetus to have baselines between 100 and 110 bpm. Brady-cardia can occur secondary to umbilical cord compression or occlusion, maternal hypotension, uterine hyperstimulation resulting in increased intrauterine pressure during contractions (as with the use of oxytocin), chronic hypoxia (fetal bradycardia is a late, ominous sign), or inadvertent measurement of the maternal pulse.

Tachycardia exists when the FHR is greater than 160 bpm for more than 10 minutes. It can be an early, immediate compensatory reaction to increased cardiac output in instances of hypoxia. Significantly less variability in heart rate usually occurs during episodes of tachydardia. Causes of tachycardia include: transient fetal hypoxia, fetal anemia, maternal fever, maternal or fetal infec-tions, maternal smoking, sympathomimetic drugs (terbutaline) and chorioamnionitis.

A sinusoidal wave pattern is a frequent, wavelike pattern of regularly occurring increases and decreases of FHR over a range of five to 20 beats from baseline. It may be appreciated in cases of fetal anemia, erythroblastosis, or hypovolemia, and is indicative of severe fetal hypoxia. Maternal use of narcotics may also result in a sinusoidal wave pattern, in which case it is not an indication of fetal distress.

Variability in baseline FHR is normal, and indicates an adequately oxygenated and normally functioning autonomic nervous system; it is associated with normal oxygenation status at deliv-ery. Variability occurs as the sympathetic and parasympathetic nervous systems alternate in exert-ing influence on the fetal heart rate and can be described as short-term and long-term. Short-term variability is beat-to-beat changes in FHR, and is usually irregular in rate and frequency. It is greatly influenced by the parasympathetic branch of the autonomic nervous system, which is more susceptible to hypoxia than is the sympathetic branch. The cessation of normal, short-term vari-ability may be the first indicator of fetal hypoxia. Long-term variability can be described as a broad waviness of the FHR tracing over time that can range from 5 to 25 beats above and below the baseline; less than five beats over one minute is considered short-term. Long-term variability differs from the sinusoidal wave pattern in that its waves occur with much less frequency or over a longer period of time. It is influenced by the sympathetic nervous system. Absent or minimal variability, both long and short term, can be the result of fetal hypoxia, maternal narcotic use, smoking, administration of magnesium sulfate, extreme prematurity, fetal neurologic insult, and normal fetal sleep cycles.

Increased variability can be an early sign of hypoxia, or the result of the use of an ultrasound (US) transducer, which is notorious for erroneously high variability readings in the critical care transport environment. Ultrasound transducers are, however, the most likely measuring devices to be used by a transport team because of their noninvasive nature. If true evaluation of FHR short-term variability is required, placement of a fetal scalp electrode by a physician is recommended.

Periodic changes that can occur in the FHR include accelerations and decelerations. Acceler-ations are obvious, abrupt increases (less than 30 seconds from onset to peak rate) in FHR with a peak rate 15 bpm above baseline that lasts for greater than 15 seconds and less than two minutes from onset to return to baseline. An acceleration that lasts greater than two minutes is considered prolonged, and greater than ten minutes is considered a change in baseline. Accelerations are usu-ally benign, can occur secondary to uterine contractions or fetal movement, and indicate that the fetus has an intact central nervous system and a normal pH. Accelerations can also indicate de-veloping fetal hypoxia before a change in pH has occurred, so the critical care transport team should ensure that fetal movement or contractions accompany all accelerations. Ask the mother if there is fetal movement or if contractions are taking place. In addition, the uterus can be palpated during the acceleration, or a tocodynamometer can be used to identify contractions.

Decelerations are an obvious, gradual (greater than 30 seconds from onset to nadir) decrease and return of FHR from baseline during a uterine contraction and are considered normal during uterine contraction. The nadir of the deceleration occurs simultaneously with the peak of the uter-ine contraction, and in most cases the progression of the deceleration is a mirror image of the contraction. Decelerations are classified as early, late, or variable. Early decelerations are not associated with fetal hypoxia or acidosis, and no intervention is required. Late decelerations are a more serious sign than early decelerations, indicating the presence of hypoxia and acidosis secondary to uteroplacental insufficiency. Late decelerations begin at the peak of a uterine contraction and then return to the FHR baseline after the contraction is finished; the degree of deceleration is proportional to the strength of the contraction. Two mechanisms are responsible for late decelerations: central nervous system-induced reflex bradycardia secondary to hypoxia, and metabolic acidosis resulting in myocardial depression. Causes of uteroplacental insufficiency include abruptio placentae and previa, uterine hypertonicity secondary to oxytocin administration, maternal hypotension, and smoking, diabetes, and postmaturity.

Variable decelerations can occur any time during a contraction or independent of contractions and are caused by umbilical cord compression and occlusion secondary to uterine contraction or fetal movement. They are characterized by an abrupt decrease in FHR below baseline greater than 15 bpm and last between 15 seconds and two minutes. Their morphology may be in the shape of an inverted **V**, or an **M**, and the short accelerations on either side of the deceleration are termed "shoulders." Smoothing out of the decelerations or loss of shoulders is indicative of fetal distress; their appearance is thought to be caused by a partial, rather than complete, cord occlusion. Variable decelerations are the most common decelerations seen in labor, and while not an ominous sign when isolated, should rouse concern when they are deep and of long duration, are accompanied by decreased FHR variability, are slow to return to baseline, or when the baseline FHR increases or becomes tachycardic.

Changes in trending patterns of FHR can be difficult to follow, and the following questions will assist the health care provider in ruling fetal distress in or out:

- Is the FHR baseline within a normal range?
  - If the baseline is between 110 and 160 bpm, the fetus is maintaining an adequate cardiac output and metabolic acidosis is not present.
- Is adequate variability present?
  - If so, the fetus is being adequately oxygenated.
  - If hypervariabilty is present, it may be due to the ultrasound transducer.
- Are accelerations present?
  - Accelerations can only occur in the absence of metabolic acidosis; therefore, their presence is reassuring.
- Is the event an early deceleration?
  - If so, it is a normal, benign event that can be expected to occur with each uterine contraction.
- If tachycardia or bradycardia is present, are accelerations and adequate variability present?
  - If so, metabolic acidosis is not present.
- If late or variable decelerations are present, are accelerations and adequate variability present?
  - If so, the fetus is tolerating the events well and metabolic acidosis is not present.

Signs that the fetus is not tolerating the event well and may be developing hypoxia and acidosis include a gradual, significant, uncorrected decrease in baseline FHR over time, a fluctuating baseline over time, tachycardia or bradycardia with reduced short- and long-term variability, reduced variability as labor progresses, and late decelerations that smooth out over time.

5. **Describe the pathophysiology, assessment, and management of various OB-GYN emergencies to include:**

   a. **Fetal distress**   **p. 857**
   When fetal distress is suspected, intrauterine resuscitation measures need to be employed promptly with the goal being the improvement of uterine blood flow and increasing fetal oxygenation. Assure patient is breathing adequately and has a pulse, and administer 100 percent oxygen via NRM. Place the patient in the left lateral recumbent position, and if hypotension is present, consider repeated fluid boluses until hypotension is corrected. Perform an external vaginal exam to ensure that there is no vaginal hemorrhage or umbilical cord prolapse, especially if the patient is at high risk for abruptio placentae or previa. If the fetal distress occurs secondary to hypertonic contractions resulting from oxytocin infusion, discontinue the infusion immediately, and

consider a tocolytic agent such as terbutaline 0.25 mg subcutaneous or 0.125 to 0.25 mg intravenous to relax the uterus. Consider the need for amnioinfusion.

b. Vaginal hemorrhage during pregnancy   **p. 857**
Vaginal hemorrhage during pregnancy can occur secondary to abruptio placentae, placentae previa, complications of labor and delivery, and premature labor. All of these pathologies are discussed individually in the text that follows.

c. Abruptio placentae   **p. 858**

Pathophysiology

Abruptio placentae is the premature separation of a normally implanted placenta from the uterine wall, and it begins with arterial hemorrhaging into the deciduas basalis. Hematoma formation and progression can result in an expanding abruption. As abruption continues, a greater number of vessels become involved, further contributing to the expanding retroplacental hematoma. The uterus will often contract during an abruptio episode, and the deciduas is rich in thromboplastin, encouraging rapid clot formation that may help attenuate the hemorrhage. Separation of the placenta can be partial (marginal) or complete. Abruption with vaginal bleeding is termed an external hemorrhage and, if no vaginal bleeding is appreciated on physical exam, the abruption is said to be concealed. Blood loss is impossible to estimate based on external observation alone, as significant amounts of blood can remain in the uterus, trapped behind the placenta. Most of the blood loss that occurs is maternal in origin, although it is possible for the fetus to hemorrhage as well. Risk factors associated with abruptio placentae include chronic or gestational hypertension (the most common factor), cocaine use, smoking, trauma, increasing maternal age (over 35 years), multiparity, uterine scarring from surgeries, past curettage, infection, or past incidence of abruptio placentae.

Complications of abruptio placentae include fetal complications, hypoxia, anoxia, anemia, and CNS compromise. Maternal complications include the development of hemorrhagic shock, the development of disseminated intravascular coagulation (DIC), and end-organ failure.

Assessment

Classic signs and symptoms of abruptio placentae are considered to be:

- Presence of abdominal pain (50 percent)
- Uterine contractions (> 90 percent)
- Vaginal bleeding (90 percent)
  - Except in cases of concealed abruptio placentae
- Uterine tenderness to palpation
- Fetal demise

Severe cases may present with a rigid, boardlike abdomen upon palpation, and signs and symptoms of hemorrhagic shock.

Ultrasound cannot diagnose the presence or absence of abruptio placentae itself although it can demonstrate a placental hematoma that is consistent with abruption (placental hematomas are recognized in 2 to 25 percent of all abruptions). Ultrasound can rule out placenta previa as a cause of vaginal bleeding by determining the location of the placenta.

Labs ordered should include:

- CBC
- Type and crossmatch
- Coagulation profile
- Renal function studies

Patients should also be assessed for signs associated with DIC, which include bleeding from IV or catheter sites, hypotension, and increased ventilatory resistance.

Management

Oxygenation and perfusion is a priority in the treatment of abruptio placentae, especially in cases where the signs and symptoms of shock are present, in which cases 100 percent oxygen should, at the very least, be supplied at 15 lpm via a nonrebreather mask. Assisted ventilations with a BVM or endotracheal intubation may be required. IV access should consist of two large bore IVs or central line placement. Volume resuscitation with crystalloid solution should be considered in cases of mild abruptio. If hemorrhagic shock is present, aggressive volume replacement should be initiated with a crystalloid solution and packed RBCs. The transport team should procure additional packed RBCs from the transporting facility for infusion during transport. A Foley catheter should be inserted to monitor urinary output, > 0.5 mL/kg/hr is desired. Administering tocolytic agents may help prevent the expansion of a developing abruption.

d. Placenta previa   p. 859

Pathophysiology
Placenta previa occurs when the placenta implants and develops in the lower third of the uterus, totally or partially covering the cervical os. Three types of presentation are possible. Marginal previa occurs when the edge of the placenta lies adjacent to, but does not cover, the cervical os. Partial previa is characterized by a placenta that partially covers the cervical os. In complete previa the placenta completely covers the cervical os.

Risk factors contributing to placenta previa include: advanced maternal age (over 35 years), smoking (doubles the risk compared to nonsmokers), cocaine use, prior history of previa, multiparity, multifetal gestations, previous cesarean section, or curettage.

Maternal complications associated with previa include the need for a cesarean delivery, postpartum hemorrhage, and the development of hemorrhagic shock. Fetal complications include hypoxia, anoxia, and death.

Assessment
The hallmark of previa is the acute onset of painless, bright red bleeding in the late second or third trimester. A history of recent vaginal exam, sexual intercourse, or onset of labor should increase suspicion, but none is necessary for previa to occur. The abdominal exam is usually benign, though uterine contractions may be present. A digital or speculum examination is to be avoided in all cases of suspected placenta previa. Diagnosis of previa is confirmed with transabdominal ultrasound, which has an accuracy of 93 to 98 percent and a false negative rate of about 7 percent.

Management
Same as abruptio placentae

e. Preterm labor   p. 860

Pathophysiology
Preterm labor is defined as frequent uterine contractions resulting in progressive cervical dilation or effacement between the 20th and 37th weeks of gestation. Numerous physiologic factors can contribute to the development of preterm and premature labor, including hormonal influences (prostaglandin release, high levels of oxytocin), decreased uteroplacental blood flow (maternal dehydration, maternal hypertension, overdistension of the uterus, smoking, cocaine use, cardiovascular disease, placental abruption, or previa) and anatomic/physiologic abnormalities that affect the cervix or uterus.

Risk factors for the development of preterm and premature labor include premature rupture of membranes (PROM), smoking, cocaine use, poor nutritional status, maternal age over 35 years or less than 20 years, previous preterm delivery, abruptio placentae, or previa, infection, dehydration, uterine abnormalities, cervical incompetence, or STDs such as chlamydia, gonorrhea, or syphilis.

Maternal complications of premature labor include endometritis, septicemia and septic shock secondary to PROM, and chorioamnionitis. Fetal consequences of premature labor include preterm birth.

Assessment
Assess for evidence of the numerous etiologies of preterm labor, including the presence of fever, dehydration, vaginal hemorrhaging, and PROM. An exploration of the patient's history will identify risk factors such as age, previous history of preterm labor, and social history. A cervical exam should be performed by an appropriately trained health care provider to assess for cervical dilation or membrane rupture. The identification of suspected amniotic fluid can be performed with nitrazine paper, although the presence of blood will render this test useless. In

addition, the fundal height should be determined, fetal weight estimated, and FHR and contractions monitored via EFM.

Lab studies to be evaluated include:

- CBC to evaluate for leukocytosis and low hematocrit
- Urinalysis to assess the degree of dehydration and rule out infection
- Cervical cultures for chlamydia, gonorrhea, and group B streptococci
- Urine toxicology screen can be considered if substance abuse is suspected
- Serum glucose and potassium should be determined prior to the initiation of β-adrenergic agonists for tocolysis

Pay attention to the pattern of contractions, the status of membranes, and the degree of cervical dilation to determine the stage of labor. This allows for an informed decision on the part of the transport crew as to whether the transport should be delayed to allow delivery at the transporting facility.

Management
Management goals during transport include maintaining uteroplacental perfusion and suppressing labor. The patient should be placed in the left lateral recumbent position and 100 percent oxygen administered at 15 lpm via nonrebreather mask. Peripheral IV access should be obtained and volume replacement initiated if dehydration is suspected. Tocolytic agents can be used to delay birth up to 2 days, allowing time for corticosteroid administration to hasten fetal lung development. β-adrenergic agonists, magnesium sulfate, calcium channel blockers, and prostaglandin synthetase inhibitors are the agents most commonly used for tocolysis, with IV terbutaline or magnesium sulfate commonly utilized by critical care transport teams.

f. Breech presentation   **p. 862**

Pathophysiology
Breech presentation is the term used to describe the situation in which the fetus' buttocks or legs present first. Frank breech presentation, the most common type, occurs when both legs are extended upward with both hips flexed and both knees extended. Complete breech occurs when the buttocks descend first, both hips are flexed, and one or both knees are flexed, resulting in one or both feet presenting with the buttocks. Maternal trauma is common during breech birth, and fetal complications include prolapsed cord, cord compression, cord entanglement, and birth trauma.

A breech fetus is at higher risk for hypoxia, acidosis, and anoxia than an infant delivered in the cephalad position is.

Management
The fetus should be allowed to deliver on its own, with no traction applied to the fetus. Once the umbilical cord has delivered, the CCP can assist in freeing the legs, if necessary. At this point the fetus can be wrapped in a towel and rotated so the shoulders are in an anterior-posterior position. As the shoulders become visible, a finger can be used to hook each arm and apply gentle downward traction to remove each one. In addition, upward traction can be applied to facilitate the delivery of the posterior shoulder, and downward traction for the anterior shoulder. After the shoulders have been delivered, the body is rotated so the back is anterior; flexion of the head is maintained by placing the index and middle fingers over the fetus' maxilla. With the body resting on the forearm of the same arm and the opposite hand supporting the head and shoulders, upward traction can be applied to the body while an assistant applies suprapubic pressure to encourage the delivery of the head with as little traction as possible.

g. Dystocia   **p. 863**

Pathophysiology
Dystocia occurs when delivery of the fetal head is followed by impaction of the fetal shoulders against the pubic symphysis and sacrum, within the pelvis. Risk factors that contribute to dystocia include a birth weight greater than 4,000 grams, maternal diabetes, maternal obesity, operative delivery, and contracted maternal pelvis.

Assessment

The classic finding associated with dystocia is the turtle sign, which occurs when the fetal head retracts slightly as it is pulled down against the perineum.

Management

Upon recognition of dystocia, immediately drain the urinary bladder with a Foley catheter. A generous mediolateral episiotomy may facilitate delivery. Pressure to the fetus' anterior shoulder should be applied to dislodge the anterior shoulder from the pubic symphysis; the anterior shoulder can be palpated in the maternal suprapubic area. DO NOT apply pressure to the fundal area, as this will further impact the shoulders on the pelvic rim. At the same time, gentle downward traction can be applied to the fetal head. If this maneuver is unsuccessful, other maneuvers can be attempted, such as McRobert's maneuver, the Woods corkscrew maneuver, the Rubin maneuver, or the Zavanelli maneuver.

h. Umbilical cord prolapse   p. 865

Pathophysiology

Two types of umbilical cord prolapse can occur; overt and occult. Overt umbilical cord prolapse occurs when the cord enters the vaginal canal or presents externally prior to the fetus. Occult cord prolapse occurs when the cord slips into or near the pelvis and is occluded by a presenting part so that the cord is not visible or palpable on exam. Risk factors for umbilical cord prolapse include PROM, transverse lie of the fetus in the uterus, breech presentation, large fetus, multiparity, multiple gestations, preterm labor, and a long cord.

The major concern with a prolapsed cord is cord compression and occlusion that may lead to fetal complications including hypoxia, acidosis, anoxia, and death.

Assessment

While the assessment findings of an overt umbilical cord prolapse are straightforward, the occult prolapse can be much more insidious and requires a careful examination on the part of the critical care transport team. Clinical signs revolve around evidence of fetal distress, including:

- Absence of short- and long-term variability
- Fetal bradycardia
- Recurrent variable decelerations that do not respond to maternal positioning, oxygen administration, or fluid administration

Management

If the umbilical cord presents externally or can be visualized in the vagina, two fingers of a gloved hand should be used to prevent any presenting part of a delivering fetus from occluding the cord. The presenting cord should never be either pulled or replaced into the uterus, though it should be allowed to retract if it does so spontaneously. The exposed cord should be kept free of pressure for the duration of transport; a Trendelenburg or knee-chest position can help achieve this. One hundred percent oxygen should be administered at 15 lpm via a nonrebreather mask, and an IV of normal saline started and kept at a KVO rate. Administration of a tocolytic agent such as terbutaline can be used to alleviate pressure on the umbilical cord. Definitive treatment for unresolved prolapse is cesarean section.

i. Uterine rupture   p. 865

Pathophysiology

Uterine rupture is the complete disruption of all layers of the uterine wall, allowing communication between the uterine and abdominal cavities. The majority occur in women who have undergone previous cesarean section. Risk factors include: previous cesarean section, overdistension of the uterus, grand multiparity, previous rupture, and trauma.

Fetal complications include hypoxia, acidosis, anoxia, and death.

Assessment

Common clinical findings of uterine rupture include:

- Acute onset of sharp, severe abdominal pain
- Signs and symptoms of hypovolemic shock

- Rebound tenderness and distension
- Palpation of extrauterine fetal parts
- Vaginal bleeding may be present

Palpation of the uterus can reveal hypertonic contractions, normal contractions, or cessation of contractions. Laboratory studies of immediate use include a CBC, type and crossmatch, and a coagulation profile. If uteroplacental blood flow is compromised, evidence of fetal distress may be evident and includes:

- Absence of short- and long-term variability
- Fetal bradycardia
- Recurrent variable decelerations that do not respond to maternal positioning, oxygen administration, or fluid administration

Management

The primary goal in the treatment of uterine rupture is to maintain ABCs in order to preserve uteroplacental perfusion. The patient should be placed in the left lateral recumbent position and administered 100 percent oxygen at 15 lpm via a nonrebreather mask. Large bore IV access should be initiated and fluid volume resuscitation provided if the patient is in shock. A Foley catheter should be inserted to monitor urine production, an output of 0.5 mL/kg/hr is desired. Definitive treatment is surgical repair.

j. Postpartum hemorrhage   p. 866

Pathophysiology

A postpartum hemorrhage (PPH) is said to exist when there is greater than 500 mL of blood loss after a vaginal delivery or greater than 1,000 mL of blood loss after a cesarean section. Normally, postlabor platelet aggregation and clot formation in the decidua is complimented by myometrial contraction that constricts and occludes blood vessels torn when the placenta disassociates from the uterine implantation site, preventing serious bleeding. As the blood flow to the uteroplacental boundary is about 600 mL/min, the potential for significant hemorrhage exists if uterine contraction does not take place (uterine atony). As uterine contractions are prevented, blood accumulates and clots within the uterus, further preventing uterine contraction and worsening bleeding.

Common causes of PPH include uterine atony, retained placental fragments, and birth canal trauma.

Risk factors for uterine atony and PPH include: retention of placental fragments, overdistension of the uterus, multiparity, polyhydramnios, chorioamnionitis, prolonged or obstructed labor, use of general anesthesia, and magnesium tocolysis.

In addition, a major risk factor for retained placenta is the development of placenta accreta.

Assessment

Uterine atony can be identified by a lack of uterine contractions and a flaccid uterus upon palpation. Vaginal bleeding should be apparent, but external blood loss may not be representative of total blood loss, much of which may be sequestered in the uterus. Signs and symptoms of shock, rather than estimates of total blood loss, should be assessed to evaluate the patient's hemodynamic status.

Laboratory results useful to the critical care transport paramedic include:

- CBC
- Type and crossmatch
- Hematocrit
- Coagulation studies

Management

The primary goal in the management of postpartum hemorrhage is to preserve uteroplacental perfusion through the maintenance of the ABCs. The patient should be placed in the left lateral recumbent position and administered 100 percent oxygen at 15 lpm via NRM. Large bore IV access should be initiated and the need for fluid volume resuscitation anticipated if bleeding is significant. If hypovolemic shock is present, initiate aggressive volume replacement with a crystalloid and packed RBCs via a central venous catheter. A Foley catheter should be inserted to monitor urine production; an output of 0.5 mL/kg/hr is desired. Uterine fundal massage and the administration of oxytocin can help stimulate uterine contractions and control bleeding, as can carboprost tromethamine (Hemabate).

k. Hypertension in pregnancy p. 867; l. Preeclampsia p. 867; m. Eclampsia p. 869

Pathophysiology

Four categories of hypertension during pregnancy are recognized: chronic hypertension, gestational hypertension, preeclampsia, and chronic hypertension with preeclampsia. Chronic hypertension is hypertension that predates pregnancy or is identified prior to 20 weeks gestation. Gestational hypertension occurs after 20 weeks gestation and is not accompanied by proteinuria. Preeclampsia is recognized when hypertension and proteinuria coexist. Chronic hypertension with preeclampsia exists when a female with known hypertension develops worsening hypertension and proteinuria during pregnancy. A pregnant female is considered hypertensive when she has a systolic blood pressure above 140 mmHg or a diastolic blood pressure above 90 mmHg.

Preeclampsia occurs in 6 to 8 percent of all live births, and the exact cause or causes of preeclampsia are unknown, although theoretical models exist that include immunologic responses, increased sensitivity to endogenous vasoconstrictors, endothelial damage with prostacyclin and thromboxane A2 production, chronic DIC, and genetic predisposition.

A common thread among practically all of these models is an increase in vasoconstriction, peripheral vascular resistance, and subsequent hypertension. Known risk factors for preeclampsia include: age over 35 years and less than 15 years, history of preeclampsia in a previous pregnancy, multiparity, preexisting renal or cardiovascular disease, diabetes, family history of preeclampsia, African-American descent.

Maternal risks include renal failure, hepatic failure, DIC, seizures and strokes, and death. Fetal risks associated with preeclampsia include uteroplacental hypoperfusion, placental infarction, abruptio placentae, inhibited fetal growth, oligohydramnios, and fetal demise.

The HELLP syndrome is an acronym for Hemolysis, Elevated Liver function tests, and Low Platelets, and is thought to be a subcategory of severe preeclampsia. Patients exhibiting the HELLP syndrome often experience a rapid, degenerative course, and many physicians elect for prompt delivery before the onset of eclampsia. Eclampsia, the most serious manifestation of pregnancy-induced hypertension, is said to be present when the patient has a seizure.

Assessment

Signs and symptoms of preeclampsia include:

- Headaches, nausea and vomiting, seizures, and cerebral edema
- Decreased urine output, proteinuria, decreased kidney function
- Decreased liver function

Laboratory findings associated with preeclampsia include:

- Elevated serum uric acid, urea nitrogen, and creatinine
- Elevated liver function tests
- Proteinuria

Severe preeclampsia is said to exist when any of the following clinical or laboratory exam findings are present:

- SBP > 160 mmHg or DBP > 110 mmHg two times at least six hours apart.
- Proteinuria > 5 g in 24 hours
- Cerebral or visual symptoms
- Oliguria, 500 mL over 24 hours
- Pulmonary edema
- Right upper quadrant pain
- Elevated liver enzymes
- Low platelet count ($< 100,000/mm^3$)
- Restricted fetal growth

Management

The primary goal in the treatment of preeclampsia is to maintain ABCs in order to preserve utero-placental perfusion. The patient should be placed in the left lateral recumbent position, and 100 percent oxygen administered at 15 lpm via nonrebreather mask. IV access can involve large bore peripheral IVs or central venous access, depending on the patient's condition. Monitoring of urinary output ($>$ 0.5 mL/kg/hr is desired) is accomplished with the insertion of a Foley catheter, and a urine dipstick is used to assess for proteinuria. IV magnesium sulfate should be administered for seizures, and morphine or furosemide for pulmonary edema. Antihypertensives utilized for severe elevations in blood pressure include magnesium sulfate, hydralazine, or labetalol.

N. Gestational diabetes **p. 869**

Pathophysiology

The term gestational diabetes mellitus (GDM) describes those cases of diabetes, regardless of severity or insulin requirements, which initially present during pregnancy. GDM can be a true initial onset of Type I or Type II diabetes, or may represent a previously unrecognized case, worsened by the increased demand placed on the mother by the developing fetus. The pathogenesis of GDM mimics that of Type II non-insulin dependent diabetes; impaired insulin secretion and increased insulin resistance are present in both. Most cases of GDM resolve after pregnancy, though there is a 32 percent lifetime risk of developing Type II DM after GDM. Risk factors for developing GDM include maternal obesity, previous infant over 4,000 g birthweight, history or family history of DM, history of preeclampsia, maternal age over 30 years, excessive weight gain during pregnancy (more than 40 lbs.).

Maternal complications include preterm labor, preeclampsia, pyleonephritis, and the need for cesarean section. Fetal complications include increased perinatal morbidity and mortality, shoulder dystocia, stillbirth, operative delivery, and macrosomia.

Assessment

Blood glucose determination should be performed every hour for patients with GDM in active labor. Patients with preterm labor being controlled with β-adrenergic agonists are at a higher risk for hypoglycemia and should be monitored carefully.

Management

The management of GDM is the same as for nonpregnant patients. If hypoglycemia is present, administer 25 to 50 g of dextrose IV, and if hyperglycemia is present, administer insulin subcutaneously. If blood glucose levels drop below 80 dL/mg, a continuous infusion of D5W, 125 mL/hour can be initiated. For insulin dependent patients in labor, a continuous insulin infusion can be considered.

O. Embolism **p. 870**

Pathophysiology

Pregnancy results in a hypercoagulable state that is secondary to an increase of clotting factors and a decrease in fibrinolytic activity, and to an increase in platelet activation and venous stasis. As such, pregnant women have two components of Virchow's triad, hypercoagulability and venous stasis. As a result, a pregnant female has an increased risk of DVT formation and a five times increase in risk of venous thromboembolism, which is the most common cause of maternal mortality in the United States. Trauma to a pregnant female provides the third component of Virchow's triad, vascular injury, further increasing the risk of thromboembolism. Childbirth is considered a traumatic event.

Amniotic fluid embolism (AFE) is rare, but when it occurs it is associated with mortality rates between 80 percent and 90 percent. The majority of those deaths occur within the first few hours of the event. Risk factors associated with AFE include large fetus, maternal age over 32 years old, multiparity, premature separation of the placenta, tumultuous labor, and placental abruption.

The pathophysiology behind AFE shares many of the same features as anaphylactic and septic shock. There is a release of cellular chemical mediators such as prostaglandins, histamines, and leukotrienes, which are associated with many of the manifestations of AFE. It is believed that when the amniotic sac tears, there is a release of fluid into the maternal venous circulation, which then travels to the lungs. Vasospasm occurs, which causes transient pulmonary hypertension and subsequent right ventricular failure, pulmonary edema, and severe hypoxia. DIC is a common process with this emergency and is thought to be the result of activation of the fibrinolytic system by the amniotic fluid.

Assessment
Signs and symptoms of pulmonary embolism include:

- Acute onset of respiratory distress, dyspnea
- Tachycardia, tachypnea
- Hypotension, JVD
- Cardiovascular arrest, PEA

Laboratory tests useful in the diagnosis of pulmonary embolism include D-dimer assay, and nuclear V/Q scanning offers diagnostic information.

Management
Airway maintenance and adequate ventilation with 100 percent oxygen are a priority; endotracheal intubation and mechanical ventilation may be necessary. Large bore peripheral IV access or central venous catheterization should be performed early, and fluid volume resuscitation should be initiated if shock is present. Fibrinolysis and/or heparin therapy is the standard of care.

Case Study

You have never taken a transfer directly out of an operating room before, but you always say that there's a first time for everything. Your critical care ground transport team has been called to a community acute care hospital to transport an obstetrical patient for admission to the ICU at the hospital where your unit is based. The dispatcher told you that the patient just delivered a baby by caesarean section and is now experiencing "complications." The OR circulating nurse meets your team at the main doors of the surgical suite and gives you a report. The patient is a 39-year-old woman, who is G_3P_3. She was at 36 weeks gestation when she was brought to the OR for an emergent C-section due to severe preeclampsia. Shortly after the delivery of a healthy boy, the patient became very hypotensive, dyspneic, and hypoxic. She quickly required intubation and a small amount of blood-tinged fluid was suctioned from the tube. She had significant perioperative blood loss and received 2 units of packed RBCs and 3 L of lactated ringers IV without improvement in blood pressure. The patient was given platelets via IV infusion and was started on a dopamine drip of 10 mcg/kg/min upon stabilization of her blood pressure. Although laboratory tests are still pending, the patient is diagnosed with disseminated intravascular coagulation (DIC) secondary to an amniotic fluid embolism (AFE).

Your patient presents lying on the operating table, intubated, sedated, and chemically paralyzed. The surgical drapes have been removed, the surgical wounds have been dressed, and the patient is ready to be moved to the ambulance stretcher. The anesthesiologist, with occasional input from the obstetrician, gives you an update on the patient's condition. The patient's heart rate and blood pressure have stabilized. The heart rate is currently 122 and the monitor is showing a sinus tachycardia. Her blood pressure is 102/86. Her oxygenation has improved significantly since intubation and her SpO_2 is now 96 percent. Bleeding from the surgical wound has slowed and, other than a small amount of vaginal bleeding, there have been no other areas of bleeding. She was just given an IV bolus of vecuronium and midazolam for continued paralysis and sedation during transport and the physicians both feel that although the patient remains critical, she should not deteriorate during transport.

The patient does very well during the 40-minute transport and the dopamine infusion is titrated and then discontinued because of continued improvement in her blood pressure. You arrive at the receiving hospital and she is transferred to the ICU staff without further change. Later, you learn that she continued to improve quickly and was extubated and moved to the step down unit the next day.

DISCUSSION QUESTIONS

1. Describe the pathophysiology, assessment, and management of the following OB-GYN emergencies:
   a. preeclampsia/eclampsia
   b. embolism

Content Review

MULTIPLE CHOICE

_____ 1. Gestation is the time between:
   A. ovulation and birth.
   B. ovulation and fertilization.
   C. fertilization of the oocyte and birth.
   D. fertilization of the egg and implantation in the uterus.

_____ 2. Gestation in a human averages _____.
   A. one week   C. 252 days
   B. two weeks   D. 266 days

_____ 3. A gestation less than _____ weeks is considered preterm.
   A. 35   C. 40
   B. 37   D. 42

_____ 4. A gestation less than _____ weeks is considered post-term.
   A. 35   C. 40
   B. 37   D. 42

_____ 5. Fertilization, if it takes place, most commonly occurs in the:
   A. distal third of the fallopian tube.
   B. in the uterus.
   C. in the proximal half of the fallopian tube.
   D. none of the above.

_____ 6. The blastocyst usually implants in the uterus at the level of the:
   A. cervical os.   C. base.
   B. body or fundus.   D. isthmus.

_____ 7. The trophoblast erodes a path through the endometrial wall and develops within the _____ zone.
   A. functional   C. perimetrium
   B. basilar   D. none of the above

_____ 8. An embryo is termed a fetus by the end of week:
   A. 7.   B. 8.
   C. 9.   D. 10.

_____ 9. The placenta has fully developed by the end of week:
   A. 28.   C. 30.
   B. 29.   D. 31.

_____ 10. During the first few days of implantation, _____ is produced and stimulates the release of _____ by the corpus leuteum.
   A. human growth hormone, estrogen
   B. estrogen, progesterone
   C. human chorianic gonadotropin, progesterone
   D. human growth hormone, estrogen

_____ 11. The placenta's primary function is to:
   A. produce hormones necessary for the maintenance of pregnancy and fetal development.
   B. facilitate the exchange of nutrients and wastes between the mother and fetus.
   C. both A and B.
   D. none of the above.

_____ 12. A fetus can be expected to be moving by the end of week:
  A. 16.   C. 18.
  B. 17.   D. 19.

_____ 13. A baby born between weeks _____ is considered full term.
  A. 36–37   C. 36–40
  B. 36–38   D. 37–40

_____ 14. Which of the following is not a change of the maternal cardiovascular system typical during pregnancy?
  A. Rennin and erythropoietin production increase.
  B. Maternal blood volume increases by 40 to 50 percent.
  C. There is a decrease in maternal PaO_2 and an increase in $PaCO_2$.
  D. Fluid shifting into the intravascular space results in peripheral edema.

_____ 15. _____ occurs when the gravid uterus obstructs blood return to the heart via compression of the inferior vena cava.
  A. Vena cava compression syndrome   C. Lateral vena cava syndrome
  B. Supine hypotensive syndrome   D. None of the above

_____ 16. Changes in the maternal respiratory system during pregnancy include all of the following except:
  A. creation of a mild, compensatory respiratory alkalosis.
  B. increased oxygen consumption.
  C. stiffening of the costal cartilages.
  D. increased tidal volume.

_____ 17. Which of the following is a change that occurs in the maternal digestive system during pregnancy?
  A. Peristalsis increases.
  B. Maternal nutritional requirements increase by 10 to 30 percent.
  C. Gastric emptying is delayed.
  D. Liver and splenic function is decreased.

_____ 18. Which of the following is not a normal change in maternal physiology associated with pregnancy?
  A. Clotting factor activity, fibrinolytic activity, and platelet activation increase.
  B. Glomerular filtration rate increases by 50 percent.
  C. The uterus receives up to 15 percent of cardiac output.
  D. Decreased peripheral vascular resistance results in slight decrease in blood pressure during the first and second trimesters.

_____ 19. Why is maternal age an important part of the patient history?
  A. Underage mothers will need an adult's consent for treatment.
  B. Patient age is required for insurance reimbursement.
  C. Extremes of age predispose the obstetrical patient to complications.
  D. Chronic disease can be assumed with advanced age.

_____ 20. A patient's gravida/para (G/P) status is commonly followed with the acronym T-P-A-L, which stands for:
  A. number of term pregnancies, number of preterm infants, number of abortions, and number of living children.
  B. number of full-term infants, number of preterm infants, number of abortions, and number of living children.
  C. number of full-term infants, number of postterm infants, number of abortions, and number of living children.
  D. number of full-term infants, number of preterm infants, number of abortions, and last menstrual period.

_____ 21. A dilation and curettage involves:
  A. dilation of the cervix and taking an endometrial tissue sample.
  B. dilation of the vaginal canal and curettage of the cervical os.
  C. dilation of the fallopian tube and inspection of the ovary.
  D. none of the above.

_____ 22. EDC is a common acronym that stands for:
  A. emergency dilation and curettage.
  B. estimated date of confinement.
  C. estimated date due.
  D. none of the above.

_____ 23. A tocodynamometer is an:
  A. extrauterine monitoring device used to detect and monitor the fetal heart rate (FHR).
  B. extrauterine monitoring device used to detect and record uterine contractions.
  C. intrauterine monitoring device used to detect and monitor the fetal heart rate (FHR).
  D. intrauterine pressure-monitoring catheter used to detect and record the intensity of uterine contractions.

_____ 24. Each cm of fundal height corresponds to roughly the:
  A. gestational age in days.
  B. gestational age in weeks.
  C. gestational age in months.
  D. number of weeks remaining in gestation.

_____ 25. Palpation of the uterus can reveal:
  A. length of uterine contractions.
  B. intensity of uterine contractions.
  C. frequency of uterine contractions.
  D. all of the above.

_____ 26. Which of the following regarding examination of the genitalia is false?
  A. The external genitalia should be assessed for trauma, infection, or discharge.
  B. The external genitalia should be assessed for prolapsed cord and crowning.
  C. An internal vaginal exam should be performed by the transport paramedic on every patient suspected of being in labor.
  D. Blood on the external genitalia may indicate intraabdominal or intrauterine hemorrhage.

_____ 27. During transport, fetal heart rate (FHR) is best evaluated with:
  A. a cardiac monitor.
  B. a stethoscope.
  C. doppler auscultation.
  D. a tocodynamometer.

_____ 28. Indications for the sustained use of a fetal heart rate monitor include all of the following except:
  A. maternal diabetes, chronic hypertension, and preeclampsia.
  B. multiple gestation.
  C. meconium staining, prematurity, suspected abruptio placentae or placenta previa.
  D. normal, active labor.

_____ 29. The baseline FHR is the:
  A. average FHR during a 10-minute period rounded off to the nearest 5 bpm.
  B. average FHR during a 5-minute period rounded off to the nearest 10 bpm.
  C. average FHR during a 5-minute period rounded off to the nearest 5 bpm.
  D. average FHR during a 10-minute period rounded off to the nearest 10 bpm.

_____ 30. For baseline FHR to be established, there must be at least 2 minutes out of the 10 minute period where there are no:
  A. periods of significant FHR variability.
  B. instances of episodic changes.
  C. segments of the baseline with differences greater than 25 bpm.
  D. all of the above.

_____ 31. Normal baseline FHR is:
  A. 100–160 bpm.   C. 110–150 bpm.
  B. 110–140 bpm.   D. 110–160 bpm.

_____ 32. Bradycardia is said to exist when the FHR is less than:
  A. 100 bpm for greater than 5 minutes.
  B. 100 bpm for greater than 10 minutes.
  C. 110 bpm for greater than 10 minutes.
  D. 110 bpm for greater than 5 minutes.

_____ 33. It is not uncommon for a term or postmature fetus to have a baseline FHR between 100 and 110 bpm secondary to their more mature neurologic and cardiovascular systems.
  A. True.
  B. False.

_____ 34. Fetal bradycardia can occur secondary to all of the following except:
  A. umbilical cord compression or occlusion.
  B. maternal smoking.
  C. maternal hypotension.
  D. chronic hypoxia.

_____ 35. Tachycardia is defined as FHR of greater than:
  A. 160 bpm for more than 10 minutes.
  B. 150 bpm for greater than 10 minutes.
  C. 170 bpm for greater than 5 minutes.
  D. none of the above.

_____ 36. Causes of fetal tachycardia include:
  A. sympathomimetic drugs, chorioamnionitis, and erythroblastosis.
  B. maternal hypotension, uterine hyperstimulation, and increased intrauterine pressure.
  C. transient fetal hypoxia, fetal anemia, and maternal fever.
  D. all of the above.

_____ 37. A sinusoidal FHR wave pattern is characterized by:
  A. a wavelike pattern created as heart rate repeatedly fluctuates from nadir to trough over 20 to 30 seconds.
  B. a frequent, wavelike pattern of regularly occurring increases and decreases of FHR over a range of 5 to 20 beats from baseline.
  C. short, 5- to 20-second periods of alternating tachycardia and bradycardia.
  D. none of the above.

_____ 38. All of the following statements about FHR variability are true except:
  A. variability in baseline FHR is normal.
  B. variability indicates an adequately oxygenated and normally functioning autonomic nervous system.
  C. variability of FHR occurs as the sympathetic and parasympathetic nervous systems alternate in exerting influence on the fetal heart rate.
  D. short-term variability is greatly influenced by the sympathetic branch of the autonomic nervous system.

_____ 39. The cessation of normal, short-term variability may be the first indicator of fetal hypoxia.
  A. True.
  B. False.

_____ 40. Absent or minimal variability, both long and short term, can be the result of:
A. fetal hypoxia.
B. administration of magnesium sulfate, maternal narcotic use, and smoking.
C. fetal neurologic insult, extreme prematurity, normal fetal sleep cycles.
D. all of the above.

_____ 41. Accelerations and decelerations in FHR always indicate fetal distress.
A. True.
B. False.

_____ 42. An acceleration is best defined as:
A. a gradual increase in FHR with a peak rate 15 bpm above baseline that lasts for greater than 15 seconds and less than 2 minutes from onset to return to baseline.
B. an acute increase in FHR with a peak rate 20 bpm above baseline that lasts for greater than 10 seconds and less than 2 minutes from onset to return to baseline.
C. an acute increase in FHR with a peak rate 15 bpm above baseline that lasts for greater than 15 seconds and less than 2 minutes from onset to return to baseline.
D. none of the above.

_____ 43. An acceleration that lasts greater than _____ minutes is considered prolonged, and greater than _____ minutes is considered a change in baseline.
A. 2, 10   C. 2, 15
B. 3, 10   D. 3, 15

_____ 44. FHR accelerations can:
A. occur secondary to uterine contractions or fetal movement.
B. be an indication that the fetus has an intact central nervous system and a normal pH.
C. signal developing fetal hypoxia.
D. all of the above.

_____ 45. FHR decelerations can be classified as:
A. early or late.   C. mild or severe.
B. early, late, or variable.   D. none of the above.

_____ 46. An obvious, gradual (greater than 30 seconds from onset to nadir) decrease and return of FHR from baseline during a uterine contraction is termed a(n):
A. early deceleration.
B. late deceleration.
C. variable deceleration.
D. none of the above.

_____ 47. The nadir of an early deceleration occurs simultaneously with the:
A. beginning of a uterine contraction.
B. peak of a uterine contraction.
C. end of a uterine contraction.
D. entire uterine contraction.

_____ 48. Decelerations observed during uterine contraction most likely represent:
A. a response to hypoxia secondary to umbilical cord compression.
B. developing acidosis secondary to uteroplacental insufficiency.
C. a vagal response secondary to fetal head compression.
D. all of the above.

_____ 49. A late deceleration is characterized by:
   A. an onset at the peak of a uterine contraction, and then a return to the FHR baseline after the contraction is finished.
   B. an onset at the beginning of a uterine contraction, and then a return to the FHR baseline after the contraction is finished.
   C. an onset at the end of a uterine contraction, and then a return to the FHR baseline about 20 to 30 seconds later.
   D. an onset at the end of a uterine contraction, and then a return to the FHR baseline sometime before the next contraction.

_____ 50. Late decelerations can occur secondary to:
   A. abruptio placentae and previa.
   B. uterine hypertonicity secondary to oxytocin administration, postmaturity.
   C. maternal hypotension, smoking, and diabetes.
   D. all of the above.

_____ 51. Variable decelerations are typically characterized by an:
   A. acute decrease in FHR below baseline greater than 20 bpm and lasting between 1 and 2 minutes.
   B. abrupt decrease in FHR below baseline greater than 15 bpm and lasting between 15 seconds and 2 minutes.
   C. abrupt decrease in FHR below baseline greater than 15 bpm and lasting between 30 seconds and 1 minute.
   D. abrupt decrease in FHR below baseline greater than 20 bpm and lasting between 15 seconds and 2 minutes.

_____ 52. Variable decelerations can occur:
   A. any time during a contraction.
   B. independent of contractions.
   C. secondary to umbilical cord compression and occlusion.
   D. all of the above.

_____ 53. Which of the following situations would be most indicative of fetal distress?
   A. FHR baseline is 134 bpm, variability and accelerations are present, early decelerations are present with contractions.
   B. FHR baseline is 152 bpm, variability and accelerations are present, early decelerations are present with contractions.
   C. FHR baseline is 110 bpm, late decelerations occur with contractions, and variability and accelerations are not present.
   D. FHR baseline is 110 bpm, late decelerations, short-term variability and accelerations all occur with contractions.

_____ 54. Management of fetal distress may include all of the following except:
   A. discontinuation of oxytocin administration.
   B. terbutaline administration.
   C. amnioinfusion.
   D. internal vaginal exam.

_____ 55. Which of the following would best treat fetal distress secondary to hypertonic uterine contractions?
   A. administration of 100 percent oxygen via a nonrebreather mask.
   B. placing the patient in the left lateral recumbent position.
   C. administration of terbutaline.
   D. administration of a fluid challenge.

400 CRITICAL CARE PARAMEDIC

©2007 Pearson Education, Inc.
Critical Care Paramedic

_____ 56. Which of the following statements regarding abruptio placentae is true?
   A. Most of the blood loss that occurs is fetal in origin.
   B. Blood loss can be effectively estimated on external observation alone.
   C. Abruption begins with arterial hemorrhaging into the endometrium.
   D. Thromboplastin released from the deciduas basalis may encourage rapid clot formation, which may attenuate the hemorrhage.

_____ 57. All of the following are common physical finding associated with abruptio placentae except:
   A. fever.
   B. abdominal pain, uterine tenderness to palpation.
   C. uterine contractions.
   D. vaginal bleeding.

_____ 58. Ultrasound is an extremely useful tool for identifying the presence or absence of abruptio placenta.
   A. True.
   B. False.

_____ 59. Labs useful in the assessment and treatment of a patient with abruptio placentae include:
   A. CBC, type, and cross-match.   C. renal function studies.
   B. coagulation profile.   D. all of the above.

_____ 60. A fibrinogen level below 150 mg/dL accompanying abruptio placentae indicates:
   A. DIC.   C. hemodynamic stability.
   B. hemorrhagic shock.   D. none of the above.

_____ 61. Management of a patient with severe abruptio placentae is most likely to include:
   A. administration of oxygen, small-bore peripheral IV insertion, volume infusion with crystalloids and packed RBCs, insertion of Foley catheter, administration of a tocolytic.
   B. administration of oxygen, central line insertion, volume infusion with crystalloids, insertion of Foley catheter, administration of an anxiolytic.
   C. administration of oxygen, central line insertion, volume infusion with crystalloids and packed RBCs, insertion of Foley catheter, administration of a tocolytic.
   D. administration of oxygen, peripheral IV initiation, volume infusion with crystalloids, monitoring of urine output.

_____ 62. Advanced maternal age, smoking, cocaine use, multiparity, and uterine scarring are risk factors associated with:
   A. abruptio placentae.
   B. placenta previa.
   C. both A and B.
   D. none of the above.

_____ 63. Placenta previa occurs when:
   A. a normally implanted placenta prematurely separates from the uterine wall.
   B. the placenta implants and develops in the lower third of the uterus, totally or partially covering the cervical os.
   C. a fertilized egg implants and develops in the fallopian tube.
   D. none of the above.

_____ 64. Complications occur with placenta previa when:
   A. cervical effacement and dilation takes place, prior to the onset of labor.
   B. the fetal head enters the birth canal during the expulsion stage of labor.
   C. the placenta tears away from the uterine wall and arterial hemorrhaging occurs into the decidua basalis.
   D. hematoma formation and progression result in an expanding retroplacental injury.

_____ 65. The hallmark of placenta previa is:
A. the acute onset of abdominal pain and dark red bleeding in the second or third trimester.
B. gradual onset of painless bright red bleeding in the late second or third trimester.
C. the acute onset of painless, bright red bleeding in the late second or third trimester.
D. none of the above.

_____ 66. The management of placentae previa includes all of the following except:
A. administration of a tocolytic.
B. volume infusion with crystalloids and packed RBCs.
C. insertion of Foley catheter.
D. administration of morphine.

_____ 67. Preterm labor is defined as:
A. frequent uterine contractions occurring between the 20th and 37th weeks of gestation.
B. frequent uterine contractions resulting in progressive cervical dilation or effacement between the 20th and 37th weeks of gestation.
C. uterine contractions resulting in progressive cervical dilation or effacement between the 30th and 37th weeks of gestation.
D. the premature rupture of the amniotic membranes occurring between the 20th and 37th weeks of gestation.

_____ 68. Physiological factors that can contribute to development of preterm and premature labor include:
A. decreases in uteroplacental blood flow.
B. maternal dehydration.
C. maternal hypertension.
D. all of the above.

_____ 69. Lab studies useful in the assessment of preterm labor include:
A. CBC, urine culture, serum glucose, ABG.
B. coagulation studies, ABG, urinalysis, renal function tests.
C. CBC, urinalysis, cervical cultures, serum glucose, and potassium.
D. serum glucose, urine culture, renal function tests, coagulation studies.

_____ 70. Which of the following best describes the management goals of preterm labor?
A. Support the ABCs, maintain uteroplacental perfusion, and suppress labor.
B. Support the ABCs, suppress labor.
C. Suppress labor, correct hypoxia, deliver fetus in surgery.
D. Oxygenate, ventilate, suppress labor.

_____ 71. Medications used for tocolysis in the management of preterm labor include:
A. β-adrenergic agonists, magnesium sulfate.
B. calcium channel blockers.
C. prostaglandin synthetase inhibitors.
D. all of the above.

_____ 72. A (An) _____ breech occurs when the buttocks descend first, both hips are flexed, and one or both knees is flexed, resulting in one or both feet presenting with the buttocks.
A. frank   C. incomplete
B. complete   D. vertex

_____ 73. Risk factors that predispose a fetus for breech presentation include:
A. prostaglandin release associated with bacterial infections, abdominal trauma, and PROM.
B. advanced maternal age (over 35 years), smoking (doubles risk compared to nonsmokers), cocaine use.
C. grand multiparity, multiple gestation, placenta previa, and hydrocephaly.
D. chronic or gestational hypertension and uterine scarring from surgeries, past curettage, or infection.

_____ 74. Management of a breech birth may include all of the following except:
  A. refraining from touching the fetus and letting the delivery happen on its own.
  B. administration of a tocolytic.
  C. applying upward traction to facilitate the delivery of the posterior shoulder, and downward traction for the anterior shoulder.
  D. applying upward traction to the body while an assistant applies suprapubic pressure to encourage the delivery of the head.

_____ 75. Dystocia occurs when:
  A. delivery of the fetal head is followed by impaction of the fetal shoulders against the maternal pubic symphysis and sacrum, within the pelvis.
  B. both legs are extended upward, with both hips flexed and both knees extended.
  C. delivery of the fetal head is impeded by impaction of the fetal skull against the maternal pubic symphysis and sacrum, within the pelvis.
  D. none of the above.

_____ 76. Management of dystocia may include all of the following except:
  A. immediate draining of the urinary bladder and a mediolateral episiotomy.
  B. application of pressure to the fetus' anterior shoulder.
  C. application of gentle downward traction to the fetal head.
  D. application of pressure to the maternal fundal area.

_____ 77. The McRobert's maneuver involves:
  A. rotating the posterior shoulder of the fetus 180 degrees in a corkscrew fashion in an attempt to free the posterior shoulder.
  B. displacing the anterior shoulder toward the chest of the fetus within the pelvis.
  C. sharply flexing the maternal legs against the abdomen in an attempt to stretch the pelvic joints and increase the diameter of the pelvis.
  D. flexing the fetal head and placing the fetus back into the uterine cavity and then removing the fetus via emergent cesarean section.

_____ 78. Clinical signs of occult prolapsed cord include:
  A. the absence of short- and long-term variability in FHR.
  B. fetal bradycardia.
  C. recurrent variable decelerations in FHR.
  D. all of the above.

_____ 79. Of the following, the most appropriate management of prolapsed cord is:
  A. immediate administration of 100 percent oxygen, placing mother in knee-chest position, IV initiation, prevention of cord occlusion, transport.
  B. prevention of cord occlusion, placing mother in knee-chest position, administration of 100 percent oxygen, IV initiation, administration of a tocolytic agent, cesarean section if cord does not resolve spontaneously.
  C. immediate administration of 100 percent oxygen, placing mother in knee-chest position, prevention of cord occlusion, IV initiation, application of gentle traction on cord to facilitate delivery.
  D. prevention of cord occlusion, placing mother in knee-chest position, administration of 100 percent oxygen, cesarean section.

_____ 80. The four recognized categories of hypertension during pregnancy are:
  A. chronic hypertension, gestational hypertension, preeclampsia, and chronic hypertension with preeclampsia.
  B. hypertension, chronic hypertension, preeclampsia, and chronic hypertension with preeclampsia.
  C. hypertension, gestational hypertension, preeclampsia, and chronic hypertension with preeclampsia.
  D. chronic hypertension, gestational hypertension, preeclampsia, and gestational hypertension with preeclampsia.

©2007 Pearson Education, Inc.
Critical Care Paramedic   CHAPTER 28 *Obstetrical/Gynecological Emergencies* **403**

_____ 81. Preeclampsia is said to exist when:
   A. a hypertensive and pregnant patient experiences a seizure.
   B. a systolic blood pressure above 140 mmHg or a diastolic blood pressure above 90 mmHg develops.
   C. hypertension and proteinuria coexist.
   D. none of the above.

_____ 82. Proteinuria is present when:
   A. greater than 300 mg of protein is present in a 24-hour urine collection.
   B. a urine dipstick tests positive for protein.
   C. either A or B.
   D. none of the above.

_____ 83. Risk factors for gestational diabetes include:
   A. prostaglandin release associated with bacterial infections, abdominal trauma, and PROM.
   B. an age over 35 years or under 15 years, history of preeclampsia in a previous pregnancy, multiparity, preexisting renal or cardiovascular disease, diabetes, family history, and African-American descent.
   C. advanced maternal age (over 35 years), smoking (doubles risk compared to non-smokers), cocaine use.
   D. grand multiparity, multiple gestation, placenta previa, and hydrocephaly.

_____ 84. Severe preeclampsia is said to exist when which of the following clinical or laboratory exam findings are present:
   A. proteinuria >5 g in 24 hours, cerebral or visual symptoms.
   B. oliguria 500 mL over 24 hours, pulmonary edema.
   C. right upper quadrant pain, elevated liver enzymes, low platelet count (< 100,000/mm^3).
   D. all of the above.

_____ 85. The HELLP syndrome is an acronym for:
   A. Hematocrit, Elevated Liver function tests, and Low Platelets.
   B. Hemorrhage, Elevated Lactate, and Low-lying Placenta.
   C. Hemolysis, Elevated Liver function tests, and Low Platelets.
   D. Hemolysis, Elevated Lactate, and Low-lying Placenta.

_____ 86. Lab studies useful in the evaluation of preeclampsia include:
   A. liver function tests, CBC, urinalysis, serum glucose.
   B. CBC, urinalysis, coagulation studies, electrolytes.
   C. ABG, CBC, urine dipstick, serum amylase, serum lipase.
   D. ABG, liver function tests, coagulation studies.

_____ 87. Management of preeclampsia may include:
   A. administration of oxygen, morphine, furosemide, hydralazine, magnesium sulfate, and benzodiazepines.
   B. administration of oxygen, monitoring of urine output, morphine, judicious use of furosemide, and hydralazine.
   C. administration of oxygen, nitrates, bed rest in a low-lit, quiet environment.
   D. none of the above.

_____ 88. Risk factors for gestational diabetes include:
   A. maternal obesity, previous infant over 4,000 g birthweight, and excessive weight gain during pregnancy.
   B. history or family history of DM, history of preeclampsia, maternal age over 30 years.
   C. both A and B.
   D. none of the above.

_____ 89. Maternal complications of gestational diabetes include:
   A. preterm labor and preeclampsia.
   B. Pyleonephritis.
   C. need for cesarean section.
   D. all of the above.

_____ 90. The treatment of gestational diabetes may include:
   A. administration of 100 percent oxygen via nonrebreather mask at 15 lpm, IV of normal saline established, blood glucose determined, administration of dextrose IV if hypoglycemia present.
   B. administration of 100 percent oxygen via nonrebreather mask at 15 lpm, IV of normal saline established, blood glucose determined, administration of insulin SQ if hyperglycemia present.
   C. both A and B.
   D. none of the above.

Chapter 29

Neonatal Emergencies

Review of Chapter Objectives

Upon completion of this chapter, the student should be able to:

1. Appreciate the physiological differences between the adult and the neonate. p. 876

Neonates have significant physiological differences compared to an adult; differences that affect assessment, management, and transport decisions. Many of these differences are the same as for the pediatric patient, covered in Chapter 27, and will be reviewed again here. Specific areas of concern are the cardiovascular and pulmonary systems, airway anatomy, metabolism and thermoregulation, and glucose requirements.

The majority of physiologic change that occurs with the shift from intrauterine to extrauterine life occurs in the first few minutes after delivery and includes the change in circulation from the placenta to the pulmonary system with the clamping of the umbilical cord. This change in circulation occurs as a result of the interruption of low-resistance, placental blood flow from the umbilical cord, which causes an increase in systemic vascular resistance (SVR). Increased SVR forces closure of the ductus venosus, which results in increased renal perfusion.

The neonatal heart is capable of increasing its rate in order to improve cardiac output, but is unable to increase contractile force. As such, cardiac output may be drastically reduced with bradycardia. In addition, the neonate's first breaths result in lung expansion. Expansion of the lungs causes a reduction in pulmonary vascular resistance. Reduced pulmonary vascular resistance results in an increase in pulmonary blood flow and a reduction in pulmonary artery pressures. The left side of the heart assumes higher pressures then the right, resulting in closure of the foramen ovale; closure of the ductus arteriosus occurs in the first hours to weeks after birth, driven by changes in arterial oxygen content.

While still in utero, the fetus is oxygenated through the placenta. Any disturbance to alveolar ventilation and gas exchange following birth must be identified and dealt with immediately to ensure adequate respiration.

Neonate patients have unique airway anatomy and physiology compared to adults that greatly affects their response to disease and trauma and also your approach to airway control. Specific differences in pediatric airway anatomy include:

- Larger tongue in relation to oropharynx
- Nares are proportionally smaller
- Trachea is more narrow and pliable
- Epiglottis is larger, less supported, and omega-shaped
- Larynx is more superior and anterior
- Production of larger amounts of oral secretions
- Narrowest part of pediatric airway is at the level of the cricoid ring

A tongue that is larger in comparison to the oropharynx results in less room for airway swelling and a greater risk of airway occlusion. The smaller external nares may occlude easier from edema, mucus or blood accumulation, or tissue hypertrophy. The more narrow and pliable pediatric trachea is subject to occlusion from hyperextension/hyperflexion, and from occlusion secondary to swelling, mucus and blood accumulation, and neoplasm. The neonatal epiglottis may be difficult to identify and/or control during intubation. The neonatal larynx is located at the level of the first or second cervical vertebrae, compared to the adult, where it is found at the level of the fourth or fifth cervical vertebrae; it is superior and anterior compared to the adult. The narrow, neonatal cricoid ring acts as a physiological cuff when the endotracheal tube is in place, and can also be the site of occlusion secondary to foreign body aspiration.

The neonatal rib cage, being incompletely calcified, is more flexible than that of an adult and is unable to support the lungs during times of great negative intrathoracic pressure that is typical of large-volume ventilation attempts. In such instances, accessory muscles are recruited to aid in ventilation. However, due to the more horizontal position of the ribs, the leverage achieved during intercostal muscle contraction in a neonate is less than that of an adult, resulting in less lift of rib during inspiration. In addition, the accessory muscles of neonates are less developed; the younger the patient, the less developed the muscles. This, combined with decreased rigidity of the chest wall, contributes to diaphragmatic breathing in the neonate. During inspiration, the neonate experiences less increase in anterior/posterior chest diameter, less increase in intrathoracic volume, and a smaller tidal volume. Neonates have a lower pulmonary reserve capacity than an adult, as the relatively large heart decreases the room available for lung expansion. Neonates are also primarily abdominal breathers, which means that they rely heavily on diaphragmatic motion (a consequence of immature intercostal muscles and pliable ribs) for the work of breathing. In addition, a small abdominal cavity filled with relatively large abdominal organs tends to impede diaphragmatic movement; decompressing the stomach can increase diaphragm motility.

Neonates have a higher metabolic rate than adults, and they consume oxygen in the bloodstream at nearly double the rate of an adult. Their smaller pulmonary reserve capacity, coupled with a higher metabolic demand for oxygen, leaves the neonate more predisposed to hypoxemia at the cellular level, even with spontaneous respirations. Hypoxemia in the neonate is a problem that can develop rapidly with disastrous effects should the critical care paramedic not stay attuned to the pulmonary functioning of the patient.

A summary of the airway, pulmonary, and metabolic differences that impact ventilation and respiration in a neonate can be summarized as follows:

- The larger tongue and pliable epiglottis allow for the development of airway occlusion in the obtunded neonate very easily. In addition, they both serve as a formidable challenge when providing orotracheal intubation.
- The pliancy of the thoracic bony structure fails to provide needed lift and support to the lung tissue to allow inhalation, especially in situations of heightened ventilatory effort.
- The nature of the neonate being primarily an abdominal breather is diminished by any situation in which intra-abdominal pressure is elevated, thereby limiting diaphragmatic motion.
- Because the neonatal musculature is still relatively weak, muscle fatigue will occur quickly in situations where ventilatory effort is markedly higher.
- The higher metabolic consumption of oxygen at the cellular level in neonates will result in faster onset of hypoxemia from an airway or ventilatory deficit.

All of these differences contribute to the tendency of the neonate to rapidly decompensate from hypoxemia and hypercapnia induced by pulmonary dysfunction.

Neonates are at greater risk for developing hypoglycemia secondary to decreased glycogen stores, immature hepatic development (decreased glycogenolysis), increased metabolic rate (increased glucose requirements), and pre-existing diabetes.

Thermoregulation in the neonate is effected by the increased surface area-to-volume ratio, which is four times that of an adult. With heat production only 1½ times that of an adult, a pediatric patient has a greater risk of hypothermia. Heat loss can occur as a result of convection, radiation, evaporation, and conduction.

Convective heat loss, secondary to drafts and/or cold environments, is perhaps the most likely cause of the development of hypothermia in the neonatal patient in the transport environment.

2. Discuss the pathophysiology of respiratory complications in the neonate. p. 880; 3. Discuss the pathophysiology of meconium aspiration. p. 882

Prior to a review of respiratory complications in the neonate, it is worth taking a moment to review the terms commonly used to describe respiratory distress. Preciseness in the use of terms describing respiratory distress, respiratory failure, and respiratory arrest are necessary, as the distinction between the three dictates the aggressiveness of the management of the acutely ill neonate. In cases of respiratory distress, the patient still has the ability to compensate and maintain adequate minute ventilation spontaneously. Respiratory failure is considered to be present when the patient has exhausted all of his compensatory mechanisms, and the respiratory effort present is insufficient in meeting the body's metabolic oxygenation and carbon dioxide elimination demands. Respiratory arrest occurs when the patient is apneic.

Respiratory complications seen in the neonate include persistent pulmonary hypertension, meconium aspiration syndrome, transient tachypnea of the newborn (TTN), infant respiratory distress syndrome (IRDS) and congenital diaphragmatic hernia.

Persistent pulmonary hypertension of the newborn (PPHN)

PPHN is a clinical syndrome in which pulmonary vascular resistance is elevated in the presence of changes in pulmonary vessel reactivity. The end result is sustained fetal circulation and the failure of the ductus arteriosus and foramen ovale to close. Right-to-left shunting occurs, resulting in inadequate pulmonary perfusion and the development of respiratory distress, hypoxemia, and acidosis. PPHN is commonly associated with meconium aspiration syndrome, perinatal hypothermia, hypoglycemia, congenital diaphragmatic hernia, hyaline membrane disease, hypoxia, sepsis, and pneumonia.

The clinical presentation mirrors many of the signs and symptoms seen with congenital heart diseases:

- Cyanosis
- Tachycardia, tachypnea

The management of PPHN may include:

- Minimal stimulation: limit handling, suctioning
- Airway/breathing
  - Endotracheal intubation, mechanical ventilation often necessary to maintain oxygenation
  - Use of NMBAs, or sedatives if patient is mechanically ventilated
  - High-frequency, oscillatory, and jet ventilation is sometimes utilized
  - Continuous pulse oxymetry
- Pharmacological intervention:
  - Alkalinizing agents
    - Sodium bicarbonate: correct metabolic acidosis
  - Pulmonary vasodilating agents
    - Decrease pulmonary vascular resistance
    - Nitric oxide: inhaled
    - Adenosine, magnesium sulfate
  - Vasopressors
    - Increase systemic blood pressure to greater than pulmonary blood pressure, decreasing right-to-left shunt
    - dopamine
- Lab studies
  - Serum glucose
  - ABG
    - Assessment of pH, $PaCO_2$, PaO_2
    - Rule out acidosis
  - Serum lactate
  - CBC

- WBC and differential: detect underlying sepsis, pneumonia
- Platelets are commonly low
- Evaluate for elevated hematocrit, rule out polycythemia
  - Imaging studies
    - Chest radiograph
      - Rule out congenital diaphragmatic hernia
      - Detect underlying lung disease as cause
        - Meconium aspiration syndrome
        - Pneumonia
    - Cardiac ultrasound
      - Detect congenital heart abnormalities
      - Assess for presence and severity of right-to-left shunt and pulmonary hypertension

Meconium aspiration syndrome

Meconium is the first gastrointestinal discharge from a newborn, consisting of intestinal secretions, epithelial cells, mucus, and lanugo, and having a viscous, dark green appearance. While meconium is expelled prematurely in 10 to 15 percent of all deliveries, only 2 to 10 percent of neonates will aspirate meconium into their lower airways. Meconium reduces the antibacterial ability of the amniotic fluid, increase the risk of bacterial infection, and is irritating to fetal skin, thereby increasing the risk of erythema toxicum. The most severe complication of meconium passage is aspiration of meconium-stained amniotic fluid before, during, and after birth. Aspiration can result in airway obstruction, chemical pneumonitis, and inactivation of alveolar surfactant leading to neonatal respiratory distress. A right-to-left shunt and ventilation-perfusion (V/Q) mismatch is common with significant aspiration. Factors that contribute to the passing of meconium include placental insufficiency, maternal hypertension, maternal drug abuse (cocaine, tobacco), oligohydramnios, and preeclampsia.

Signs and symptoms present on clinical exam include:

- Respiratory distress: grunting, nasal flaring, cyanosis
- Tachycardia, tachypnea
- Presence of meconium in oropharynx, airway

There are no known prevention strategies, though nasopharyngeal and endotracheal suctioning prior to delivery of the thorax may limit the extent of meconium aspiration into the lower airways. Common management of meconium aspiration may include:

- Airway/breathing
  - Suctioning of meconium
  - Endotracheal intubation
  - Mechanical ventilation
    - Use of NMBAs, sedatives if patient mechanically ventilated
    - High-frequency, oscillatory, and jet ventilation sometimes utilized
  - Continuous pulse oxymetry
- Pharmacological intervention
  - Pulmonary vasodilating agents
    - Decrease pulmonary vascular resistance
    - Nitric oxide: inhaled
  - Vasopressors
    - Increase systemic blood pressure to greater than pulmonary blood pressure, decreasing Right-to-Left shunt
    - Dopamine
- Lab studies
  - ABG
    - Assessment of pH, $PaCO_2$, PaO_2 necessary to assess for V/Q mismatch
    - Rule out acidosis
  - Serum lactate
  - CBC

- Rule out infection
- Rule out thrombocytopenia
- Ensure adequate hemoglobin and hematocrit
- Serum glucose
- Imaging studies
  - Chest radiograph
    - Determine extent of meconium contamination
    - Identify atelectasis, air blockage
  - Cardiac ultrasound
    - Assess for presence and severity of right-to-left shunt and pulmonary hypertension
    - Ensure normal cardiac development
- Extracorporeal membrane oxygenation (ECMO) if all other therapy unsuccessful

Transient tachypnea of the newborn (TTN)

Also known as "wet lung" or "Type II Respiratory Distress Syndrome," TTN occurs secondary to a delay in the clearance of fluid in the fetal lungs after birth. Neonates with TTN will present within the first few hours of extrauterine life with tachypnea; ABG analysis reveals occasional or mild hypoxia without CO_2 retention (due to CO_2's ability to more readily dissolve in, and pass through, water), and increased O_2 demand. Risk factors for TTN include cesarean delivery, prolonged labor, maternal asthma, and smoking.

TTN is a self-limiting process that usually resolves within 48 to 72 hours from birth, though admission to an ICU is warranted. It is important to monitor a neonate with TTN closely, should the patient deteriorate due to an undiagnosed pathology or fatigue develop.

Management of TTN may include:

- Airway/breathing
  - Supportive care to assure adequate oxygenation and ventilation
  - Oxygen hoods for mild TNN
  - Rarely, CPAP, endotracheal intubation may be necessary
  - Continuous pulse oxymetry
- Pharmacological intervention
  - Antibiotics
    - Usually administered for 36 to 48 hours after birth, until sepsis ruled out
- Lab studies
  - ABG
    - assessment of pH, $PaCO_2$, PaO_2
    - rule out acidosis
  - Serum lactate
  - Serum glucose
- Imaging studies
  - Chest radiograph
  - Characteristic findings of TTN include patchy infiltrates, perihilar streaking, and fluid in the interlobular fissures

Infant respiratory distress syndrome (IRDS)

Affecting about 10 percent of all preterm infants, IRDS, also known as hyaline membrane disease (HMD), is rarely seen in full-term infants. IRDS occurs secondary to a deficiency of pulmonary surfactant and results in atelectasis, decreased lung compliance, decreased functional residual capacity, and increased dead air space. As a result, the neonate's lungs are more difficult to inflate (requiring the neonate to work hard at breathing) and gas exchange is limited in collapsed alveoli. R-to-L shunting may occur through a patent ductus arteriosus and/or a patent foramen ovale. The incidence and severity of IRDS are inversely related to the gestational age, as maturation of the lung parenchyma and surfactant production are some of the last processes to take place in fetal development, at around 32 weeks or more. Risk factors of IRDS include maternal diabetes, premature birth, and a family history of IRDS.

Signs and symptoms of IRDS include:

- Tachypnea, shortness of breath
- Accessory muscle use, sternal retractions, grunting, nasal flaring
- Respiratory arrest from muscle fatigue, hypoxemia, and acidosis

The management of IRDS may include:

- Airway/breathing
  - Assure adequate oxygenation and ventilation
  - Oxygen hoods for mild IRDS
  - CPAP, endotracheal intubation
  - Mechanical ventilation
    - Use of NMBAs, sedatives if patient mechanically ventilated
    - High-frequency, oscillatory, and jet ventilation sometimes utilized
  - Continuous pulse oxymetry
- Pharmacological intervention:
  - Pulmonary surfactant
    - Beractant, calfactant, poractant, colfosceril
- Lab studies:
  - ABG
    - Assessment of pH, $PaCO_2$, PaO_2
    - Rule out acidosis
  - Serum glucose
  - Serum lactate
- Imaging studies
  - Chest radiograph
    - Characteristic finds include atelectasis, air bronchograms

Congenital diaphragmatic hernia (CDH)

CDH is a complication in which the bowel protrudes into the thoracic cavity through an interruption of the diaphragm, usually as the result of congenital abnormality. There are three basic types of CDH; Morgagni hernia, hiatus hernia, and Bochdalek hernia. A Morgagni hernia occurs at the sternocostal hiatus of anterior diaphragm, at the midline. A hiatus hernia occurs at the esophageal hiatus. A Bochdalek hernia is a posterolateral defect in the diaphragm. Left-sided Bochdalek hernia accounts for about 85 percent of all cases of CDH, and allows small and large bowel and solid organ herniation into the thorax.

The main insult resulting from CDH is pulmonary hypoplasia, thought to result from the prolonged intrauterine compression of the developing lung. In addition, the herniated abdominal viscera prevents full lung expansion in the affected hemithorax; both complications contribute to pulmonary compromise. Gastric volvulus, gastric blockage, and intestinal perforation are possible and can lead to complications. PPHN and R-to-L shunting often complicates CDH. Mortality ranges from 40 to 60 percent.

Signs and symptoms of CDH include:

- Respiratory distress
- Unequal lung sounds
- Scaphoid-shaped abdomen
- Cyanosis

Management of CDH may include:

- Airway/breathing
  - BVM ventilation should be avoided
  - Endotracheal intubation
    - As soon as severe CDH identified
    - NMBAs, sedation
    - Mechanical ventilation

- Orogastric tube to decompress stomach
- Pulse oxymetry monitoring on all patients
- Pharmacological intervention
  - Pulmonary surfactant
    - Beractant, calfactant, poractant, colfosceril
  - Pulmonary vasodilators
    - Nitric oxide: inhaled
  - Vasopressors
    - Dopamine
    - Dobutamine
- Lab studies:
  - ABG
    - Assessment of pH, $PaCO_2$, PaO_2
    - Rule out acidosis
  - Serum lactate
  - Serum glucose
- Imaging studies
  - Chest radiograph
    - Orogastric tube may assist in locating stomach
    - Findings charateristic of Bochdalek hernia include loops of bowel in thorax, right shift of cardiac silhoutte, and pneumothorax
  - Cardiac ultrasound
    - Rule out congenital defect
- Definitive treatment is surgical repair

4. Discuss the step wise procedure used to manage a neonate who presents with meconium aspiration. pp. 882, 883; 5. Discuss the pathophysiology of congenital heart disease in the neonate. p. 884

Congenital heart disease (CHD) occurs in approximately eight per 1,000 live births, equal to about 40,000 neonates born each year with a heart defect. Many congenital heart defects are subclinical and are not identified until they affect hemodynamic status. CHDs can result in abnormalities in volumes and/or pressures in the atria or ventricles, in the mixing of venous and arterial blood, and inadequate cardiac output and poor systemic perfusion.

Specific defects include left-to-right shunt defects such as atrial septal defect (ASD), ventricular septal defect (VSD), and patent ductus arteriosus; obstruction defecta (aortic and pulmonary stenosis, coarchtation of the aorta), and cyanotic defects such as transposition of the great vessels (TGV) and tetralogy of Fallot.

Left-to-right shunt defects are conditions in which oxygenated blood is shifted from the left side of the heart to the right side. The defect is said to be acyanotic, as deoxygenated blood does not enter the aorta and get distributed to the body because higher pressures on the left side of the heart prevent unoxygenated blood from the right side of the heart from entering the aorta and systemic circulation. Specific examples of left-to-right defects are ASDs, VSDs, and PDAs.

Atrial Septal Defect (ASD)
ASD is commonly the result of nonclosure of the foramen ovale, referred to as a "patent" foramen ovale. Oxygenated blood from the pulmonary vein enters the left atria in a higher left atrial pressure compared to right. This pressure difference produces a volume shift from the left atria to the right, and atrial and ventricular enlargement.

Signs and symptoms associated with ASD include:

- Commonly subclinical
  - Clinical significance related to size of defect
- Transient or persistent episodes of cyanosis may develop
- Rarely, CHF might develop

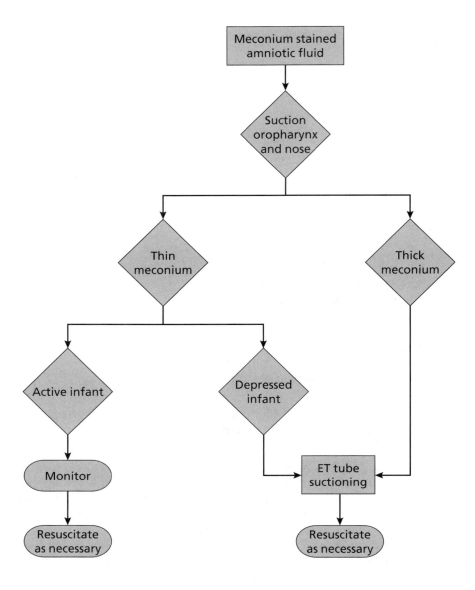

Management of ASD may include:

- Supportive care
  - Oxygen administration
  - Anticoagulatnts to eliminate risk of embolus in specific situations
- Lab studies
  - ABG analysis
  - Serum lactate
  - Serum glucose
- Imaging studies:
  - Echocardiography: will identify ASD
- Surgical repair is the definitive treatment

Ventricular septal defect (VSD)
A VSD is a defect in the ventricular septum that allows blood to flow between the ventricles. VSD can result in left-to-right shunting of blood, pulmonary hypertension, changes in the pulmonary vascular bed, and decreased systemic cardiac output.

The size of the defect determines the clinical significance:

- Small VSD
  - Produces a small left-to-right shunt
  - Little pulmonary vascular congestion, chamber enlargement
  - More difficult to diagnose
  - Chest radiograph:
    - Normal heart size
    - Normal pulmonary vascularity
  - ECG:
    - Findings usually normal
- Large VSD
  - Produces large amounts of pulmonary blood flow
  - Initially, pulmonary vascular resistance (PVR) and systemic vascular resistance (SVR) are nearly equal
    - Little left-to-right shunting
  - With drop in PVR (about two to 12 weeks of age), pulmonary blood flow increases
    - Pulmonary hypertension develops
    - Signs of left ventricular overload, CHF develops
  - Chest radiograph shows
    - Right ventricular hypertrophy
    - Prominent pulmonary artery
    - Decreased pulmonary vasculature in outer lung fields

Again, a VSD can present early or late in extrauterine life; early presentation is typified by global ventricular enlargement, while late presentation is typified by equal left-to-right and right-to-left shunting/mixing of blood, a result of equal/near-equal PVR and SVR.

Signs and symptoms of VSD include:

- Respiratory distress, fatigue, diaphoresis at feedings
- History of poor weight gain or weight loss
- CHF
- Squatting, in infants with large defects

Management of VSD includes:

- Supportive care
  - Oxygen administration
- Lab studies:
  - ABG analysis
  - Serum lactate
  - Serum glucose
- Pharmacological management
  - Treat CHF if present
  - Furosemide, Captopril
- Surgical management
  - Large VSDs often are corrected surgically

Patent ductus arteriosus (PDA)

PDA is a condition characterized by failure of the ductus arteriosus to close after pulmonary circulation has been established in the neonate, allowing blood to flow from the aorta to the pulmonary artery. Flow through the PDA is greatest when systemic vascular resistance (pressure) is high and/or pulmonary vascular resistance (pressure) is low. The blood flow through a typical PDA follows a path into the pulmonary artery, then through the pulmonary capillaries, the pulmonary veins, the left atrium, the left ventricle, and then the aorta.

As a result of this increased blood flow, PDA can cause pulmonary hypertension and left-sided myocardial hypertrophy.

The size of the defect and amount of blood flow determine the clinical significance of the PDA.

Signs and symptoms of PDA include:

- The typical patient with PDA is asymptomatic
- Difficulty breathing, tachypnea, tachycardia
- Bounding pulses, widening pulse pressures
- Failure to thrive, fatigue at feedings

Management of PDA may entail:

- Supportive care
  - Oxygen administration
- Lab studies
  - ABG analysis
  - Serum lactate
  - Serum glucose
- Imaging studies
  - Chest radiograph
    - Prominent pulmonary artery and veins
    - Left artial and ventricular enlargement
  - Echocardiography
    - Diagnostic for PDA
- ECG
  - Usually normal
  - May show left ventricular enlargement
  - Neonates may present with T-wave inversion and ST depression
- Pharmacological management
  - Indomethacin
    - Prostaglandin inhibitor
- Surgical management
  - Cardiac catheterization

Obstructive defects occur when a structural deformity completely or partially blocks blood flow from the heart. Signs and symptoms are secondary to the cardiovascular structures involved. Examples of obstructive defects are aortic and pulmonary valve stenosis and coarctation of the aorta.

Aortic and pulmonary valve stenosis

Aortic or pulmonary valvular narrowing is the hallmark of stenosis. In both cases, blood flow is impeded, resulting in increased intraventricular pressure, ventricular enlargement, and post-stenotic vessel dilation.

Signs and symptoms of valvular stenosis include:

- Respiratory distress, tachypnea, tachycardia
- Weak pulse, hypotension, and fatigue at feedings

Management includes:

- Supportive care
  - Oxygenation
- Lab studies
  - ABG analysis
  - Serum lactate
  - Serum glucose
- Imaging studies
  - Echocardiography
    - Diagnostic
- Pharmacological management
  - Antibiotics
    - Prophylaxis prior to procedures that may result in bacteremia

- Prostaglandin E$_1$
  - Keeps ductus arteriosus patent
  - Allows blood from pulmonary artery to enter aorta and maintain systemic circulation
- Surgical management
  - Balloon angioplasty/valvuloplasty

Coarctation of the aorta (CoA)

CoA is characterized by narrowing of the aorta near the distal aspect of the aortic arch, impeding blood flow from the left ventricle and resulting in increased left ventricular pressures, increased left ventricular workload, and left ventricular hypertrophy.

Signs and symptoms of CoA include:

- Tachycardia, tachypnea
- Bounding pulses in the upper extremities with thready or absent pulses in the lower extremities
- Fatigue at feedings
- CHF and shock may develop

Management of CoA may include:

- Supportive care
  - Oxygen administration
- Lab studies
  - ABG analysis
  - Serum lactate
  - Serum glucose
- Pharmacological management
  - Prostaglandin E$_1$
    - Keeps ductus arteriosus patent
    - Allows blood from pulmonary artery to enter the aorta to maintain systemic circulation
  - Treatment of CHF
    - Furosemide, inotropic agents
- Surgical management
  - Balloon angioplasty/surgical resection is the definitive treatment

Cyanotic defects are characterized by poor pulmonary blood flow resulting from one or more of the following:

- Difficulty in pumping blood out of the right side of the heart
- Greater pressure gradient from the right to the left side of the heart that promotes a shunting of blood to the left side
  - This results in unoxygenated blood being returned to the left side of the heart
- Blockage of pulmonary blood flow or structural deformity

Specific examples of cyanotic defects include complete transposition of the great vessels and tetralogy of Fallot.

Complete transposition of the great vessels (TGV)

TGV is characterized by abnormal positioning of the aorta and pulmonary arteries, resulting in a pulmonary artery that leaves the left ventricle and an aorta that leaves the right ventricle. TGV is associated with ASD, VSD, and PDA up to 80 percent of the time, and has to be for the patient to survive as parallel, closed circulations are created without them. Without these defects, no intracardiac mixing of oxygenated and deoxygenated blood occurs, and the child dies from systemic hypoxia. The degree of cyanosis and acidosis depends on number and size of intracardiac and extracardiac shunts. Signs and symptoms include:

- Difficulty breathing
- Tachypnea, tachycardia
- Cyanosis

Treatment of TGV involves supportive care until surgical repair (arterial switch) is performed.

Tetralogy of Fallot

Tetralogy of Fallot is a condition characterized by four criteria: VSD, pulmonary stenosis, rightward displacement of aortic valve that overrides the VSD, and right ventricular hypertrophy.

The degree of cyanosis secondary to mixing of oxygenated and deoxygenated blood is determined by the degree of pulmonary stenosis. The greater the pulmonary stenosis, the greater the right side intraventricular pressure, the greater the right-to-left shunt, and the more deoxygenated blood reaches systemic circulation via the aorta. Signs and symptoms include tachypnea, tachycardia, and fatigue at feedings. Treatment is supportive, ensuring adequate oxygenation, and prostaglandin should be adminstered.

Transport guidelines for congenital heart defects:

- Ensure patent airway
- Ensure adequate ventilation, oxygenation
- Treat CHF
- Correct circulatory compromise
  - Fluid volume resuscitation
  - Vasopressors
- Keep patient warm

6. **Describe the initial steps and ongoing management in the assessment and management of the neonate. (p. 891); 7. Discuss the importance of, and how to assure, normothermia in the neonatal patient during transports.** (p. 892)

Several assessment findings are common in the neonate that are not frequently seen in older patient populations. Cyanosis is the most common finding, and is insignificant when the neonate is crying. Jaundice, a result of high serum bilirubin levels, is typical for most neonates in the first week of extrauterine life and usually resolves without intervention. Treatment, if necessary, is phototherapy, in which the neonate is exposed to ultraviolet light. Bilirubin undergoes structural isomerization, and the photoisomers are excreted in bile and in urine. Blood transfusion is necessary if fluorescent light treatment proves unsuccessful. Neonatal vital signs are extremely variable in neonates, and deviate from what is generally considered the norm. Access to reference material, such as a pediatric Broselow tape or pocket guide, is advisable. In addition to respiratory rate, blood pressure, and heart rate, consider blood glucose level a vital sign in the neonate, with 70–80 mg/dL considered nonhypoglycemic.

General treatment considerations in the neonate include airway, vascular access, temperature regulation, and blood glucose regulation. The airway should be secured and maintained as soon as possible. RSI is not as common in the neonatal population as in the adult, but should be used when necessary. Accidental extubation is a frequent respiratory complication during transport, and useful prevention measures include sedation, the use of NMBAs and C-collars, and lateral immobilization of the head.

Obtaining vascular access can be difficult even for experienced providers, but multiple access options should be available on all neonatal patients including IV, IO, and umbilical routes.

Temperature regulation is critically important and should be consistently reassessed and assured during transport. Temperature regulation is initially provided by preventing heat loss (drying the neonate, wrapping him in a blanket, covering his head) while promoting strategies for aggressive warming. Prior to transport, radiant warmers, insulated blankets, and heated blankets can be utilized. Transport incubators are industry standard for the transport environment.

Serum glucose levels should be checked frequently and hypoglycemia managed aggressively with the infusion of D10W 0.5–1.0 g/kg (or 5–10 mL/kg of D10W) IV. Maintenance infusion, if necessary, is typically 80cc/kg/day. Administration of D25W or D50W is contraindicated, as significant increases in plasma osmolarity resulting in hypernatremia and cerebral edema can occur.

8. **Discuss the pathophysiology of hypoglycemia in the neonate.** p. 876

Newborns are at significant risk for the development of acute hypoglycemia because of poor glucose stores and the inability to stimulate the release of glucose stores from the immature

©2007 Pearson Education, Inc.
Critical Care Paramedic

neonatal liver. An increased metabolism results in the utilization of large quantities of available glucose.

Neonatal glucose levels should be assessed within one to two hours after birth and repeated every 30 minutes to one hour thereafter until normal glucose levels have been attained. Normal blood glucose levels (BGLs) in the neonate should be maintained above 70–80 mg/dL.

Case Study

Your team has been activated to intercept a BLS ground ambulance for a "high risk" OB patient. The patient was being transported to the medical center where your program is based from a rural community approximately 70 miles away. The hospital closest to the scene is a small community hospital without an OB service, lying approximately 30 miles in the opposite direction. An update in flight advises you that the patient is a 15-year-old female who has had no prenatal care and whose due date is unknown. She began crowning, so the ambulance has stopped to prepare for imminent delivery at a high school parking lot frequently used by your service as an LZ.

After departing the aircraft, you and your partner are met at the edge of the LZ by the local fire chief, who informs you that the ambulance crew has just delivered the baby and tells you, "It doesn't look good." Climbing into the side door of the ambulance, you note the look of fear in the eyes of the EMTs. On the stretcher is a small female who is being attended by two EMTs. She appears distraught and keeps repeating over and over, "I can't be pregnant, I can't be pregnant . . . " Looking at the girl's abdomen, you note a very small, limp, female infant being suctioned by another EMT. The baby is lying on a towel, is blue in color, and appears premature. She is covered with amniotic fluid, but there does not appear to be any meconium present. While the EMT continues to suction the neonate's mouth and nose, you begin towel drying the baby. Your partner clamps and cuts the cord and instructs one of the EMTs attending to the mother to administer blow-by oxygen to the baby. Even though the infant's airway is clear now and its skin is dry, she remains blue and has no apparent respiratory effort. You move the infant to the bench seat and onto a dry towel with a slight rolled edge under her shoulders to assist in maintaining an airway. While your partner continues to stimulate the baby, you begin to ventilate her with a BVM attached to high flow oxygen at a rate of 60 breaths per minute. Your partner assesses the infant's brachial pulse at 80 beats per minute, but agrees that there is good chest rise and that compressions should be withheld for now. Thirty seconds later, while reassessing the pulse, your partner's face splits into a wide grin and he says, "It's fast and strong . . . it's . . . uh . . . 22 times 6, that's 132, the heart rate is 132 and strong." You note that the baby is now moving her arms and is becoming pink. You stop ventilations and note that she is breathing on her own at a rate of 42 breaths per minute. Keeping the mask of the BVM near her face to administer blowby oxygen, you continue to reassess her. She now has a strong cry and is moving her arms actively. Your partner tests her blood glucose with a glucometer and a sample from her heel. Wrapping her in a dry towel, you then cover the towel with a plastic reflective infant swaddling blanket. Your partner reports that the baby's blood sugar is 68 mg/dL, allaying your concerns about hypoglycemia. With the baby stable, you turn your attention to her mother. The EMT in charge of her care advises you that mom's vital signs are stable and other than being insistent about the fact that she could not be pregnant, is doing just fine. Your partner takes the baby from your arms and lays her on her mother's chest, while you advise the pilot that everything is under control and you're going to ride in with the ambulance. Throughout the transport, reassessment of the infant is without change and the mother delivers the placenta without complication. On arrival at the medical center, you bypass the emergency department and deliver both of your patients directly to the labor and delivery floor.

DISCUSSION QUESTIONS

1. What are the initial steps in the assessment and management of a neonatal patient?
2. What is the procedure used to manage a neonate with meconium aspiration?
3. What is the importance of blood glucose assessment in neonatal patients?

Content Review

MULTIPLE CHOICE

_____ 1. Common potential complications associated with a neonate born at 43 weeks gestation include:
   A. thermoregulation, IRDS, sepsis.
   B. pneumonia, birth asphyxia, meconium aspiration, sepsis.
   C. IRDS, meconium aspiration, sepsis, asphyxia-related complications.
   D. asphyxia-related complications, sepsis.

_____ 2. Factors that place a neonate at risk for hypothermia include:
   A. inability to shiver.
   B. reduced fat stores.
   C. heat production that is only one-half that of an adult.
   D. all of the above.

_____ 3. Methods of thermoregulation of the neonate during transport include all of the following except:
   A. use of transport incubator.
   B. placing heat packs in contact with neonate.
   C. swaddling the neonate in blankets.
   D. covering the neonate's head with a cap.

_____ 4. Which of the following reasons why the neonate is at risk for the development of acute hypoglycemia is false?
   A. The neonate has poor glucose stores.
   B. The neonate is unable to stimulate the release of glucose stores from its immature liver.
   C. Decreased metabolism utilizes large quantities of available glucose.
   D. Increased metabolic demand utilizes large quantities of available glucose.

_____ 5. All of the following are characteristic of the neonatal airway except:
   A. large tongue in relation to oropharynx.
   B. trachea is narrow and pliable.
   C. epiglottis is large, less supported, and omega-shaped.
   D. larynx is inferior, anterior.

_____ 6. Neonates utilize diaphragmatic breathing during periods of respiratory distress to:
   A. overcome the disadvantage of a lack of accessory muscles.
   B. increase antero-posterior chest diameter.
   C. increase intra-abdominal pressure.
   D. increase intrathoracic pressure.

_____ 7. Factors that contribute to a neonate's relatively diminished pulmonary reserve capacity include:
   A. a large heart.
   B. limited availability of intrathoracic space for lung expansion.
   C. limited ability to increase intrathoracic volume.
   D. all of the above.

_____ 8. Which of the following statements regarding neonatal pulmonary anatomy and physiology is true?
   A. A stiff neonatal sternum contributes to the ability to create a strong negative intrathoracic pressure during inspiration.
   B. Neonatal ribs are more horizontal than they are rounded, producing little leverage to increase the anterior and posterior diameter of the chest.
   C. Neonates develop hypoxemia and hypercapnia slower than adults owing to their reduced oxygen consumption.
   D. All of the above.

_____ 9. The neonate can increase cardiac output by which of the following mechanisms?
   A. increasing heart rate
   B. increasing heart rate and peripheral vascular resistance
   C. increasing heart rate and stroke volume
   D. none of the above

_____ 10. The change in circulation from the placenta to the pulmonary systems occurs with:
   A. birth.   C. cutting of the umbilical cord.
   B. clamping of the umbilical cord.   D. none of the above.

_____ 11. Closure of the ductus arteriosus occurs as a result of:
   A. increased left ventricular pressures.
   B. increased systemic vascular resistance.
   C. increased PaO_2.
   D. decreased $PaCO_2$.

_____ 12. Which of the following correctly lists, in order, the series of physiological changes that occur in the first moments of extrauterine life?
   A. Lungs expand, pulmonary blood flow increases, pulmonary vascular resistance decreases, pulmonary artery pressures decrease.
   B. Lungs expand, pulmonary vascular resistance decreases, pulmonary blood flow increases, pulmonary artery pressures increase.
   C. Lungs expand, pulmonary blood flow increases, pulmonary vascular resistance decreases, pulmonary artery pressures increase.
   D. Lungs expand, pulmonary vascular resistance decreases, pulmonary blood flow increases, pulmonary artery pressures decrease.

_____ 13. The term _____ describes the time period where fetal life and growth occur outside the uterus.
   A. intrauterine   C. extrauterine
   B. birth   D. extraplacental

_____ 14. Which of the following is a structure that allows, during intrauterine development, for the flow of blood from the right to the left atrium?
   A. foramen ovale   C. artial septal defect
   B. ductus arteriosus D. ductus venosus

_____ 15. The situation in which a patient's respiratory effort is insufficient in meeting the body's metabolic oxygenation and carbon dioxide elimination demands is termed:
   A. respiratory distress.   C. respiratory failure.
   B. difficulty breathing.   D. respiratory arrest.

_____ 16. Which of the following patients would be considered to be in respiratory distress, rather than respiratory failure or arrest?
   A. a four-month-old with difficulty breathing, tachypnea, retractions, $PaO_2 = 80$, $PaCO_2 = 46$, $pH = 7.34$
   B. a three-month-old with difficulty breathing, tachypnea, $PaO_2 = 100$, $PaCO_2 = 40$, $pH = 7.36$
   C. a two-month-old with apnea
   D. a five-month-old with bradypnea, nasal flaring, head bobbing, and decreased tidal volume

_____ 17. Which of the following conditions can lead to sustained fetal circulation?
   A. transient tachypnea of the newborn
   B. neonatal respiratory distress syndrome
   C. congenital diaphragmatic hernia
   D. persistent pulmonary hypertension of the newborn

_____ 18. Treatment of persistent pulmonary hypertension of the newborn (PPHN) may include the administration of all of the following except:
   A. sodium bicarbonate.   C. magnesium sulfate.
   B. inhaled nitric oxide.   D. prostaglandin E_1.

_____ 19. Risks associated with the use of nitroprusside as a pulmonary vasodilator in the treatment of persistent pulmonary hypertension of the newborn (PPHN) include:
   A. significant systemic hypotension.
   B. hemodynamically significant bradycardia.
   C. respiratory arrest.
   D. none of the above.

_____ 20. Aspiration of meconium by the neonate may result in:
   A. airway obstruction.
   B. inactivation of alveolar surfactant.
   C. chemical pneumonitis.
   D. all of the above.

_____ 21. Which of the following is least likely to be part of the management of a neonate with transient tachypnea of the newborn (TTN)?
   A. endotracheal intubation
   B. administration of diuretics
   C. administration of inotropic agents
   D. administration of antibiotics

_____ 22. Management of infant respiratory distress syndrome (IRDS) may include all of the following except:
   A. endotracheal intubation and mechanical ventilation.
   B. administration of prostaglandin E_1.
   C. administration of exogenous surfactant.
   D. administration of 100 percent oxygen.

_____ 23. A one-day-old neonate presents with respiratory distress. Upon exam, you find decreased lung sounds on the left and a schaphoid-shaped abdomen. Based on the clinical exam findings, which of the following is the most likely cause of the patient's respiratory distress?
   A. congenital diaphragmatic hernia (CDH)
   B. infant respiratory distress syndrome (IRDS)
   C. meconium aspiration syndrome
   D. persistent pulmonary hypertension of the newborn (PPHN)

_____ 24. A neonate is born at 42 weeks gestation with obvious staining of the amniotic fluid with thin meconium. After suctioning the mouth and nares and drying the neonate's body, you note that he has a vigorous cry, is moving his extremities, his skin is blue, and his heart rate = 108. Based on the clinical exam findings, which of the following would be the most appropriate care?
  A. suctioning the trachea with an endotracheal tube
  B. direct laryngoscopy to examine the trachea for meconium
  C. ensure thermoregulation and monitor the patient
  D. suctioning the trachea with a bulb syringe

_____ 25. Which of the following would be the least desirable management modality for a neonate with respiratory distress secondary to congenital diaphragmatic hernia?
  A. endotracheal intubation and mechanical ventilation
  B. endotracheal intubation and manual ventilation with a BVM
  C. BVM ventilations with a face mask
  D. insertion of a nasogastric tube and gastric decompression

_____ 26. Which of the following is the most common congenital heart defect affecting neonates in the United States?
  A. atrial septal defect
  B. pulmonary stenosis
  C. ventricular septal defect
  D. coarctation of the aorta

_____ 27. Which of the following congenital heart diseases is least likely to have an asymptomatic presentation?
  A. atrial septal defect
  B. patent ductus arteriosus
  C. ventricular septal defect
  D. complete transposition of the great vessels.

_____ 28. Which of the following congenital heart defects does not result in the mixing of oxygenated and deoxygenated blood?
  A. coarctation of the aorta
  B. vetricular septal defect
  C. tetralogy of Fallot
  D. patent ductus arteriosus

_____ 29. Which of the following congenital heart diseases must coexist with a PDA, VSD, or ASD for the patient to survive?
  A. coarctation of the aorta
  B. complete transposition of the great vessels
  C. tetralogy of Fallot
  D. patent ductus arteriosus

_____ 30. The various congenital heart defects that result in a decrease in pulmonary blood flow are collectively known as:
  A. obstructive heart defects.
  B. cyanotic heart defects.
  C. left-to-right shunt defects.
  D. none of the above.

_____ 31. _____ is a serious gastrointestinal disease of unknown etiology seen in neonatal patients and is characterized by intestinal necrosis.
  A. Congenital diaphragmatic hernia
  B. Sepsis
  C. Necrotizing enterocolitis
  D. Jaundice

_____ 32. Which of the following best describes the management of necrotizing enterocolitis?
  A. keep patient NPO, nasogastric tube insertion and gastric decompression, administration of IV fluids, and antibiotic therapy
  B. endotracheal tube insertion and mechanical ventilation, nasogastric tube insertion and gastric decompression, and prostaglandin E_1 administration
  C. oxygen administration, deep tracheal suctioning, IV fluid therapy, and antibiotic administration
  D. none of the above

_____ 33. The presentation of sepsis in the neonate may be subtle and difficult to distinguish from noninfectious pathology.
  A. True.
  B. False.

_____ 34. _____ is a clinical exam finding that results from the collection of unconjugated bilirubin in the neonatal blood.
  A. Bilirubinemia   C. Scleratitis
  B. Jaundice   D. Hypotension

_____ 35. Treatment of bilirubinemia may include all of the following except:
  A. monitoring only.   C. blood transfusion.
  B. phototherapy.   D. all of the above.

_____ 36. All of the following are complications associated with umbilical vein catheterization except:
  A. liver failure.   C. renal failure.
  B. hepatic necrosis.   D. infection.

_____ 37. Which of the following correctly lists the correct concentration and dose of glucose utilized for maintenance infusion?
  A. D10W 0.5–1.0 g/kg   C. D5W 8 cc/kg/hr
  B. D10W 80 cc/kg/day   D. D5W 5–10 g/kg

_____ 38. A neonate presents with a serum glucose of 78 mg/dL. Based only on the serum glucose, which of the following correctly states the concentration and dose of glucose that should be administered?
  A. no glucose administration is required   C. D10W 5–10 g/kg
  B. D10W 0.5–1.0 g/kg   D. D10W 80 cc/kg/day

_____ 39. NMBAs should never be used in the neonatal population.
  A. True.
  B. False.

_____ 40. Which of the following abnormalities is not characteristic of tetralogy of Fallot?
  A. right ventricular infundibular stenosis
  B. right ventricular hypertrophy
  C. aortic valve positioned over the right ventricle
  D. atrial septal defect

©2007 Pearson Education, Inc.
Critical Care Paramedic

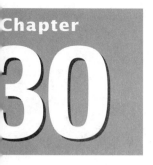

Environmental Emergencies

Review of Chapter Objectives

Upon completion of this chapter, the student should be able to:

1. Describe the pathophysiology associated with the varying levels of heat-related emergencies.   **p. 897**

Temperature management in the human body is a process of balancing heat loss with heat production. When heat production exceeds heat loss a hyperthermic condition results, and a hypothermic condition results when heat loss exceeds heat production.

Human body temperature is usually maintained between 35.6–37.8°C, with an average of 38.6°C. At elevated temperatures enzymes cease to function, proteins denature, and cellular metabolism is hampered. A "critical thermal maximum" is said to exist when the core temperature is greater than 43°C.

The hypothalamus, part of diencephalons, is responsible for, among many other things, temperature regulation and water balance and thirst. The preoptic region of hypothalamus is the principle center for thermoregulation, analyzing input from thermoreceptors that monitor body temperature from locations in the skin (peripheral thermoreceptors), body core, blood vessel walls (central thermoreceptors) and hypothalamus.

Based on the hypothalamic set point (which refers to the internal temperature that the body wants to maintain) versus the relative temperature of the body, certain compensatory mechanisms are set in motion.

As long as these feedback mechanisms for heat gain and heat loss are working properly, a stable internal temperature will be maintained. However, certain conditions can alter the normal functioning of the regulatory process and predispose the patient to temperature-related emergencies.

2. List the factors that contribute to the heat-related emergencies.   **p. 898**

Factors that effect temperature regulation include patient age, patient health, medications, and exposure time.

3. Describe the methods of thermoregulation in the body.   **p. 900**

Methods of thermoregulation, both to increase and decrease body temperature, include voluntary and involuntary methods. Involuntary methods of heat loss that occur during periods of increased body temperature include the activation of sweat glands and the production of sweat, capillary dilation, and the inhibition of mechanisms that result in heat production.

Voluntary methods of heat loss that occur during periods of increased body temperature include the limitation of activity, moving to a cooler environment, and removing clothing.

Involuntary methods of heat production that occur during periods of decreased body temperature include the constriction of peripheral blood vessels, piloerection, release of thyroxine from the thyroid gland, and increased production and release of epinephrine.

Voluntary methods of heat production are the addition of heavier clothing, increased activity, and the reduction of exposed skin.

4. **Determine, based on clinical presentation, the different levels of heat-related emergencies.**   p. 903

Heat tetany

Heat tetany is characterized by the use of hyperventilation as a cooling mechanism, similar to panting in a dog. Hyperventilation can lead to respiratory alkalosis and resultant carpopedal spasms.

Heat cramps

Brief, painful muscle cramping that occurs secondary to salt depletion and electrolyte abnormalities. It is common in athletes and outdoor workers, and is also a frequent complication of heat exhaustion.

Heat syncope

Heat syncope usually occurs in persons unacclimatized to heat. It is a form of postural hypotension characterized by massive peripheral vasodilation and dehydration.

Heat exhaustion

Heat exhaustion is an ill-defined syndrome associated with hot air temperatures and excessive sweating. Particular populations at risk include athletes, outdoor workers, the elderly, and the young. Signs and symptoms include:

- Dizziness, fatigue, irritability, anxiety
- Headache, chills, nausea, vomiting
- Heat cramps
- Tachycardia, hyperventilation, hypotension, syncope

Heatstroke

Heatstroke is defined by a core temperature greater than 40.5°C with altered mental status and anhydrosis, though anhydrosis does not have to be present for heatstroke to occur. Heatstroke represents a total failure of the thermal regulatory mechanisms and can be rapidly fatal. Two categories of heatstroke are recognized; exertional and nonexertional. Metabolic breakdown and irreversible organ death occurs at 43°C. A "critical thermal maximum" is reached, cellular respiration impaired, cellular membrane permeability is increased, and protein denaturing and tissue necrosis occur.

Signs and symptoms of heat exhaustion include:

- Altered mental status, altered level of consciousness, unconsciousness
- Anhydrosis: may or may not be present
- Hyperventilation, hypoventilation, tachycardia
- Pulmonary edema, seizures, posturing

5. **Describe the appropriate treatment modalities for heat exhaustion.**   p. 904

The treatment for heatstroke involves removing the patient from the hot environment, allowing them to rest, and replacing lost fluids and electrolytes. Patients can be cooled with ice packs to the axillae, neck, and groin. In cases of mild heat exhaustion, fluid and electrolyte replacement can be accomplished by having the patient drink a 0.1 percent isotonic NaCl solution. For more severe cases, IV replacement is warranted.

6. **Describe the appropriate treatment modalities for heatstroke.**   p. 905

Patients with heatstroke have a greater likelihood to have issues with airway and oxygenation, so support of ABCs are a prime concern. At a minimum, the patient should be administered

100 percent oxygen via a nonrebreather mask. Fluid and electrolyte replacement should be accomplished via the IV route, and the judicious use of fluids is encouraged, as hypotension may correct once peripheral vasodilation occurs with cooling. Hydration status can be monitored via CVP, PWP, SVR, and CI. Immediate cooling to a temperature of 40°C can be accomplished with the use of cold packs, cold water immersion, evaporative cooling with lukewarm water, and thoracic and peritoneal lavage. Placement of an indwelling rectal or esophageal thermometer will provide accurate feedback on the effectiveness of your cooling efforts. Lorazepam or chlorpromazine can be administered to control shivering. If rhabdomyolysis present aggressive hydration and mannitol administration is recommended to increase GFR, and alkalization of the urine can be accomplished with the administration of sodium bicarbonate.

7. Describe the pathophysiology of hypothermia.   **p. 906**

Hypothermia is said to exist when a person's core temperature falls to less than 35°C, and severe hypothermia is said to exist when a person's core temperature falls to less than 32.2°C.

The speed of onset of hypothermia is influenced by temperature, degree of exposure, wind chill factor, and the presence of comorbidities.

The onset of mild and severe hypothermia follows a fairly predictable progression. Mild hypothermia results in the activation of heat conserving and generating mechanisms. Heart rate, blood pressure, and cardiac output (CO) rise, and patients typically exhibit:

- Shivering
- Lethargy
- Lack of coordination
- Loss of fine motor control
- Cool, dry, pale skin

As severe hypothermia develops, the bodies metabolism slows, HR, BP, and CO fall, and patients typically exhibit:

- ECG abnormalities
  - J wave
  - Dysrhythmia
- Lack of shivering
- Loss of voluntary muscle control
- Hypotension
- Undetectable pulse and BP
- Cardiac arrest

8. Describe the impact of hypothermia on neurologic, cardiovascular, and respiratory systems.   **p. 908**

Neurologic system

Hypothermia depresses CNS metabolism and activity in a linear fashion as core temperature drops, and an electroencephalogram taken on a patient with a core temperature lower than about 19°C may appear consistent with brain death. Cerebral oxygen requirements decrease as core temperature decreases, as much as 6 percent to 7 percent for each 1°C of decline until the temperature of 25°C (77°F) is reached. In lower temperatures the oxygen requirement of the patient can be as much as 25 percent to 50 percent less than normal. This mechanism serves to facilitate survivability by decreasing the amount of anoxic damage.

Cardiovascular system

The most profound effect on the cardiovascular system is the onset of bradycardia secondary to decreased depolarization of cardiac pacemaker cells. As it is not a result of vagal stimulation, this bradycardia will be refractory to standard ACLS therapies, such as atropine. As a result of bradycardia, cardiac output will decrease, resulting in a decrease of mean arterial pressure. ECG may show the presence of the characteristic J, or Osborne, wave.

Respiratory system

The respiratory impact of hypothermia is directly related to the overall slowing of the metabolism. A decrease in the respiratory rate decreases the amount of oxygen available to the tissues. The slowing of metabolism, the decrease in cardiac output, and the decrease in the delivery of oxygen produce anaerobic conditions that result in lactic acid production. Together this will lead to a respiratory and metabolic acidosis.

9. **Understand how hypothermic events should be addressed in the presence of other etiologies.** p. 907

The correction of hypothermia should proceed in concert with any treatment of underlying disease or trauma that poses a threat to the patient's life. In addition, a patient is not considered dead until they have been adequately rewarmed.

10. **Determine, based on clinical presentation and assessment, the appropriate treatment modalities for hypothermic patients.** p. 910

The treatment of hypothermia is dependent on the severity. All hypothermic patients should be dried and protected from additional heat loss. Avoid rough handling, as cardiac irritability may lead to dysrhythmia. Measure and monitor core body temperature. The degree of warming efforts that should be undertaken is driven by the degree of hypothermia. Warming methods for mild and severe hypothermia include:

• Mild hypothermia
  • Active external methods
    • Blankets
    • Heat packs
    • Warm water immersion
    • Warm humidified oxygen
• Severe hypothermia
  • External and internal methods
    • Warm IV fluids
      • 45–65°C
  • Thoracic, abdominal lavage

11. **Understand the various treatment modalities, applied in the critical care setting, for the management of cold-related injuries. (p. 912); 12. List the signs and symptoms of frostbite and describe the appropriate treatment. (pp. 908, 912)**

The signs and symptoms associated with frostbite aid in the classification of frostbite:

• First degree
  • Superficial freezing
  • Edema present, skin with waxy appearance
  • No blisters or vesicles
• Second degree
  • Blister formation with clear fluid
  • Erythema, edema present
• Third degree
  • Blood filled blisters present
• Fourth degree
  • Full thickness injury
  • Death of dermal tissue, extension into muscles, tendons, bones

Treatment for frostbite consists primarily of the rewarming of the affected area, though rewarming should be deferred if refreezing is possible. A warm bath of 39–42°C should be used, and analgesics such as morphine or fentanyl administered for pain, which will accompany rewarming.

13. List the different types of mechanisms for drowning and near-drowning.   p. 912

Drowning can be divided into two categories: drowning and near-drowning. Drowning is defined as death from suffocation due to submersion in a liquid within 24 hours of insult. Survival past the 24-hour point is categorized as near-drowning. Drowning and near-drowning patients can be further categorized as:

- Asymptomatic
- Symptomatic
- Cardiopulmonary arrest
- Obviously dead

14. Explain the pathophysiology associated with drowning.   p. 912

Wet drowning involves the aspiration of the liquid the drowning occurred in, and accounts for about 85 percent of all drownings. A washout of surfactant occurs from the aspiration of liquid, resulting in atelectasis, intrapulmonary shunting, and V/P mismatch. Freshwater aspiration results in hemodilution and hemolysis secondary to the movement of water from the alveoli into the pulmonary vasculature along the osmotic gradient that was created.

A dry drowning occurs when laryngospasm prevents the aspiration of liquid; dry drowning accounts for about 15 percent of all drownings. Regardless of whether a drowning is wet or dry, the principle insult is hypoxia.

**15. Discuss the short- and long-term effects of hypoxia associated
with drowning and near-drowning.**   p. 912

The short-term effects of hypoxia include cardiopulmonary and CNS depression and the development of acidosis resulting in decreased cardiac output and hypotension. In addition, hypoxia leads to increased pulmonary vascular resistance and pulmonary artery pressure. Progressive hypoxia leads to apnea, rhythm disturbance, asystole, and then death. Long-term effects of hypoxia include ischemic injury to the brain and myocardium and multiple organ failure. Posthypoxic encephalopathy, with or without cerebral edema, is the most common cause of morbidity and mortality in hospitalized drowning victims.

**16. Explain the cardiovascular, neurologic, and respiratory impact
of drowning and near-drowning.**   p. 913

Cardiac complications are usually secondary to hypoxic events. Rhythms borne out of hypoxic etiologies are common, namely, atrial fibrillation, PVCs, and in extreme cases ventricular tachycardia or fibrillation.

The hypoxia that occurs secondary to drowning may result in CNS depression. Neurologic deficit may be due to the event or the presence of another mechanism such as ETOH (alcohol) or drug use or head injury.

While much has been made about the pathophysiologic differences between fresh and saltwater drowning, there are no important differences from a clinical or management point of view. The aspiration of either results in surfactant washout and/or destruction, alveolitis, atelectasis, noncardiogenic pulmonary edema, and hypoxia.

17. List and discuss the treatment modalities for drowning and near-drowning.   p. 914

- Airway and breathing
  - Ensure airway patency
  - Ensure adequate oxygenation
    - Pulse oximetry
    - Blood gas analysis (BGA)
    - PEEP
- Circulation
  - CPR if necessary

- Insertion of NG/OG tube
  - Evacuate stomach of water, chyme
- Pharmacological management
  - Diuretics
    - If hemodilution present
  - Beta blockers
    - To correct bronchorrhea
- Determine need for rewarming

The treatment for drowning and near-drowning is determined largely by the patient's clinical status, as the possible effects of drowning are many. Cardiopulmonary arrest should be provided in accordance with ACLS or institutional/program guidelines. Respiratory arrest requires intubation and ventilation with 100 percent oxygen.

Patients with acute pulmonary edema and hypotension should be promptly intubated and ventilated with positive pressure and 100 percent oxygen. Additional indications that suggest the need for intubation include:

- $SaO_2 < 90$ percent
- $PaO_2 < 70$ mmHg
- $PaCO_2 > 45$ mmHg
- Tachypnea

NMBAs, sedatives, and analgesics should be used to facilitate endotracheal intubation. FiO_2 can be initiated at 1.0 but can be titrated to about 0.5, if possible, to prevent worsening the pulmonary injury with oxygen toxicity; the goal is to maintain an SpO_2 of greater than 90 percent. PEEP should be provided to achieve an intrapulmonary shunt of 20 percent or less or a PaO_2/FiO_2 of 250 or greater. If hypotension persists after administration of oxygen, administer crystalloid fluids. Patients with acute pulmonary edema without hypotension can often also require intubation and mechanical ventilation to produce SaO_2 greater than 90 percent, though administration of oxygen via a nonrebreather mask can be attempted. If hemodilution is present, diuretics can be administered to lower plasma volume.

Patients who present normotensive with rales can be treated with supplemental oxygen and beta-blocking agents, should bronchospasm be present.

Metabolic acidosis is present in a majority of patients who require hospitalization, and should be corrected if a patient on ventilatory support has a pH < 7.2 and $HCO_3^- < 12$ mEq/L.

Case Study

Your critical care ground transport team has been called to a small, two-bed, rural emergency department for a teenaged patient who has reportedly "drowned." Pulling into the parking lot, you note a large group of kids and a few adults milling around the ambulance entrance. One of the adults is in an animated conversation with a sheriff's deputy. As you park, the deputy signals the speaker to wait and walks over to the door of your ambulance. The deputy tells you that the patient is a 12-year-old boy, a "fresh air kid" from the city. The patient was climbing out of the camp pool when he slipped and struck his chin, falling back into the pool and losing consciousness. The pool was busy and by the time he was noticed and pulled from the water, he was pulseless and apneic. CPR was started by counselors and by the time the deputy arrived, approximately eight minutes after the 911 call came in, the patient was breathing on his own. Counselors estimate that CPR was performed for approximately four to five minutes before a pulse returned and the patient started breathing on his own. The patient quickly regained consciousness. The patient was transported by BLS ambulance to the closest hospital and arrived without change.

Entering the emergency room you note a muscular adolescent male sitting upright on the stretcher looking very anxious. He is bare-chested, clothed only in swimming trunks and is clearly using accessory muscles to breathe. He is receiving high flow, high concentration oxygen by nonrebreather mask and has coarse crackles audible over the hiss of the oxygen. The nurse practitioner caring for the patient escorts

©2007 Pearson Education, Inc.
Critical Care Paramedic

you to a side room and tells you that the patient needs to be transferred to the regional trauma center approximately 50 miles away. She also tells you that although the patient has remained conscious since arrival, his respiratory status has been continuously declining. Initially, he maintained a SpO$_2$ of 95 percent on a nonrebreather mask, but now it is only in the high 80s and she was considering noninvasive positive pressure ventilation as your team arrived. Returning to the bedside, the patient's nurse tells you that they have been unable to contact his parents, but that the head counselor has consented to the transfer and any care that is needed. In answer to your inquiry, she tells you that his spine was cleared of injury immediately upon arrival. The patient's current vital signs are: respiratory rate of 44 and labored with a SpO$_2$ of 86 percent, heart rate of 132 beats per minute, showing a sinus tachycardia on the monitor and blood pressure 128/78. The patient is alert and although unable to speak, moves his head to yes or no questions and tries to follow commands. He appears to be using every muscle of his chest, neck, and abdomen to breathe and auscultation of his chest reveals coarse rales bilaterally on both inspiration and expiration. Glancing over the patient at your partner, she gives you an upward hooking motion with her left hand signaling that she feels the patient needs to be intubated immediately. Nodding in agreement you explain to the NP that you feel the patient would do better in transfer if he was intubated instead of a trial with NPPV. She agrees with you and your partner prepares the intubation equipment while you explain the procedure to the patient. The patient is quickly and easily intubated using rapid sequence intubation and is ventilated with 100 percent oxygen via BVM. The patient improves quickly and, as the ambulance begins rolling toward your destination, his SpO$_2$ has increased to 96 percent, his heart rate decreased to 108 and his blood pressure has stabilized at 102/68. The rest of the transfer is uneventful and the patient remains stable en route.

DISCUSSION QUESTIONS

1. Define the terms drowning and near-drowning.
2. What are the major pathophysiologic features of drowning injuries?
3. What are the treatment modalities for drowning and near-drowning injuries?

Content Review

MULTIPLE CHOICE

_____ 1. The temperature of the human body is maintained:
   A. at 98.2°F.
   B. between 35.6°–37.8°C.
   C. between 95°–101°F.
   D. B and C.

_____ 2. A critical thermal maximum is said to exist when a person's core temperature reaches:
   A. 43°C.
   B. 104.9°F.
   C. 41°C.
   D. 103.9°F.

_____ 3. Temperature regulation is controlled by which of the following structure(s)?
   A. perioptic region of the pituitary gland
   B. central and peripheral thermoreceptors
   C. preoptic region of the hypothalamus
   D. none of the above

_____ 4. Central thermoreceptors are located in the:
   A. skin.
   B. perioptic region of the hypothalamus.
   C. body core and blood vessel walls.
   D. organs, hypothalamus, and skin.

_____ 5. The difference in temperature between two objects is termed the:
   A. thermal equilibrium.   C. thermal differential.
   B. thermal gradient.   D. basal metabolic rate.

_____ 6. The amount of energy needed to maintain homeostasis while at rest is termed:
   A. basal metabolic rate.   C. thermal equilibrium.
   B. futile cycle.   D. chemical thermogenesis.

_____ 7. _____ is the loss of heat from the body through direct contact of the skin with another, cooler, solid object.
   A. Conduction   C. Evaporation
   B. Radiation   D. Convection

_____ 8. High relative humidity diminishes the effectiveness of which of the following types of heat loss?
   A. conduction   C. evaporation
   B. radiation   D. convection

_____ 9. Voluntary mechanisms that will reduce the amount of heat in the body include all of the following except:
   A. moving to a cooler environment.   C. limiting activity.
   B. removing heavy clothing.   D. cessation of shivering.

_____ 10. On average, males have a higher basal metabolic rate than do women.
   A. True
   B. False

_____ 11. Unopposed, the basal metabolic rate can raise the temperature of the body about:
   A. 0.5°C/hr.   C. 2.0°C/hr.
   B. 1.1°C/hr.   D. 10.1°C/hr.

_____ 12. Which of the following statement regarding thermogenesis is false?
   A. Epinephrine release promotes the creation and retention of heat by causing shivering and producing peripheral vasoconstriction.
   B. Activation of sweat glands and peripheral vasodilation are examples of involuntary methods of heat loss.
   C. Thyroxine, released from the thyroid gland, acts directly on human cells to increase cellular metabolism and basal metabolic rate.
   D. Cooling may be accomplished via the inhibition of shivering and chemical thermogenesis.

_____ 13. Mechanisms used to decrease body temperature include all of the following except:
   A. vasodilation.   C. decreased heat production.
   B. sweating.   D. piloerection.

_____ 14. Hyperthermia, like fever, is a normal physiological response to changes in the internal and external environment.
   A. True
   B. False

_____ 15. Signs and symptoms of heat tetany include:
   A. hyperventilation and muscle cramping.
   B. orthostatic blood pressure changes, diaphoresis.
   C. hyperventilation and carpopedal spasm.
   D. altered mental status, loss of consciousness, hypotension.

_____ 16. An elderly patient who has been exposed to hot ambient temperatures for four days and presents with a core temperature of 39.5°C, fatigue, irritability, and signs and symptoms of dehydration is most likely experiencing:
   A. heat cramps.   C. heat exhaustion.
   B. heat syncope.   D. heatstroke.

©2007 Pearson Education, Inc.
Critical Care Paramedic

_____ 17. The term anhydrosis refers to:
   A. a state of not sweating, or the inability to sweat.
   B. a state of dehydration.
   C. decreased intravascular fluid volume.
   D. the inability to maintain fluid homeostasis.

_____ 18. Heatstroke is always accompanied with anhydrosis.
   A. True
   B. False

_____ 19. Heatstroke is characterized by:
   A. a core temperature greater than 40.5°C, CNS dysfunction, anhydrosis.
   B. a core temperature greater than 45°C, coma, anhydrosis.
   C. a core temperature greater than 43°C and altered mental status.
   D. none of the above.

_____ 20. A conscious, alert, and disoriented football player experiencing headache, chills, nausea, vomiting, and heat cramps after a hard practice on a warm day is most likely experiencing:
   A. heat cramps.   C. heat exhaustion.
   B. heat syncope.   D. heatstroke.

_____ 21. Specific patient populations at risk for heat exhaustion include:
   A. athletes.   C. pediatric.
   B. geriatric.   D. all of the above.

_____ 22. A patient who presents with acute onset of confusion, lethargy, warm and diaphoretic skin, and hypotension after participating in an athletic event on a hot and humid day is most likely suffering from:
   A. exertional heatstroke.   C. heat exhaustion.
   B. nonexertional heatstroke.   D. heat syncope.

_____ 23. The treatment of heat exhaustion will most likely include:
   A. removal of the patient from the environment and observation only.
   B. oral administration of an electrolyte solution, rest, and removal from the environment.
   C. IV administration of an electrolyte solution and active cooling measures.
   D. none of the above.

_____ 24. The treatment of heatstroke will most likely include:
   A. removal of the patient from the environment and observation only.
   B. oral administration of an electrolyte solution, rest, and removal from the environment.
   C. IV administration of an electrolyte solution and active cooling measures.
   D. none of the above.

_____ 25. Acceptable methods of active cooling include:
   A. ice water immersion.
   B. use of ice packs.
   C. use of cool, wet sheets to increase evaporative heat loss.
   D. all of the above.

_____ 26. A patient who presents with an altered mental status, warm and dry skin, and hypotension after prolonged exposure in a hot environment is most likely suffering from:
   A. heat cramps.   C. heat exhaustion.
   B. heat syncope.   D. heatstroke.

_____ 27. _____ increase the risk of heatstroke secondary to the inhibition of sweating.
   A. Beta blockers   C. Antihypertensives
   B. Tricyclic antidepressants D. Diuretics

_____ 28. Mild hypothermia is defined as a core temperature less than:
  A. 34°C.   C. 36°C.
  B. 35°C.   D. 37°C.

_____ 29. A patient with mild hypothermia will exhibit all of the following except:
  A. shivering.   C. lack of coordination.
  B. lethargy.   D. dysrhythmia.

_____ 30. Severe hypothermia is defined as a core temperature less than:
  A. 31.1°C.   C. 32.2°C.
  B. 31.2°C.   D. 33.3°C.

_____ 31. Active methods of rewarming a patient in the prehospital environment include all of the following except:
  A. administration of warmed IV fluids.   C. use of warm blankets.
  B. application of heat packs.   D. warm-water immersion.

_____ 32. The biggest potential life threat for a hypothermic patient who is being actively rewarmed is:
  A. ventricular fibrillation.   C. hypotension.
  B. ventricular tachycardia.   D. cerebral anoxia.

_____ 33. Groups of patients at high risk for hypothermia include all of the following except:
  A. elderly patients.   C. athletes.
  B. pediatric patients.   D. trauma patients.

_____ 34. A patient wearing wet jeans and a tee shirt, lying in a snow bank on a 23°F, windy night would be susceptible to heat loss via which of the following mechanisms?
  A. evaporation, conduction, radiation, and convection
  B. evaporation, radiation, and convection
  C. conduction, radiation, and convection
  D. convection and conduction

_____ 35. Atropine is unlikely to correct bradycardia associated with hypothermia because:
  A. hypothermia decreases the bioavailability of atropine.
  B. bradycardia associated with hypothermia does not occur secondary to vagal stimulation.
  C. biotransformation in hypothemic blood renders atropine inactive.
  D. hypothermia-induced structural changes to the ACh receptors on the postsynaptic membrane prevent atropine from binding.

_____ 36. In hypothermia, cerebral oxygen requirement decrease about _____ for each 1°C drop in core temperature.
  A. 4–6 percent   C. 6–8 percent
  B. 5–7 percent   D. 4–8 percent

_____ 37. The characteristic ECG finding associated with hypothermia is:
  A. ventricular fibrillation.   C. the presence of an Osborne wave.
  B. bradycardia.   D. tachycardia.

_____ 38. Initial treatment for patients with hypothermia, regardless of the severity, includes:
  A. removal of cold and wet garments, removing the patient from the cold environment, and beginning passive external warming techniques.
  B. IV access, cardiac monitoring, active internal warming techniques.
  C. removal of cold and wet garments, IV access, cardiac monitoring, and beginning active external warming techniques.
  D. removal of cold and wet garments, IV access, cardiac monitoring, endotracheal intubation, and beginning active internal warming techniques.

_____ 39. Hypothermic patients in cardiac arrest should be resuscitated until their core temperature is greater than:
A. 30°C.   C. 32°C.
B. 31°C.   D. 33°C.

_____ 40. An endotracheal tube should never be placed in a patient with severe hypothermia and a pulse, as it can induce ventricular fibrillation.
A. True
B. False

_____ 41. A patient with a core body temperature of 31°C who is 30 minutes away from the destination facility should receive which type of rewarming?
A. passive rewarming only
B. active external rewarming only
C. active external and active internal rewarming
D. active internal rewarming only

_____ 42. Frostbite that presents with blood or fluid-filled blisters would be considered:
A. first degree.   C. third degree.
B. second degree.   D. fourth degree.

_____ 43. Frostbite always occurs as a component of moderate to severe hypothermia, it never presents as a sole event.
A. True
B. False

_____ 44. Rewarming of an area affected by frostbite can be accomplished by:
A. immersing the part in a warm bath of temperature 39°C–45°C.
B. immersing the part in a warm bath of temperature 39°C–48°C.
C. exposing the affected part to radiant heat, as from a fire or heater.
D. active internal rewarming with the administration of warm IV fluids.

_____ 45. The treatment of frostbite may include the administration of narcotic analgesics for pain control.
A. True
B. False

_____ 46. Effective methods of heat reduction in a hyperthermic patient include all of the following except:
A. spraying the patient with lukewarm water.
B. fanning the patient.
C. ice water immersion.
D. application of ice packs to the chest and legs.

_____ 47. Active cooling techniques utilized on a hypothermic patient should be ceased when the patient's core temperature reaches:
A. 36°C.   C. 39°C.
B. 37°C.   D. 40°C.

_____ 48. The situation in which hypothermia is induced in a previously hyperthermic patient who is receiving active cooling measures is termed:
A. reverse hypothermia.   C. iatrogenic hypothermia.
B. accidental hypothermia.   D. secondary hypothermia.

_____ 49. A hyperthermic patient who is being actively cooled starts to shiver. What should be done?
A. Nothing, the patient should be allowed to shiver.
B. The patient should be passively warmed with blankets until shivering stops.
C. Active cooling measures should be stopped.
D. Active cooling measures should be continued and a benzodiazepine utilized to control shivering.

_____ 50. Which of the following statements regarding the physiology associated with drowning is false?
   A. Activation of the mammalian dive reflex results in apnea, bradycardia, and vasoconstriction.
   B. Prognosis is determined by the type of drowning (wet versus dry), type of fluid aspirated (fresh versus salt water), and degree of pulmonary vasodilation.
   C. Freshwater drowning may result in hemodilution.
   D. Both freshwater and saltwater drowning result in surfactant abnormalities.

_____ 51. Indications for endotracheal intubation in a patient who has suffered a near-drowning event include:
   A. a PaO_2 of 70 mmHg while on 100 percent oxygen.
   B. altered mental status.
   C. decreased level of consciousness.
   D. all of the above.

31

Diving Emergencies

Review of Chapter Objectives

Upon completion of this chapter, the student should be able to:

1. Describe physical laws that affect gas pressure and depth (physics of diving).   **p. 919**

The pressure exerted by the weight of the column of water above a diver can result in physiologic strain. Pressure (P) is the relationship between force (F) and area (A) and is represented by the equation P = F/A. Units of pressure can be measured in pounds per square inch (psi), pascals (Pa), Newtons/meter^2, kilopascals (kPa), millimeters of mercury (mmHg)/torr, centimeters of water (cm/H_2O), and perhaps most frequently in diving, atmospheres (atm). The air pressure at sea level = 1 atm. 1 atm = 14.7 lbs/in = 760 mm Hg = 760 torr = 101.3 kPa = 1,033 cm/H_2O. As a diver descends, he reaches an increase in pressure equal to 1 atmosphere at about 33 feet. The rate of pressure accumulation is constant, so at about 99 feet of depth a diver is experiencing a pressure equal to about 3 atm.

As a diver is breathing gas while diving, the gas laws play a role in diving physiology. These laws should be reviewed at this time. See Chapter 4 (Altitude Physiology) for a review of the important gas laws.

2. Describe the effects on the body at depth in an underwater environment (physiology of depth).   **p. 920**

Both oxygen and nitrogen have toxic effects on the body when under pressure. Oxygen, necessary for normal metabolism, is toxic at pressures above 0.21 atmospheres of absolute pressure (ATA) for long periods of time. Deep divers breathe a mixture of oxygen with nitrogen or helium aimed at reducing the percentage of oxygen in the total mixture. Nitrogen, considered an "inert gas" on the body at the surface, has specific dangers at depth. Under pressure, nitrogen has narcotic effects that can lead to dangerous behavioral changes underwater. The absorption of nitrogen at depth can lead to problems, including decompression sickness, upon surfacing. To avoid this, divers are now adding oxygen to regular air to allow for a lengthier dive with a reduced risk of decompression sickness. However, this practice increases the risks of oxygen toxicity if deep depths are reached.

3. Identify diving environments.   **p. 920**

Diving is often differentiated into coastal diving, where a diver can enter the water from land, and open water diving, where a boat is utilized to get to a water entry point. Specialty and technical diving includes wreck, ice, cave, deep water, or high altitude situations.

4. Identify diving equipment.   p. 921

Common diving equipment includes a pressurized air tank, a regulator, a depth gauge, an air pressure gauge, a watch or some other timing device, and an exposure suit.

Air tanks are commonly constructed of aluminum, steel, or even carbon fiber, and are filled with compressed atmospheric air. Other air mixtures can be used such as oxygen/nitrogen mixtures (nitrox), nitrogen/helium mixtures, or oxygen mixed with other inert gases. Rebreather devices are air "scrubbers" that recycle the oxygen contained in exhaled breaths after removing the carbon dioxide.

A regulator, connected to the air tank with a length of high-pressure hose, allows the diver to breathe the air contained in the tank. It is a one-way valve that controls the release of air from the tank only when the diver initiates a breath.

An air pressure gauge lets a diver know how much air is left in his tank, which is often reported in psi. The air pressure gauge has an open line to the air tank, and it is connected with a high-pressure hose. A depth gauge keeps the diver informed as to his depth below the surface. The depth gauge and air pressure gauge are commonly located together, secured to each other by a rubber or plastic housing.

Exposure suits may be of either the wet suit or dry suit variety, the use of one or the other is usually determined by the temperature of the water.

5. Describe the pathophysiology, assessment, management, and critical care considerations of:

a. Ear, sinus, pulmonary, and other significant barotrauma   p. 922

Tympanic membrane (TM) rupture can occur when pressure in the middle ear is lower than the pressure in the ear canal, the situation that just happens to exist as a diver descends to depth. This situation can be avoided by utilizing techniques that equalize the pressure in the middle ear, preventing the TM from pushing inward. Of course, the opposite occurs on ascent. Signs and symptoms include the acute onset of pain, hearing loss (which may be permanent), and vertigo. Management of a ruptured TM is supportive only, and a ruptured TM will often heal on its own. Needless to say, diving is on hold until the membrane heals.

Sinus squeeze occurs when air trapped in sinus cavities shrinks in volume with descent. Pain is often felt above the upper teeth, above and behind eyes, and deep within the skull. The pain often resolves during the dive but returns on ascent. Capillary and tissue leakage may result in nasal hemorrhage and contribute to sinus infection. Management includes the administration of decongestants and possibly antibiotics.

"Face squeeze" may occur when the shrinking volume of air inside a facemask sucks the face into the collapsing mask. Facial bruising and conjunctival hemorrhage are common results, and management is not necessary.

Pulmonary barotrauma occurs when a diver holds his breath on ascent, resulting in a trapping of expanding air volume within the lungs and overexpansion injury. Pneumomediastinum and pneumothorax are possible results. Management is identical as for nondiving etiology.

b. Nitrogen narcosis   p. 923

Nitrogen narcosis is a situation in which pressurized nitrogen has euphoric effects on the central nervous system that are similar to narcotics or alcohol. The subsequent loss of reasoning skills and lack of judgment can lead to injuries or death. Treatment is immediate ascent from depth.

c. Decompression sickness   p. 923

Decompression sickness is also known as Caisson's Disease or "the bends." Normally when at depth, nitrogen is absorbed into the bloodstream and tissues. During ascent, it desaturates from the tissues into the bloodstream, and is exhaled. If ascent is too rapid, nitrogen expands in the bloodstream and forms bubbles. Gas collects in joint spaces and emboli may form, occluding blood vessels. Signs and symptoms include:

- Joint pain
  - Shoulder
  - Knee
  - Wrist
  - Hip

- Headache, vertigo, sensory impairment
- Dyspnea, pulmonary edema
  - Secondary to pulmonary emboli

Management considerations include:
- Transport at low altitude
  - Air transport may prove problematic
- Airway and ventilatory support
  - 100 percent oxygen
- Fluid replacement
  - Correct dehydration
- Hyperbaric recompression

d. High-pressure neurologic syndrome (HPNS) p. 925

HPNS can occur with the breathing of helium mixtures at depths greater than 400 feet. Signs and symptoms include loss of muscular coordination, tremors, confusion, altered mental status, loss of consiousness (LOC), and seizures. Treatment is immediate ascent.

e. Hypoxia and gas toxicity p. 926

Mixed gases are used by divers to increase their bottom time. The greatest risk associated with mixing gases is hypoxia. Most gases inhaled at depth can have unpredictable physiologic effects, and errors such as the failure to include sufficient oxygen or the introduction of contaminants can occur during the filling of air tanks. Signs and symptoms and management of hypoxia secondary to diving injury are the same as for any other etiology.

6. Discuss aquatic concerns associated with diving.

a. Drowning p. 927

A frequent misconception by nondivers is that divers can swim, and a misconception by divers is that swimming is not necessary. Realizing this, drowning then seems less out of place than it first appears. Although divers enter the water with a presumably full scuba cylinder, a wide range of factors can make that cylinder simply a fashion accessory. Running out of air at depth, medical emergencies underwater, panic, euphoria, and stupidity are all on the list of reasons divers drown. Of these, panic is probably the biggest contributor. Functioning in an alien environment can be a frightening experience for even the most avid diver. When underwater conditions make the diver uneasy, panic often takes over and obscures rational thought. Without quick action of fellow divers or a sudden focus on the problems at hand, the panic can turn deadly.

b. Saltwater aspiration syndrome p. 927

Faulty regulators or leaking seals can allow small amounts of water to enter the diver's lungs, leading to a condition known as saltwater aspiration syndrome. This condition can produce pneumonia-like symptoms including dyspnea, cough, hemoptysis, and even radiographic changes. A similar condition can be expected from diving is freshwater that is not "fresh," such as stagnant ponds, pools, and sediment-rich runoff areas. Rest, oxygen, and occasionally antibiotics are included in the treatment of these patients.

c. Cold and hypothermia p. 927

Hypothermia is a condition that can occur in relatively warm water. Because water conducts heat 20 times faster than air, divers who are not properly insulated can experience hypothermia in water we would normally consider warm. This is a factor that should be considered in the care and transport of every diver experiencing an emergency.

d. Infection p. 927

Divers may come into contact with agricultural, industrial, or sewage runoff containing contaminants that can cause local or systemic infection.

e. Dangerous animals p. 927

Animals that may bite and cause trauma include large predators such as sharks, barracuda, and moray eels. Other animals, some seemingly harmless and even "friendly," include sea lions, seals, octopi, dolphins, and smalltoothed whales. The initial life threat from hemorrhagic shock and infection is a secondary concern.

Animals that may bite and envenomate include sea snakes, the blue-ringed octopus, and cone snails. These animals inject a neurotoxin, which results in muscle rigidity and respiratory paralysis. Airway and breathing are obviously a priority. Treatment is immersion in water as hot as the patient can stand, about 105-115°F, as warm water deactivates venom. In addition, pressure immobilization techniques can be employed in an attempt to contain the venom locally.

Animals that puncture include lionfish, scorpionfish, stonefish, catfish, and sea urchins. If puncture envenomation occurs, treatment is the same as for biting envenomation.

Stinging animals belong to the phylum Cnidaria and include jellyfish (box jellyfish are considered the most deadly animal in the world), hydroids, fire coral, and anemones. The stinging apparatus is known as a nematocyst, a small harpoonlike structure designed to ensnare prey and in some species, deliver venom. Management consists of removing the remaining tentacles. Fresh water should not be used to irrigate, as it will result in discharge of remaining nematocysts. Deactivate remaining nematocysts with vinegar or a $\frac{1}{4}$ strength ammonia or baking soda solution.

7. **Identify causes of medical emergencies related to diving.**

   a. **Hearing loss** p. 930

   Hearing loss is a frequent complication seen in avid divers. Repeated damage to the tympanic membrane and the round or oval windows can result in the development of scar tissue, which disrupts sound determination. A single incident of tympanic rupture or disruption of cochlear function can lead to permanent damage in the affected ear.

   b. **Disorientation** p. 930

   Disorientation underwater occurs when the vestibular system fails to compensate for the effects of pressure and buoyancy. Vertigo is often the result, causing the diver to lose the ability to maintain a straight and level swim pattern. This can have disastrous consequences if the diver swims down instead of up, ending up below safe depths.

   c. **Unconsciousness** p. 930

   Divers who experience unconsciousness while underwater are unlikely to reach the surface alive. When this condition occurs on land, the victim maintains the ability to breathe as long as the airway stays open. While underwater, however, the diver's regulator will most likely not remain in the mouth. Even if the regulator remains in place, the natural breathing tendency would be unlikely to pull air from the scuba system. A dive buddy with enough presence of mind to remain calm and slowly ascend while using the purge system on the unconscious diver's regulator may be the only hope of survival. Even so, the risks of pulmonary barotrauma would be extremely high. The role of the critical care paramedic in the care of these patients would be rapid transport to a recompression chamber.

   d. **Diver deaths** p. 930

   Recreational diving has an incidence of death of about one in every 100,000 dives made. Women make up 25 percent of all divers, but account for only 10 percent of deaths. Diving death factors include human error, environmental causes, and equipment failure. Human error causes include diving with a disqualifying medical condition, panic, fatigue, buoyancy problems, and improper use of equipment. Environmental causes include adverse sea conditions, water movement, and extreme temperatures.

   Professional diving has an incidence of death of about one in every 5,000 dives, and 30 percent are related to decompression sickness or arterial gas embolism.

   e. **Sudden death syndrome** p. 931

   As divers age, the possibility of sudden death syndrome becomes greater. Approximately 20 percent to 25 percent of diver deaths are related to heart disease and related conditions. Divers who exhibit significant cardiac risk factors should reconsider their future in diving.

8. **Understand hyperbaric medicine.** p. 931

A hyperbaric chamber allows for the repressurization of the patient to "depth," and then the patient is slowly brought back to surface pressure. Transport hyperbaric chambers are bulky and used primarily in utility helicopters and fixed-wing aircraft. Hyperbaric medicine is also used to treat CO and cyanide poisoning, wounds, and burns.

9. Identify concerns for females who dive and for stress associated with diving.   p. 932

Women have a smaller muscle mass compared to men, which allows for longer bottom times and increases the risk of decompression sickness. In addition, women have greater fat stores, resulting in increased adipose absorption of nitrogen and an increased risk of decompression sickness.

10. Discuss the role of the CCP in diving emergency support situations.   p. 933

Simply put, the role of the critical care paramedic in a diving emergency is one of support. He will most likely not be taking place in the rescue or recovery efforts, but will be waiting in a predetermined area for the rescue team to deliver the patient, at which point advanced care would be initiated.

Considerations that the critical care paramedic should be advised of other than the number of potential patients include the characteristics of the diving emergency. Is the situation a search and rescue or a body recovery? Is the water deep or shallow? Is the water temperature warm, cold, or icy? Is the scenario one of fast water diving, hazardous materials diving, or black-water diving? Does it involve underwater cave diving or underwater vehicle extrication? Are those participating in the dive novice or experienced? How long was the person(s) underwater? Remember too that you may be waiting for the recovery of one person, but one of the divers involved in the recovery process may experience a diving emergency and become your patient.

Case Study

It is a beautiful, cloudless August day but, in 15 years of working in EMS, you can't remember a more disturbing call. A tour boat has capsized on a large freshwater lake with 35 senior citizens on board, many with significant disabilities. Twenty-one of the passengers were rescued by nearby pleasure boats and transported to local hospitals or treated and released, but 14 people are still missing. It has been four hours since the incident and the water is about 75°F, so the rescue has been downgraded to a recovery operation. Your aeromedical team was initially called for medevac of victims from the scene, but all recoverable patients were transported before your arrival, and now you have been requested to standby on scene for the safety of the massive recovery effort. Although this is a fairly unusual request for your service, your dispatcher approves it, explaining to you that the incident is so large, and in such a remote area that on-site air assets are appropriate. You're standing by the unified command post when a distraught voice comes over the radio requesting EMS to respond to the shoreline staging area. You arrive at the shoreline just as an inflatable boat plows roughly onto the shore. Lying on the floor of the boat is a wet, middle-aged man wearing a dry diving suit, holding his chest and slumped to his right side. His suit is open at the chest and he is moaning. The rest of his gear is lying by his side in the boat and another diver in the boat is cutting away the remains of his suit and other equipment with his diver's knife. "What happened?" you ask the apparently uninjured diver. He tells you that they were searching inside the boat that lies on its side on the bottom of the lake in about 80 feet of water when something went wrong. "It was our first dive of the day and Dave's first recovery ever," he continues, referring to his partner. "We came across a body inside the boat and he just took off for the surface," he says, "I think he freaked out." The boat operator adds, "He just kind of blasted out of the water with his suit all puffed out like the Michelin Man!" The patient is complaining of right-sided chest pain and shortness of breath as he is lifted and carried to a waiting ambulance. You climb into the side door of the ambulance and begin to assess the patient. The patient remains alert and, speaking in two- to three-word sentences, complains of severe right-sided chest pain and mild difficulty breathing. He is intermittently coughing up foamy, blood-tinged sputum. His breath sounds are slightly diminished on the right, but are normal on the left and no adventitious sounds are heard. His vital signs are: respiratory rate 36 and shallow with a SpO_2 of 96 percent on high flow oxygen via nonrebreather mask, heart rate of 122 and regular and a blood pressure of 128/66. While your partner establishes an IV and attaches the cardiac monitor, you discuss with the incident commander the location of the nearest hyperbaric chamber. You learn that the ground transport time to the closest chamber is over an hour and a half but is less than 30 minutes by air. You decide the patient should be transported by air and as your partner packages the patient to prevent hypothermia during transport, you advise the pilot and your communications center. You advise the pilot of the need to keep as low an altitude as possible during the flight. Your pilot tells you that staying low should not present much of a problem, as the hospital you will be transporting to is located within the same valley as the lake, making it unnecessary to climb over the surrounding mountains. With the patient packaged and the rotors spinning, the patient is "hot loaded" into the helicopter. During the transport you closely monitor the patient's airway and breathing status with particular concern for the development of a tension pneumothorax on the right. The transport is uneventful and you arrive at the destination facility without change in the patient's condition. He is moved directly into a large multiplace hyperbaric chamber and care is turned over to the chamber staff.

DISCUSSION QUESTIONS

1. What are the pathophysiology, assessment, and management considerations of the following diving emergencies?
    a. Pulmonary overexpansion
    b. Decompression sickness

Content Review

MULTIPLE CHOICE

_____ 1. _____ is a type of diving in which divers are placed in an underwater habitat for extended periods of time at depths often exceeding 1,000 ft.
   A. Open water diving   C. Deep water diving
   B. Saturation diving   D. Habitat diving

_____ 2. Why do some divers elect to create mixtures of oxygen, nitrogen, helium, and other gases rather than use atmospheric air?
   A. Using gas mixtures reduces the risk of decompression sickness, nitrogen narcosis, and other conditions.
   B. Gas mixtures are often cheaper than atmospheric air.
   C. Gas mixtures allow for increased strength, reducing the risk of injury.
   D. Gas mixtures repel potentially harmful underwater predators, such as sharks and orcas.

_____ 3. _____ is a condition leading to the death of bone tissues, resulting in unexpected fractures, bone degeneration, and devastating arthritis.
   A. Deep water bone necrosis   C. Dysbaric osteonecrosis
   B. Dysbaria osteoimperfecta   D. Barotraumatic osteonecrosis

_____ 4. Which of the following correctly states the formula for pressure (P)?
   A. P = Force × Mass   C. P = Force/Area
   B. P = Mass × Area   D. P = Mass/Force

_____ 5. 1 atm is equal to:
   A. 760 torr.   C. 17.4 lb/in.
   B. 1,066 cm/H_2O.   D. none of the above.

_____ 6. The type of force experienced by a diver at depth is:
   A. atmospheric pressure.   C. air pressure.
   B. hydrodynamic pressure.   D. hydrostatic pressure.

©2007 Pearson Education, Inc.
Critical Care Paramedic

_____ 7. Which of the following gases can have narcoticlike effects on the CNS when inhaled under pressure?
A. oxygen
B. helium
C. carbon dioxide
D. nitrogen

_____ 8. _____ is determined by the density of an object and the specific gravity of the liquid in which it is suspended.
A. Weight
B. Buoyancy
C. Mass
D. Area

_____ 9. "Normal" sport diving is diving that occurs at depths not exceeding how many feet?
A. 80
B. 100
C. 120
D. 140

_____ 10. All of the following are injuries associated with descent to depth except:
A. tympanic membrane rupture.
B. sinus squeeze.
C. round window injury.
D. pulmonary overpressure injury.

_____ 11. _____ is a condition caused by the expansion of nitrogen in the body tissues and bloodstream following a dive of significant depth and duration.
A. Decompression sickness
B. Nitrogen narcosis
C. Pneumomediastinum
D. None of the above

_____ 12. The best treatment for nitrogen narcosis is:
A. immediate descent.
B. immediate ascent.
C. treatment in a decompression chamber.
D. airway control, oxygenation, and ventilation.

_____ 13. The definitive treatment for decompression sickness is:
A. immediate descent.
B. immediate ascent.
C. treatment in a decompression chamber.
D. airway control, oxygenation, and ventilation.

_____ 14. A diver who experiences joint pain, vertigo, paralysis, and seizures soon after ascent is most likely experiencing which of the following?
A. tympanic membrane rupture
B. nitrogen narcosis
C. high-pressure neurologic syndrome
D. decompression sickness

_____ 15. Management for a diver experiencing decompression sickness may include all of the following except:
A. administration of IV benzodiazepines.
B. administration of an IV fluid bolus.
C. placement of the patient in a right-sided Trendelenburg position.
D. advanced airway management.

_____ 16. _____ can occur as a result of breathing pressurized helium and oxygen at depths exceeding 400 feet.
A. Nitrogen narcosis
B. High-pressure neurologic syndrome
C. Decompression sickness
D. Hypoxia

_____ 17. Injuries associated with ascent from depth include all of the following except:
   A. pneumomediastinum.   C. arterial gas embolism.
   B. tympanic membrane rupture.   D. mask squeeze.

_____ 18. Signs and symptoms of high-pressure neurologic syndrome include:
   A. tremors, impaired muscle coordination, altered mental status, unconsciousness.
   B. joint pain, vertigo, paralysis, seizures.
   C. difficulty breathing, decreased lung sounds, decreased SaO_2.
   D. seizures, increased ICP, tympanic membrane rupture, coma.

_____ 19. Definitive treatment for high-pressure neurologic syndrome is:
   A. immediate ascent.
   B. recompression in a hyperbaric chamber.
   C. decompression in a hyperbaric chamber.
   D. IV benzodiazepines or other sedatives.

_____ 20. _____ occurs secondary to the aspiration of sea water, and can produce pneumonia-like symptoms including dyspnea, cough, and hemoptysis.
   A. Saltwater pneumonia   C. Saltwater aspiration syndrome
   B. Saltwater pneumonitis   D. Drowning

_____ 21. Treatment of marine organism envenomation may include all of the following except:
   A. hot water (105–115°F) immersion of the effected part, if practical.
   B. administration of antivenom.
   C. utilization of "pressure immobilization" techniques.
   D. application of a tourniquet.

_____ 22. Treatment of jellyfish or Portuguese man-of-war stings may include irrigation of the affected area with all of the following except:
   A. vinegar.   C. baking soda solution.
   B. water.   D. urine.

_____ 23. Which of the following is a toxin that accumulates in the flesh of large, reef-dwelling fish?
   A. Shigella   C. scombroid
   B. ciguatera   D. Nematocyst

_____ 24. Women make up about 25 percent of the diving population but account for only about 10 percent of the deaths.
   A. True
   B. False

_____ 25. About what percentage of diver deaths is related to heart disease and related conditions?
   A. 10 percent   C. 35–40 percent
   B. 20–25 percent   D. 50 percent

_____ 26. A spear-fisherman presenting with nausea, abdominal pain, skin rash, extremity pain, cardiac dysrhythmia, and the reversal of hot and cold perception is most likely suffering from:
   A. nitrogen narcosis.   C. ciguatera poisoning.
   B. scombroid poisoning.   D. decompression sickness.

_____ 27. Transportation by which of the following methods has the greatest risk of complicating decompression sickness?
   A. ground ambulance   C. pressurized aircraft
   B. rotor-wing aircraft   D. personal vehicle

_____ 28. Hyperbaric chambers can be utilized to treat all of the following diseases except:
   A. burns.
   B. decompression sickness.
   C. carbon monoxide poisoning.
   D. all of the above.

_____ 29. Which of the following statements regarding diving considerations in females is false?
   A. Females have a lower oxygen consumption rate than do men.
   B. Females have a higher risk of decompression sickness than do men.
   C. Women tend to be more buoyant than are men.
   D. Women cannot dive as deep or for as long as men.

32 Toxicological Emergencies

Review of Chapter Objectives

Upon completion of this chapter, the student should be able to:

1. Describe the epidemiology of toxic emergencies.   **p. 938**

Almost 2.4 million human toxin exposures were reported to U.S. poison control centers in 2003. This number includes accidental and intentional drug use, drug abuse, and environmental exposures. Emergency Medical Services were involved in over 90 percent of exposures that occurred at residences. Over 125,000 cases resulted in a moderate or major medical effect, and 1,106 fatalities were reported. The breakdown of the reported cases reveals that over 75 percent of cases involved ingestion, 7.5 percent were dermal exposure, 5.8 percent were inhalational exposure, and 3.5 percent involved an envenomation.

2. Briefly describe the role of the poison control center (PCC) to include how to contact them in case of emergency.   **p. 938**

One of the many roles of a U.S. poison control center is to assist with the triage and management of patients with potential toxic exposures. They can be contacted at 800-222-1222.

3. Define the following:

Drug or substance abuse   **p. 938**

The United States Department of Health and Human Services defines substance abuse as a maladaptive pattern of substance use leading to clinically significant impairment or distress, as manifested by the occurrence of one or more of the following within a 12-month period:

- Recurrent substance use resulting in a failure to fulfill major role obligations at work, school, or home.
- Recurrent substance use in situations in which it is physically hazardous.
- Recurrent substance-related legal problems.
- Continued substance use despite having persistent or recurrent social or interpersonal problems caused or exacerbated by the effects of the substance.

Drug addiction   **p. 938**

Drug addiction is a condition characterized by one or more of the following behaviors: impaired control over drug use, compulsive drug use, continued drug use despite harm, and drug craving. The condition's development and manifestations are influenced by genetic, psychosocial, and environmental factors.

Drug dependency (physical and psychological)   p. 938

Physical dependency is a state of adaptation that is manifested by a drug-class specific physical withdrawal syndrome that can be produced by abrupt cessation, rapid dose reduction, decreasing blood level of drug, or administration of an antagonist.

Psychological dependency is another state of adaptation manifested by psychological withdrawal symptoms upon abrupt cessation, rapid dose reduction, decreasing blood level of drug, or administration of an antagonist.

Drug withdrawal   p. 938

Patients experiencing drug withdrawal typically present with a characteristic withdrawal syndrome. Withdrawal syndrome requires two things: a pre-existing physical adaptation (tolerance) to a specific drug with continued exposure necessary to prevent withdrawal, and decreasing concentrations of that drug to cause the withdrawal. Specific clinical manifestations of withdrawal syndrome are determined by the drug's underlying physiologic actions. Withdrawal syndrome usually manifests symptoms opposite those that the drug manifests.

4. **Discuss the presentations of the following toxidromes:**

Hallucinogens   p. 939

Hallucinogens are compounds that typically involve serotonergic effects and lead to distorted sensorium, hallucinations, and entactogenic effects. Commonly abused agents include lysergic acid diethylamide (LSD), psilocybin (mushrooms), mescaline (from the peyote cactus), and 3,4, methylenedioxy-amphemtamine (MDMA or ecstasy). Signs and symptoms of toxicity include altered sensorium, ataxia, bruxism, and labile emotions. Agents that also produce sympathomimetic effects (like hallucinogenic amphetamines) may produce diaphoresis, tremor, tachycardia, and hypertension.

Sympathomimetics   p. 939

Sympathomimetics are a class of drugs that mimic the effects of the endogenous catecholamines epinephrine and norepinephrine. They produce effects by stimulating adrenergic receptors in the nervous system. Examples include illicit drugs such as cocaine, amphetamines, and methamphetamines, as well as over-the-counter prescription medications such as ephedrine and phenylpropanolamine. Signs and symptoms of toxicity include tachycardia, hypertension, delirium, and agitation. Toxic effects can include intracranial hemorrhage, seizure, myocardial infarction, and hyperthermia.

Opiates   p. 939

Opiates are a group of naturally occurring compounds derived from the poppy plant (*Papaver somniferum*), which stimulate opiate receptors in the central and peripheral nervous systems. Examples include morphine and codeine. The classic opiate toxidrome involves myosis, respiratory depression, and sedation. Other signs and symptoms of toxicity include apnea, noncardiogenic pulmonary edema, and seizures (associated with meperidine, propoxyphene, or tramadol abuse). The antidote for opiate toxicity is naloxone.

Sedative   p. 940

Sedative-hypnotics include a wide range of medications used for the treatment of anxiety and insomnia. Also included are several subgroups, each with different mechanisms of action. The largest group includes agents that increase concentrations of gamma-aminobutyric acid (GABA), the main neuroinhibitory transmitter in the central nervous system. Examples include benzodiazepines, barbiturates, gamma-hydroxybutyrate (GHB), chloral hydrate, propofol, and meprobamate. Other subgroups of the sedative-hypnotics include antihistamines (diphenhydramine), skeletal muscle relaxants (methocarbamol and cyclobenzaprine), and certain antidepressants used for their sedating effects (trazodone). Signs and symptoms of toxicity include drowsiness, coma, ataxia, nystagmus, respiratory depression, bradycardia, hypotension, and respiratory arrest.

5. **Describe the clinical manifestation and basic management techniques for the following toxic emergencies by prescription class:**

Cardiac medications p. 940

Classes of cardiac medications include calcium channel blockers (CCBs), beta blockers (BBs), and digitalis glycosides. There are three main types of CCBs; dihydropyridines (nifedipine, amlodipine), benzothiapines (diltiazem), and phenylalkylamines (verapamil). Signs and symptoms of CCB toxicity include hypotension, bradycardia or other bradydysrhythmias, metabolic acidosis, pulmonary edema, and coma. Signs and symptoms of BB toxicity include bradycardia, hypotension, dysrhythmias, and hypoglycemia with severe toxicity in children. In addition, propranolol toxicity can lead to QRS widening and seizures secondary to sodium channel blockade.

The digitalis glycosides are a widely used cardiac medication class with a narrow therapeutic window; minimal elevations in blood concentrations can lead to toxicity. Digoxin produces toxicity by poisoning the sodium-potassium pump and allowing more sodium and calcium to enter the myocardial muscle cell, therefore increasing excitability; PVCs and tachydysrhythmias can result. Digoxin also increases vagal tone, leading to heart blocks and bradydysrhythmias. Signs and symptoms of toxicity include nausea and vomiting, generalized malaise, visual disturbances, mental status changes, and ECG changes.

The initial management of cardiac medication toxicity should focus on supporting cardiac function with airway maintenance, IV fluids for hypotension, and cardiac dysrhythmia control with ACLS medications. CCB and BB toxicity can be treated specifically with the administration of IV calcium as calcium gluconate or calcium chloride bolus or continuous infusion. Calcium administration should be avoided in any patient who may be dig toxic, as digitalis toxicity increases intracellular calcium concentrations; additional calcium may encourage dysrhythmia and ventricular fibrillation. Positive inotropes such as epinephrine and dopamine can increase cardiac output by increasing myocardial contractility and have the added advantage of vasoconstrictive properties that can help correct hypotension. Administration of glucagon will increase intracellular cAMP levels, promoting calcium entry into the cells.

Sodium bicarbonate IV can be administered for dysrhythmia and hypotension associated with QRS widening and propranolol-induced seizures.

Psychiatric medications p. 941

Pathophysiological effects of tricyclic antidepressants (TCAs, cyclic antidepressants) include sodium channel blockade, alpha-adrenergic blockade, inhibition of neuronal catecholamine uptake, and anticholinergic effects. Specific examples of TCAs are amitriptyline, nortriptyline, desipramine, and amoxapine. Signs and symptoms of toxicity include anticholinergic effects (manifested by agitation and delirium), tachydysrhythmias, hypotension, seizures, and coma. Treatment consists of supportive care, glucagon administration, IV sodium bicarbonate for QRS widening, and benzodiazepine administration for seizures.

Monamine oxidase inhibitors (MAO-Is) are rarely used because of numerous food and drug interactions and severe toxicity in overdose. MAO-Is can adversely interact with selective serotonin reuptake inhibitors (SSRIs), amphetamines, and tyramine-containing foods such as certain wines, cheeses, and beer. Signs and symptoms of toxicity include neurologic manifestations such as lethargy, ataxia, headache, confusion, disorientation, mumbling speech, seizures, and coma. Autonomic instability can lead to flushing, diaphoresis, hypertension, tachycardia, and ventricular dysrhythmias. Neuromuscular complications include tremor, nystagmus, myoclonus, fasciculations, and generalized rigidity. Treatment consists of supportive care, IV benzodiazepines for severe agitation and seizures, and ACLS protocols for cardiac toxicity.

Selective serotonin reuptake inhibitors (SSRIs) are widely used agents for the treatment of psychiatric illness. They act by increasing the availability of serotonin and other neurotransmitters such as dopamine and norepinephrine in the central nervous system. Examples include venlafaxine, trazadone, buproprion, olanzapine, and mirtazapine. Signs and symptoms of toxicity can vary with the severity of the overdose. Mild overdose is characterized by nausea, lethargy, tremor, and mild to moderate hypotension typically associated with reflex tachycardia. Severe overdoses are characterized by hypotension, severe agitation, tremor, and seizures.

Serotonin syndrome occurs as the result of the coingestion of several different pro-serotonergic medications such as SSRIs, MAO-Is, lithium, amphetamines, dextromethorphan, and meperidine. Signs and symptoms include delirium, agitation, seizures, autonomic instability (fever, tachycardia, hypertension, or hypotension), myoclonus, and rigidity. Treatment involves supportive care (airway control and NMBAs if necessary), IV hydration, active control of hyperthermia, and IV benzodiazepines for muscular rigidity.

Lithium is a common drug used to treat bipolar disease and other psychiatric disorders, and it has a narrow therapeutic window. Toxicity can develop with minimal changes in blood concentrations, and lithium toxicity is also possible despite normal lithium levels. Toxicity is caused by excessive levels in tissue, particularly the brain, and is not caused by elevated blood levels. Signs and symptoms of toxicity vary with severity. Mild toxicity typically presents with nausea, tremor, ataxia, and rigidity; moderate toxicity with delirium, vomiting, diarrhea, and myoclonus; and severe toxicity with hypotension, seizures, and coma. Treatment revolves around supportive care, IV hydration, and hemodialysis.

Anticonvulsants   p. 942
Benzodiazepines and barbiturates stimulate gamma-aminobutyric acid (GABA) receptors in the central nervous system (CNS), leading to depression of neuronal activity. Signs and symptoms of toxicity include CNS depression, decreased respiratory effort and motor activity, hypothermia, and progressive stupor and coma.

Phenytoin, used to treat generalized and partial complex seizures and cardiac dysrhythmias, undergoes slow and erratic absorption following oral ingestion. Toxic effects can occur from chronic, excessive ingestion or IV administration. Signs and symptoms of toxicity include nausea, tremor, nystagmus, ataxia, delirium, and sedation. Massive overdose can lead to stupor, coma, and seizures. Rapid IV administration can lead to hypotension, bradycardia, or cardiac arrest.

Carbamazepine (Tegretol) has numerous clinical indications for use, including seizures, chronic pain, and psychiatric illness. Systemic absorption can be delayed for over 24 hours following the acute overdose of an extended-release formulation. Carbamazapine has a similar structure to tricyclic antidepressants, and can lead to anticholinergic effects in overdose. Signs and symptoms of toxicity include ataxia, nystagmus, myoclonus, and respiratory depression. Massive overdose can lead to seizure, coma, and hypotension. During recovery, patients may experience cyclic coma with recurrent symptoms.

Valproic acid (Depakote) is commonly used to control seizures, bipolar disorder, migraines, and chronic pain syndromes. Signs and symptoms of toxicity include nausea, vomiting, pancreatitis, confusion, coma, encephalopathy, respiratory failure, and paradoxical seizures.

Treatment of anticonvulsant-induced toxicity centers around supportive care, IV hydration, blood glucose determination and correction, and benzodiazepines for seizure control.

Over-the-counter (OTC) medications   p. 943
In toxicity, acetaminophen (APAP or Tylenol) overwhelms normal hepatic metabolism and leads to cellular toxicity and possible fulminant hepatic failure. The clinical effects can be divided into four stages, with significant overlap. Stage one develops one-half to 24 hours after ingestion, and patients develop nausea, vomiting, and abdominal pain. Stage two occurs 24 to 48 hours after ingestion and is associated with an improvement of gastrointestinal symptoms. Upper right quadrant pain may develop. Stage three occurs two to three days after ingestion, and is characterized by hepatic and renal failure, coagulopathy, jaundice, and hypoglycemia; shock may develop. Stage four develops two days to eight weeks after ingestion and is associated with either recovery or fulminant hepatic failure and potential death. Definitive treatment is administration of n-acetylcysteine.

Salicylates (aspirin or ASA) are found in numerous OTC and prescription medications as well as other compounds, including oil of wintergreen and Pepto Bismol. In overdose, ASA acts as a cellular poison, disrupting energy production and causing metabolic acidosis. Signs and symptoms of toxicity vary with severity. Mild toxicity characteristically presents with dehydration secondary to tachypnea, vomiting, diaphoresis, tinnitus, nausea, tachycardia, and tachypnea. Moderate toxicity presents with marked tachypnea and tachycardia, diaphoresis, agitation, severe toxicity with delirium, hyperthermia, cardiac dysrhythmias, pulmonary edema, and seizures. Treatment for

ASA toxicity includes supportive care, glucose determination and maintenance, IV hydration, IV sodium bicarbonate, and hemodialysis.

Nonsteroidal anti-inflammatory drugs (NSAIDs) are common agents used in intentional overdose. Most patients develop only minimal symptoms, and there are myriad signs and symptoms including metabolic acidosis. Severe toxicity can lead to coma, respiratory depression, and renal insufficiency. Treatment consists of supportive care, ventilation to treat metabolic acidosis, and IV hydration.

Dextromethorphan is a common ingredient in numerous OTC medications, and is metabolized to a compound that activates glutamate receptors, leading to central nervous system excitation. A commonly abused drug, it produces altered sensorium and hallucinations. Signs and symptoms of toxicity include ataxia, dizziness, nystagmus, mydriasis, seizures, hyperthermia, rhabdomyolysis, and serotonine syndrome. Treatment includes supportive care, IV rehydration, and benzodiazepines to control seizures.

Herbal medications   p. 944

The availability of herbal medications has rapidly increased since the passage of the Dietary Supplement Health and Education Act in 1994. Dietary supplements (including herbal medications) are not stringently regulated by the FDA or any other government agency. As such, these products do not undergo any scientific testing and are potentially dangerous for several reasons: there is no verification of ingredients, no testing for biological effects, and no knowledge of drug interactions. Common prescription drugs with herbal interactions include warfarin, digoxin, and several anticonvulsants. Commonly used herbal medications in the United States include: aloe, bilberry, echinacea, *Ginkgo biloba*, ginseng, grape seed extract, saw palmetto, and St. John's wort. It is nearly impossible to predict what medical effects or toxicity can be expected from either acute or chronic use of herbal medication, though expected toxic effects can include gastroenteritis with nausea, vomiting, and diarrhea, and additional toxic effects can involve hepatic or renal dysfunction. Some Chinese herbal medications have been found to contain digoxin-like compounds, which can lead to cardiac dysrhythmias that are treated with digoxin-specific Fab antibodies.

6. Explain how caustic injuries can affect the body.   p. 944

When an alkali compound comes into contact with tissue, proteins and cell membranes are emulsified in a process termed liquefaction necrosis, and deep tissue penetration is possible. Eschar formation (secondary to coagulation necrosis) resulting from exposure to acids such as hydrofluoric acid and phenol limits the extent of deep tissue injury.

7. Discuss ethanol and toxic alcohol emergencies.   p. 945

The toxic alcohols are common ingredients in many commercial and industrial products, and include methanol, ethylene glycol, and isopropanol. Shared clinical effects of all alcohols include gastritis, altered sensorium (euphoria, inebriation, coma), impaired judgment, and ataxia.

The effects of ethanol depend on several factors including the amount ingested, the rate of ingestion, coingestions, and tolerance. After ingestion and absorption, ethanol is metabolized by the enzyme alcohol dehydrogenase. In addition to those listed above, signs and symptoms of toxicity include nystagmus, loss of social inhibitions, agitation, and aggressive behavior. Coma, respiratory depression, and loss of airway reflexes can occur in severe intoxication. Chronic ethanol abuse can lead to liver disease, coagulopathy, gastrointestinal bleeding, cardiac dysrhythmias, and central or peripheral neural disorders. Treatment for ethanol toxicity centers around supportive care, with airway control and ventilation a priority. A glucose determination should be made, and blood glucose levels can be maintained with the IV administration of D_5W, which can also serve to address any fluid volume deficits. IV fluid administration in the absence of fluid volume deficit is unnecessary, as increased glomerular filtration rate (GFR) does not increase ethanol elimination.

Isopropanol (isopropyl alcohol), found in rubbing alcohol, is occasionally abused as a substitute for ethanol. It is metabolized to acetone, which can prolong the duration of central nervous system and respiratory depression but does not cause a metabolic acidosis. Additional signs and symptoms of toxicity include significant gastritis, CNS depression, respiratory depression, and coma. Treatment priorities include airway maintenance, ventilation, and support of intravascular volume. Dehydration can be managed with IV fluid administration. Hypotension unresponsive to treatment indicates the need for hemodialysis, as does hemodynamic instability and a predicted peak isopropanol level of greater than 400 mg/dL.

Methanol is found in windshield washer fluid or as a contaminant in the production of moonshine. Initial signs and symptoms include an ethanol-like intoxication with gastritis, ataxia, and inebriation. Methanol is metabolized by alcohol dehydrogenase to formaldehyde and formic acid. Formic acid accumulation is responsible for the clinical manifestations of toxicity, which include metabolic acidosis, blindness, seizure, coma, and death. Because folate is a cofactor in the metabolism of formic acid to carbon dioxide and water, patients who are folate-deficient (alcoholics, for example) may exhibit higher degrees of methanol toxicity because of greater formic acid accumulation. Treatment of methanol poisoning centers around supportive care, correcting acidosis, preventing the metabolism of methanol into its harmful metabolites, and hemodialysis. Prevention of methanol metabolism and the production of formic acid can be accomplished with the administration of fomepizole, a competitive inhibitor of alcohol dehydrogenase. Alternatively, IV ethanol can be administered, which will also act as a competitive inhibitor to alcohol dehydrogenase. And yes, oral ethanol, in the form of alcohol, can be administered with the same effect, if the situation requires it, though it is of questionable validity in the transport environment.

Ethylene glycol initially presents with inebriation and ataxia, but is metabolized to acidic compounds that lead to metabolic acidosis, respiratory distress, seizures, and renal failure. Severe acidosis develops and death occurs in the absence of appropriate interventions. Treatment is the same as for methanol toxicity.

8. **Discuss toxic emergencies regarding industrial exposure.**   **p. 946**

Carbon monoxide (CO) is a colorless, odorless, nonirritating gas that when inhaled is rapidly absorbed into blood and tissue. It is the result of incomplete combustion and can be encountered near any source of combustion such as fires, generators, space heaters, and automobiles. The amount of CO absorbed depends on the ambient CO concentration and the length of exposure. CO binds to hemoglobin, preventing oxygen from binding, thus inhibiting the delivery and cellular utilization of oxygen, and leads to hypoxia. Signs and symptoms of toxicity include headache, dizziness, nausea, and confusion; the clinical effects moderately correlate with blood levels. Pulse oximetry is, of course, useless in CO poisoning and will generate false high readings. Treatment centers around supportive care and the administration of high flow, 100 percent oxygen; intubation may be necessary. Hyperbaric oxygen therapy is indicated in patients with persistent acidosis or neurologic symptoms unrelieved with 100 percent oxygen, concurrent burns, pregnancy, and a history of loss of consciousness, myocardial infarction (MI), seizure, hypotension, or coma during or after the episode.

Hydrogen sulfide (HS) is the byproduct of the natural breakdown of organic material. It is a highly lethal gas that smells like rotten eggs. Heavier than air, HS accumulates in low-lying pits, trenches, or containers, and is rapidly absorbed after inhalation and inhibits the cellular use of oxygen, leading to hypoxia, lactate accumulation, and metabolic acidosis. Its mechanism of toxicity is very similar to that of cyanide. Signs and symptoms of toxicity include burning eyes, cough, headache, nausea, dizziness, and the rapid development of coma. Massive or prolonged exposure can lead to seizures, cardiovascular shock, and death. Treatment includes supportive care such as high flow, 100 percent oxygen and intubation, if necessary, and hyperbaric oxygen therapy may be of benefit. In addition, administration of the sodium nitrate and amyl nitrate from a cyanide antidote kit may encourage the conversion of sulfide to considerably less toxic sulfmethemoglobin.

Cyanide's cellular toxicity is similar to hydrogen sulfide and leads to similar clinical effects. Treatment consists of supportive care, the treatment of seizures, and the administration of a cyanide antidote kit.

Hydrofluoric (HF) acid is a highly reactive corrosive commonly found in commercial and industrial products such as rust removers and glass etching compounds, and is also used in the manufacturing of semiconductor chips. Clinical effects vary depending on the route of exposure, HF acid concentration, and the amount of tissue exposed. Exposure to a low concentration of HF acid may not produce symptoms for over 12 hours. Signs and symptoms of toxicity vary depending on exposure route. Inhalation exposure presents with mucous membrane irritation, bronchospasm, and chemical pneumonitis or pulmonary edema. Dermal exposure results in burning pain with or without signs of dermal burn, erythema or blanching, or edema. Treatment for dermal burns includes irrigation with water and the topical application of calcium-containing gels. Ocular exposure can be managed with irrigation, and airway exposure with airway support, oxygen, and bronchodilators. Patients with intact airways after ingestion exposure can receive oral calcium or magnesium-containing substances such as milk or calcium carbonate. General treatment includes supportive care, IV calcium for cardiac dysrhythmia, and the administration of intra-arterial calcium gluconate.

9. Explain the two major categories of warfare agents. p. 948

There are two general groups of modern warfare agents; biological agents and chemical agents. Biological agents produce toxicity by causing infectious disease. Organisms utilized as biological agents include anthrax, botulinum toxins, plague, smallpox, and tularemia.

Chemical agents include nerve agents, vesicants, lacrimators, and incapacitating agents. Nerve agents are considered organophosphate (OP) compounds, and include tabun, sarin, soman, VX, and carbamate insecticides like Malathion and Chlormephos. Vesicants are substances such as mustard and lewisite gases, which produce dermal toxicity and lead to vesicle formation and tissue corrosion. Lacrimators are irritant gases and solutions that cause mucus membrane irritation. They are typically used as riot control agents and are substances such as tear gas and capsaicin (pepper spray).

10. List common findings seen in a toxic emergency involving plants and mushrooms. p. 951

- Gastroenteritis
- Dermal and mucus membrane irritation
- Multiple-system organ failure
- Seizures
- Anticholinergic poisoning
- Hallucinations
- Hepatic failure

11. What are some common findings in toxic emergencies from envenomations and stings? p. 952

The clinical findings associated with snake bites vary with specific snakes. Rattlesnake and copperhead envenomations result in significant pain, edema, myonecrosis, and coagulopathy. Coral snake and cobra envenomations result in pain and neurologic effects that include fasciculations and weakness.

Hymenoptera envenomation is characterized by localized pain, edema, and erythema. Systemic effects such as urticaria, wheezing, hypotension, airway compromise, or anaphylaxis are also possible.

Black widow spider bites are often initially unrecognized. Inspection of the bite site may reveal two small puncture wounds with minimal erythema or inflammation, and the development of a target lesion is possible. Localized effects typically begin within 60 minutes of the envenomation and include pain, diaphoresis, and piloerection isolated to the bite site. Severe envenomation will progress to include diffuse pain, muscle cramps (typically of the abdomen or back), tachycardia, and hypertension. Additional effects include nausea, headache, fever, tremor, and weakness. Rarely reported are periorbital edema or ecchymosis, priapism, cardiac dysrhythmias (including reflex bradycardia), or paralysis.

Brown recluse spider envenomation can lead to varying amounts of local vascular injury and dermonecrosis. Classically, the bite site develops into a necrotic wound within four days of envenomation. Eschar forms, falls off, and the wound heals slowly over several weeks. Systemic effects, termed loxoscelism, are rare but possible and typically develop one to two days after the envenomation. Clinical findings include nausea, fever, and myalgias. Serious effects include significant skin deterioration, exudates from the bite site, systemic hemolysis, renal failure, and death.

The clinical effects of scorpion envenomation include immediate pain and paresthesias at the sting site. Large envenomations may progress to involve diffuse pain, paresthesias, and muscle fasciculations. Severe envenomations progress to involve cranial nerve dysfunction and cause rotatory nystagmus, hypersalivation, difficulty swallowing, and possible airway compromise.

Marine animal envenomations include a wide variety of organisms and clinical presentations. Poisonous species include jellyfish, fire coral, sea urchins, sea snakes, stingrays, and various fishes, and envenomation can occur through several mechanisms including bites, barbs, and nematocysts. Sea snake envenomation results in pain and muscle weakness that may progress to paralysis and respiratory failure. The majority of other envenomations lead to local pain, erythema, and edema and the extent of pain can be overwhelming and contribute to weakness, nausea, and autonomic instability.

12. Recognize scene and environmental indicators that may identify that a toxicological emergency has occurred or may occur.   **p. 955**

An in-depth scene survey is paramount to initiating optimal care while ensuring rescuer safety. Prehospital providers may be the only health care professionals capable of uncovering important information necessary to determine the cause for the patient's condition and its impact on the treatment plan. Items such as pill bottles, product containers (e.g., antifreeze bottles), suicide notes, or bystander interviews can provide immediate information relevant to patient care that would otherwise be missed. The need to gather as much information from the scene without delaying transport cannot be overemphasized.

13. Describe such issues as initial evaluation, toxin decontamination, and transportation issues as they pertain to toxicological emergencies.   **p. 955**

Issues involving the initial evaluation are discussed above, in Objective 12. The initial steps in decontamination involve removing the patient(s) from the source of toxicity. While rescuer safety can never be compromised, decontamination techniques should not delay life-saving interventions. Mechanical decontamination involves attempts to remove any toxins from physical contact with the patient. Solid substances should be removed by carefully wiping them off, and care should be taken not to scrub the patient's skin, as small abrasions can allow increased dermal absorption. All contaminated clothing should be removed and bagged for proper disposal. Copious irrigation with water or saline can remove contaminants not removed by brushing or the removal of clothing. Gross decontamination can take place in a shower or under a hose. Finer decontamination can be accomplished with irrigation with water or saline from IV bags or small containers. Contact lenses should be removed from the patient's eyes prior to irrigation with low-pressure water, and care should be taken to avoid runoff from surrounding skin into the patient's eyes, ears, or mouth.

A few general principles are worth keeping in mind with regard to the transport of a poisoned patient. Consider intubation prior to transport if history suggests the potential for increasing CNS depression and airway compromise, or if there is a concern for severe agitation. The judicious use of naloxone in intubated patients suffering opiate coma is recommended to prevent the agitation typical after naloxone administration. Consider the use of sedative agents for agitated patients rather than physical restraints. Gravid patients are managed the same as nongravid patients; treatment and support are focused on the mother. Fetal compromise is the result of maternal compromise in the vast majority of toxicological emergencies. Some toxins are associated with metabolic derangements and can lead to a severe metabolic acidosis (salicylates, methanol, ethylene glycol). Patients may benefit from IV fluid administration, sodium bicarbonate administration, and hyperventilation to maintain a low-to-normal $PaCO_2$.

Case Study

Your critical care ground transport unit has been called to a small rural emergency department to transport a 35-year-old male patient to the regional medical center for admission. The dispatch information is that the patient has altered mental status secondary to a "medication reaction." On arrival at the facility, you and your partner find yourselves waiting to get a report and meet your patient but the department receptionist informs you that both the PA and the RN are busy in the only other exam room, splinting a tib/fib fracture. She hands you a packet containing a photocopy of the patient's chart and other transfer paperwork. Reviewing the chart, you become confused since the chief complaint is clearly documented as "right flank pain, possible kidney stone." Reading further, you note that the patient had a kidney stone on the right two years ago. He came to the emergency department complaining of right-side low back pain radiating to his abdomen and right testicle. The pain is associated with nausea and reportedly is exactly like the onset of his previous stone. Your confusion has only deepened and you skip to the end of the chart, where it lists a diagnosis of renal colic, but it is listed below the primary diagnosis of serotonin syndrome. Looking at the patient's medication list, you see that he is taking the selective serotonin reuptake inhibitor (SSRI) fluoxetine, 120 mg a day, for depression. The PA steps out from behind the other curtain and introduces himself to you and your partner. He tells you that the patient came in with severe right flank pain, nausea, abdominal and right CVA tenderness, and hematuria. He was presumptively given a diagnosis of right renal stone. He received IV fluids and 50 mg of meperidine IV push with significant relief of his pain. A technician was called in to perform an abdominal CT, which had to be abandoned in favor of a plain X-ray of the abdomen because the patient became anxious and diaphoretic. It was presumed that the patient was claustrophobic in the CT scanner but his symptoms worsened after the X-ray, which showed a small calcification at the right vesico-ureteral junction. When his unexplained anxiety and diaphoresis became associated with tremor and coordination difficulties, it was determined that the patient was most likely suffering from serotonin syndrome secondary to the administration of meperidine. The patient was given 5 mg of diazepam IV with significant relief of his anxiety and tremor and is resting comfortably at this time. Other than the hematuria, his labs are normal and he has stable vital signs. You gently awaken the patient, introduce your partner and yourself and explain that you are here to take him to the medical center for further care. The patient says "OK" and quickly resumes sleeping. You awaken him again to question him about how he's feeling and assess his mental status and he tells you the name of the hospital he's at, that he is comfortable, and just wants to go back to sleep. You note that the patient is very somnolent, but his airway is self-maintained without difficulty and his SpO_2 on room air is 98 percent. He is gently moved to the ambulance stretcher and then to the ambulance for transport. During the transfer the patient continues to sleep but remains stable at each reassessment. By the end of the 45-minute transport, the patient is more easily aroused and as the ambulance starts backing up the ramp at your destination, he awakens by himself, looks around, stretches, and tells you that he feels much better.

DISCUSSION QUESTIONS

1. What is the role of the poison control center in the management of toxicological emergencies, and how can they be reached?
2. Describe the clinical appearance and basic management of a patient suffering from serotonin syndrome.

Content Review

MULTIPLE CHOICE

_____ 1. About how many human toxin exposures were reported to U.S. poison control centers in 2003?
A. 755,000   C. 2.4 million
B. 1.2 million   D. 3.8 million

_____ 2. The vast majority of toxin exposures take place via which of the following exposure routes?
A. dermal   C. envenomation
B. inhalation   D. ingestion

_____ 3. _____ can be defined as an adaptation to a specific class of drugs, the cessation of which can produce a withdrawal syndrome.
   A. Drug abuse
   B. Addiction
   C. Physical dependence
   D. Tolerance

_____ 4. A patient who takes morphine regularly for pain finds that she requires larger doses to produce the same effect is experiencing _____ to the drug.
   A. an addiction
   B. physical dependence on
   C. tolerance
   D. none of the above

_____ 5. Which of the following is/are a collection of signs and symptoms that, together, reliably suggest an exposure to a particular drug class?
   A. toxidrome
   B. warning signs
   C. chief complaint
   D. withdrawal syndrome

_____ 6. Psilocybin, mescaline, and 3, 4, methylenedioxy-amphemtamine are examples of which of the following drug classes?
   A. narcotics
   B. hallucinogens
   C. sympathomimetics
   D. sedative-hypnotics

_____ 7. Which of the following toxidromes presents with headache, nausea, confusion, ataxia, tachycardia, and syncope?
   A. opioid withdrawal
   B. anticholinergic
   C. GABA-agonist withdrawal
   D. hypoxia/hypoxemia

_____ 8. _____ are a class of drugs that mimic the effects of endogenous catecholamines.
   A. Epinephrine and norepinepherine
   B. Sympathomimetics
   C. CNS depressants
   D. Dopaminergics

_____ 9. Which of the following are examples of sedative-hypnotics?
   A. ephedrine and phenylpropanolamine
   B. meperidine and propoxyphene
   C. chloral hydrate, propofol, and meprobamate
   D. lysergic acid diethylamide and psilocybin

_____ 10. Which of the following are examples of sympathomimetics?
   A. meperidine and tramadol
   B. chloral hydrate, propofol, and meprobamate
   C. barbiturates, gamma-hydroxybutyrate
   D. ephedrine and phenylpropanolamine

_____ 11. Ingestion of toxic amounts of which of the following medications is least likely to result in sedation, respiratory depression, and apnea?
   A. propofol
   B. morphine
   C. phenylpropanolamine
   D. barbiturates

_____ 12. Ingestion of toxic amounts of which of the following medications is least likely to result in tachycardia and hypertension?
   A. choral hydrate
   B. mescaline
   C. ephedrine
   D. methamphetamine

_____ 13. Coingestion of cocaine should be suspected in a patient who presents with an opioid toxidrome but:
   A. does not respond to the administration of naloxone.
   B. responds to the administration of beta blockers.
   C. becomes severely agitated and develops a hyperadrenergic state after the administration of naloxone.
   D. develops immediate cardiopulmonary arrest after the administration of naloxone.

_____ 14. Which of the following correctly identifies the three main types of calcium channel blockers?
   A. benzothiapines, dihydropyridines, and phenylalkylamines
   B. diphenhydramines, benzodiazepines, and phenylalanines
   C. slow channel blockers, fast channel blockers, and nonspecific channel blockers
   D. phase I blockers, phase III blockers, and phase IV blockers

_____ 15. A patient complaining of nausea, vomiting, malaise, and visual disturbances is found to have a new-onset second-degree (Wenckebach) heart block. This patient has most likely overdosed on a(n):
   A. beta blocker.   C. digoxin.
   B. calcium channel blocker.   D. ACE inhibitor.

_____ 16. Management of beta-blocker toxicity consists of all of the following except:
   A. administration of IV calcium.
   B. administration of a beta-agonist.
   C. administration of 100 percent oxygen.
   D. administration of IV sodium bicarbonate.

_____ 17. Management of severe digitalis toxicity consists of all of the following except:
   A. administration of IV Digibind.
   B. administration of IV calcium.
   C. transcutaneous pacing.
   D. administration of antidysrhythmics.

_____ 18. The treatment of dysrhythmia secondary to heart medication toxicity should include normal ACLS cardiac medications.
   A. True
   B. False

_____ 19. Which of the following psychiatric medications is considered the least toxic?
   A. tricyclic antidepressants (TCAs)
   B. monoamine oxidase inhibitors (MAO-Is)
   C. selective serotonin reuptake inhibitors (SSRIs)
   D. all are equally toxic

_____ 20. Which of the following toxidromes presents with tremor, agitation, delirium, seizure, tachycardia, hyperthermia, and hypertension?
   A. GABA-agonist withdrawal   C. hypoxia/hypoxemia
   B. cholinergic   D. sympathomimetic

_____ 21. The hypotension associated with tricyclic antidepressant overdose occurs as a result of:
   A. alpha-adrenergic blockade.
   B. anticholinergic effects.
   C. sodium channel blockade.
   D. inhibition of neuronal catecholamine uptake.

_____ 22. Which of the following medications can interact with certain wine, beer, and cheeses to create toxic effects?
   A. TCAs   C. SSRIs
   B. MAO-Is   D. none of the above

_____ 23. Which drug class's toxidrome can be remembered by the mnemonic "three Cs and an A"?
   A. TCAs   C. SSRIs
   B. MAOIs   D. narcotics

_____ 24. What are the signs represented in the mnemonic "three C's and an A"?
   A. Confusion, congestion, constipation, and apnea
   B. Convulsions, coma, cardiac dysrhythmias, and acidosis
   C. Confusion, coma, cardiac dysrhythmias, and apnea
   D. Loss of consciousness, coma, cardiopulmonary arrest, and acidosis

_____ 25. Due to its narrow therapeutic window, _____ toxicity can occur with minimal changes in serum drug levels, and can manifest with ataxia, muscular rigidity, seizures, and coma.
   A. digitalis   C. SSRI
   B. bupropion   D. lithium

_____ 26. Hemodialysis is a management consideration in which of the following medication overdoses?
   A. lithium   C. A and B
   B. salicylates   D. none of the above

_____ 27. Serotonin syndrome can occur with:
   A. the ingestion of a single serotonergic medication.
   B. the co-ingestion of a single serotonergic medication and alcohol.
   C. the co-ingestion of a single serotonergic medication and a sympathomimetic.
   D. the co-ingestion of several different pro-serotonergic medication.

_____ 28. Agents that increase GABA activity include all of the following except:
   A. benzodiazepines.   C. diphenhydramine.
   B. barbiturates.   D. cocaine.

_____ 29. Which of the following toxidromes presents with salivation, diarrhea, urinary incontinence, ataxia, seizures, miosis, and abdominal cramping?
   A. sympathomimetic   C. cholinergic
   B. anticholinergic   D. opioid withdrawal

_____ 30. Toxicity with which of the following psychiatric medications is specifically associated with tremor, tachycardia, and seizures?
   A. bupropion   C. MAO-Is
   B. TCAs   D. lithium

_____ 31. Which of the stages of acetaminophen toxicity is characterized by the onset of hepatic and renal failure?
   A. Stage 1   C. Stage 3
   B. Stage 2   D. Stage 4

_____ 32. Definitive treatment of acetaminophen toxicity includes the administration of which of the following medications?
   A. Digibind   C. ethanol
   B. n-acetylcyctine   D. sodium nitrate and amyl nitrate

_____ 33. Common sources of methanol include which of the following?
   A. beer, wine, and liquor
   B. rubbing alcohol and disinfectant solutions
   C. automotive antifreeze
   D. windshield washer fluid and paint remover

_____ 34. Toxicity with all of the following can result in metabolic acidosis _except_:
   A. salicylates.   C. isopropanol.
   B. NSAIDs.   D. methanol.

_____ 35. All of the following are considered "toxic alcohols," even when present in the blood at nontoxic levels, _except_:
   A. ethylene glycol.   C. isopropanol.
   B. ethanol.   D. methanol.

_____ 36. Which of the following is a metabolite of methanol responsible for the clinical manifestations of methanol toxicity?
A. formic acid
C. formalin
B. formaldehyde
D. alcohol dehydrogenase

_____ 37. A Material Safety Data Sheet (MSDS) must contain specific information about a product, including:
A. chemical name, brand name, signs and symptoms of toxicity, treatment, and Chemical Abstracts Service number.
B. chemical name, brand name, signs and symptoms of toxicity, available antidotes, and Chemical Abstracts Service number.
C. chemical name, signs and symptoms of toxicity, OSHA phone number, and Chemical Abstracts Service number.
D. chemical name, brand name, health effects, and Chemical Abstracts Service number.

_____ 38. Specific examples of solvents that are considered industrial hazards include which of the following?
A. ethylene oxide, glycol ethers
B. hexavalent chromium, vinyl chloride, benzene
C. hydrocarbons, acetone, xylene, toluene
D. n-Hexane, acrylamide

_____ 39. Which of the following gases is colorless, odorless, and can cause asphxia at toxic levels?
A. carbon monoxide
C. hydrofluoric acid
B. hydrogen sulfide
D. none of the above

_____ 40. The amyl and sodium nitrate from a cyanide antidote kit may be used to treat which of the following poisonings?
A. hydrogen sulfide
C. carbon monoxide
B. hydrofluoric acid
D. ethylene glycol

_____ 41. A patient may, if removed from the toxic environment, spontaneously recover from debilitation secondary to which of the following toxins?
A. hydrofluoric acid
C. carbon monoxide
B. hydrogen sulfide
D. cyanide

_____ 42. The management of a patient with cyanide poisoning may include all of the following _except_:
A. intubation and mechanical ventilation.
B. the administration of vasoconstrictors.
C. the administration of benzodiazepines.
D. the administration of sublingual nitrates.

_____ 43. Inhalation of hydrogen fluoride gas can result in:
A. bronchospasm.
C. pulmonary edema.
B. chemical pneumonitis.
D. all of the above.

_____ 44. Small dermal exposures to highly concentrated hydrofluoric (HF) acid solutions can lead to systemic toxicity.
A. True
B. False

_____ 45. Exposure to a low concentration of HF acid may not produce symptoms for more than 12 hours.
A. True
B. False

_____ 46. Management of HF acid exposure may include all of the following except:
   A. topical application of a calcium-containing gel.
   B. administration of nebulized albuterol.
   C. ingestion of sodium bicarbonate.
   D. administration of nebulized calcium.

_____ 47. _____ are examples of warfare agents classified as vesicants.
   A. Tear gas and capsaicin
   B. Mustard gas and lewisite
   C. Sarin and soman
   D. Botulinum toxin and tularemia

_____ 48. Management of a patient exposed to a lacrimating agent is least likely to include which of the following treatments?
   A. decontamination
   B. administration of atropine
   C. irrigation with water or saline
   D. administration of oxygen

_____ 49. Which of the following warfare agents is least likely to respond to the administration of atropine?
   A. VX   C. Tabun
   B. Chlormephos®   D. Capsaicin

_____ 50. The primary concern after the ingestion of a hydrocarbon is:
   A. aspiration and the development of respiratory distress.
   B. systemic absorption and hepatic failure.
   C. systemic absorption and renal failure.
   D. esophageal and gastric burns.

_____ 51. A chronic hydrocarbon abuser is being transported to a regional health care facility for evaluation of frequent episodes of hemodynamically significant tachycardia. Which of the following medications should be avoided should the patient experience cardiac arrest during transport?
   A. atropine   C. epinephrine
   B. sodium bicarbonate   D. lidocaine

_____ 52. Which of the following is least likely to occur with heavy metal toxicity?
   A. hepatic failure   C. renal failure
   B. cardiomegaly   D. neuropathy

_____ 53. The classic symptoms of food poisoning are:
   A. nausea, vomiting, dehydration, and hypotension.
   B. dehydration, hypotension, tachycardia, and diaphoresis.
   C. abdominal pain, diarrhea, dehydration, and hypotension.
   D. nausea, vomiting, abdominal pain, and diarrhea.

_____ 54. The use of antibiotics and antidiarrheal agents is routinely indicated in cases of food poisoning.
   A. True
   B. False

_____ 55. Clinical manifestations of botulinum poisoning include which of the following?
   A. nausea, vomiting, abdominal pain, and fatigue
   B. abdominal pain, diarrhea, malaise, and dehydration
   C. gastritis, muscle weakness, and descending paralysis
   D. gastritis, paresthesias, weakness, and myoclonus

_____ 56. The development of gastroenteritis, and a rash covering the face, neck, and chest is most likely caused by which of the following?
A. scombroid toxin
B. *C. botulinum* toxin
C. *Shigella* toxin
D. tularemia toxin

_____ 57. Management of *C. botulinum* toxin poisoning may include which of the following?
A. administration of an antitoxin
B. aggressive IV fluid replacement
C. administration of electrolytes
D. all of the above

_____ 58. The onset of gastroenteritis within six hours of a mushroom ingestion is a good sign, generally speaking, as it is a good indicator that effects will be limited to gastroenteritis and not include systemic involvement.
A. True
B. False

_____ 59. Which of the following best details the initial treatment of all mushroom or plant ingestions?
A. oxygenation, rehydration, and gastric emptying
B. airway support, rehydration, and control of nausea
C. airway support and oxygenation, correction of hemodynamic instability, and administration of antidote
D. airway support and oxygenation, maintenance of blood pressure, control of nausea, and gastric emptying

_____ 60. Identification of the specific species involved is required for optimal management of a bite from a venomous snake.
A. True
B. False

_____ 61. Which of the following is contraindicated in the management of a patient with a bite from a venomous snake?
A. elevation of the affected limb
B. immobilization of the affected limb
C. application of ice or cold packs to the affected area
D. administration of antivenin

_____ 62. Antivenom is available for all of the following except:
A. brown recluse spiders.
B. rattlesnakes.
C. black widow spiders.
D. coral snakes.

_____ 63. Encounters with all of the following marine animals may leave a "retained barb" in a wound, resulting in deep tissue infection and necrosis, except:
A. lionfish.
B. sea urchins.
C. stingrays.
D. jellyfish.

_____ 64. Treatment of jellyfish envenomation includes immediate irrigation of the contact site with copious amounts of water or saline.
A. True
B. False

_____ 65. Management of marine animal envenomation may include all of the following except:
A. administration of IV analgesics.
B. treatment of an anaphylactic reaction.
C. immersion of the envenomation site in ice water.
D. IV fluid administration.

_____ 66. Which of the following statements about decontamination procedures is false?
   A. A patient's contact lenses should be immediately removed in any contamination involving the eye.
   B. Care should be taken to ensure that runoff from surrounding skin does not contaminate the patient's eyes, ears, or mouth.
   C. Decontamination should always precede treatment, even of potential life threats.
   D. Solid substances such as powders should be carefully brushed off of a patient.

_____ 67. Which of the following is an example of a gastric decontamination technique?
   A. administration of syrup of ipecac
   B. administration of activated charcoal
   C. gastric lavage
   D. all of the above

_____ 68. Gastric decontamination is often a life-saving intervention.
   A. True
   B. False

33 Weapons of Mass Destruction

Review of Chapter Objectives

Upon completion of this chapter, the student should be able to:

1. **Discuss how to ensure personal protection in situations involving weapons of mass destruction.**   **p. 963**

   All patients must be thoroughly decontaminated prior to the assessment, management, and transport of a patient by a critical care crew so that there is no risk for off-gasing from chemicals on the patient's body or trapped in his clothing. Rarely, off-gasing can occur from the GI/pulmonary tract secondary to toxic substance ingestion. Caution from chemical elimination via exhalation, perspiration, lacrimation, defecation, urination, or vomiting should be taken at all times.

   A small number of toxicants are so toxic that metabolism and excretion do not alter the chemicals before they are eliminated. In such cases, the critical care provider must wear the appropriate chemical protective equipment and treat the patient as though he is still contaminated. Following care all personnel, equipment, supplies, and vehicles must be free of contamination before being returned to service.

2. **Define CBRNE agents.**   **p. 962**

   CBRNE agents are defined as chemical, biological, radiological, nuclear, and explosive agents or substances that possess the ability to cause illness or injury to exposed victims.

3. **Describe the concept and importance of decontamination.**   **p. 963**

   The first priority for the critical care paramedic is the safety of the crew and the patient. To ensure safety, the patient must be thoroughly and completely decontaminated prior to interaction with the medical crew, medical equipment, and transport vehicle. A contaminated crew or equipment poses many problems. First, if the contamination is identified, the crew and/or equipment must be pulled from transport service, possibly hindering operations if a situation of limited resources is at hand. Second, if the contamination is unidentified, additional patients, care providers, and laypersons may become contaminated with the offending agent.

4. **Describe the characteristics, clinical effects, and critical care interventions for the following chemical agents:**

   Nerve agents   **p. 964**
   Nerve agents are chemical warfare or industrial chemicals that affect the ability of the nervous system to function properly by inhibiting the actions of acetylcholinesterase (AChE), causing a disturbance in normal neural activity. Examples include tabun (GA), sarin (GB), soman (GD), cyclosarin (GF), and V nerve agents.

Acetylcholine (ACh) is a neurotransmitter that has its effects on the nicotinic and muscarinic receptors within the nervous system. Nicotinic receptors are responsible for skeletal muscle movement; muscarinic receptors control function of glands and the smooth muscles of the gut. AChE is an enzyme that performs the deactivation and breakdown of ACh in the synapse after it has performed its function. During the normal propagation of a nerve impulse, ACh leaves the presynaptic neuron and crosses the synaptic cleft to the postsynaptic cholinergic receptor site. Binding of ACh to this site results in the transmission of the appropriate neural impulse. AChE, present on the postsynaptic membrane, breaks down ACh into acetic acid and choline. As such, ACh is effectively removed from the receptor site, thereby ceasing transmission of the neural impulse and resetting the cholinergic receptor to its pre-stimulated condition. ACh is immediately regenerated and prepared for the next signal transmission opportunity.

Nerve agents bind with the AChE, rendering it unable to function, thereby inhibiting its ability to deactivate and degrade the ACh present in the synapse. ACh then remains in the synaptic cleft and continues to interact with the cholinergic receptor, resulting in a constant, uncontrolled stimulation of the receptor site. If binding of the nerve agent to the AChE is not reversed through timely treatment, a process known as "aging" can occur. Aging is a biochemical process that results in a permanent binding of the nerve agent to the AChE and causes a situation that is refractory to all clinical intervention attempts. Once aging occurs, the AChE is rendered permanently useless, and the clinical effects of the resultant ACh overstimulation will remain until new AChE enzyme is produced. The aging time for CW nerve agents is relatively short:

- Soman (GD)—2 to 6 minutes
- GA (tabun)—14 hours
- GB (sarin)—5 hours
- VX—48 hours

The aging process is an important difference between organophosphate compounds (including nerve agents) and carbamate pesticides. Organophosphate pesticides function in a similar manner to the military nerve agents, and aging will occur at rates that vary depending on the specific pesticide used. In carbamate casualties, AChE aging does not ever completely occur and the agent's effects are almost always reversible.

Exposure to organophosphorus compounds results in clinical effects associated with the resultant uncontrolled stimulation of the smooth muscles, the skeletal muscles, the central nervous system, and the exocrine glands. Increased perspiration, lacrimation, increased salivation and drooling, miosis, skeletal muscular fasciculation, rhinorrhea, bronchorrhea, bronchoconstriction, and associated respiratory distress, nausea, vomiting, diarrhea, and altered level of consciousness are characteristic of poisoning with organophosphorus compounds. Patients exposed to higher doses of the substance will experience more significant CNS effects including loss of consciousness, seizures, and respiratory arrest.

Treatment for organophosphate compound poisoning revolves around whether or not aging has occurred. If aging has not occurred, the primary goals are airway maintenance and prevention of acetylcholine (ACh) receptor site overstimulation. Atropine competitively inhibits the effects of the uncontrolled ACh stimulation at the receptor site; it is very effective in reducing the muscarinic effects of organophosphate toxicity, but less effective on the nicotinic effects. Pralidoxime chloride (2-PamCl), an oxime, is effective in breaking the bond between the nerve agent and the AChE, effectively reactivating AChE , which can continue hydrolyzing ACh. Oxime therapy should be initiated within the first 48 hours following the exposure, and is not effective once aging has occurred. Benzodiazepines may be administered to control seizure activity, and may also be effective in reducing the long-term central nervous system effects that result from the hypoxic episodes that occur during seizure activity. The remainder of care is supportive.

If aging has occurred, oximes will be ineffective, and it will be necessary to maintain a therapeutic dose of atropine for a prolonged period of time, until new AChE is generated. The dose of atropine in these cases is based upon clinical presentation, and may be as high as 2.0 mg IV every 5 to 15 minutes. Extreme cases of exposure to organophosphorous compounds may result in the need for IV dosages as high as 5 mg every 10 minutes for the first 24 hours. Atropine infusions may need to be continued for several weeks, with doses ranging from 0.5–2.4 mg/kg/hr. The remainder of care is supportive.

©2007 Pearson Education, Inc.
Critical Care Paramedic

Pulmonary agents
p. 967

Pulmonary agents are commonly distributed as a vapor and may be lethal in relatively low concentrations as they are readily absorbed across the pulmonary tissue. Chlorine is considered to be immediately dangerous to life or health in concentrations as low as 1.0 parts per million (ppm). The degree of injury that a pulmonary agent casualty receives is based upon the concentration, solubility, and reactivity of the specific chemical involved. Chemical vapor reacts with the water present in the respiratory tract, causing direct damage to the affected structures.

Chlorine rapidly reacts with water to form both hypochlorous and hydrochloric acids, resulting in chemical burns to the airway. At low concentrations, most of the chlorine reaction will occur in the upper airways, resulting in damage to the nasopharynx, oropharynx, and trachea. At higher concentrations, damage will occur to both the upper and lower airways, with extensive damage to the structures of the central and peripheral airways, including the bronchi, bronchioles, and alveoli. Direct damage to the alveoli may cause an increase in pulmonary capillary permeability and the development of noncardiogenic pulmonary edema.

Phosgene causes sequelae to the alveolar-capillary membrane similar to chlorine, though the chemical reaction converting phosgene to hydrochloric acid is much slower, delaying the onset of airway and respiratory symptoms in comparison to those exposed to chlorine.

The treatment for both pulmonary agents centers around airway support, oxygenation, and ventilation. A SaO_2 of greater than 95 percent should be strived for, and endotracheal intubation and the application of PEEP might be required to achieve this. The use of diuretics is contraindicated, and the pulmonary edema accompanying pulmonary agent exposure is noncardiogenic in nature. Beta agonists such as albuterol, metaproterenol, and aerosolized terbutaline should be utilized to treat bronchospasm, and the administration of corticosteroids may help prevent short-term airway inflammation.

Cyanide
p. 967

Cyanide inactivates the cellular enzymes necessary for normal aerobic metabolism, resulting in a disruption of cellular respiration within the mitochondria despite the presence of adequate oxygen levels. In such a situation, cells can no longer produce ATP, and all biochemical processes depending upon ATP cease to function. The resulting anaerobic cellular respiration will produce severe lactic acidosis and cellular degradation. Widespread cellular degradation leads to tissue and organ failure, which will ultimately result in death.

The clinical signs and symptoms of cyanide poisoning can progress rapidly. The initial presentation includes tachypnea, hypertension, and tachycardia, which may progress quickly to seizures, respiratory arrest, and cardiac arrest.

Treatment of cyanide poisoning requires the ubiquitous cyanide antidote kit. 0.3 cc/kg of a 3 percent sodium nitrite solution is administered slow IV push (maximum 10cc), followed by 12.5g of sodium thiosulfate administered very slow IV push over ten minutes.

Sodium nitrite converts hemoglobin into methemoglobin, which cyanide has a strong affinity for. Methemoglobin irreversibly binds the cyanide to form a compound known as cyanmethemoglobin. The sodium thiosulfate reacts with the newly formed cyanmethemoglobin to form thiocyanate, which is then excreted by the kidneys. Additional treatment includes supportive care to ensure that the airway is patent and protected and that adequate oxygenation and ventilation is provided.

Vesicants
p. 968

Vesicants are agents that form blisters on the skin after contact and include the agents mustard and lewisite. They are relatively easy to synthesize and manufacture, and are a likely choice for groups who decide to develop a capacity for chemical weapons. Vesicants can be delivered by a variety of methods including liquid spray or aerosolization, and represent both a vapor and a liquid threat to all exposed skin and mucous membranes.

After exposure, mustard penetrates the skin and distributes to other tissues of the body. Within minutes, the mustard agent forms a highly reactive substance that binds to DNA, RNA, and proteins, causing cellular damage. Despite the speed of its damage, clinical effects are not typically observed for four to six hours, and can be delayed for as much as 48 hours.

At high doses, systemic mustard distribution can affect the kidneys, liver, lungs (significant damage to the airway epithelium), GI tract (severe vomiting and diarrhea), and bone marrow precursor cells (can lead to significant compromise of the immune system).

There is no specific treatment or antidote for mustard casualties; treatment is largely supportive and symptomatic. Eye damage is the most common injury. Effort should be made to maintain ophthalmic moisture, and ophthalmic antibiotics can help prevent infection. Skin damage caused by these agents will also leave these patients prone to secondary infection, necessitating the use of prophylactic antibiotics. Frequent flushing of the wounds and debridement of damaged skin is necessary during long-term treatment. In addition, IV fluid replacement and the administration of analgesics can be considered on an as-needed basis.

Lewisite exposure will result in many of the same clinical features as mustard exposure, though lewisite will cause immediate severe pain in exposed areas. In large doses, it can cause an increase in the permeability of systemic capillary beds, which may result in significant intravascular fluid loss and the development of hypovolemic shock. Lewisite has more prominent GI effects than mustard exposure and may lead to hepatic or renal necrosis. Unlike mustard, lewisite does not cause immunosuppression.

Treatment for lewisite toxicity is the antidote British Anti-Lewisite (Dimercaprol), also know as BAL. An IM injection of .04cc/kg (up to 4cc) of a 10 percent solution in oil may be repeated up to three times in four-hour intervals. The antidote is available in extremely limited quantities across the United States. Additional treatment is supportive and aimed at patient comfort and maintenance of normal hemodynamic status.

Signs and symptoms of phosgene oxime exposure will not differ greatly from those of mustard. Immediate pain on contact and spontaneous blanching of the skin is followed by the development of an erythematous ring within the first minute of exposure. Wheals form within the first hour of exposure, and associated extreme pain may persist for days. No specific antidotes are known, and treatment is supportive.

Incapacitating and irritant agents   p. 970

Incapacitating and irritant agents are commonly employed throughout society for both defensive and law enforcement purposes. Examples include tear gases such as chlorobenzylidenemalononitrile (CS) and chloroacetophenone (CN), and pepper spray (oleoresin capsicum [OC]). These agents produce transient local pain and involuntary eye closure and render an exposed patient temporarily incapable of normal activity. Signs and symptoms include immediate pain and burning sensation of exposed mucous membranes and skin and bronchospasm. Exacerbation of restrictive airway disease may occur. Treatment is supportive only.

5. **Describe the characteristics, clinical effects, and critical care interventions for the CDC Category A biological agents:**

   a. **Bacterial agents**

      i. **Anthrax**   p. 972

         Anthrax is caused by the bacterium *Bacillus anthracis*. Historically, this was transmitted by exposure to contaminated wool, hides, or tissues of infected cattle, sheep, or goats. There are three potential presentations of anthrax infection: cutaneous form, gastrointestinal form, or inhalational form.

         Cutaneous anthrax occurs when the bacteria breeches the skin barrier, and is characterized by sores or blisters that form at the site of inoculation, which is typically on the hands or forearms. Infection is often associated with fever and malaise and may progress to cause systemic septicemia. Standard infection controls and precautions are of paramount importance, as direct contact with the lesions may result in dermal contamination and subsequent secondary infection. The cutaneous form is typically successfully treated with antibiotics.

         Gastrointestinal anthrax, rare in humans, is typically caused by the ingestion of meat from an infected animal. The disease typically presents with nausea, vomiting, and fever, which may be followed by severe abdominal pain with hematemesis, ascites, and diarrhea. Patients may present with associated oropharyngeal lesions and sore throat, and systemic symptoms may include fever, chills, and malaise. Gastrointestinal anthrax is not considered

©2007 Pearson Education, Inc.
Critical Care Paramedic

to be transmissible from person to person, though the strict use of standard precautions is still recommended. Treatment includes supportive care, IV fluid replacement therapy, vasopressors, and IV antibiotics.

Inhalational anthrax is the result of the inhalation of anthrax spores. Eight thousand to 10,000 anthrax spores are typically required to cause a case of inhalational anthrax. The disease is uncommon, and standard precautions are recommended to prevent transmission. The clinical progression is initially characterized by malaise, fatigue, myalgia, and fever, followed by nonproductive cough and mild chest discomfort persisting for two or three days. There may be a prodromal phase before the patient experiences an acute onset of increasing respiratory distress with dyspnea, stridor, cyanosis, increased chest pain, and diaphoresis, sometimes associated with edema of the chest and neck. The disease can progress very rapidly, often resulting in the rapid onset of shock and death within 24 to 36 hours. Meningitis may be associated with up to 50 percent of the inhalational cases, causing an initial presentation of seizures. Treatment is supportive in nature with particular concern for airway control and assuring adequate oxygenation and ventilation, and IV antibiotic and corticosteroid administration are routine.

ii. Plague   p. 973
Plague is caused by the bacteria *Yersinia pestis*, and was the causative agent of the Black Death of fourteenth-century Europe. Plague is a naturally occurring disease, and is still endemic to certain portions of the United States to this day. In North America plague is found from the Pacific Coast eastward to the western Great Plains and from British Columbia and Alberta, Canada, southward to Mexico.

Forms of plague include bubonic and pulmonic. Bubonic plague (so-named because of the formation of "buboes") is typically transmitted to humans from the bite of infected fleas. It is characterized by the abrupt onset of high fever and headache, followed by the development of painful, swollen regional lymph nodes known as buboes. If untreated, bubonic plague can lead to bacteremia, and can eventually progress to full systemic septicemia. Septicemic plague is not considered transmissible, and patients with septicemic plague may also develop a secondary pneumonic plague, which *is* transmissible. Therefore, all patients with septicemic plague should be considered communicable.

Pneumonic plague is characterized by high fever, cough, chills, chest pain, and hemoptysis, and it appears clinically similar to a pneumonia or acute tuberculosis. Treatment is supportive in nature, with particular concern for airway control and assuring adequate oxygenation and ventilation. IV hydration should be considered in all patients with evidence of dehydration or hypotension; invasive hemodynamic monitoring can help in ascertaining fluid status. Antibiotic therapy with gentamicin, streptomycin, tetracyclines, chloramphenicol, or doxycycline is typical.

iii. Tularemia   p. 974
Tularemia is caused by the bacteria *Francisella tularensis*, is endemic to the majority of the northern hemisphere, and has been reported in every U.S. state except Hawaii. It exists in a wide variety of animal and arthropod hosts including ticks, rabbits, hares, mice, and squirrels. Tularemia is one of the most infective agents known, requiring as few as ten organisms to cause disease. It is not considered contagious, so isolation is unnecessary, though universal precautions are advised.

Tularemia presents in several different forms. Ulceroglandular tularemia occurs when bacteria are introduced through breaks in the skin or through the mucous membranes of the eye or mouth. It is characterized by the formation of a lesion at the site of exposure and the enlargement of associated regional lymph nodes.

Oculoglandular tularemia occurs when bacteria are introduced through the conjunctiva; the progression is similar to ulceroglandular tularemia. Pneumonic tularemia occurs when bacteria are contracted through the primary inoculation of the respiratory tract. This form typically presents in a manner similar to pneumonia; patients experience a dry or mildly productive cough, and less commonly will present with pleuritic chest pain, shortness of breath, or hemoptysis. Thyphoidal (septicemic) tularemia is a possible endpoint for all forms of tularemia infection. Regardless of the form, typical symptoms of infection with tularemia include: an abrupt onset of fever, chills, rigors, myalgia, cough, and headache.

Treatment is supportive, with airway control, oxygenation, IV hydration, and the administration of IV antibiotics being the cornerstone. Streptomycin is generally considered the antibiotic of choice, though ciprofloxacin, gentamicin, chloramphenicol, or tetracycline may also be used.

b. Viral agents

i. Smallpox   p. 975

Smallpox, caused by the *variola* virus, is a highly contagious disease spread primarily through direct contact with body fluids, including respiratory droplets. The disease has an incubation period of 7 to 17 days, and patients initially present with malaise, fever, rigors, vomiting, headache, and backache. Two to four days later, a discrete rash will begin to appear about the face and extremities and spread centrally to the trunk. Lesions found in higher concentrations on the extremities and face, termed centrifugal distribution, are an important diagnostic feature of the disease. There is also synchronous lesion development, in which all lesions appear in the same stage of development. Care providers should utilize contact and respiratory isolation practices, as patients are considered contagious until all scabs separate. Treatment for smallpox consists of supportive care, administration of viral agents such as cidofovir, and antibiotic therapy for secondary infections.

ii. Viral hemorrhagic fevers (VHFs)   p. 975

Viral and hemorrhagic fevers (VHFs) are a diverse group of illnesses caused by a multitude of different viruses. The incubation period varies depending on the specific infective agent and can range from days to months. Hemorrhagic fever viruses are highly contagious and spread through contact with body fluids, respiratory droplets, and contact with secondarily contaminated surfaces. Special caution must be exercised in handling sharps, needles, and other potential sources of parenteral exposure. Strict adherence to standard precautions is effective in preventing nosocomial transmission of most VHFs. All caregivers must wear gloves, gowns, and eye protection, and respiratory protection should consist of a mask or respiratory protection device capable of 100 percent HEPA filtration.

Specific diseases include Argentine hemorrhagic fever, Bolivian hemorrhagic fever, Venezuelan hemorrhagic fever, Lassa fever, Congo-Crimean hemorrhagic fever, Rift Valley fever, ebola, marburg, dengue, and yellow fever.

Initial presenting symptoms may include fatigue, fever, myalgia, and prostration. Physical examination may reveal conjunctival injection, periorbital edema, petechial rash, flushing, and mild hypotension. As the disease progresses, the patient may develop generalized mucous membrane hemorrhage, disseminated intravascular coapulation (DIC), shock, multiple organ system failure, or death. Signs of pulmonary, hematopoietic, and neurologic involvement may be appreciated.

Treatment consists of supportive care, fluid resuscitation, vasopressors, management of electrolyte imbalance, and administration of antivirals.

c. Toxins

i. Botulinum   p. 977

Botulinum toxin is produced by the bacteria *Clostridium botulinum*, and is considered the most toxic substance known; it is 15,000 times more toxic by weight than VX nerve agent and 100,000 times more toxic than Sarin. Transmission occurs via the ingestion of contaminated foods (toxin), wound infection, or by respiratory exposure. Botulinum toxin inhibits the release of acetylcholine from cholinergic nerves that control both autonomic and skeletal muscle function, causing cranial nerve and skeletal muscle paralysis. Symptoms usually begin 12 to 36 hours following intoxication, and can vary depending on the dose and route of exposure. Motor complications of botulism feature a descending bilateral paralysis that usually begins with cranial nerve palsies leading to blurred vision, diplopia, dysphonia, and dysphagia. Flaccid skeletal muscle paralysis follows in a symmetrical, descending, and progressive manner. Collapse of the upper airway may occur due to weakness of the oropharyngeal musculature, and respiratory failure may occur as the descending motor weakness involves the diaphragm and accessory muscles of respiration. Treatment is supportive care with attention to respiratory support, IV hydration, administration of Botulinum antitoxin, and IV antibiotics for secondary infections.

©2007 Pearson Education, Inc.
Critical Care Paramedic

6. Identify CDC Category B biological agents. p. 977

CDC Category B biological agents include Q fever, typhus fever, brucellosis, Glanders and Melioidosis, alphaviruses, ricin, and Staphylococcal enterotoxin B. Q fever is a rickettsial disease found in sheep, cattle, and goats. Humans acquire the disease by inhalation of contaminated particles. The disease is typically self-limiting and causes a febrile illness with headache, general malaise, and myalgia, and typically lasts two days to two weeks. Complications of the disease include pneumonia and endocarditis. Typhus fever is another rickettsial disease and is characterized by severe headaches, sustained high fever, generalized muscle aches, and skin rash.

Brucellosis is a bacterial disease acquired through broken skin while handling infected animals or through the ingestion of nonpasteurized dairy products. The acute form typically presents as an acute, nonspecific febrile illness with chills, sweats, headache, fatigue, myalgia, arthralgia, and anorexia.

Glanders and Melioidosis are bacterial diseases that cause similar human disease complexes and are highly communicable. Infection produces fever, rigors, sweating, myalgia, headache, and pleuritic chest pain. Glanders may present with generalized papular/pustular rash that may be mistaken for smallpox. Both are almost always fatal without treatment.

Alphaviruses (VEE, EEE, WEEa) include Venezuelan, Eastern, and Western Equine Encephalitis, and are transmitted by mosquitoes. They cause generalized malaise, spiking fever, severe headache, photophobia, and myalgias. Nausea, vomiting, cough, sore throat, and diarrhea are also associated with illness, and severe cases progress to encephalitis.

Ricin is a toxin generated as a by-product of castor bean processing. Ingestion can cause nausea, vomiting, abdominal cramps, severe diarrhea, and vascular collapse. Inhalation may cause more nonspecific symptoms such as weakness, fever, cough, and hypothermia, which are then followed by hypotension and cardiovascular collapse.

Staphylococcal enterotoxin B (SEB) is one of several exotoxins produced by Staphylococcus aureus, the causative agent in typical food poisoning. If inhaled, SEB may cause sudden onset of fever, chills, headache, myalgia, nonproductive cough, dyspnea, retrosternal chest pain, and pulmonary edema.

7. Describe ionizing radiation. p. 979

Types of ionizing radiation include alpha, beta, and gamma particles. Alpha particles are massive, charged particles that travel only a few inches in air. Intact skin and clothing provide adequate shielding from alpha particles. Beta particles are very small charged particles that can travel several feet in air. The energy released is able to penetrate the first few layers of intact skin, causing "beta burns," a condition very similar to a thermal burn. Both alpha and beta particles pose their most significant hazard if inhaled or ingested. Gamma rays are high-energy waves of ionizing radiation similar to X-rays. Highly penetrating, they can cause whole-body exposure. Shielding is accomplished through the use of lead or other very dense substances.

8. Identify the difference between internal and external contamination. p. 979

External contamination may result from direct contact with radioactive material. Internal contamination results from the inhalation, ingestion, or direct absorption of these materials through either the skin or open wounds.

9. Identify acute radiation syndrome. p. 980

Acute radiation syndrome (ARS) can develop following exposure to high doses of ionizing radiation. It presents as a sequence of phased symptoms. The specific onset and severity of symptoms will vary and are dependent upon the total radiation dose received. The prodromal phase may begin within hours of exposure and is characterized by nausea, vomiting, diarrhea, fatigue, weakness, fever, and headache. During the latent period, the patient is relatively symptom-free for a period of days to weeks. The latent period is followed by a manifest illness phase, which is characterized by numerous physiologic changes. Bone marrow function is often affected, causing decreased resistance to infection and anemia. Gastrointestinal system degradation occurs, causing diarrhea, hemorrhage, and severe fluid loss. Neurovascular changes are associated with very high radiation doses and result in a steadily deteriorating state of consciousness with eventual coma and death.

10. Describe the characteristics, clinical effects, and critical care interventions for patients suffering medical consequences related to radiation exposure. (p. 981); 11. Describe the management steps for radiation illness. (p. 982)

The clinical effects of raditation exposure vary depending on the dose, and are summarized in Table 33-2 from the text, Table 33-1 below.

Management of radiation illness is supportive, and the need for ventilatory support and IV fluid administration should be expected. In addition, the administration of antiemetics, antibiotics, and analgesics may be required. There are several pharmacological agents that promote the dilution or blocking of internal contaminants, including ferric ferrocyanide (Prussian blue), stable iodine compounds (potassium iodide), diethylenetriaminepentaacetic acid (DTPA), and calcium edetate (caEDTA).

12. Discuss the importance of explosives as a weapon of mass destruction (WMD) and detail the pathophysiologic processes associated with explosives use.   p. 983

Explosive devices are the most widely used WMD. An explosion occurs with the ignition of fuel that burns extremely rapidly; the resultant shock wave displaces hot gases outward. The blast

Table 33-1 Dose-Effect Relationships to Ionizing Radiation

Whole Body Exposure	
Dose (RAD)	Effect
5–25	Asymptomatic. Blood studies are normal.
50–75	Asymptomatic. Minor depressions of white blood cells and platelets in a few patients.
75–125	May produce anorexia, nausea, and vomiting, and fatigue in approximately 10 to 20 percent of patients within 2 days.
125–200	Possible nausea and vomiting. Diarrhea, anxiety, tachycardia. Fatal to less then 5 percent of patients.
200–600	Nausea and vomiting, diarrhea in the first several hours, weakness, fatigue. Fatal to approximately 50 percent of patients within 6 weeks without prompt medical attention.
600–1,000	Severe nausea and vomiting, diarrhea in the first several hours. Fatal to 100 percent of patients within 2 weeks without prompt medical attention.
1,000 or more	"Burning sensation" within minutes, nausea and vomiting within 10 minutes, confusion ataxia, and prostration within one hour, watery diarrhea within 1–2 hr. Fatal to 100 percent within short time without prompt medical attention.
Localized Exposure	
50	Asymptomatic.
500	Asymptomatic (usually). May have risk of altered function of exposed area.
2,500	Atrophy, vascular lesion, and altered pigmentation.
5,000	Chronic ulcer, risk of carcinogenesis.
50,000	Permanent destruction of exposed tissue.

wave typically moves out in concentric circles from the blast at a sonic speed. Structures or shielding devices can channel a shock wave in a specific direction. The greater the distance from the center of the explosion a person is situated, the lesser the injuries sustained as a result. The presence of barriers such as protective clothing, walls, or vehicles may offer some protection from the shock wave or blast. An absence of barriers or the presence of an explosive in a closed room or space results in an amplification of the shock wave and an increase in the number and severity of the injuries.

The initial phase of a blast is the actual detonation of the explosive material, and involves the sudden and violent release of energy in the form of rapidly moving molecules. The rapid expansion of hot gases causes a pressure wave to move outward in all directions; this initial movement of air from the epicenter is termed the "overpressure," and while it may be violent near the epicenter of the explosion it rapidly loses its strength as it travels outward. Overpressure results in a drastic but brief increase, and then decrease in the air pressure as it passes. The blast wind is a slower moving (less violent) wave of air traveling behind the pressure wave. It has less strength and a longer duration compared to the pressure wave, and may result in victims being propelled or showered with thrown debris such as the casing which held the explosive, building components, or nearby objects picked up and thrown by the blast. Personal displacement occurs when the pressure wave and blast wind physically propel the victim from his original location when the bomb detonates. Personal displacement causes the individual to become a projectile that can impact the ground or other nearby objects such as walls, trees, or vehicles, or strike other objects in flight.

The injuries sustained by the victims of an explosion can be classified into three types: primary blast injuries, secondary blast injuries, and tertiary blast injuries. Primary blast injuries are caused by the heat of the explosion and the overpressure wave, which typically result in burn injuries as well as damage to hollow organs of the body (tympanic membranes, lungs, GI tract, and so on). Secondary blast injuries are injuries that occur from projectiles striking the body, which may cause extensive blunt, penetrating, and burn injuries. Tertiary blast injuries result from the person being thrown away from the explosion and striking other objects, and may also occur in a structural collapse. Injuries sustained may be blunt, penetrating, or a mix.

Incendiary devices include napalm, thermite, magnesium, and white phosphorous. Agents of opportunity include gasoline, propane, and natural gas, all of which burn at an extremely high temperature and can result in severe burns.

13. Identify additional information resources.   p. 984

Additional information resources are:

- Centers for Disease Control and Prevention (CDC): http://www.cdc.gov
- World Health Organization (WHO): http://www.who.int
- U.S. Department of Homeland Security: www.dhs.gov
- Virtual Naval Hospital: http://www.vnh.org

Case Study

Your critical care ground transport team serves as the medical coverage for law enforcement incidents. You and a few of the other paramedics on your service have been trained as tactical medics and serve as members of the local special response team (SRT) during tactical insertions. Arriving on scene, you check in at the command post, while the rest of your crew waits with the ambulance at the secure staging area. Entering the command post, you're greeted by one of the other team medics, who fills you in on the details of the incident. A 911 call was received from a distraught woman reporting an assault by her husband. Responding units were greeted at the door by gunshots within and retreated to the cover of their vehicles. The address is known to the patrol officers for repeated domestic dispute complaints associated with alcohol, but there are no children in the household and in the past no weapons have been involved. Communication attempts with the inside of the residence and the suspect have been unsuccessful and the team is preparing to assault the building. You are told that you will be on the secondary team and will be staged just outside the hot zone. Donning your protective gear, you join the rest of the team behind the building next door to the suspect's building. Monitoring the radio traffic, you hear the assault team getting approval from command to use riot agents on the building. Shortly thereafter, you hear the dull thud of launchers and the breaking of glass as the tear gas grenades are propelled through widows on all sides of the structure. You can hear yelling and gagging inside the building and commands being shouted at the perpetrator by the assault team. You tense up as you wait expectantly for the sound of gunshots, which never come. There is a collective sigh as the radio announces "Building is secure, two in custody." As your team heads back to staging, the radio squawks again, "Command to team two, medic up, assist team one medic on A side of building!" As you acknowledge the command post, you are advised that the gas has dispersed, and that respiratory protection is no longer necessary. Your cover officer leads the way to the front of the building, where you see a medic with his gas mask pushed up on to the top of his head, crouching behind a car and moving quickly between a male and female lying next to each other on the ground. "What have you got?" you ask as you slide up next to your colleague. "Both got a good shot of CS gas. He's going to be fine, but I'm worried about her," he says, pointing to the female patient. A middle-aged woman is lying on her side, with her arms handcuffed behind her back and her head is being held off the ground by an officer. She is coughing incessantly, gagging intermittently and, as you get closer, you hear audible wheezes. A quick initial assessment shows that her airway is open and self-maintained, but there is a copious amount of clear mucus discharging from both nares. Her respiratory rate is approximately 44, with shallow, gasping breaths, and auscultation of her chest has equal air entry with coarse expiratory wheezes bilaterally. Her pulse is 128 and strong at the radial and she has no obvious signs of bleeding. You request that the manacles be switched to the arms-in-front position to help ease her breathing as you administer high-flow oxygen via a nonrebreather mask. With her hands now cuffed in front of her, the patient is assisted to a sitting position against the car. You put a hand on the patient's shoulder, look directly into her eyes and tell her in a commanding tone, "Just breathe deeply, slow your breathing down, you're going to be fine." Reassessing the patient, you note that although there are now less airway secretions and her respiratory rate has slowed slightly, she continues to cough and wheeze. You ask the patient, "Do you have asthma?" Your suspicions are confirmed as she nods her head in the affirmative. At your request, the cover officer advises command that a suspect will need emergency department treatment, and as you begin to administer a nebulized beta-agonist breathing treatment, you hear your ambulance being ordered to advance to the scene. After loading the patient in the ambulance, reassessment shows that her respiratory rate has slowed to 20 breaths per minute and she looks more comfortable. She continues to have expiratory wheezes, but is now able to speak in short sentences. Her pulse is 100 beats per minute and her blood pressure is 138/98. As your partner establishes an IV of normal saline, you administer a second breathing treatment. By the time you arrive at the closest emergency department ten minutes later, she is speaking in full sentences and complaining only of a mild tightness in her chest.

DISCUSSION QUESTIONS

1. Define CBRNE agents.
2. What are some general methods to ensure personal protection in situations involving weapons of mass destruction?
3. What are the characteristics, clinical effects, and critical care interventions for exposure to incapacitating and irritant agents?

Content Review

MULTIPLE CHOICE

_____ 1. The acronym CBRNE stands for:
- A. combustable, biological, radiological, nuclear, and explosive.
- B. chemical, biological, radiological, nuclear, and engineered.
- C. chemical, biological, radiological, nuclear, and explosive.
- D. chemical, biohazard, radiological, nuclear, and explosive.

_____ 2. _____ are common and unusual industrial agents and toxic chemicals that may be used as weapons and are readily available.
- A. Weaponized substances
- B. Potential hazards
- C. Weapons of opportunity
- D. Agents of opportunity

_____ 3. _____ is the emanation of chemical vapors trapped in a patient's clothing or on the patient's body.
- A. Fuming
- B. Fumigation
- C. Off-gasing
- D. Vaporization

_____ 4. There are relatively few chemicals that can be utilized as a chemical weapon.
- A. True
- B. False

_____ 5. Which of the following best describes how a nerve agent affects the human body?
- A. Nerve agents bind acetylcholinesterase receptors on the postsynaptic cell membrane, producing an accumulation of acetylcholine in the synapse.
- B. Nerve agents bind to and irreversibly inhibit the action of acetylcholine, producing an accumulation of acetylcholinesterase in the synapse.
- C. Nerve agents bind to acetylcholine receptors on the postsynaptic cell membrane, producing extended stimulation of the receptor sites.
- D. Nerve agents bind to and irreversibly inhibit the action of acetylcholinesterase, producing an accumulation of acetylcholine in the synapse.

_____ 6. Administration of which of the following is least likely to be part of the management of a patient with nerve agent toxicity?
- A. benzodiazepines
- B. atropine
- C. an oxime
- D. sodium thiosulfate

_____ 7. Nerve agents include all of the following except:
- A. soman.
- B. cyclosarin.
- C. cyanide.
- D. tabun.

_____ 8. _____ is a biochemical process that results in a permanent binding of the nerve agent to AChE.
- A. Aging
- B. Biotransformation
- C. Irreversible binding
- D. Permanent bonding

_____ 9. Which of the following statements regarding the treatment of cyanide toxicity is true?
- A. Continuous oxime administration may be required during transport.
- B. Intubation and mechanical ventilation may be necessary to correct metabolic acidosis.
- C. Continuous sodium nitrate infusion may be required during transport.
- D. An atropine infusion will be necessary in patients who have undergone the cyanide aging process.

_____ 10. Carbamate toxicity is unique among nerve agents in that AChE aging occurs incompletely and the effects of poisoning are almost always reversible.
  A. True
  B. False

_____ 11. A significant exposure to organophosphate compounds will result in:
  A. bronchospasm, noncardiogenic pulmonary edema, muscle tetany, and seizures.
  B. skeletal and smooth muscle flaccidity, respiratory failure, cardiopulmonary arrest.
  C. uncontrolled skeletal and smooth muscle, CNS, and exocrine gland stimulation.
  D. none of the above.

_____ 12. Sodium nitrate is administered in the treatment of cyanide poisoning in order to:
  A. convert hemoglobin into methemoglobin.
  B. convert methemoglobin into thiocyanate.
  C. convert theocyanate into methemoglobin.
  D. none of the above.

_____ 13. The clinical manifestations of exposure to a vesicant are immediately observable.
  A. True
  B. False

_____ 14. Which of the following therapies would be least effective if initiated after aging of a nerve agent has occurred?
  A. Administration of 100 percent oxygen   C. Administration of 2-PamCl
  B. Administration of atropine   D. Administration of an oxime

_____ 15. Which of the following best lists the likely treatment in the management of severe chlorine toxicity?
  A. airway control, oxygenation and ventilation, application of PEEP, judicious fluid administration, and administration of a diuretic
  B. airway control, oxygenation and ventilation, application of PEEP, and administration of beta 2-agonists
  C. airway control, oxygenation and ventilation, administration of atropine, and administration of an oxime
  D. airway control, oxygenation and ventilation, application of PEEP, and aggressive fluid administration

_____ 16. Treatment for exposure to oleoresin capsicum is least likely to include which of the following?
  A. administration of bronchodiltors
  B. flushing of exposed tissue with copious amounts of water
  C. administration of oxygen
  D. intubation and mechanical ventilation

_____ 17. Which of the following best describes the pathophysiology of a phosgene inhalation?
  A. Inhaled phosgene rapidly reacts with water to form hydrochloric acid, resulting in upper airway burs, necrosis, and inflammation.
  B. Inhaled phosgene easily crosses the alveolar-capillary membrane and enters the bloodstream, resulting in widespread dissemination of the toxin and eventual multi-system organ failure.
  C. Inhaled phosgene crosses the alveolar-capillary membrane, enters the bloodstream, and accumulates.
  D. Inhaled phosgene reacts slowly with water to form hydrochloric acid, resulting in lower airway burning, necrosis, and inflammation.

_____ 18. Which of the following correctly describes cyanides mechanism of action on the human body?
  A. Cyanide interferes with cellular utilization of ATP, resulting in anaerobic respiration and lactic acidosis.
  B. Cyanide interferes with cellular utilization of ATP, resulting in aerobic respiration and lactic acidosis.

©2007 Pearson Education, Inc.
Critical Care Paramedic

C. Cyanide disrupts normal mitochondrial function, interferes with normal cellular respiration, and decreases ATP production.

D. Cyanide reacts with water in the lungs to produce hydrochloric acid, disrupting the alveolar-capillary membrane and decreases gas exchange. Anaerobic respiration and lactic acidosis result.

_____ 19. Humans have physiologic mechanisms in place to metabolize and eliminate low levels of cyanide and survive low-concentration exposures.
A. True
B. False

_____ 20. Which of the following is an example of a vesicant?
A. chlorine
B. lewisite
C. chloroacetophenone
D. VX

_____ 21. In the management of cyanide poisoning, _____ is administered, which reacts with the cyanide metabolite cyanmethemoglobin to form _____, which is then excreted by the

_____.
A. sodium thiosulfate, cyanatehemoglobin, kidneys
B. sodium thiosulfate, thiocyanate, kidneys
C. sodium nitrate, thiocianate, GI tract
D. sodium nitrate, thiocyanethmoglobin, lungs

_____ 22. _____ are chemical agents that produce severe blistering of human and animal tissue upon contact.
A. Incapacitating agents
B. Irritating agents
C. Vesicants
D. Biological agents

_____ 23. Treatment for exposure to mustard gas is least likely to include which of the following?
A. administration of bronchodilators
B. topical and IV antibiotic administration
C. flushing and debridement of wounds
D. hemodialysis

_____ 24. Which of the following forms of anthrax is has the highest mortality?
A. inhalational
B. cutaneous
C. gastrointestinal
D. gastrourinary

_____ 25. Which of the following would be least likely to be included in the management of a patient with inhalational anthrax?
A. endotracheal intubation and mechanical ventilation
B. administration of vasopressors
C. administration of antiviral medications
D. IV hydration

_____ 26. Which of the following is not a characteristic of smallpox infection?
A. centrifugal distribution of lesions
B. synchronous development of lesions
C. patient complains of malaise, vomiting, backache, and headache
D. the appearance of a rash after healing of lesions has begun

_____ 27. Which of the following statements regarding botulinum poisoning is true?
A. A single organism is capable of causing disease in a human.
B. Botulinum poisoning is often associated with improper food preservation.
C. Botulism is caused by the virus _B. clostridium_.
D. None of the above.

_____ 28. Which of the following is a disease caused by infection with _Yersinia pestis_?
A. botulism
B. plague
C. Q fever
D. yellow fever

_____ 29. As septicemic plague is not transmissible, personal protective equipment other than gloves is unnecessary with a patient diagnosed as such.
A. True
B. False

_____ 30. Pneumonic plague is transmitted via:
A. the bite of an arthropod.
B. mammals such as squirrels or rats.
C. respiratory droplets.
D. contact with blood or body fluids.

_____ 31. Which of the following is a possible vector for tularemia?
A. ticks
B. squirrels
C. mice
D. all of the above

_____ 32. Which of the following diseases or agents are commonly treated with antibiotics?
A. smallpox
B. tularemia
C. lassa fever
D. ricin

_____ 33. For which of the following is there an antitoxin available?
A. botulinum toxin
B. Staphylococcal enterotoxin B
C. Brucellosis toxin
D. ricin toxin

_____ 34. Which of the following diseases would not respond to antibiotic therapy?
A. ebola
B. Glanders
C. Brucellosis
D. plague

_____ 35. Which of the following diseases initially presents petechial rash, flushing, and mild hypotension followed by mucous membrane hemorrhage, shock, multisystem organ failure (MSOF), and death?
A. plague
B. botulism
C. Marburg disease
D. melioidosis

_____ 36. Which of the following is relatively contraindicated during the management of a viral hemorrhagic fever?
A. administration of blood or blood products
B. administration of electrolytes
C. use of vasopressor agents
D. transport by aircraft

_____ 37. Transmission of a viral hemorrhagic fever can occur via:
A. respiratory droplets.
B. contact with body fluids.
C. contact with contaminated surfaces.
D. all of the above.

_____ 38. Characteristics of botulinum poisoning include which of the following?
A. septicemia, multi-system organ failure, severe hypotension, and death
B. initial descending bilateral paralysis followed by skeletal muscle paralysis and respiratory failure
C. cranial nerve palsy, slowed neuronal impulses, and coma
D. peripheral paralysis, progressing central paralysis, cranial nerve dysfunction, and death

_____ 39. Which of the following organisms is not considered a Category A biological agent by the CDC?
A. bacillus anthracis
B. ebola virus
C. variola major
D. rickettsia prowazekii

_____ 40. _____ are high-energy waves of ionizing radiation similar to X-rays.
A. Gamma rays
B. Beta particles
C. Alpha particles
D. Delta rays

_____ 41. Which of the following forms of ionizing radiation can travel several feet in air, are able to penetrate the first few layers of skin, and can cause injuries similar to thermal burns?
A. X-rays
B. beta particles
C. alpha particles
D. delta rays

_____ 42. What is said to have occurred when irradiation from a radioactive source has come into proximity with the body?
A. exposure
B. internal contamination
C. external contamination
D. radioactivity

_____ 43. Which phase of acute radiation syndrome is characterized by nausea, vomiting, diarrhea, fatigue, and fever?
A. prodromal phase
B. latent period
C. manifest illness phase
D. terminal phase

_____ 44. Management of radiation illness may include all of the following except:
A. administration of calcium edetate.
B. administration of antiemetics and antibiotics.
C. IV fluid replacement.
D. administration of ferric acid.

_____ 45. Which of the following types of blast injuries result from a patient being thrown away from an explosion and striking other objects?
A. primary blast injury
B. secondary blast injury
C. tertiary blast injury
D. blast wave injury

Organ Donation and Retrieval

Review of Chapter Objectives

Upon the completion of this chapter, the student should be able to:

1. Describe the indications for organ transplantation and the need for solid organ donors.   pp. 990, 991

Critical care paramedics (CCPs) may find themselves involved in organ procurement and transplantation process, and therefore must be familiar with the issues and procedures involved. Organ transplant is primary therapy for end-stage failure of the heart, lungs, liver, kidneys, pancreas, and small intestine. Only a small percentage of patients are suitable for transplant, and very few ever receive an organ. Since 1995, over 400,000 patients have been listed for transplant, and about 223,000 transplants have been performed; a lack of organs is the primary reason for this disparity. Out of about 10,500 to 13,800 suitable organ donors per year, only about 42 percent of these become organ donors. Organ procurement organizations (OPOs) work on improving organ donation consent rates and removing barriers to organ donation.

2. List the clinical indications to notify the organ procurement organization of a potential donor.   p. 991

The Centers for Medicare and Medical Services (CMS) requires OPOs and hospitals to establish mutually agreed-upon triggers for referral of potential organ donors. Generally agreed-upon triggers for referral to OPO include ventilator dependency, neurological devastation, and a GCS greater than 5. Criteria for organ donation can vary widely, and hospital staff are discouraged from making further clinical judgments about a potential donor's suitability. The OPO will immediately dispatch a staff member to the hospital for a review of the patient's medical record. The OPO staff works with the hospital staff to include brain death and organ donation assessment into the patient's plan of care. The critical need for organs has encouraged many transplant centers to expand criteria for organ donor suitability, and patients with a history of hepatitis, drug use, or chronic disease may be considered suitable organ donors.

3. Define neurologic death and identify signs that neurologic death may be impending.   p. 991

Neurologic death is defined as complete, irreversible cessation of all brain and brain stem activity. Critical findings in a brain death examination that suggest impending brain death include unexplained loss of consciousness, no motor response to painful stimuli, no brainstem reflexes, and apnea.

©2007 Pearson Education, Inc.
Critical Care Paramedic

479

4. Identify the hallmarks of neurologic death testing.   p. 991

An examination of a brain-dead patient should demonstrate the following:

- Coma
  - Lack of motor response to painful stimuli
- Absence of pupillary reflexes
  - Pupils should be dilated and unresponsive to light
- Absence of ocular movement
  - No eye movement occurs when the head is turned or when ice water is injected into the ear canal
- Absence of response to corneal stimulation
  - No blink or other response when a cotton swab touches the cornea
- Absence of pharyngeal/tracheal reflex
  - No gag reflex is noted when the posterior pharynx is stimulated, nor any cough reflex during bronchial suctioning

An apnea test is performed to verify the complete cessation of brain stem function. In this procedure, a patient is oxygenated with 100 percent FiO_2, and a baseline ABG demonstrating normocarbia ($pCO_2 > 40$ mmHg) is obtained. The ventilator is disconnected and oxygen administered at 6 lpm via nasal cannula placed into the endotracheal tube to the level of the carina. The patient is observed for respiratory effort. If respiratory effort is observed, the test is terminated and the patient is placed on a ventilator. If no respirations are witnessed over the course of several to eight minutes, an ABG sample is taken and the patient reconnected to the ventilator. A pCO_2 greater than 60 mmHg in the absence of respiratory effort is considered consistent with loss of brain stem function.

Additional tests can be performed in cases where a clinical exam is impossible or when patient condition prevents exam. Tests to confirm the absence of blood flow to the brain include four-vessel angiography, isotope angiography, and portable cerebral blood flow studies. Tests to confirm the absence of cortical brain activity include an electroencephalography and somatosensory evoked potentials.

5. Describe the systems in place for one to indicate one's wishes regarding donation prior to death.   p. 992

All states have a version of the Uniform Anatomical Gift Act (UAGA), which describes the process by which consent is granted for organ and tissue donation, including donation by donor designation on a donor document (referred to in some areas as "first-person consent"). Historically, OPOs have been hesitant to act on donor cards without consent from the donor's legal next-of-kin (LNOK). In recent years, though, many OPOs have begun to embrace the concept of first-person consent, and to date no OPO has suffered any legal action when acting in good faith on such a document. Many different states have established online registries of donors so that OPOs can establish first-person consent without the need for an actual donor card at the time of the patient's death. Some states allow anyone to register; others require that registrants be residents of the state itself. Although no formal information-sharing agreements exist among registries, OPOs will frequently check a state donor registry at the request of another OPO handling a potential donor from that state.

6. Discuss the process of obtaining consent from the patient's legal next-of-kin.   p. 992

Some OPOs employ staff members who are solely responsible for working with donor families. They are called organ procurement coordinators (OPC). The OPC will reiterate and reinforce physician reports of patient condition, help the family understand that the patient is dead, and help the family make decisions about organ donation.

Families who agree to donate sign an authorization form detailing what organs and tissues will be donated. Most authorization forms describe the testing that is performed, the fact that the OPO is responsible for the costs associated with donation, how organs and tissues are allocated (including any other organizations that may be involved in the recovery of the gifts), and that the donor family will receive information from the OPO regarding the specifics about the donated organs.

The OPC will also complete a medical, social, and behavioral history interview with the family or other appropriate historian. The interview is designed to identify donors who may be at high risk for hepatitis or HIV, as well as to identify underlying medical conditions that may affect the safety and quality of the organs and tissues. In some cases, the legal next-of-kin may not be the best historian, especially if he has been living apart from the donor for a prolonged period of time. In these cases, the OPC will attempt to locate a close friend of the donor who may be able to provide more complete information about the donor's recent history and behavior.

7. Describe the system for matching donated organs with recipients.   p. 993

The United Network for Organ Sharing (UNOS) oversees organ donation and transplantation in the United States; they are a contractor operating the organ procurement and transplantation network (OPTN) on behalf of federal government. All transplant candidates and recipients are listed and matched with matching criteria agreed upon by UNOS members, which include all transplant centers and OPOs in the United States.

Organs are matched by blood type, donor/recipient size match, and donor/recipient distance, although exact criteria varies by organ. When a donor is identified, the OPO lists donor demographic and clinical information into a UNOS computer and requests a match run for organs. The computer assigns a unique identifier to the donor and compares donor demographics against candidate demographics. Candidates are ranked according to a matching algorithm for each organ. The OPC then prints a list and contacts transplant centers in the order of the list. The center decides if the donor's clinical situation will provide a good outcome for recipient; the center may accept or decline the organ. If the center declines the organ, the next center on the list is contacted.

**8. Identify clinical management challenges encountered and the therapies
indicated when managing the organ donor.**   p. 994

Organ donors are almost by definition going to be critically ill, and must be carefully managed in order to optimize organ function for the recipient. Hypotension secondary to hypovolemia is the most common complication, and is best treated with IV fluid infusion of 0.45 percent saline, lactated ringers, albumin, or blood products; avoid the use of vasopressors.

Diabetes insipidus, secondary to loss of ADH with cerebral death, can complicate hypovolemia with increased urine output as high as 1500–2000 mL/hr. Vasopressin IV should be administered to maintain urine output of 7–10 cc/kg/hr. In hypertensive patients whom you will want to avoid using vasopressors with, desmopressin 1–2 mcg IV can be administered for the same effect.

Use of central venous or pulmonary artery catheter should be utilized to assure that CVP = 6–9 and PAWP = 8–11. Once the patient is adequately fluid resuscitated, vasopressors can be used to maintain MAP of 60 or greater. Commonly used vasopressors include dopamine, neo-synephrine, and vasopressin. Avoid the use of epihepherine and norepinephrine, as end-organ damage secondary to hypoperfusion is undesirable in patients who are donating them.

All brain-dead patients will receive mechanical ventilation to maximize end-organ oxygenation and minimize the risk of infection. Adequate pulmonary toilet should be ensured with frequent suctioning and turning of the patient.

Administration of broad-spectrum IV antibiotics is a common practice to prevent infection.

**9. List the testing and evaluations performed to assess viability
for each organ system.**   p. 995

- Heart
  - ECG
  - Echocardiogram
    - EF determination
      - EF < 40 percent = nontransplantable heart
    - Akinetic/dyskinetic wall motion abnormalities
    - Myocardial hypertrophy

- Incompetent valves
  - Coronary angiography
- Lungs
  - Assessment of pulmonary function
  - Chest radiograph
  - Bronchoscopy
  - Evaluation of respiratory secretion samples
  - Arterial blood gas
  - Oxygen challenge
- Liver
  - Liver function tests
  - Biopsy
- Pancreas
  - Pancreatic function tests
- Kidneys
  - Kidney function tests

10. Describe anesthesia requirements for the organ recovery procedure.   p. 996

No anesthesia is required for pain control during the organ recovery procedure, as there is no pain sensation experienced when the donor is brain dead.

11. Discuss the organ recovery procedure and organ preservation.   p. 996

In preparation for surgical recovery of organs, first there is dialogue between the OPC and operating room (OR) staff. The OPC explains the process to those OR staff unfamiliar with the procedure. The OPO provides the hospital with a list of required supplies, and the OPO generally supplies donor-specific items such as retractors, storage basins, and flush solutions. The hospital generally supplies standard surgical supplies such as gloves, gowns, drapes, and surgical equipment. All parties agree on OR staff needed for the procedure, and a review of the documentation of brain death, authorization for donation, and credentials of the surgical teams coming to recover the organs is done prior to the start of procurement. Organs are recovered in the OR. A preservation fluid is flushed into the organs using their arterial and venous vessels, and they are examined for gross abnormalities prior to being packaged for transport to the transplant center.

12. Identify tissues that can be donated and differences between tissue and organ donation.   p. 997

A variety of tissue can be donated from individuals who suffer cardiac arrest and have a suitable medical and social history. There are stricter criteria regarding disease for tissue donation; no disease is overlooked, and tissue is unsuitable if any possibility of disease transmission exists. Tissue donation is often life enhancing, not life saving. Tissues must be recovered within 24 hours of death if patient cooled, within 15 hours after death if patient not cooled.

Tissues harvested include the dura mater, whole eyes, cornea, mandible, skin, heart valves, bone, tendon, and veins.

Case Study

The beautiful little eight-year-old girl's picture was on the front of every local paper and you remember seeing it on the television news. The senselessness of the incident devastated the community and now, two days later, you sit in the OR waiting room recalling what you can about the accident and wait for the harvest team to finish their work. Eleanor and her father were walking home from the playground when a car driven by an intoxicated teenager jumped the curb and struck her, literally ripping her from her father's hand. Eleanor was rapidly evacuated to the regional trauma center with severe head trauma, and, although her vital signs stabilized, she was determined to be brain dead. Although the family was devastated, they consented to organ and tissue donation in the hope that something good would come of the tragedy. A coordinator from the organ procurement organization worked with the family and transplant teams from two different hospitals to obtain all useful organs and tissues. Her heart and liver were assessed as viable and removed to be transplanted immediately. Her eyes and long bones are being recovered for future tissue donations.

You're notified that the organ recovery teams are almost ready, and the driver of your rig and that of the second rig leave to bring the ambulances to the main hospital entrance. The heart team comes out of the OR carrying an insulated cooler and you secure it to the ambulance stretcher. You move quickly to the rig and ensure that the cooler and the team are well secured for the expeditious trip to the airport. On the way, you assist the leader of the procurement team with the notification of their communications center and alert their pilot as to your ETA to the airport. The team thanks you for your help and, as they are loading into their aircraft, you hear the ambulance transporting the second team calling en route to the airport. Before calling back in service, you locate that team's pilot and inform him of the team's ETA. As you call back in service, you reflect on how many lives this one little girl and her family have touched today.

DISCUSSION QUESTIONS

1. Define neurological death and identify signs that neurological death may be impending.
2. What is the procedure for organ recovery and preservation?
3. What is the main difference between tissue and organ donation and what tissues can typically be donated?

Content Review

MULTIPLE CHOICE

_____ 1. _____ are organizations that work on improving consent rates and removing barriers to organ donation.
   A. Organ procurement organizations
   B. Organ donor organizations
   C. Organ and tissue transplant organizations
   D. Organ donor procurement organizations

_____ 2. About _____ of persons suitable for organ donation actually donate organs each year.
   A. 30 percent   C. 54 percent
   B. 42 percent   D. 62 percent

_____ 3. Which of the following is not an organ commonly transplanted?
   A. liver   C. pancreas
   B. small intestine   D. spleen

_____ 4. A generally agreed-upon trigger for hospital referral to an OPO include all of the following except:
   A. ventilator dependency.   C. GCS < 5.
   B. neurological devastation. D. A, B, and C.

_____ 5. Neurologic death is defined as:
   A. a GCS of greater than 5 with neurologic injury.
   B. neurologic injury with apnea.
   C. complete, irreversible cessation of all brain and brain stem activity.
   D. neurologic injury with cessation of cerebral activity.

_____ 6. Critical findings in brain death examination include:
A. explained loss of consciousness, no motor response to painful stimuli, no brain stem reflexes, and apnea.
B. loss of consciousness secondary to brain trauma, loss of motor activity, apnea, and brain stem insult.
C. unconsciousness secondary to brain insult, loss of motor activity, and apnea
D. explained loss of consciousness, loss of reflexes, and apnea.

_____ 7. An exam positive for brain death should demonstrate all of the following *except* absence of:
A. ocular movement.
B. pharyngeal reflex.
C. papillary reflex.
D. Babinski reflex.

_____ 8. Which of the following findings in an apnea exam is considered consistent with loss of brainstem function?
A. a PaO_2 less than 90 mmHg in the absence of respiratory effort
B. a $PaCO_2$ greater than 60 mmHg in the absence of respiratory effort
C. a $PaCO_2$ greater than 30 mmHg
D. a PaO_2 less than 70 mmHg

_____ 9. The _____ is a state-specific legal act that describes the process by which consent is granted for organ and tissue donation.
A. Organ Donor Assurance Act (ODAA)
B. Tissue and Organ Gift Act (TOGA)
C. Uniform Anatomical Gift Act (UAGA)
D. Gift of Life Act (GLA)

_____ 10. First-person consent for organ or tissue donation can be established by:
A. a patient's legal next of kin.
B. carrying an organ donor card.
C. registering with a state donor registry.
D. all of the above.

_____ 11. A(n) _____ is often utilized by donor organizations to ease donor families through the organ and tissue donation process.
A. organ procurement coordinator
B. organ donor assistant
C. tissue and organ facilitator
D. none of the above

_____ 12. The _____ is the organizational contractor responsible for operation and oversight of the Organ Procurement and Transplantation Network (OPTN) on behalf of the U.S. Government.
A. Organ Sharing Network (OSN)
B. United Network for Organ Sharing (UNOS)
C. Organ Sharing and Transplant Service (OSTS)
D. United States Organ Network (USON)

_____ 13. Hypotension secondary to hypovolemia in a brain-dead organ donor should be managed with:
A. the administration of vasopressors.
B. the administration of IV fluids or blood products.
C. supportive care only; hypovolemia is desirable in brain-dead organ donor patients.
D. the administration of desmopressin.

_____ 14. Should vasopressors be utilized in brain-dead patients who will be donating their organs?
A. Yes, but only to maintain a MAP of 60 mmHg or greater after adequate fluid resuscitation.
B. No, organ donors should never be administered vasopressors.
C. Yes, but only after fluid resuscitation has failed to correct hypovolemic shock.
D. Yes, vasopressors can be used to maintain a MAP of 60 mmHg or greater.

_____ 15. Use of which of the following medications should be avoided with the brain-dead organ donor because of the possibility of decreased end-organ perfusion?
- A. dopamine
- B. vasopressin
- C. neosynephrine
- D. norepinephrine

_____ 16. Hemodynamic status in a brain-dead patient may be complicated by excessive water loss that occurs secondary to which of the following complications?
- A. the overadministration of diuretic medications
- B. increased GFR
- C. diabetes insipidus
- D. vasodilation

_____ 17. Which of the following medications would be the best to administer to a brain-dead patient with hypertension who requires a decrease in urine output?
- A. vasopressin
- B. epinephrine
- C. desmopressin
- D. dopamine

_____ 18. Urine output in a brain-dead organ donor should be maintained at:
- A. 5–15 mL/kg.hr.
- B. 7–10 mL/kg/hr.
- C. 8–12 mL/kg/hr.
- D. 15–20 mL/kg/hr.

_____ 19. To be considered suitable for transplant, a heart must have an ejection fraction greater than which of the following?
- A. 65 percent
- B. 55 percent
- C. 40 percent
- D. 30 percent

_____ 20. Which of the following is least likely to be administered by an anesthesiologist during an organ procurement surgery?
- A. anesthesia
- B. vasopressor agents
- C. fluids
- D. heparin

_____ 21. Which U.S. government organization regulates the transplantation of human tissue in the United States?
- A. Food and Drug Administration
- B. American Medical Association
- C. College of American Surgeons
- D. none of the above

_____ 22. Which of the following statements regarding tissue donation is true?
- A. Tissue donors can always be organ donors also.
- B. Tissue donation only requires death secondary to a cardiac event.
- C. Tissues must be transplanted immediately or the tissue will perish.
- D. Tissue retrieval can take place in an nonsterile environment such as the emergency department.

_____ 23. Tissues that can be transplanted include all of the following except:
- A. whole eyes.
- B. bone.
- C. skin.
- D. pia mater.

_____ 24. When initiating an on-scene death referral to an OPO, which of the following information should be obtained on scene by the paramedic?
- A. location of the deceased, brief medical history
- B. name, age, and sex of deceased, next-of-kin contact information
- C. mechanism of injury, name of next-of-kin
- D. all of the above

_____ 25. Which of the following statements regarding the management of the brain-dead organ donor patient is false?

    A. Lasix may be administered to correct developing pulmonary edema.

    B. Broad-spectrum IV antibiotics are often administered as prophylaxis against infection.

    C. Vasopression can be administered to patients experiencing brain-injury induced diabetes insipidus in order to maintain a urine output of 15 mL/kg/hr.

    D. All of the above.

Chapter 35

Quality Improvement in Critical Care Transport

Review of Chapter Objectives

Upon completion of this chapter, the student should be able to:

1. Describe why quality improvement processes and practices are essential for any EMS operation.   p. 1007

Simply put, quality improvement processes and practices are essential for any EMS operation to assure that the greatest efficiency and accuracy of patient care is delivered.

2. Describe the importance of ongoing monitoring of key performance indicators in EMS and critical care practice.   p. 1017

A successful QI program requires data so that informed decisions can be made about system performance, including clinical care and operational processes. Key performance indicators should be developed and monitored to detect any unusual variations in an organization's process.

3. Detail items and information that can be gleaned from environmental scanning.   p. 1007

Environmental scanning is the process of reviewing the clinical literature for information which might affect the protocols and clinical management of patients in the system. Examples of information that can be gleaned from environmental scanning include:

- The use of paralytics for intubation
- HEMS utilization
- Basic CPR technique
- The use of CPAP in respiratory compromise
- Fluids resuscitation in hypotensive trauma patients

4. List and define some of the key performance indicators in critical care transport medicine.

Some key performance indicators (KPIs) tracked in the critical care environment include:

- Was the treatment rendered required?
- Was the treatment rendered appropriate?
- Was appropriate care withheld?
- Was the patient's chief complaint documented?
- Were scene times recorded?
- Were at least two sets of vital signs recorded?

5. Describe the QCDSM model of information analysis. p. 1009

QCDSM stands for quality, cost, delivery, safety, and morale. Each component consists of a subset of KPIs that tell you how you are doing. Each one of the following indicators should be reviewed on a scheduled basis in order that management can determine where best to implement improvements.

Quality: can be described as a degree of excellence. Some examples of quality measurements for a critical care transport program are:
- Customer satisfaction
- IV or intubation success rates
- Medication or documentation errors

Cost: sustaining a critical care transport program requires managers to understand where the money is being spent. Some examples of cost measurements that may be helpful are:
- Fleet maintenance (tire wear, brake wear, fuel usage)
- Payroll (unscheduled overtime)
- Supplies (both disposable and durable medical supplies)

Delivery: usually refers to cycle times:
- Time from call received until critical care team arrival (response time)
- Time from arriving on scene to departure (bedside time)
- Time from arrival at destination to available (turnaround time)
- Miles between ambulance breakdowns (mission failures)

Safety: may describe incidents or accidents. May also be used as a subjective measurement to determine compliance with policies. Some examples of measurements of safety in critical care service:
- Days between injury
- Lost workdays due to injury
- Cost per injury
- Compliance with safety goggle use
- Compliance with ear protection use (for helicopters)

Morale: a measurement of the employee's well-being:
- Annual employee satisfaction surveys
- Attendance and tardiness

6. Discuss the advantages and disadvantages of various schemes for reporting data and trends including:

a. Flowcharts p. 1011

A flowchart is used to document a given process. The goal when creating your flowchart is to understand what the current process looks like, then find inefficiencies and remove them. A flowchart allows everyone to view the system and understand his role. A good method to try is to document how you think a process should work, then document how the process actually works presently. Most often, you will find redundancies and inefficient practices when you see the system in a simplified flowchart.

b. Cause-and-effect (fishbone) diagrams p. 1011

Cause-and-effect charts, otherwise known as Ishikawa or fishbone diagrams, are often used during brainstorming sessions when a group is trying to understand all of the variables that cause a problem. Some groupings that are common in the service industry are policies, procedures, equipment, and personnel, but you can use as many others as you need. Each bone can have as many "bones" as needed to document the variables.

c. Run (trend) charts p. 1011

Run, or trend, charts are perhaps the simplest of all the charts to understand. A run chart simply charts data points over a given period of time to see if there is any detectable trend. For example, one EMS agency found that there were not enough ambulances on duty during the midday hours. After creating a run chart they were able to determine their cycles of higher volume and staff accordingly.

d. Histograms p. 1012

A histogram is used to see how frequently something occurs. Perhaps your local mayor wants to know your response time to a specific area of town. A histogram is a good type of chart to use to display the information.

e. Scatter diagram p. 1012

A scatter diagram is used to show the relationship between two variables. Suppose your system's intubation success rate is not very good and you wonder if it is because of the experience level of your paramedics. A scatter diagram would be a good tool to determine that information.

f. Pareto charts p. 1013

In any given process you most likely want to investigate problems that keep occurring. A Pareto chart is a vertical bar–based chart that visually demonstrates which problem occurs most frequently. Understanding the true root cause of the problem will allow you to focus on the larger problem so you will have a greater potential for system improvement. The proven Pareto principle states that 20 percent of the sources cause 80 percent of the problem.

g. Control charts p. 1013

A process control chart is simply a graph that plots data points in a timeline. All process control charts have the same basic structure; they have a centerline (the mean), an upper control limit (UCL), and a lower control limit (LCL). A control chart is used to improve process performance by viewing it over a period of time and studying its variation. Control charts are very powerful and will show you whether a process is in statistical control or out of statistical control.

7. Discuss the traits of an effective leader. p. 1015

Leadership is not necessarily supervision. When identifying problems, leaders focus on the system as a whole and not on individuals. A leader recognizes that employees have strengths and weaknesses. A leader recognizes when an employee needs help, and facilitates that help. A leader excels at ensuring that all parts of the system work seamlessly. A leader removes obstacles that prevent employees from being proud of their work.

8. Contrast the difference between common cause and special cause variations. p. 1015

Common cause variation is fluctuation from the norm caused by unknown factors resulting in a steady but random distribution of output around the average of the data. Since the factors are unknown, it is difficult to correct common cause variation.

Common cause variation is a measure of the process's potential, or how well the process can perform when special cause variation is removed. Therefore, it is a measure of how the process normally works, without special circumstances. Common cause variation is the normal variation that occurs when many employees contribute small variations in performance that have little affect on the overall system performance.

Unlike common cause variation, special cause variation is caused by known factors that result in a nonrandom distribution of output. In other words, it is not caused by something that is normally part of the system. It may be caused by factors such as changes in environmental conditions, introduction of new procedures, or an increase in inexperienced employees. As such, a special cause variation in performance can be identified and corrected. Special cause variation is the normal variation that occurs when a few employees contribute large variations in performance that have a large effect on the overall system performance.

Case Study

The coffee had just finished brewing when Julia, one of the night shift paramedics, enters the room. "I smell it!" she exclaims, making straight for the coffee urn and drawing chuckles from everyone else in the room. Today, like every other Wednesday morning you, Julia, your assistant medical director, and two other paramedics formally meet as your service's quality improvement committee. During the first half of the meeting, all charts will be reviewed and, using a printed worksheet, certain data collected. The criteria for which data will be recorded at this meeting were determined at previous meetings and often vary, although some is continuously collected. The data collected on an ongoing basis includes such things as individual and service-wide success rates for procedures, response times, and customer satisfaction surveys. Any specific deviations from accepted standards of operation or medical practices are noted and discussed later in the meeting. These are then analyzed for possible causes and either the system is changed or service-wide training is initiated to alleviate the concerns. The specific deviation previously found is then re-evaluated to determine whether an appropriate change was accomplished or if further changes are necessary. Currently the committee is also collecting data relating to the use of a new rescue airway device protocol. A separate evaluation tool was created to assess the effectiveness of this recently updated guideline. Earlier studies had determined that the rescue device in use previously was too complicated to use successfully. The committee researched devices and, with medical director's input, selected and trained on a new device. That was three months ago and all indications are that the change has been a great success. You recall that the service you previously worked at had a quality improvement program that was punitive in nature and it's now very clear to you that your current service provides much higher quality service.

Discussion Questions

1. Why are quality improvement processes and practices essential to any critical care transport operation?
2. What is the importance of ongoing monitoring of key performance indicators in critical care transport?

Content Review

Multiple Choice

_____ 1. The concept of total quality management varies based upon the service or product provided.
   A. True
   B. False

_____ 2. All of the following are components of the Deming Cycle except:
   A. consumer research is performed and used to plan the product.
   B. assure the product was produced in accordance with the plan.
   C. develop a system of delivering the product.
   D. analyze the reception of the product by the consumers in terms of quality, cost, and other criteria.

_____ 3. The _____ is a statistic that tells you how tightly all the various examples are clustered around the mean in a set of data.
   A. flowchart   C. six sigma system
   B. standard deviation   D. confidence level

_____ 4. Which of the following quality plans would assure the fewest number of defective products?
   A. σ C. 4σ
   B. 2σ D. 6σ

_____ 5. Which of the following is not a component of the Six Sigma Road Map?
   A. Select a cross-functional team.
   B. Develop quantifiable goals.
   C. Develop an implementation plan that stresses disciplinary action for those employees not meeting standards.
   D. Coordinate the roadmap.

_____ 6. The goal of quality improvement in a critical care transport service is:
   A. to develop strategies that will increase the efficiency and accuracy of patient care.
   B. to assure that quality care and service are being provided.
   C. to identify employees who are performing at subpar levels.
   D. none of the above.

_____ 7. _____ is an operation that looks for changes in clinical literature that might affect the protocols and clinical management of patients in a system.
   A. Chart review   C. Morbidity and Mortality report
   B. Environmental scanning   D. Clinician feedback

_____ 8. Which of the following is least likely to be a key result area for a transport organization?
   A. employee satisfaction   C. financial performance
   B. clinical performance   D. individual performance

_____ 9. _____ is fluctuation from the norm caused by unknown factors resulting in a steady but random distribution of output around the average of the data.
   A. Special cause variation   C. Common cause variation
   B. Distribution   D. Environmental variation

_____ 10. A (An) _____ is an information and analysis model that assesses quality, cost, delivery, safety, and morale.
   A. QCDSM model   C. Pareto chart
   B. environmental scan   D. quality improvement plan

_____ 11. Which of the following is not a tool utilized to analyze data:
   A. scatter diagram   C. chart review
   B. histogram   D. cause-and-effect chart

_____ 12. A data analysis tool that helps employees view the system they work in and better understand their role is the:
   A. fishbone diagram.   C. Pareto chart.
   B. flowchart.   D. histogram.

_____ 13. _____ charts data points over a period of time to better visualize detectable trends.
   A. A cause-and-effect chart   C. A run chart
   B. A scatter diagram   D. None of the above

_____ 14. A _____ is used to show the relationship between two variables.
   A. control chart   C. histogram
   B. flowchart   D. scatter diagram

_____ 15. A _____ is a vertically oriented chart that demonstrates which problem is the most frequent.
   A. flowchart   C. control chart
   B. pie chart   D. Pareto chart

_____ **16.** Your critical care transport organization has purchased a new style of IV catheter that is very different from the style you had been using. As a result, you and many of your colleagues have been missing more IV attempts than usual, and the overall success rate for the organization falls from 96 percent to 72 percent in one month. This variation from the norm would be considered:

A. common cause variation.

B. special cause variation.

C. acceptable.

D. incidental variation.

36 Communications and Documentation

Review of Chapter Objectives

Upon completion of this chapter, the student should be able to:

1. **Understand the importance of verbal, written, and electronic communication to the success of any critical care mission.** p. 1031

   Communication and documentation for the critical care paramedic (CCP) is just as important as for those working as a prehospital care provider. The CCP will interact with a myriad of other professionals, including other health care providers (crew members, hospital staff, physicians), laypersons (patient and/or patient's family), and other emergency service providers (law enforcement, fire department, hospital security personnel, and possibly air traffic controllers). Whether written or verbal, the communication that occurs must be concise, timely, objective, and interpretable.

   Your patient care report is the sole document that commits to record what occurred during transport. As such, it must be factual, comprehensive, well written, and appropriately completed. The old prehospital adage "If it wasn't written, it wasn't done" certainly carries over to the critical care transport environment.

   To summarize, effective communication and documentation optimize patient care and transport, provide the needed information to ensure quality care progresses at the receiving facility, and allow the transport service to know that patient care decisions and interventions meet the expected standard of care.

2. **Identify current technology used to collect and exchange information in the critical care environment.** p. 1036

   Equipment used to collect and exchange information in the critical care environment includes, but is not limited to: telephones, radios, logging recorders, computers, cameras, radar, mapping systems, and facsimile machines.

3. **Explain the responsibility of the FCC in the licensing and use of communication equipment and radio frequencies.** p. 1037

   Radio frequencies utilized by the critical care organization are assigned by the Federal Communications Commission (FCC) in conjunction with the state's chapter of Associated Public Safety Communications Officers. The FCC is an independent U.S. government agency, directly responsible to Congress. The FCC was established by the Communications Act of 1934 and is charged with regulating interstate and international communications by radio, television, wire, satellite, and cable. The FCC also issues frequency licenses and assigns call letters to be utilized on one of several radio bands. The FCC sets aside several UHF frequency ranges for the exclusive use of EMS.

4. **Understand dispatch center considerations and the dynamics of verbal communication as they pertain to the:**

   a. **Communications specialist**   **p. 1032**

   The communications specialist is an individual who answers the phone and/or dispatches missions out to the critical care transport units; they are commonly referred to informally as "dispatchers."

   b. **Aeromedical pilot**   **p. 1039**

   The aircraft (aeromedical) pilot regularly communicates with the communications center, the air medical crew, air traffic control, and the emergency medical services on the ground. After confirmation of acceptance of flight, pilot, crew, and dispatch prepare for the mission. The communications specialist relays the destination heading and coordinates to the pilot and crew. The onboard autopilot and GPS unit are programmed with the flight information. Prior to liftoff, the pilot will typically communicate with crew via the internal headset communications of the aircraft to assure all personnel and equipment are prepared for liftoff.

   After liftoff, the communications specialist is notified and given the direction of travel. The aircraft's departure location and general heading announced over "ship to air" frequency, which alerts any aircraft in vicinity of the air medical aircraft's presence and route of travel. The pilot then contacts the local air traffic control to advise them of the travel plan. During flight, latitude and longitude coordinates given to dispatch every ten minutes.

   Air traffic controllers are responsible for the safe and efficient flow of air traffic throughout the nation's airspace. Monitoring and communication of the flight is passed from tower controllers to an En Route Center when the aircraft leaves a specific airspace. En Route controllers regulate flights between airports and contact the pilot by radio and control the pilot's position in the airways between tower jurisdictions. They maintain a progressive check on aircraft and issue instructions, clearance, and advice to the pilot.

   A "lifeguard status" declaration to the air traffic controller identifies that the aircraft's mission is one of patient care, which generally gives priority status for your flight plans over all other flights. A phonetic alphabet and numeric system, created by the International Civil Aviation Organization (ICAO), is used by air traffic controllers and aircraft pilots for consistency and accuracy in radio communications.

   The pilot will also communicate with the on-scene emergency service agencies landing zone (LZ) coordinator. Communication typically takes place directly between the pilot and LZ coordinator via a predetermined radio frequency, though coordinates may also be passed through the communications center or a flight crew member.

   c. **Critical care team members**   **p. 1041**

   The critical care paramedic should be efficient with using the onboard radio systems employed by the flight program, and should also be familiar with the methods of programming all radios on the aircraft. The critical care team should also be familiar with the phases of the transport in which the pilot will communicate with the traffic control tower so as not to unnecessarily distract the pilot during these times. Specific situations include after lifting off when the pilot advises the tower of the direction of travel and altitude, when the aircraft is passing from one tower airspace into another, and when landing at the airport following a mission (returning to base) or for refueling. The pilot can isolate his communication procedures from the crew with a flip of a switch. Crew members are not responsible for communicating with air traffic controllers.

   Crew members should also be intimately familiar with the flight program's requirements about when to contact the dispatch center during the various phases of a mission. This allows the communications specialist to time-stamp these phases of the mission to ensure accurate documentation. Times that the communications center should be contacted during a mission include:

   - When the mission is accepted by the pilot
   - When the aircraft lifts off
   - Every ten minutes or so during flight (to give coordinates)
   - Upon final descent for landing
   - Upon aircraft landing
   - At patient contact (on scene or in hospital)
   - When lifting off with the patient loaded

©2007 Pearson Education, Inc.
Critical Care Paramedic

- During final descent at destination
- Upon landing at final destination
- When patient transfer of care has occurred and the aircraft is back in service
    Other times when the dispatch center should be contacted include:
- When the aircraft is in need of refueling
- If a warning light illuminates or a sensor alarms
- If the aircraft suddenly encounters significant weather turbulence
- If the mission needs to be abandoned due to inclement weather conditions
- When the flight heading is changed by the air traffic control tower
- When unable to land at a designated LZ or hospital helipad
- Any other unique or uncharacteristic incidence during a flight

Crew members will interface with a much wider array of health care providers than is probable when working as prehospital providers. The critical care team will find themselves in many hospital departments that routinely a prehospital provider will not commonly access. Communication with other health care providers should incorporate appropriate medical terminology so that clarity in the message is maintained. Because of the specialization of departments within a hospital, the staff may have a specific way of assessing and treating the patient; this may translate into the department's unfamiliarity with procedures that the flight crew considers routine.

d. Sending and receiving health care facilities   **p. 1043**

Sending facilities will often arrange for transport by contacting the communications center. At this time, basic patient information, patient and facility location, receiving facility, and any additional required information will be exchanged. It is not uncommon for a medical crew member to call the sending facility prior to liftoff or while en route to get a more formal patient report to anticipate any special needs. Examples of specific information medical crew members might be interested in include:

- MOI / NOI
- Current vitals
- Specific airway, breathing, and circulatory parameters
- Significant medical history, allergies, and medications
- Current therapies (medications, IV fluids)
- Important physiologic or hemodynamic findings relative to the medical/traumatic condition the patient is experiencing
- Any unusual or uncommon medical technology being used on the patient (IABP, VAD, and so on)

The critical care team should call ahead to the receiving facility either prior to departure or while en route to provide a patient update and allow the receiving facility time to make preparations to receive the patient. The following information should be ready prior to establishing phone or radio contact with the facility:

- Age, gender, ethnicity
- Chief complaint, purpose of transport
- Significant medical history and history of the chief complaint
- Current mental status
- Airway and breathing status
- Invasive / noninvasive assessment of hemodynamics
- Care being provided currently (meds, fluids, vent settings, and so on)
- Patient response to current therapy
- Confirmation of medical records/documentation
- Estimated arrival at the emergency department
- Requests for additional personnel or equipment upon arrival

The final component of the communication needs of the critical care paramedic would include oral transmission of patient information. The staff at the receiving facility will expect an oral report, and organizing the patient data prior to communicating it will enhance this verbal exchange of information. A suggested method of organization is as follows:

- Age, gender
- Primary medical / traumatic condition

- Significant physical findings
  - Head
  - Neck
  - Thorax
  - Abdomen
  - Pelvis
  - Extremities
- Last set of vitals
- Current interventions
- Response to therapy
- Significant treatment limitations

Always end this verbal exchange of information with the following question: "Is there anything else you need or are there questions I can answer?"

5. **Identify and differentiate between the following communication system components:**

a. **Simplex**   **p. 1037**

A simplex system can only send and receive on the same frequency, it cannot simultaneously transmit in both directions.

b. **Half-duplex and full duplex**   **p. 1037**

A half-duplex system uses two different frequencies for transmitting and receiving, and typically uses UHF high bands. Its hardware only allows for one direction of communication flow at a time.

A full duplex can transmit and receive simultaneously by employing one frequency for transmitting and a different one for receiving, usually using UHF bands. They also allow the transmission of voice or data.

c. **Multiplex**   **p. 1037**

Multiplex systems provide the capability of transmitting data and voice simultaneously, and allow ongoing conversation between individuals while sending data information concurrently.

d. **Trunking systems**   **p. 1037**

A trunking system uses a computer to pool all available frequencies and assign an arriving transmission to an open frequency. When transmission ends, the frequency is added back into the pool of available frequencies.

e. **Digital systems**   **p. 1037**

Digital systems translate voice (analog) into digital code for broadcast, and are much faster and accurate than other systems. They are not detectable by scanners, and therefore allow transmitted data to remain secure.

f. **Logging recorders**   **p. 1038**

Emergency agencies routinely utilize some type of recording technology for archiving incoming and outgoing transmissions, with the dictaphone being an often-utilized method. The Dictaphone is a reel-to-reel recorder that records all activity for up to 24 hours on a single reel. Full reels can then either be stored or reused after a given number of days. A short-term option is a "callbox," which records about four hours of information and is useful for immediate retrieval of information.

g. **Computer terminals**   **p. 1038**

Common software applications as well as computer aided dispatch (CAD) software are capable of integrating patient information, map directions, latitude and longitude, trip times, and paging into one seamless program.

h. **Camera monitors**   **p. 1038**

Allows the communications specialist to have visual contact with the crew during downtimes, loading, liftoff, or landing procedures.

i. **Weather radar**   **p. 1038**

Weather radar is available for the pilot to consult prior to the acceptance of any aeromedical mission, and allows the communications specialist the ability to monitor the meteorological conditions that the aircraft may be flying into or away from. Radar is especially beneficial for programs that do not have aircraft equipped with weather radar.

j. Mapping systems
p. 1039

Mapping systems can be as elaborate as a large flat screen monitor that shows the terrain covered by each unit or as simple as a large geographical map with the radius of each base drawn on it. These systems allow the communications specialist to quickly determine the headings for any aeromedical mission that originates in the base's service area. Street maps should also be available that show the street index of locales in that service area.

k. Facsimile
p. 1039

Fax machines allow for rapid transmission of printed material across phone lines.

6. Properly use the phonetic alphabet and numbering system for verbal communication.

The single most important thought in pilot–controller communications is mutual understanding. To help achieve this, pilots and air traffic controllers use a unified vocabulary for certain words or numbers. The International Civil Aviation Organization (ICAO) has created a phonetic alphabet and numeric system to be used by air traffic controllers and aircraft pilots for consistency and accuracy in radio communications (Table 36-1). All air crew members should be familiar with the use of this system.

7. Discuss additional documentation needs and strategies as they pertain to the critical care paramedic.
p. 1047

The documentation of every mission and every patient contact is expected, and the documentation needs of the critical care paramedic mirrors the documentation procedures seen in the prehospital environment, with a few exceptions.

One component in the completion of a patient care report (PCR) by the critical care paramedic is the documentation of information that is not normally collected in the prehospital environment. This includes the documentation of electrolytes, certain laboratory values, and often ventilator settings. This documentation is usually performed in a conventional manner that the critical care paramedic should be familiar with. One such method for documenting patient variables uses a

Table 36-1 Phonetic Alphabet for Use in Aircraft Communications

Letters:	
Alpha	November
Bravo	Oscar
Charlie	Papa
Delta	Quebec
Echo	Romeo
Foxtrot	Sierra
Golf	Tango
Hotel	Uniform
India	Victor
Juliet	Whiskey
Kilo	Xray
Lima	Yankee
Mike	Zulu

Numbers:			
0	Zero	6	Six
1	Wun	7	Seven
2	Too	8	Ait
3	Tree	9	Niner
4	Fower		(decimal) Point
5	Fife		

fishbone diagram. This diagram allows the rapid documentation of the following variables: sodium, chloride, blood urea nitrogen (BUN), glucose, creatinine, bicarbonate, and potassium. The "fishbone" is completed as follows:

$$\frac{Na^+ \mid Cl^-}{K^+ \mid HCO_3^-} < \begin{array}{l} BUN \\ Glucose \\ Creatinine \end{array}$$

Other electrolytes may be documented as well (calcium, magnesium, phosphate, and so on) in the appropriate space on the report. Other values, however, are documented in a specific fashion and include the following: the white blood cell count, hemoglobin level, hematocrit, and platelet level. The format utilized is as follows:

$$WBC > \frac{Hgb}{Hct} < Platelets$$

8. Identify and properly use medical terminology, medical abbreviations, and acronyms.

The CCP should become familiar with the common medical terminology, abbreviations, and acronyms used in the critical care arena. The use of medical terms transforms your patient report into a universally accepted medical document, and verbal command of the spoken language ensures that you can communicate effectively with other health care providers. Ensure that your spelling and use of medical terms is accurate.

9. Describe the desired characteristics of a properly completed patient care report.   p. 1045

Good documentation includes the following characteristics:

- Appropriate medical terminology used throughout
  - Use of medical terms transforms your report into a universally accepted medical document
  - Ensure your spelling and use of medical terms is accurate
- Medical abbreviations and acronyms used when appropriate
  - Allows for an increase in the amount of information present on the PCR
  - Only use abbreviations or acronyms that have a specific, widely accepted meaning
- Only objective language is used
- Events are recorded in military time
- The PCR is completed in its entirety
- The information recorded is accurate and legible
- The PCR is submitted in a timely fashion
- The PCR must be devoid of mistakes, and it should be submitted as complete and not needing additional addendums or alterations
- The PCR should have all appropriate diagnostic and imaging exam results and treatments recorded

10. Describe at least one effective system for providing thorough documentation on a patient care report.   p. 1048

It has been alluded to numerous times that PCRs take a multitude of forms. The first and most traditional is the narrative report. With a narrative report, the call is described at length and there is less structure with this type of written documentation because of the absence of check boxes. The narrative format provides the critical care team with the freedom to describe the mission events and a patient's condition as they deem necessary. The narrative reporting style is favored by many practitioners because of the freedom in documentation; this freedom, though, comes with a trade-off of time. This type of report typically takes a great deal longer to complete, and is more prone to missing information.

    Patient care reports can also be prepared with a series of check-off boxes or fill-in-the-bubble spaces, also called "bubble sheets," to denote the patient's care. The great advantage of this type of format is that it consumes very little time, and often the PCR can be scanned into an organization's computer system to allow the generation of research data. This mode of documentation fails in that it is less specific in nature. The use of bubble sheets inherently reduces the depth and breadth of information gathered.

The final type of PCR is the style that uses technology to its advantage. The availability of electronic clipboards for documenting allows a PCR to be designed to meet an organization's specific needs. It could be a combination of fill-in boxes and narrative sections that can be uploaded immediately to the organization's mainframe computer system by way of a wireless link. The use of PDA (personal digital assistant) technology is also gaining favor in EMS and critical care realms due to the size, cost effectiveness, and availability of software programs. Also gaining increased popularity is specific computer software used for generating patient care reports. Like electronic clipboards and PDAs, the availability of software programs that can be modified to meet program needs makes this option extremely attractive. Many times this software can also be dovetailed into the agency's mainframe computer system so that the information entered by the critical care paramedic can also be used for quality assurance, administrative, and billing purposes automatically.

11. Describe the potential complications of illegible, incomplete, or inaccurate documentation in the critical care transport realm. p. 1048

Inappropriate documentation carries with it both medical and legal consequences. Of these two, the medical consequences are naturally most severe since care decisions may be made based on your submitted patient care report, and if there are errors or omissions, the consequences can be poor subsequent patient care. From a legal standpoint, there are significant ramifications of poor documentation as well. In a court of law, what you document is many times what is debated, not what you actually did. Even though your patient care may have been exemplary on a particular mission, if the documentation does not bear this out, you may be found libel or negligent for the damages the plaintiff is claiming. Additionally, poor documentation practices will lead your program's administration, quality assurance committees, and billing departments to become more aware of your practices. These aforementioned intraorganizational departments rely heavily on the quality of the documentation provided by the critical care teams and progressive correctional action (up to and including dismissal) may be taken against the critical care provider who continually fails to document appropriately.

Case Study

Your text pager vibrates against your hip, alerting you to your next call. Walking to the nearest house telephone, you dial the number to your communications center. As the communications specialist finishes giving you the details of the transfer, she informs you that your pilot has also been advised and will meet you on the helipad. Arriving at the roof top office, you note the pilot sitting at the weather computer terminal. "How does it look, Jim?" you ask him as you walk to the fax machine on the other side of the room. "It looks like clear sailing," he says, adding, "there was a band of T-storms over the area earlier, but they have pushed a long way east now and there should be no problems." The fax machine has finished spitting out copies and a quick review of the paperwork shows that the transfer is for a stable trauma patient located in a small rural emergency department who will be coming back to your base hospital. While waiting for the pilot and your partner to finish a final preflight check on the aircraft, you pick up the phone and call the sending facility for an updated report and to confirm landing zone information. You are told that the patient has an unstable C-spine fracture following a rollover MVA, but has no neurological deficits and otherwise is completely stable. You are also informed that the LZ will be the small, paved heli-spot next to the ED entrance and that the local volunteer fire department will be on scene to serve as LZ coordinator. Confirming that the radio frequencies for the fire department and hospital remain the same, you advise the facility that your estimated time of arrival (ETA) will be 30 minutes. Climbing into the helicopter, you update your partner and the pilot and within three minutes the aircraft is airborne. Contacting the fire department on their frequency approximately five minutes out from the LZ, you are advised that there are no hazards to landing and after one reconnaissance orbit the pilot takes the aircraft straight in for an uneventful landing. While you receive a full report and ensure that the transfer paperwork is in order, your partner assesses the patient and packages him for transport. Before moving the patient to the aircraft, you phone your communications center and give them an update. As you do not require medical direction, you ask the communications specialist to update your emergency department on the condition of the patient and your ETA. After the patient is gently loaded in to the helicopter, you are quickly airborne and en route to the receiving hospital. After an uneventful flight, you use the simplex radio to advise the emergency department of your impending arrival in approximately five minutes. With the aircraft shut down on the rooftop helipad, the patient is gently transferred to a waiting emergency department stretcher, and you and your partner accompany the patient to the emergency department. While you assist the ED staff in assessing the patient, your partner finishes writing and files the patient care report (PCR).

DISCUSSION QUESTIONS

1. What communication devices may be used before, during, and after critical care transports?
2. What are the potential complications of illegible, incomplete, or inaccurate documentation in the critical care realm?

Content Review

MULTIPLE CHOICE

_____ 1. The _____ is an individual who answers the phone and dispatches missions to the critical care transport units.
   A. communications specialist
   B. communications center
   C. dispatcher
   D. A and C

_____ 2. Of the following, the most ideal location for a transport agency's communications center would be:
   A. in the same building as the marketing, billing, and administrative offices.
   B. in an offsite location independent of all other organization operations.
   C. in the same building as the transport aircraft or vehicles.
   D. at an offshore location in India.

_____ 3. Desirable characteristics for communications center personnel include:
   A. critical thinking skills.
   B. computer skills.
   C. even temperament.
   D. all of the above.

_____ 4. Which of the following is not a task routinely assigned to a communications specialist?
   A. monitoring video cameras that may be installed in ground unit garages or helipads
   B. pre-shift checks on transport vehicles and aircraft
   C. helping to coordinate the flow of patient care information for internal uses such as quality assurance, billing, or administration
   D. answering phone calls and routing them internally as needed

_____ 5. Which of the following describes a desirable attribute that every dispatch center should have?
   A. separate heating and cooling controls from the rest of the building
   B. soft but sufficient lighting
   C. an emergency backup power supply
   D. all of the above

_____ 6. Radio frequencies used by emergency services are assigned by the:
   A. FCC
   B. ECC
   C. VHF
   D. SEC

_____ 7. The radio band located between 30 to 50 MHz is:
   A. VHF high-band.   C. VHF AM.
   B. VHF low-band.   D. UHF.

_____ 8. Which of the following radio systems uses two different frequencies for transmitting and receiving, but only allows for one direction of communication flow at a time?
   A. half-duplex system   C. simplex system
   B. multiplex system   D. trunking system

_____ 9. Which of the following radio systems uses a computer to pool all available frequencies, assigning frequencies as the need arises?
   A. digital system   C. trunking system
   B. full duplex system   D. multiplex system

_____ 10. Which of the following radio systems allows for the transmission of data?
   A. full duplex system   C. digital system
   B. multiplex system   D. all of the above

_____ 11. A _____ is a short-term data-recording device used by communications specialists for immediate retrieval of information from a recent phone call.
   A. callbox   C. tape recorder
   B. dictaphone   D. call back

_____ 12. A _____ can be utilized to allow any person in the dispatch area to quickly review the status and location of each ground and airborne unit at any time.
   A. radar   C. tracking board
   B. mapping system   D. all of the above

_____ 13. Which members of the critical care transport team are required to be "rated" for particular aircraft utilized by the organization?
   A. medical crew members   C. aircraft mechanics
   B. pilots   D. all of the above

_____ 14. Which of the following should not have any part in a pilot's decision to accept a mission?
   A. weather   C. patient information
   B. total flying distance of mission   D. time of day

_____ 15. Information that is typically communicated between the aircraft pilot and the communications center includes all of the following except:
   A. weather status.   C. landing time.
   B. aircraft location.   D. patient information.

_____ 16. The practice of "flight tracking" involves which of the following?
   A. monitoring an aircraft's location by local air traffic control personnel
   B. the pilot, or some other crew member, relaying aircraft location coordinates to the communications center every ten minutes.
   C. being aware of other aircraft located in the immediate area
   D. none of the above

_____ 17. Which of the following is a typical task performed by the aircraft pilot prior to landing at an emergency scene?
   A. She will perform an "orbit" of the landing zone.
   B. The pilot will communicate with a LZ coordinator via an agreed-upon radio frequency.
   C. The pilot will attempt to identify any potential hazards that surround the landing zone.
   D. All of the above.

_____ 18. Which of the following is a correct representation of a letter pronounced using the phonetic alphabet used in aircraft communications?
A. pizza
B. whiskey
C. indian
D. quiz

_____ 19. Air medical crew members are often responsible for communicating with air traffic controllers.
A. True
B. False

_____ 20. Points in a mission where the communications center should be contacted include all of the following except:
A. on aircraft landing.
B. during final descent at destination.
C. at patient contact (on scene or in hospital).
D. when a patient report is given to a receiving facility.

_____ 21. Which of the following is the least important information that can be given to a receiving facility in a report delivered while en route?
A. estimated time of arrival at department
B. care being provided by the transport crew
C. type of aircraft/vehicle being utilized for transport
D. airway and breathing status

_____ 22. All of the following are persons who may utilize the information recorded on a PCR except:
A. lawyers.
B. billing department personnel.
C. researchers.
D. reporters.

_____ 23. All of the following are considered standard for the completion of a patient care report except:
A. documenting important events utilizing the 12-hour clock system.
B. using appropriate abbreviations and acronyms.
C. using appropriate medical terminology.
D. completing the report in its entirety in a timely fashion.

_____ 24. How will an aircraft pilot keep from being distracted by talking between medical crew members over the aircraft communication system?
A. The pilot will ask the medical crew not to talk.
B. The pilot can isolate himself from the crew cabin with a door or curtain.
C. The pilot can isolate himself and air traffic control from the channel being utilized by the medical crew.
D. None of the above.

_____ 25. A fishbone diagram can be utilized to organize which of the following patient information?
A. sodium, chloride, blood urea nitrogen (BUN), glucose, creatinine, bicarbonate, and potassium
B. PaO_2, $PaCO_2$, HCO_3^-, pH
C. past medical history, medications, and allergies
D. hemoglobin, hematacrit, platelets, and glucose

Chapter 37

The Critical Care Paramedic in the Hospital Environment

Review of Chapter Objectives

Upon completion of this chapter, the student should be able to:

1. **Understand the evolution of the paramedic in both the prehospital and hospital environment.** **p. 1052**

   In the not-so-distant past, an ambulance was staffed by an untrained person who simply picked up the ill or injured and provided them transport to a hospital. However, in a scant 40 years or so, these early services have grown into a well organized and sophisticated system of certified health care providers who provide care in the emergency environment with the assets of enhanced education, improved clinical competence, sophisticated medical technology, and liberal protocols that literally bring the emergency department to the patient. Likewise, all signs indicate that there is no slowing down in the future trends for the critical care paramedic.

   In fact, both the paramedic and the critical care paramedic are finding additional employment opportunities with differing responsibilities within the hospital environment. Hospital departments that have employed critical care paramedics include the emergency department (ED), critical care units (CCU), and special procedure units such as the cardiac catheterization lab, stress lab, and radiologic suite. Although the idea of using paramedics in the hospital environment is not a new idea (some hospital systems have been using paramedics for more than ten years now), the idea is not yet widespread, but it is gaining acceptance.

2. **Value the importance of skills and knowledge that the critical care paramedic brings into the hospital environment.** **p. 1053**

   Simply put, the paramedic brings a skill set and knowledge base that allows him to correct potential life-threatening insults to patient airway, breathing, and circulation. This skill and knowledge base, when combined with the nurse's skill and knowledge base that centers around more long-term care issues, makes for a well-rounded health care team.

3. **Discuss how state law and medical direction can influence the critical care paramedic's role in the hospital.** **p. 1053**

   States typically issue the scope of practice for CCP through EMS regulations, and the scope of practice is usually defined in a medical practice act. Specific medical practice acts govern the practice for specific health care professions. Medical practice acts may also govern the extent to which a physician may delegate additional authority to a CCP. In addition, standards regarding certification and licensure are determined by the state, and serve as the mechanism by which the state regulates health care practice. It is the responsibility of the health care provider to understand the limits of their certification or licensure.

©2007 Pearson Education, Inc.
Critical Care Paramedic

503

Additional state laws and regulations that affect the CCP in the hospital environment are familiar from the prehospital and include: Mandatory reporting requirements, negligence and medical liability, confidentiality, HIPAA law, defamation of character, obtaining patient consent, patient withdrawal of consent (refusal of care), advanced directives, and potential crime and/or accident scenes.

A CCP is only allowed to provide care under the auspices of a physician medical director under direct physician oversight or under an RN with the responsibility of delegating to the CCP.

4. Understand and be able to discuss the common pros and cons of paramedics working in the hospital as maintained by political entities involved with this ongoing debate. p. 1054

CCPs should be aware of the various entities opposed to their presence in the hospital environment; understanding the opposition better prepares the CCP to interface with them in the work environment and helps to bridge the divide between health care team members.

The role of the CCP in the hospital is not to replace other health care team members; rather, it is an issue of integration and enhancement of existing health care levels. The best patient care is delivered when all involved agree on the role of the CCP, including hospital administration, physicians, nurses, ancillary allied health professionals, and CCPs themselves.

There remain longstanding issues with nursing professionals over the role of the CCP in the hospital. From the CCP perspective, the CCP thought process is akin to a physician's. As such, paramedics should flourish in the emergency department and in the critical care unit. Paramedics have proven assessment and intervention skills for airway, breathing, circulatory compromise, ECG interpretation, and pharmacologic management.

From the nursing perspective, the CCP is an unlicensed provider who lacks the breadth of knowledge base offered in nursing school. The CCP is concerned with skill provision, not holistic long-term management. The American Nursing Association, a professional nursing organization, issued a position statement in 1992 critical of the practice of using paramedics in the emergency department. The statement refers to paramedics as unlicensed personnel, and states that the use of paramedics is "not in the interest of the health, safety, and welfare of the public." Their position remains the same over a decade later, that the paramedic should be an assistant to the RN in the emergency department.

The best position is probably one that recognizes that each profession has its strengths and weaknesses, and together they can best provide excellent patient care.

5. Name common hospital departments where the critical care paramedic may work alongside other health care providers. p. 1056

Paramedics commonly work in the emergency department (ED), critical care unit (CCU), and special procedure units such as the cardiac catheterization lab, stress lab, and radiological suite. In addition, CCPs may work in a surgical intensive care unit (SICU), medical intensive care unit (MICU), cardiovascular intensive care unit (CVICU), pediatric intensive care unit (PICU), or neonatal intensive care unit (NICU).

6. Name the most common skills the critical care paramedic is already familiar with that may be employed in the hospital setting. p. 1058

Skills employed in the hospital setting that are familiar to the CCP include:

- Patient assessment and reassessment
- Airway skills (suctioning, OPA/NPA, BVM, ETT, ETC, LMA)
- ECG monitoring (3-lead and 12-lead)
- Patient movement and handling
- Charting and documentation tasks (some hospitals utilize a fully computerized system which is integrated with the hospital's mainframe system).
- Medication administration (IVP, IM/SQ, IO, infusions)
- IV initiation

- Immobilization
- Equipment preparation (central lines, suturing, ECG, EEG, IABP, casting and splinting, and wound dressing)
- Venous blood sampling
- Bedside cardiac enzyme testing
- Capnography, bedside BGL determination, and pulse oximetry
- Aerosolized and nebulized bronchodilitation therapy

In 1999, the American College of Emergency Physicians conducted a survey and determined that about 20 percent of hospitals employed paramedics. The survey also reported the following with regard to the skills that paramedics and EMTs were allowed to perform in the ED:

- Performing basic skills (94 percent)
- Intermediate skills (89 percent)
- Advanced level skills (50 percent)
- Administering ACLS drugs (51 percent)
- Administering non-ACLS drugs (38 percent)
- Administering medications via IM/SubQ (48 percent)
- Administering medications IV (46 percent)
- Administering medications oral (45 percent)

Type of patient encounters:

- Wound care (86 percent)
- Medical emergencies (79 percent)
- Suturing (23 percent)
- Rape intervention (17 percent).

Sixty-seven percent of EDs reported that paramedics performed triage.

7. **Discuss additional skills beyond those of the critical care paramedic that may be used within the hospital.** p. 1058

Less frequently utilized paramedic skills in the emergency department include:

- Foley catheter insertion
- NG/OG tube insertion
- Tracheal airway replacement
- Sterile techniques (tracheal suctioning, surgical procedures)
- ABG blood draw
- Setting up equipment (central lines, chest tubes, and so on)
- Conscious sedation monitoring
- Monitoring critical patients during transport to other departments
- Billing procedures if task is done by the critical care paramedic

8. **Discuss common techniques aimed at smoothing the transition of patient care from prehospital to emergency department (ED) care, as well as between hospital departments.** p. 1056

The critical care paramedic working in the emergency department is also commonly called on to be part of "special teams" such as trauma alerts or cardiac arrests. In either scenario, the critical care paramedic has a wealth of knowledge and experience to draw from while care is being provided simultaneously by a number of care providers. The paramedic can also serve as a go-between between EMS crews and the trauma staff, because paramedics understand the situational dynamics and the equipment common to prehospital care. Although rare, a transporting EMS crew may arrive with some type of immobilization device or automatic CPR compression device that may be unfamiliar to the emergency department providers. In this situation, the critical care paramedic can help make the transition from the EMS cot to the hospital bed more fluid while facilitating a seamless transition from care being rendered by the prehospital crew to the emergency department staff. Likewise, if a patient is being transported from the emergency department to another facility by an EMS crew, and the EMS crew is unfamiliar with the type of medication infusion pump being used, the critical care paramedic can ease this transition by assisting with the transfer of care to the EMS equipment.

Case Study

"Code Blue, outpatient clinic parking lot," the pager announces for the second time as you grab the AED and jump bag and head out the door toward the parking lot. Turning your portable radio to the hospital security frequency, you advise the communications specialist that you are en route from the ED. She advises you that a security officer is on the scene and that a female patient is on the ground and is complaining of pain in her hip after a fall. Arriving on the scene, you are presented with a distressed elderly woman who was walking to a doctor's appointment when she tripped and fell and now is complaining of right hip and lower back pain. Her right leg is shortened and externally rotated and with the assistance of other hospital staff, you supervise her immobilization to a long spine board and transport her via stretcher to the ED for evaluation. A short time later, while performing a preoperative EKG on this same patient, you reflect on how differently that situation would have been handled a few years ago. Either an ambulance would have been called while the patient continued to wait or, worse, staff without emergency experience would have tried to get the patient into the ED for evaluation. Now, not only does the critical care paramedic staff respond to "Code Blue" calls on the hospital grounds, but they also assist the ED staff with patient care. Many procedures that were performed in the past by nurses, respiratory therapists, and technicians are now regularly performed by paramedics. Although there was initially some resistance to paramedics working in the hospital, it is now clear to everybody involved that they are a great complement to the staff already present. You recently heard that there are plans to expand the program to include the use of critical care paramedics in the critical care and postoperative recovery units. Although political debate about their use may continue to rage, it's obvious that in this hospital the use of critical care paramedics is here to stay.

DISCUSSION QUESTIONS

1. What are some common hospital departments where the critical care paramedic may work alongside other health care providers?
2. What are the most common skills the critical care paramedic is already familiar with that may be employed in the hospital setting?

Content Review

MULTIPLE CHOICE

_____ 1. _____ is (are) state-level EMS legislation that clearly defines what a prehospital care provider can and cannot do as well as where and when they can do it.
  A. Scope of practice   C. Certification
  B. EMS regulations   D. Licensure

_____ 2. _____ is (are) a mechanism by which a state regulates health care within the states boundaries.
  A. EMS regulations   C. Scope of practice
  B. Certification and licensure   D. Medical practice acts

_____ 3. The CCP is able to practice medicine independent of a medical control physician.
  A. True
  B. False

_____ 4. Which of the following skills is the CCP least likely to perform in the hospital environment?
   A. charting and documentation
   B. ECG monitoring
   C. advanced airway maintenance
   D. central venous catheterization

_____ 5. The _____ is a powerful professional nursing organization that serves the nursing profession in the United States.
   A. National Association of American Nurses (NAAN)
   B. Association of American Nurses (AAN)
   C. American Nurse's Association (ANA)
   D. United States Nursing Association (USNA)

_____ 6. A 1999 survey by the American College of Emergency Physicians found that about _____ of hospital employed paramedics.
   A. 10 percent
   B. 15 percent
   C. 20 percent
   D. 25 percent

_____ 7. A 1999 survey by the American College of Emergency Physicians found that the most frequently utilized skill by EMTs and paramedics in the emergency department was (were):
   A. basic EMT skills.
   B. administering ACLS medications.
   C. advanced level skills.
   D. administering PO medications.

_____ 8. Which of the following is least likely to be a responsibility of a paramedic working in an interventional radiology suite?
   A. initiating IV access
   B. administering IV contrast material
   C. providing care should an anaphylactic reaction of full cardiac arrest occur
   D. interpretation of MRI or CT scans

_____ 9. Which of the following is least likely to be a responsibility of a paramedic working in a noninvasive cardiology lab?
   A. initiation of IV access
   B. talking with the patient about test results
   C. prepping the patients chest fore ECG monitoring
   D. monitoring patient vital signs during the exam

_____ 10. A CCP is commonly able to perform skills outside the scope of practice of prehospital paramedics.
   A. True
   B. False

CRITICAL CARE PARAMEDIC
WORKBOOK ANSWER KEY

Chapter 1: Answer Key

CASE STUDY

1. Due to decreases in funding and in Medicare reimbursements, many small rural and community hospitals began closing in the 1980s. At the same time, larger hospitals began to specialize in only a few treatment areas. Some specialized in areas such as neurosurgery or cardiac care, while others specialized in fields like cancer care or obstetrics. This specialization allowed them to maintain high quality services and keep costs down. This shift from general hospitals to specialized hospitals meant that patients would often need to be moved from one hospital to another to receive the best possible care.

2. Professionalism is an attitude, not a matter of pay. Health care professionals promote quality patient care and always perform their duties to the very best of their ability. They set high standards for themselves, their crew, and their system, and take pride in their profession. Health care professionals maintain an ethical standard in all their interactions, placing the patient's welfare above everything but their own safety. It takes constant effort to attain and maintain professionalism.

3. The role of the critical care paramedic before, during, and after a critical care transport varies significantly with the program structure for which the paramedic works. Before taking on the role of a critical care paramedic, it is recommended that a paramedic have three to five years of experience in a busy advanced life support system. This assures initial mastery of routine advanced life support skills. Critical care paramedics often perform procedures not commonly used in the prehospital environment, and these skills must also be mastered.

   During the transport, the role of the critical care paramedic is primarily that of a direct patient care provider. Whether in the role of the primary care giver, or assisting another health care professional, the critical care paramedic must always be cognizant of what is in the patient's best interest. In addition to knowledge of direct patient care, experienced paramedics have a great deal of familiarity with the effective packaging of patients for safe transport. They are also used to working in the tight quarters typical of the critical care transport environment. This experience can often be essential to the safe, efficient transfer of patients.

   Directly after the transport, the critical care paramedic should assure that he can respond to the next request without delay. This may require the restocking of equipment and supplies, cleaning and disinfecting equipment, as well as completing records and reports. An excellent time to pursue continuing education and quality improvement activities is between transports.

CONTENT REVIEW
MULTIPLE CHOICE

1. C	*p. 3*	7. C	*p. 4*	13. A	*p. 7*
2. A	*p. 4*	8. D	*p. 5*	14. D	*p. 8*
3. D	*p. 4*	9. B	*p. 5*	15. C	*p. 11*
4. A	*p. 4*	10. D	*p. 7*	16. A	*p. 12*
5. B	*p. 4*	11. B	*p. 7*	17. A	*p. 12*
6. D	*p. 4*	12. C	*p. 7*	18. B	*p. 12*

Chapter 2: Answer Key

CASE STUDY

1. The advantages of ground ambulances over air ambulances for critical care transports include lower operating costs, short departure times, large patient compartments, the ability to travel in any weather, and safety. The main disadvantage of ground ambulances compared to air ambulances is the increased transport time.

2. Crew configurations can vary significantly depending upon patient needs and local practice. Legislation dictates crew configurations in some states. Configurations might include, but are not limited to: critical care paramedic (CCP)/CCP with an EMT driver, CCP/Critical Care Registered Nurse (CCRN) with an EMT driver, CCP/Respiratory Therapist (RT) with an EMT driver, and CCP/Resident Physician or Physician Assistant (PA) with an EMT driver. The advantages of CCP/CCP patient care teams include a high degree of proficiency with the most commonly encountered critical care transfer patient needs, the relative availability of critical care paramedics, and their cost effectiveness. One disadvantage is that both team members are trained with the same curriculum, so they bring the same perspective and education to the transport. One main advantage of a team configuration which uses a CCP in combination with a CCRN, an RT, or an MD/PA and an EMT driver, is that these providers add a greater depth of training and experience, as well as a different perspective on the care of the patient. The main disadvantages of this type of team configuration are the cost and the relative scarcity of these providers to go on a transfer.

3. Typically, a critical care ground ambulance is a large Type I or Type III unit. Larger units are

utilized due to the need for additional equipment and staff and the ability to access the patient from both sides. Although most of the equipment used by critical care paramedics is the same as what is used on routine calls, some specialized equipment is needed for critical care interfacility transfers. Some of this specialized equipment includes: single, triple, or syringe medication pumps, automatic ventilators with fully adjustable parameters, automatic blood pressure monitors, hemodynamic monitors, and intra-aortic balloon pumps.

CONTENT REVIEW

MULTIPLE CHOICE

1.	A	*p. 18*	5.	A	*p. 20*	9.	C	*p. 20*
2.	B	*p. 19*	6.	C	*p. 21*	10.	D	*p. 20*
3.	C	*p. 20*	7.	D	*p. 18*			
4.	D	*p. 20*	8.	C	*p. 20*			

Chapter 3: Answer Key

CASE STUDY

1. Indications for air medical transport can include trauma emergencies, medical emergencies, and search-and-rescue missions. Air transport can provide access to remote locations, access to specialty teams or medical centers, and access to personnel with specialized skills. When trying to determine the best method of transportation to a facility, consider the clinical status of the patient, the mechanism of injury, and the transport time to the appropriate facility. Although air transport provides higher transport speeds when compared to ground transport, do not forget to factor in the time necessary for ground transport in the event that the receiving facility does not have an onsite helipad.

2. Rotor-wing transport has the advantage of highly trained crews with specialized equipment, a generally decreased response time to the patient, and a decreased transport time. Fixed-wing transports also provide highly trained crews with specialized equipment. Fixed-wing aircraft can have a decreased response time to the patient when transport distances exceed 100 miles. They also have less susceptibility to weather constraints when compared to rotor-wing aircraft.

3. Packaging a patient for air transport varies slightly from packaging for ground transport. Tubing, wires, and hoses should be coiled and secured with tape. Patients should be wrapped in material that keeps blood and body fluids from contaminating the aircraft, and that protects them from the cold. Patients may also need to wear hearing protection. Equipment in the aircraft must be organized and readily accessible. Any equipment stored in areas accessible only from the outside must be moved to the interior of the aircraft before takeoff.

CONTENT REVIEW

MULTIPLE CHOICE

1.	B	*p. 27*	5.	C	*p. 29*	9.	B	*p. 46*
2.	D	*p. 28*	6.	B	*p. 45*	10.	A	*p. 46*
3.	A	*p. 28*	7.	C	*p. 46*			
4.	D	*p. 29*	8.	A	*p. 45*			

Chapter 4: Answer Key

CASE STUDY

1. Altitude places various stresses on the human body. Stressors in flight directly related to altitude are referred to as "stressors of altitude." These stressors include: hypoxia, barometric pressure, fatigue, dehydration, and thermal concerns. In many ways, the cause of these stressors can be traced to gas physics and physiology. As altitude increases, barometric pressure, temperature, and the partial pressures of the gases in the ambient air decrease. The decrease in barometric pressure at altitude causes air-filled spaces, such as, the cuff of endotracheal tube or the inner ear, to increase in volume, which may cause injury. The decrease in the partial pressures of the gases in the ambient air creates a relative decrease in oxygen. This contributes to the very real possibility of hypoxia with increasing altitude. With increasing altitude, the temperature and humidity of the ambient air decreases, creating an environment which can easily lead to water and heat loss. All of the above issues can increase the fatigue experienced by the patient and crew.

2. The physiological effects of "stressors of altitude" are predictable and can be compensated for. The effects of barometric pressure on closed spaces can usually be mitigated by venting those spaces which can be vented, monitoring and adjusting the pressure in spaces which can't be vented, and refraining from flying with ear or sinus inflammation. Crew hypoxia would be a concern in the event of a sudden cabin depressurization. Assuring the presence of emergency equipment and regularly training on its use, can limit the risk from this rare in-flight emergency. Patient hypoxia is a much more common concern. Transfusing patients with red blood cells can help eliminate anemic hypoxia. Monitoring the patient's SpO_2 and adjusting the FiO_2 as necessary will help decrease the concern for hypoxic hypoxia. Dehydration can be offset by early and judicious fluid replacement, as well as by humidifying any oxygen that is administered. Thermal concerns can be alleviated by assuring proper protection from the elements. Fatigue can quickly set in for both patients and crew members when they are physically distressed. Proper diet and rest before flights can help decrease the effects of fatigue.

3. "Stressors of flight" are those stressors placed on patients and air crew related to the flight, but not related to altitude per se. These stressors include: noise, vibration, gravitational forces, third spacing, spatial disorientation, and flicker vertigo.

4. Although noise and vibration are a fact of life in flight, steps can be taken to decrease their effects on crew and patient. The increased use of monitors, both invasive and noninvasive, can help decrease the effect these factors have on patient assessment. Whenever possible, hearing protection with an intercom system should be used for both crew and patients. Gravitational forces can worsen the process of third spacing or the deposition of fluid into the extravascular space. However, G-forces may be used to the patient's advantage if the

greatest average force is considered in relation to the patient's condition and their placement within the aircraft. With cardiac patients, consider positioning the patient with their head toward the aft position of the aircraft so that, on ascent, the G-forces will pool blood in the upper body and improve myocardial perfusion. Reversing this arrangement will help patients with fluid overload or head injuries by causing blood to pool in the lower extremities. Spatial distortion and flicker vertigo may affect both air crew and patients. Spatial distortion is a phenomenon in which an individual cannot determine his position, attitude, or degree of motion relative to the surface of the earth. The possibility of spatial distortion can be decreased by always using visual reference points, putting trust in the instruments, avoiding fatigue, never staring at lights, and providing tactile references for patients. Flicker vertigo is an unpleasant reaction which may include nausea, dizziness, migraines, unconsciousness, and even seizures. It occurs in some people with exposure to flickering lights. The effects of flicker vertigo can be minimized by avoiding looking at flickering lights and ensuring adequate rest and hydration.

CONTENT REVIEW

MULTIPLE CHOICE

1. D	*p. 50*	19. D	*p. 53*	37. C	*p. 67*
2. A	*p. 50*	20. C	*p. 56*	38. B	*p. 67*
3. B	*p. 50*	21. C	*p. 57*	39. A	*p. 67*
4. C	*p. 51*	22. A	*p. 59*	40. C	*p. 68*
5. D	*p. 51*	23. B	*p. 60*	41. B	*p. 68*
6. C	*p. 51*	24. C	*p. 60*	42. C	*p. 68*
7. D	*p. 51*	25. B	*p. 60*	43. D	*p. 69*
8. D	*p. 52*	26. C	*p. 60*	44. A	*p. 69*
9. B	*p. 53*	27. D	*p. 61*	45. D	*p. 69*
10. A	*p. 53*	28. A	*p. 60*	46. A	*p. 69*
11. B	*p. 53*	29. C	*p. 61*	47. C	*p. 69*
12. C	*p. 55*	30. A	*p. 62*	48. A	*p. 69*
13. D	*p. 56*	31. D	*p. 63*	49. C	*p. 70*
14. C	*p. 57*	32. C	*p. 64*	50. D	*p. 70*
15. C	*p. 57*	33. D	*p. 64*	51. D	*p. 73*
16. A	*p. 58*	34. A	*p. 65*	52. A	*p. 73*
17. B	*p. 58*	35. D	*p. 66*	53. B	*p. 68*
18. A	*p. 59*	36. A	*p. 66*	54. C	*p. 69*

Chapter 5: Answer Key

CASE STUDY

1. Flight safety consists of plans that are incorporated into the operations of aeromedical transport systems to reduce risks or eliminate them entirely. Programs should have a mechanism in place to assess for risks, prioritize those risks, develop procedures to minimize or eliminate the risks, and assess the effectiveness of the procedures implemented in reducing the risk.

2. It is important to remember that flight safety is the responsibility of each and every crew member. Crew members must be alert to potential hazards at all times and not allow themselves to be distracted. Flight safety starts long before an aircraft takes off on a mission. First, policies and procedures related to flight safety should be in place and crews should be intimately familiar with them. Pilot safety briefs are conducted at the start of each pilot's shift, and many times, before each mission. All crew members are required to attend regular safety training which ideally includes classroom training, field training in the hangar, and field training in the mission environment. Crew members are expected to be attentive to hazardous areas of helicopter operations, such as, the main rotor system, the tail rotor, rotor wash, landing zones, approaching and departing the aircraft, perimeter guards, and other air traffic. Crew members should maintain high levels of physical fitness and should be well-rested before their shift. Proper personal protective equipment should be utilized at all times.

3. Proper preparation through training and education should have a flight crew well prepared for the tasks that need to be accomplished after an unplanned landing. The crew needs to remain calm and prioritize their needs. The aircraft's survival kit should be located and inventoried for usable supplies and equipment. The immediate medical needs of any surviving personnel should be attended to first. If the accident is in a remote area where rescue may be delayed, attention should be turned to providing shelter, then to building a fire to provide heat and to allow for the boiling of water and, lastly, to finding food.

   Shelter can, in some cases, be crafted from the fuselage of the aircraft. If the fuselage is not suitable, shelter can be made from other aircraft parts and from natural resources found around the crash site, such as, tree branches, rocks, or snow. When using aircraft parts, it is important to remember that they are made from metal and will rapidly conduct body heat. Use layered clothing, dry blankets, and upholstered material from the aircraft to help minimize loss of body heat. The shelter should be constructed within the site of the wreckage, if possible.

   Fire can often be made using the fire starter kit found in the aircraft survival kit. If the fire starter kit is destroyed, preplanning will ensure that a crew knows how to start a fire and what materials are best to use.

   Water can be secured by trapping condensation, melting ice or snow, or purifying available water by boiling or using water purification tablets. If IV fluids are available, they may be utilized for hydration.

CONTENT REVIEW

MULTIPLE CHOICE

1. B	*p. 79*	7. D	*p. 88*	13. B	*p. 92*
2. A	*p. 79*	8. B	*p. 89*	14. A	*p. 94*
3. C	*p. 79*	9. B	*p. 90*	15. C	*p. 98*
4. C	*p. 83*	10. A	*p. 90*	16. D	*p. 99*
5. D	*p. 84*	11. C	*p. 90*	17. A	*p. 100*
6. A	*p. 86*	12. D	*p. 91*		

Chapter 6: Answer Key

CASE STUDY

1. One of the most important skills a paramedic can have, and the one most often used, is that of

patient assessment. A paramedic must be able to perform a rapid, detailed, and accurate patient assessment whether they are working in the prehospital environment or in the critical care transport environment. In the prehospital environment, the paramedic formulates a care plan that is based primarily on the findings from his or her clinical assessment. In the critical care transport area, there is often a working diagnosis in place prior to the arrival of the paramedic. When transporting patients between facilities, there is often additional information that needs to be integrated into the assessment of the patient, such as lab values, X-rays, and results from other diagnostic studies. In the prehospital environment, the availability of patient information can be limited, whereas transports between facilities typically provide a greater scope of information.

2. Obtaining patient assessment data begins when you are assigned a mission. Use the data you receive to start formulating your plan of treatment and thinking about what equipment you will need. Upon arrival to the patient, determine the history of present illness/injury. Review what has already been done for the patient and decide if it has worked, or if you will need to formulate a new plan of action. Anticipate any interventions that may need to be performed during the transport. If you are doing an interfacility transport, review the results of any diagnostic studies done. Perform an initial assessment of the patient, looking for loss of function in airway patency, breathing adequacy, circulatory status, or an acute alteration in mental status. If any critical findings are made, support the lost function until you can do a rapid physical exam to determine the cause of the lost function. A detailed physical exam should then be performed. Once the data from all of these steps are integrated, the critical care paramedic should have a good baseline from which to work. Do not forget the need for ongoing assessment of your patient as his condition can change rapidly.

3. Complications during a critical care transport can be minimized by proper training on equipment, having the needed equipment available, performing a thorough patient assessment, and having proper documentation for transport, including EMTALA/COBRA paperwork, consent for transfer, evidence of acceptance by the receiving facility, and all treatment records. Patients should be packaged in an organized fashion, allowing for easy access to any IV lines and minimizing the tangling of cables or tubing. If time allows, it is also helpful to update the patient's immediate family on the patient's condition, and establish firm safety rules if a family member will be accompanying you.

CONTENT REVIEW

MULTIPLE CHOICE

1. D	*p. 107*	6. B	*p. 112*	11. D	*p. 114*
2. C	*p. 108*	7. C	*p. 116*	12. B	*p. 111*
3. A	*p. 111*	8. C	*p. 116*	13. C	*p. 121*
4. B	*p. 120*	9. A	*p. 117*	14. A	*p. 113*
5. A	*p. 121*	10. A	*p. 113*		

Chapter 7: Answer Key

CASE STUDY

1. There are a number of options available to the critical care paramedic for placing an endotracheal tube. Tubes are most commonly placed orally under direct visualization with a laryngoscope. In the event that the cords cannot be visualized directly, or space does not allow proper patient positioning, patients can be intubated digitally. Sitting patients may be intubated using the sky hook technique outlined in the chapter. Retrograde intubation is a method that can be used when routine endotracheal intubation is not possible. In some cases, patients who are still breathing can be nasally intubated.

2. Rapid sequence intubation is a safe way to protect the airway of a patient who is not able to, or will not be able to, protect his own airway due to impending respiratory failure, acute airway disorder, or altered mental status with accompanying risk of vomiting and aspiration. The patient should be preoxygenated with 100 percent oxygen while you prepare your equipment, supplies, and patient. Along with the usual intubation equipment, prepare back-up devices such as the CombiTube® or LMA and have the equipment available for a surgical airway. Sedate the patient adequately. Apply Sellick's maneuver and premedicate according to your local protocols. Administer a paralytic agent and intubate once adequate relaxation has been achieved. Confirm tube placement, release Sellick's maneuver, and secure the tube. Continue sedation and paralysis during transport if the situation warrants. Do not administer paralytics without adequate sedation.

3. In the event of the failure of endotracheal intubation, including RSI, critical care paramedics must be well versed in alternative, or rescue, airways. There are many devices available on the market, each with their advantages and disadvantages. Some of the devices available include the CombiTube®, the pharyngotracheal lumen (PtL) airway, the laryngeal mask airway (LMA), intubating laryngeal mask airway (LMA Fastrach®), the Cobra perilaryngeal airway (PLA), the Ambu laryngeal mask (ALM), and the King LT airway. Surgical airway procedures available to critical care paramedics include needle cricothyrotomy and open cricothyrotomy.

4. Noninvasive monitors will help you measure the effectiveness of oxygenation and ventilation. Pulse oximetry and waveform capnography are two of the most common measurements used in critical care transport. Pulse oximetry measures hemoglobin oxygen saturation in peripheral tissues. It provides a continuous readout that reflects any changes in peripheral oxygen delivery, and can often detect problems with oxygenation faster than assessment of other vital signs. Remember, that the pulse oximetry readings can be false or misleading in cases of carbon monoxide poisoning, hypovolemia, severe anemia, pulselessness, high intensity lighting, and certain hemoglobin abnormalities.

   End-tidal carbon dioxide ($ETCO_2$) monitoring measures the levels of carbon dioxide in exhaled breath. In EMS, $ETCO_2$ monitoring was initially used only to confirm placement of endotracheal tubes. Today, this monitoring is used to provide the paramedic with information about the status of systemic metabolism, circulation, and ventilation.

CONTENT REVIEW

MULTIPLE CHOICE

1.	D	*p. 127*	21.	C	*p. 151*	41.	B	*p. 174*
2.	A	*p. 129*	22.	B	*p. 151*	42.	D	*p. 174*
3.	A	*p. 131*	23.	A	*p. 154*	43.	A	*p. 174*
4.	B	*p. 129*	24.	C	*p. 155*	44.	C	*p. 174*
5.	C	*p. 131*	25.	D	*p. 156*	45.	B	*p. 176*
6.	D	*p. 133*	26.	D	*p. 160*	46.	C	*p. 177*
7.	A	*p. 132*	27.	C	*p. 161*	47.	D	*p. 177*
8.	B	*p. 133*	28.	B	*p. 165*	48.	A	*p. 177*
9.	D	*p. 140*	29.	A	*p. 165*	49.	D	*p. 177*
10.	A	*p. 142*	30.	C	*p. 168*	50.	B	*p. 177*
11.	C	*p. 142*	31.	C	*p. 169*	51.	C	*p. 177*
12.	B	*p. 142*	32.	B	*p. 168*	52.	A	*p. 178*
13.	B	*p. 143*	33.	D	*p. 167*	53.	B	*p. 178*
14.	D	*p. 145*	34.	A	*p. 168*	54.	D	*p. 178*
15.	C	*p. 145*	35.	C	*p. 168*	55.	B	*p. 179*
16.	A	*p. 145*	36.	C	*p. 172*	56.	C	*p. 179*
17.	B	*p. 146*	37.	B	*p. 172*	57.	A	*p. 179*
18.	A	*p. 146*	38.	A	*p. 172*	58.	D	*p. 179*
19.	D	*p. 147*	39.	D	*p. 172*	59.	D	*p. 179*
20.	B	*p. 148*	40.	C	*p. 173*	60.	B	*p. 179*

Chapter 8: Answer Key

CASE STUDY

1. Shock is a state in which perfusion to the body tissues is not adequate enough to meet the cellular demands of the body. When the body's demand for oxygen exceeds the available supply, the energy yield from glucose drops dramatically, causing a change in organ function.
2. Shock can be classified into four categories: cardiogenic, obstructive, hypovolemic, and distributive. Cardiogenic shock occurs when the heart is unable to maintain sufficient cardiac output. Obstructive shock occurs from the impedance of the circulatory flow by such problems as cardiac tamponade, pericarditis, pulmonary embolism, and aortic dissection, among others. Hypovolemic shock occurs from a reduction in intravascular volume. Distributive shock occurs when there is a decrease in vascular resistance or an increased venous capacity from a vasomotor dysfunction. It can be broken down into the three subclassifications: septic shock, anaphylactic shock, and neurogenic shock.
3. Stages of shock include compensated, decompensated, and irreversible. Compensated shock occurs when the body is able to compensate for the decreased cardiac output through the activation of baroreceptors and neurotransmitters. These cause vessels in the periphery to vasoconstrict, shunting blood to vital organs and increasing cardiac output. Blood pressure usually remains normal, while the heart rate and respiratory rate increase. Mental status usually remains at the patient's baseline. Decompensated

shock occurs when the body is no longer able to compensate for the decrease in cardiac output. When the vessels constrict further, blood gets trapped in the capillary beds causing a mottled appearance. There are decreased levels of oxygen in the blood and tissues. The heart has an increase in contractility and rate, but there is a decrease in preload, leading to an eventual decrease in blood pressure. Patients exhibit a decreased level of consciousness, cool, clammy skin, tachycardia, tachypnea, delayed capillary refill, and decreased urine output. If there is no interruption in this downward trend, damage at the cellular level will occur, ultimately causing multiple organ dysfunction syndrome. The patient usually is unresponsive, and has a decreasing pulse rate. Dysrhythmias will develop and the blood pressure may be unobtainable. Prognosis is poor if a patient reaches this stage.
4. Management of the shock patient largely involves providing supportive care to the patient while the cause of the shock is identified. As with every patient, any issues with airway, breathing, and circulation should be addressed and corrected. Body temperature should be maintained. Fluid resuscitation should be based on the patient's hemodynamic status and may include IV fluids, blood products, or vasoactive medication drips.

CONTENT REVIEW

MULTIPLE CHOICE

1.	B	*p. 188*	8.	B	*p. 191*	15.	C	*p. 198*
2.	C	*p. 188*	9.	D	*p. 192*	16.	A	*p. 201*
3.	C	*p. 188*	10.	D	*p. 193*	17.	B	*p. 201*
4.	B	*p. 189*	11.	A	*p. 193*	18.	A	*p. 201*
5.	A	*p. 189*	12.	B	*p. 198*	19.	D	*p. 199*
6.	D	*p. 189*	13.	C	*p. 198*	20.	A	*p. 201*
7.	A	*p. 189*	14.	D	*p. 198*	21.	C	*p. 199*

Chapter 9: Answer Key

CASE STUDY

1. Invasive arterial monitoring provides a continuous, accurate, direct measure of arterial pressure. This is particularly useful with patients for whom you are titrating vasoactive medications. Arterial access is also indicated for patients who will need frequent blood gas samples. Central venous pressure reflects the blood pressure within the vena cava or right atrium. It provides information about intravascular blood volume, right-ventricular diastolic pressure and right ventricular function. Central venous catheters are used in patients with hypotension who are not responding to treatment, in hypovolemia, and in patients who need large volumes of fluids or infusions of inotropic drugs. They are also used for patients who need total parenteral nutrition. Pulmonary artery pressure monitoring with a catheter such as a Swan-Ganz, among others, measures right ventricular function, pulmonary vascular status, and indirectly measures left ventricular function. Other parameters that can be obtained are cardiac output, right atrial pressure, right ventricular pressure, pulmonary artery pressure, and pulmonary artery wedge

pressure. PA catheters are used in the diagnosis of shock, pulmonary edema, assessment of vascular tone, myocardial contractility, intravascular fluid balance, mixed venous oxygen saturation, management of complicated AMI, and management of hemodynamic instability after cardiac surgery. Intra-aortic balloon pumps provide mechanical circulatory support of a heart that is failing. In cases where patients have significant myocardial injury and the IABP has failed, a ventricular assist device may be inserted to provide circulatory support.

2. In order to get the most accurate reading from an invasive line, the transducer must be placed at a level corresponding to the right atrium, or the phlebostatic axis. The phlebostatic axis is located at the fourth intercostal space and the midaxillary line. Once the transducer is level, the stopcock proximal to the transducer should be turned off to the patient. Take the cap off the sideport of the stopcock and press the "Zero" button on the monitor. Allow the monitor to reset at zero. When the monitor says that zeroing is complete, replace the cap and turn the stopcock back to the sideport. This will open the line to the patient. Flush the line and check for the proper waveform. If the transducer is not leveled and zeroed correctly, inaccurate pressure readings will result.

3. The most common complications with arterial lines are pain during placement, bleeding, and

vasospasm. Complications during insertion of a central venous catheter can include bleeding, pneumothorax, dysrhythmias, and accidental cannulation of an artery. Complications after insertion can include infection, bleeding, accidental dislodgement, and extravasation of fluids. Pulmonary artery catheterization can cause pneumothorax, ventricular dysrhythmias, infection, and pulmonary artery rupture. Advancement of the PA catheter can cause coiling of the catheter in the right side of the heart, valvular damage, or pulmonary arteriole hemorrhage or infarction if the balloon is inadvertently left inflated. The most common complications of intra-aortic balloon pumps are leg ischemia and infection. IABPs and VADs can be difficult to transport due to their bulkiness.

CONTENT REVIEW

MULTIPLE CHOICE

1. A	p. 206	8. B	p. 226	15. C	p. 241
2. C	p. 211	9. D	p. 215	16. B	p. 242
3. B	p. 211	10. D	p. 231	17. A	p. 242
4. D	p. 216	11. B	p. 231	18. B	p. 238
5. A	p. 224	12. D	p. 234	19. D	p. 238
6. C	p. 228	13. C	p. 226	20. B	p. 238
7. B	p. 226	14. A	p. 240	21. D	p. 239

MATCHING

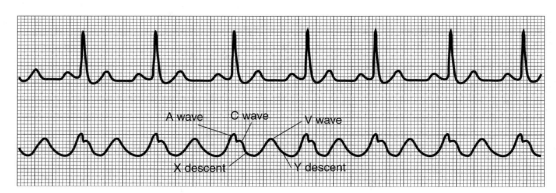

22. E p. 221	24. A p. 221	26. D p. 221
23. B p. 221	25. C p. 221	

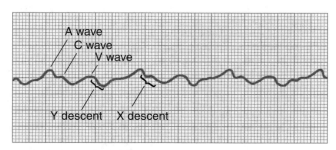

27. E p. 225	29. A p. 225	31. D p. 225
28. C p. 225	30. B p. 225	

Chapter 10: Answer Key

CASE STUDY

1. An infarct of the right ventricle can have a significant effect on systemic preload. If there is muscle damage to the right ventricle, there can be a decrease in the amount of blood available for the left ventricle to pump. The cardiovascular system will attempt to compensate for a decreased preload by increasing peripheral vascular resistance and the patient could present with a normal blood pressure.

2. A right ventricular infarct can be diagnosed by performing a 15-lead ECG and observing for other clinical signs, such as, jugular vein distention, hypotension, and clear lung sounds. The V4R lead of the 15-lead ECG will show ST segment elevation in the presence of a right ventricular infarct.

3. To acquire a 15-lead ECG, first obtain a 12-lead ECG as usual. Then place an electrode on the midclavicular line at the fifth intercostal space on the patient's right side (V4R lead). On the right side of the patient's back, place one electrode in the fifth intercostal space, midscapular line (V8 lead), and another between the V8 lead and the spine, still in the fifth intercostal space (V9 lead). Use the electrode wires from V4, V5, and V6, attaching V4 to V4R, V5 to V8, and V6 to V9. Run another 12-lead ECG, making sure to label it to reflect the new lead placements.

CONTENT REVIEW

MULTIPLE CHOICE

1. B	p. 248	10. B	p. 253	19. D	p. 264
2. C	p. 248	11. C	p. 255	20. B	p. 266
3. D	p. 248	12. D	p. 255	21. A	p. 266
4. C	p. 249	13. C	p. 258	22. A	p. 266
5. B	p. 249	14. B	p. 258	23. D	p. 260
6. A	p. 250	15. A	p. 264	24. C	p. 266
7. C	p. 250	16. B	p. 262	25. A	p. 264
8. D	p. 252	17. C	p. 262		
9. A	p. 252	18. D	p. 264		

Chapter 11: Answer Key

CASE STUDY

1. Factors such as the patient's hemodynamic status, metabolic processes, and elimination capacity should be considered prior to the administration of critical care medications. Also, factors such as a patient's medical history, allergies, regular medications, and medications already or concurrently being administered should be considered.

2. Proper pharmacologic care of a patient cannot be provided unless the critical care paramedic has a solid understanding of a drug's mechanism of action, or pharmacodynamics. By integrating the knowledge of pathophysiology of diseases with the pharmacodynamics of a drug, the critical care paramedic will be able to choose the appropriate agent to achieve the desired outcome.

3. Alteration of normal cellular activity of the body can significantly alter the body's response to a given medication. The body's ability to transport a drug to a specific target site can be altered if the patient has poor perfusion status. Metabolic changes in the body can shorten or lengthen the half-life of the drug. A lengthening of the half-life can cause an accumulative effect, making the effects of the drug last longer than anticipated. In patients who are hyperdynamic, the half-life of a drug can be shortened, leading to a shorter than anticipated effect. Bioavailability of a drug can be altered depending on a patient's protein levels. Patients in hepatic or renal failure can easily become drug toxic due to inadequate biotransformation of the drug into inactive metabolites for elimination from the body.

CONTENT REVIEW

MULTIPLE CHOICE

1. B	p. 275	11. C	p. 306	21. A	p. 280
2. A	p. 275	12. D	p. 312	22. B	p. 283
3. D	p. 275	13. B	p. 316	23. D	p. 293
4. C	p. 275	14. A	p. 320	24. C	p. 294
5. B	p. 276	15. C	p. 321	25. A	p. 297
6. A	p. 276	16. D	p. 283	26. C	p. 307
7. A	p. 281	17. B	p. 283	27. B	p. 314
8. A	p. 286	18. B	p. 291	28. A	p. 318
9. D	p. 291	19. A	p. 303	29. D	p. 320
10. B	p. 294	20. D	p. 278	30. C	p. 306

Chapter 12: Answer Key

CASE STUDY

1. Laboratory and diagnostic testing can provide valuable information to the critical care paramedic when transferring patients between facilities. Results can help determine treatment modalities and indicate if treatments already implemented are having the desired results. An example of this would be in the case of a mechanically ventilated patient. By performing serial blood gases, the critical care paramedic would be able to determine if the changes made in the ventilator settings were having the intended effects.

2. A laboratory test is a specific study or assay performed on a body tissue. These tissues can include blood, urine, and spinal fluid, among others. Examples of laboratory testing include electrolytes, complete blood counts, urinalysis, and blood glucose testing. Medical imaging uses technology to electronically visualize the body. Examples of medical imaging include X-rays, computed tomography (CT scans), magnetic resonance imaging (MRIs), fluoroscopy, and ultrasound, among others. Physiological tests are used in the diagnosis and treatment of disease. Common examples of these tests are arterial blood gas analysis, pulmonary function tests, echocardiograms, and stress testing.

3. Normal reference values are nationally established parameters of laboratory values. These are based on a large number of lab tests conducted over a period

of several years. Each lab confirms the normal reference values based on their population, and can adjust their normal reference values slightly.

4. The lab values of the patient in Case 1 represent those of a patient who is most likely in diabetic ketoacidosis secondary to an infectious process. The patient should receive adequate hydration and be placed on an insulin drip. These will lower both the blood glucose and potassium levels. Any patient on an insulin drip should have frequent monitoring of their blood glucose level in order to prevent hypoglycemia.

   The patient in Case 2 is already alkalemic as evidenced by a pH of 7.50. Following the physician's direction to hyperventilate the patient would further lower the PCO_2, making the patient even more alkalemic. Current scientific evidence does not support the routine hyperventilation of head trauma patients.

   In Case 3, the sending facility increased the heparin dosing on a patient that was already supratherapeutic. The critical care paramedic should be aware that this patient would be at increased risk for bleeding.

CONTENT REVIEW

MULTIPLE CHOICE

1. C	p. 328	10. B	p. 336	19. C	p. 345
2. D	p. 328	11. C	p. 336	20. A	p. 345
3. A	p. 329	12. A	p. 338	21. D	p. 345
4. B	p. 329	13. B	p. 337	22. B	p. 346
5. A	p. 334	14. D	p. 337	23. C	p. 346
6. B	p. 334	15. C	p. 339	24. A	p. 347
7. A	p. 334	16. A	p. 337	25. C	p. 347
8. D	p. 335	17. B	p. 341	26. D	p. 349
9. C	p. 336	18. C	p. 342	27. C	p. 335

MATCHING

28. G	30. J	32. A	34. F	36. C
29. B	31. D	33. E	35. I	37. H

Chapter 13: Answer Key

CASE STUDY

1. There are four levels of trauma center accreditation in the U.S. A Level I center provides comprehensive trauma care and can manage any type of trauma patient due to the availability of many subspecialties. Level I trauma centers are usually located at university medical centers and are active in planning and research. They must have available a certain number of operating rooms, resuscitation areas, and ICU beds. They must receive a predetermined number of severe trauma patients each year. A Level II trauma center has the resources to manage most severe trauma cases, but lacks some of the subspecialties available at Level I centers. Level III trauma center designation is given most often to community hospitals, that can provide expert initial resuscitation and stabilization, but lack surgical specialties and ICU care. Level IV designation was implemented to help guide very rural hospitals in the development of standardized plans for initial management and rapid transfer of the trauma patient. Because trauma center designation can vary slightly from state to state, it is imperative that the critical care paramedic be familiar with the capabilities of the hospitals within his coverage area.

2. The first priority when approaching a trauma scene is the safety of you and your crew. After establishing scene safety, a general impression of the mechanism of injury and potential injuries can be formulated. Evaluate the airway, breathing, and circulatory status, as well as the patient's level of consciousness. Attend to any life threats as you go. Immobilize the patient and provide rapid transport to an appropriate facility, reassessing frequently. Detailed physical exams and further interventions can be done en route. Maintain the patient's body temperature and address any pain control issues. When transporting a major trauma victim between healthcare facilities, the critical care paramedic must get a report on the patient that includes mechanism of injury, what the known or suspected injuries are, what has been done for the patient so far, and what the patient's medication allergies are, if any. The critical care paramedic must assess the patient to ensure that all life threats have been properly addressed by the sending facility. Do not assume that the sending facility has addressed or resolved all of these issues correctly. Place the patient on the transport monitors, switch IVs over to the transport pumps, and place the patient on the transport vent, if applicable. Package the patient for transport, being mindful to maintain body temperature. Closely monitor the patient during transport.

CONTENT REVIEW

MULTIPLE CHOICE

1. B	p. 359	6. D	p. 363	11. B	p. 368
2. D	p. 361	7. A	p. 363	12. B	p. 369
3. D	p. 361	8. A	p. 363	13. D	p. 369
4. B	p. 361	9. B	p. 363		
5. C	p. 362	10. D	p. 367		

MATCHING

14. F	16. D	18. B	20. A
15. E	17. G	19. C	

Chapter 14: Answer Key

CASE STUDY

1. Autoregulation is the inherent ability of the arterial system within the brain to vasoconstrict or vasodilate, as needed, in an attempt to maintain adequate cerebral perfusion, despite changes in systemic pressure. If the cerebral perfusion pressure rises, the arteries constrict to decrease the cerebral blood flow. If the cerebral perfusion pressure decreases, the arteries dilate in order to increase cerebral blood flow and ensure adequate perfusion to the tissue. This system has limitations and cannot compensate for a cerebral perfusion pressure of less than 60 mmHg or greater than 160 mmHg. Head-injured patients may lose their autoregulatory compensation mechanisms completely.

2. There are many nonpharmacological interventions that can be used by the critical care paramedic to assist in the reduction of intracranial pressure. Patients should be positioned in a semi-Fowler's position if there are no restrictions on positioning. Patients who need to have full spinal immobilization can have the head of the backboard propped up with a blanket or pillows to achieve a reverse Trendelenburg position. The head and neck of a head-injured patient should be kept in neutral alignment, and extreme flexion of the limbs should be avoided. Blood glucose should be kept within normal ranges. Use of hypotonic IV solutions should be avoided as they can be rapidly absorbed by already edematous brain tissue. Patients with known intracranial hypertension should be handled carefully and treatments should be clustered whenever possible to avoid continuous spikes in the ICP. Patients should be preoxygenated briefly before suctioning to blunt the effects of ICP spikes during the procedure. Patients should not be routinely hyperventilated in an effort to reduce ICP.

3. Pharmacological interventions to reduce intracranial pressure include mannitol, hypertonic saline, and barbiturate coma. Mannitol is an osmotic diuretic that pulls intracellular fluid from the brain and decreases cerebral edema, thereby reducing ICP. It must be administered through an in-line filter due to its tendency to crystallize. Hypertonic saline produces an osmotic draw to reduce ICP. It has been shown to reduce inflammation of the cells that line the lumens of the blood vessels, improving cerebral blood flow. Barbiturate comas can be induced with barbiturates such as pentobarbital and thiopental, if other treatments have not proven effective. One of the dangers of using barbiturates is due to their severe vasodilatory effects with subsequent hypotension. Patients need to be closely monitored to ensure that adequate mean arterial pressure and cerebral perfusion pressure are maintained.

CONTENT REVIEW

MULTIPLE CHOICE

1. C	*p. 374*	15. A	*p. 381*	29. B	*p. 389*		
2. A	*p. 374*	16. B	*p. 382*	30. A	*p. 390*		
3. D	*p. 380*	17. C	*p. 382*	31. B	*p. 392*		
4. B	*p. 380*	18. D	*p. 383*	32. B	*p. 392*		
5. B	*p. 379*	19. A	*p. 384*	33. C	*p. 392*		
6. C	*p. 392*	20. B	*p. 385*	34. D	*p. 393*		
7. C	*p. 379*	21. C	*p. 384*	35. A	*p. 393*		
8. D	*p. 379*	22. D	*p. 385*	36. C	*p. 393*		
9. A	*p. 379*	23. A	*p. 385*	37. B	*p. 395*		
10. B	*p. 379*	24. B	*p. 385*	38. A	*p. 396*		
11. C	*p. 379*	25. D	*p. 386*	39. D	*p. 397*		
12. A	*p. 381*	26. C	*p. 387*	40. C	*p. 395*		
13. B	*p. 381*	27. D	*p. 387*				
14. D	*p. 381*	28. C	*p. 389*				

Chapter 15: Answer Key

CASE STUDY

1. A closed, or simple pneumothorax, occurs when there is air in the pleural space. The affected lung may be partially or totally collapsed. Management of a closed pneumothorax depends largely on the size of the pneumothorax and the patient's clinical condition. A small pneumothorax may just require careful monitoring of the patient, while larger ones can require percutaneous evacuation of the air. The critical care paramedic should be mindful of the potential for these patients to develop a tension pneumothorax and be alert for signs and symptoms of decompensation.

An open pneumothorax, or sucking chest wound, allows atmospheric air to enter into the pleural space through the chest wall. This results in the equalization of atmospheric and pleural pressure, causing the loss of the negative intrathoracic pressure necessary for effective respirations. Treatment for an open pneumothorax focuses on preventing more air from entering into the thoracic cavity. In order to achieve this, an occlusive dressing that is taped on three sides should be placed over the open area. By leaving the fourth side open, air can escape from the chest cavity with exhalation, but is prevented from entering on inspiration. If signs and symptoms of a tension pneumothorax develop, remove the occlusive dressing to relieve the pressure.

A tension pneumothorax is a life-threatening injury that must be quickly identified and treated. It results from an accumulation of air in the plural space of one lung which causes increasing pressure. This eventually leads to the collapse of the affected lung and causes a mediastinal shift, compressing the other lung. Due to the increased pressure within the chest cavity and the mediastinal shift, venous return to the heart is decreased and perfusion is inadequate. Patients will present with severe respiratory distress and have signs and symptoms of shock. The most common method of treating a tension pneumothorax is by inserting a large-bore IV needle into the 2nd or 3rd intercostal space in the midclavicular line of the affected side, thereby releasing the pressure. This procedure may need to be performed more than once, so careful monitoring of the patient's condition is imperative. In some cases, a chest tube may need to be placed.

A hemothorax occurs when blood accumulates in the pleural space. If the hemothorax is large, this can lead to eventual respiratory compromise from compression or collapse of the affected lung. Patients may also present with signs and symptoms of hypovolemic shock due to the large loss of blood into the pleural space. Treatment of a hemothorax requires aggressive management of the airway and ventilatory status. As with all patients who present with thoracic injury, high-flow, high-concentration oxygen should be administered, and the patient should receive positive-pressure ventilatory support, if needed. A large hemothorax will require placement of a chest tube and/or open thoracotomy. Fluids should be administered in an amount necessary to maintain adequate perfusion, but must not be excessive.

A flail chest is one that has three or more broken ribs in two or more places. This causes loss of stability of the chest wall and paradoxical wall motion, where the flail segment moves in the direction opposite the rest of the chest wall during respiration. Flail segments are often associated with pulmonary contusions and can cause hypoventilation with resulting hypoxia and hypercapnia. Flail segments should be stabilized by exerting gentle pressure with a pillow or bulky dressings. A patient who is in severe respiratory distress should be intubated and manually ventilated with a BVM, unless the transport ventilator is capable of monitoring peak airway pressures. Increasing difficulty in manually ventilating a patient can indicate the development of a tension pneumothorax, which must then be treated. CPAP has also been shown to be effective in the prehospital management of flail segments.

2. Before transporting a patient with a chest tube in place, the critical care paramedic should make a thorough evaluation of both the patient and the chest tube drainage system. The drainage system should be inspected for a proper water level in the suction chamber, as this, and not the setting on the suction machine, is what determines the amount of suction. Observe the amount of bubbling, and when the bubbling occurs during the respiratory cycle. Excessive bubbling will cause rapid evaporation of the water, which will change the amount of suction being maintained. Bubbling, which indicates that air is being removed from the pleural space, should occur during expiration. Observe for fluctuations in the underwater seal chamber as these indicate a closed system. Connections should be taped, and the tubing coiled, so as to allow free flow of the drainage. Hemostats and occlusive dressings should be readily available in the event that the tubing needs to be clamped or the system becomes dislodged. The drainage container should be kept upright at all times.

CONTENT REVIEW

MULTIPLE CHOICE

1. A	p. 402	12. D	p. 408	23. A	p. 414
2. D	p. 404	13. C	p. 410	24. D	p. 414
3. D	p. 404	14. B	p. 410	25. A	p. 414
4. B	p. 405	15. B	p. 410	26. C	p. 415
5. C	p. 405	16. B	p. 410	27. C	p. 416
6. A	p. 406	17. A	p. 411	28. B	p. 416
7. B	p. 407	18. A	p. 411	29. B	p. 416
8. B	p. 407	19. A	p. 412	30. D	p. 416
9. A	p. 407	20. D	p. 413	31. A	p. 417
10. B	p. 407	21. C	p. 414	32. C	p. 418
11. D	p. 408	22. B	p. 414		

Chapter 16: Answer Key

CASE STUDY

1. Imaging studies available for evaluating abdominal trauma include sonography, computed tomography, and radiography. Sonography is the use of ultrasonic echoes that are recorded to produce an image of an organ or tissue. FAST (Focused Assessment with Sonography for Trauma) scans are used to detect blood in the pericardium and/or abdomen. These scans can be performed quickly and accurately, and are noninvasive.

Computed tomography, or CT scanning, uses a process which looks at transverse planes of tissues and forms a computerized image, allowing specific injuries to tissues, and particularly those to solid organs, to be visualized. CT scans are noninvasive and allow for the nonsurgical management of select trauma patients. They are useful for the diagnosis of retroperitoneal injuries, something that a diagnostic peritoneal lavage cannot do. CT scans have their limitations, though, and some injuries often go underdiagnosed.

Radiography, or X-ray, is most often suggestive of underlying abdominal injuries, rather than diagnostic. X-rays can detect free air in the abdomen or the presence of diaphragmatic rupture, but are unable to detect blood in the peritoneum, injuries to organs, or vascular injury.

2. Patients with abdominal trauma can be difficult to manage in the sense that intra-abdominal bleeding cannot be controlled in the usual manner of applying direct pressure. Care of the trauma patient must first focus on managing immediate life threats and then providing for the safe, rapid transport to a trauma center, providing supportive care en route. After securing the airway and ensuring proper ventilation, two large-bore IV sites should be obtained, with bloods drawn. The goal of fluid administration is not to obtain a blood pressure that would be considered normal for the patient. Rather, a lower than normal systolic pressure, approximately 75–80 mmHg should be maintained—high enough to maintain perfusion to the vital organs, but not high enough to cause greater bleeding in a patient with already uncontrolled hemorrhage. Large amounts of crystalloid fluids will cause hemodilution, so it is advisable to administer whole blood or packed red blood cells, if available. After ensuring that there is no urethral injury, a Foley catheter should be placed. In the event of bowel evisceration, the exposed bowel should be covered gently with a moist, sterile dressing. Penetrating objects should be stabilized in place and not removed during transport.

3. Retrograde cystograms are often useful in the diagnosis of urethral or bladder injury. Contrast dye is injected through the urethra and serial X-rays, or a CT scan, are taken. If dye is observed outside of the urethra or bladder, it indicates that there is a perforation of one or both of these structures. Spiral CT with contrast is diagnostic for kidney injuries and allows for the grading of injuries. Regular X-rays are unable to detect any direct injury to genitourinary structures, but may raise the index of suspicion for injury near fractures.

4. The only definitive treatment for patients with serious, life-threatening GU trauma is surgery. The critical care paramedic's role is to manage any life-threatening problems with the airway, ensure adequate oxygenation, and support the circulatory system as needed. Rapid, safe transport to an appropriate facility is required.

©2007 Pearson Education, Inc.
Critical Care Paramedic

CONTENT REVIEW

<u>MULTIPLE CHOICE</u>

1.	A	*p. 423*	22.	B	*p. 445*	43.	C	*p. 439*
2.	C	*p. 423*	23.	A	*p. 445*	44.	A	*p. 439*
3.	D	*p. 423*	24.	B	*p. 445*	45.	A	*p. 439*
4.	B	*p. 424*	25.	C	*p. 429*	46.	B	*p. 439*
5.	C	*p. 425*	26.	D	*p. 429*	47.	D	*p. 439*
6.	A	*p. 425*	27.	D	*p. 429*	48.	C	*p. 439*
7.	C	*p. 426*	28.	C	*p. 430*	49.	A	*p. 439*
8.	D	*p. 426*	29.	A	*p. 430*	50.	B	*p. 439*
9.	C	*p. 426*	30.	F	*p. 430*	51.	D	*p. 439*
10.	A	*p. 426*	31.	B	*p. 430*	52.	C	*p. 440*
11.	C	*p. 426*	32.	C	*p. 431*	53.	A	*p. 440*
12.	A	*p. 426*	33.	B	*p. 431*	54.	B	*p. 440*
13.	B	*p. 427*	34.	A	*p. 431*	55.	D	*p. 440*
14.	B	*p. 427*	35.	D	*p. 431*	56.	B	*p. 440*
15.	B	*p. 441*	36.	C	*p. 432*	57.	A	*p. 432*
16.	A	*p. 441*	37.	D	*p. 433*	58.	C	*p. 432*
17.	D	*p. 441*	38.	B	*p. 433*	59.	B	*p. 446*
18.	D	*p. 428*	39.	B	*p. 434*	60.	C	*p. 446*
19.	B	*p. 442*	40.	A	*p. 434*	61.	D	*p. 446*
20.	A	*p. 443*	41.	B	*p. 438*	62.	B	*p. 447*
21.	C	*p. 428*	42.	B	*p. 438*	63.	A	*p. 447*

Chapter 17: Answer Key

CASE STUDY

1. Assessment of airway, breathing, and circulation are extremely important in patients who present with facial trauma, as injuries can easily become life threatening. A thorough initial assessment and frequent reassessments are necessary. The most common cause of death from maxillofacial trauma is airway obstruction due to the posterior displacement of the tongue into the hypopharynx. This is generally easily remedied with BLS airway maneuvers. More advanced airway techniques may need to be employed in severely injured patients or in those patients whose airways cannot be maintained with BLS techniques. It is impossible to address every situation in this text, but the critical care paramedic must consider the advanced airway techniques available and decide, given the situation, which one would be most appropriate for the patient. Keep in mind that the anatomy of the patient may be distorted, complicating the task of airway management. Bleeding from the head should be controlled by direct pressure, and any impaled objects should be immobilized in place unless they interfere with the airway. After the primary assessment has been completed, and all life threats addressed, the critical care paramedic should perform a systematic inspection of the bony structures of the head, identifying areas of injury. The eyes, ears, nose, and throat should also be closely examined for injury.

2. In patients who present with an ocular injury, a thorough assessment of the eye and surrounding bony structures should be performed after completing a primary survey. Inspect the external eye and the anterior chamber, looking for any signs of trauma. Evaluate the patient's pupils for symmetry, accommodation, and reaction to light. Observe the patient's ability to move her eyes through all six positions of gaze. Perform a

fundoscopic exam to evaluate the retina, optic nerve, and macula. Any foreign bodies that have not penetrated the cornea may be able to be removed by irrigating the eye, or by using the corner of a 2×2 gauze. Foreign bodies that have penetrated the cornea should be removed by an ophthalmologist. Ocular globe rupture and traumatic retinal detachments are considered surgical emergencies.

CONTENT REVIEW

<u>MULTIPLE CHOICE</u>

1.	C	*p. 453*	23.	A	*p. 465*	45.	D	*p. 474*
2.	A	*p. 453*	24.	B	*p. 465*	46.	C	*p. 475*
3.	B	*p. 454*	25.	D	*p. 465*	47.	A	*p. 475*
4.	D	*p. 455*	26.	C	*p. 465*	48.	D	*p. 475*
5.	A	*p. 453*	27.	B	*p. 467*	49.	B	*p. 475*
6.	D	*p. 458*	28.	D	*p. 468*	50.	C	*p. 476*
7.	B	*p. 458*	29.	C	*p. 469*	51.	D	*p. 476*
8.	A	*p. 459*	30.	B	*p. 469*	52.	A	*p. 476*
9.	C	*p. 460*	31.	A	*p. 469*	53.	C	*p. 476*
10.	B	*p. 460*	32.	D	*p. 469*	54.	D	*p. 476*
11.	C	*p. 460*	33.	C	*p. 469*	55.	A	*p. 477*
12.	D	*p. 460*	34.	A	*p. 469*	56.	C	*p. 477*
13.	A	*p. 460*	35.	C	*p. 470*	57.	B	*p. 477*
14.	D	*p. 461*	36.	B	*p. 470*	58.	D	*p. 478*
15.	C	*p. 463*	37.	D	*p. 471*	59.	A	*p. 478*
16.	B	*p. 463*	38.	D	*p. 472*	60.	B	*p. 478*
17.	A	*p. 463*	39.	D	*p. 472*	61.	C	*p. 478*
18.	D	*p. 463*	40.	D	*p. 472*	62.	A	*p. 478*
19.	C	*p. 463*	41.	B	*p. 473*	63.	D	*p. 478*
20.	B	*p. 464*	42.	A	*p. 473*	64.	A	*p. 479*
21.	B	*p. 465*	43.	C	*p. 473*	65.	C	*p. 479*
22.	A	*p. 465*	44.	B	*p. 473*	66.	C	*p. 480*

Chapter 18: Answer Key

CASE STUDY

1. After determining that the scene is safe, the patient's airway, breathing, and circulatory status should be evaluated. Ensure a patent airway, using manual maneuvers or adjunct devices. Airway injury in a burn patient may not be immediately evident. Tissue that is exposed to superheated gases may not appear burned, but will swell quickly, constricting the airway. Give consideration to early intubation even in a patient who does not initially present with airway difficulty. Administer high-flow, high-concentration oxygen through an appropriate device. Ventilations of the patient who has circumferential burns of the chest should be carefully monitored, as the ability for chest expansion may be impaired. After ensuring the presence of a pulse, two large-bore IVs should be established, preferably in an area that has not been burned. All of the patient's clothing and jewelry should be removed in order to stop the burning process. Determine the total body surface area burned and classify the depth of the burns. Start fluid resuscitation with warmed Ringer's lactate or normal saline, using the Parkland formula. Burn victims are at high risk of hypothermia, so be sure to cover the patient, first, with a sterile sheet, and then with blankets.

2. Burns are generally classified into four categories. Superficial, or first-degree burns, involve only the

epidermis. The skin appears reddened, and inflamed, and is painful to the touch. The most common cause of superficial burns is the sun and most do not require prehospital intervention. Partial-thickness, or second-degree burns, involve the epidermis and the dermis. They are characterized by reddened areas, and blisters or open weeping areas. These burns are quite painful, and patients can show evidence of significant amounts of fluid loss. Full-thickness, or third-degree burns, involve the epidermis, dermis, and the subcutaneous tissue. The injured area will appear charred or leathery. The area of full-thickness injury is not painful due to the destruction of nerve endings. Fourth-degree burns are full-thickness burns that extend beyond the subcutaneous tissue into muscle, fascia, periosteum, or bone.

3. The most widely used standard for fluid resuscitation in burn patients is the Parkland formula. The Parkland formula uses the patient's weight, in kilograms, the percentage of total body surface area (TBSA) with partial- and full-thickness burns, and a standard fluid replacement amount. The formula is 4 mL × kg of body weight × percent TBSA burned. Half of this fluid, preferably warmed Ringer's lactate, is administered over the first 8 hours post injury, and the remaining half is given over the following 16 hours. In pediatric burn patients, resuscitation fluid replacement is based on the Parkland formula. This patient population also receives additional maintenance fluids of a dextrose-containing solution, using a standard replacement amount and the patient's weight in kilograms. For the first 10 kg of body weight, 100 mL/kg over 24 hours is administered. For the second 10 kg of body weight, 50 mL/kg over 24 hours is given. For each kilogram of body weight over 20 kilograms, an additional 20 mL/kg over 24 hours is administered. Remember, that these formulas are guidelines only; actual rates of fluid administration should be individualized based on the patient's response.

CONTENT REVIEW

MULTIPLE CHOICE

1. A	*p. 489*	16. B	*p. 503*	31. C	*p. 510*
2. C	*p. 491*	17. B	*p. 503*	32. B	*p. 511*
3. A	*p. 491*	18. A	*p. 504*	33. A	*p. 511*
4. B	*p. 492*	19. C	*p. 504*	34. C	*p. 512*
5. D	*p. 492*	20. C	*p. 504*	35. D	*p. 512*
6. C	*p. 496*	21. A	*p. 505*	36. C	*p. 513*
7. B	*p. 497*	22. B	*p. 505*	37. D	*p. 514*
8. C	*p. 498*	23. D	*p. 506*	38. A	*p. 514*
9. A	*p. 499*	24. B	*p. 507*	39. B	*p. 515*
10. B	*p. 500*	25. B	*p. 508*	40. C	*p. 515*
11. D	*p. 501*	26. A	*p. 508*	41. A	*p. 516*
12. C	*p. 502*	27. A	*p. 508*	42. A	*p. 516*
13. A	*p. 504*	28. D	*p. 509*	43. D	*p. 516*
14. B	*p. 503*	29. C	*p. 509*	44. C	*p. 519*
15. B	*p. 504*	30. D	*p. 509*		

Chapter 19: Answer Key

CASE STUDY

1. Skeletal injuries should be addressed only after assessing for, and correcting any, immediate life threats with the airway, breathing, and circulation. When doing a detailed patient assessment, evaluate circulation and neurological function in each of the extremities. Circulatory evaluation should include assessment of pain, pallor, paralysis, paresthesia, pressure, and pulses, while neurological evaluation should include assessment of sensory and motor function. Evaluation of the superficial reflexes can be helpful in determining the neurological status of a limb in an unresponsive patient. Signs of orthopedic injury include deformity, contusions, abrasions, pain, lacerations, swelling, tenderness, instability, and crepitus. Any acute deformity should be treated as a fracture until proven otherwise. Certain fractures, particularly those of long bones, can cause large amounts of blood loss. Patients should be splinted appropriately, have IV fluids administered as necessary, and receive adequate analgesia. Any patient with suspected spinal injury should be fully immobilized.

2. Orthopedic injuries most likely to cause hemodynamic instability are fractures of the long bones, which are often associated with a large amount of impact force. A fracture of the pelvis can cause extensive bleeding (1,500 mL or greater) which may go unnoticed until the patient is in the last stages of shock. Stabilization of these fractures in the field can be accomplished using a bed sheet or commercial pelvic wrap to provide circumferential compression. A fractured femur can cause the loss of up to 1,500 mL of blood and should be stabilized with a traction device, when appropriate. A fracture of the humerus can cause up to 750 mL of blood loss. The most common method of managing a fracture of this nature is with a sling and swathe. The sling should be applied so that the elbow is free, allowing some gravitational traction to be applied to the humerus.

3. There are a number of pharmacological agents available for the treatment of orthopedic injuries. Nonsteroidal antiinflammatory drugs assist in the reduction of inflammation, thus reducing the cause of the pain. Opiate analgesics, such as morphine and hydrocodone, are generally used for "breakthrough pain"—pain that is not controlled through the use of NSAIDS. Antibiotics are used for patients who have open fractures, extensive soft tissue trauma, or multi-system trauma. Muscle relaxants, such as diazepam or cyclobenzaprine, aid in the reduction of muscle spasm near the injured site that helps to reduce the pain as well. Orthopedic injury, particularly of long bones, can put patients at increased risk for deep vein thrombosis or pulmonary embolus. To mitigate the formation of these clots, patients are often put on anticoagulant therapy. Commonly administered anticoagulants include aspirin, heparin, low-molecular-weight heparin, and warfarin.

CONTENT REVIEW

MULTIPLE CHOICE

1. A	*p. 523*	3. A	*p. 253*	5. B	*p. 253*
2. A	*p. 523*	4. C	*p. 253*	6. D	*p. 523*

7. C	*p. 253*	24. C	*p. 530*	41. B	*p. 535*
8. A	*p. 524*	25. D	*p. 530*	42. A	*p. 527*
9. D	*p. 524*	26. A	*p. 530*	43. A	*p. 535*
10. C	*p. 524*	27. D	*p. 530*	44. C	*p. 536*
11. B	*p. 524*	28. B	*p. 531*	45. D	*p. 536*
12. A	*p. 524*	29. A	*p. 531*	46. B	*p. 537*
13. D	*p. 524*	30. C	*p. 532*	47. B	*p. 537*
14. D	*p. 524*	31. D	*p. 532*	48. D	*p. 537*
15. A	*p. 526*	32. B	*p. 532*	49. D	*p. 537*
16. D	*p. 526*	33. A	*p. 533*	50. D	*p. 538*
17. B	*p. 527*	34. A	*p. 533*	51. D	*p. 539*
18. C	*p. 527*	35. B	*p. 533*	52. A	*p. 538*
19. B	*p. 527*	36. B	*p. 533*	53. C	*p. 538*
20. A	*p. 528*	37. D	*p. 533*	54. D	*p. 540*
21. C	*p. 528*	38. C	*p. 535*	55. D	*p. 541*
22. D	*p. 528*	39. A	*p. 535*		
23. B	*p. 530*	40. D	*p. 535*		

Chapter 20: Answer Key

CASE STUDIES

CASE STUDY #1

Pediatrics can be among the most stressful patient populations that the critical care paramedic will encounter. There are several factors that must be taken into account when approaching an injured child. Give consideration to the age of the child and the level of his emotional and physiological development. Children, like all patients, should be shown respect. Good communication needs to be established with the child and also any caregivers present. Be honest in explaining the situation, using language and vocabulary that the child can understand. Pediatric trauma patients are managed much in the same manner as adults, but differences in anatomy and physiology will cause different patterns of injury in children. It is not until the late adolescent years that a child's vital signs are similar to those of an adult. The critical care paramedic should be familiar with, or have ready access to, parameters for normal vital signs for children of various ages. It is important that the critical care paramedic remain calm at all times.

CASE STUDY #2

Because of the many physiological changes that occur with aging, the elderly patient is more likely to die of a moderate-to-severe injury than the younger population. Changes that are considered normal in aging occur in all major body systems. It is important that the critical care paramedic be familiar with these changes so that abnormal changes can be more easily identified. Elderly people are more likely to have a host of chronic diseases for which they take a multitude of medications. Their cardiovascular, respiratory, and renal systems cannot compensate for changes as well as they once could, putting them at higher risk for CHF, fluid overload, pulmonary edema, pneumothorax, and acid-base imbalances.

CASE STUDY #3

A number of physiological changes occur in a pregnant female that the critical care paramedic must be aware of when treating obstetrical victims of trauma. Pregnant women are hypervolemic, so more blood volume may be lost before signs and symptoms of shock are evident.

As blood loss occurs, blood is shunted from the uterus first, putting the fetus at risk for hypoxia. There are also changes in cardiac output, heart rate, respiratory mechanics, and renal blood flow. The effect of trauma on a fetus depends on the gestational age of the fetus, the type and severity of the trauma, and the extent of the disruption of normal uterine and fetal physiology. The primary goal in treating a pregnant trauma victim is to stabilize the mother's condition, as this will give the fetus the best possible chance of survival. A supine pregnant female who presents with hypotension should be tilted 20 to 30 degrees on her left side, with her uterus manually displaced to the left, in order to promote venous return to her heart.

CONTENT REVIEW

MULTIPLE CHOICE

1. B	*p. 546*	19. A	*p. 555*	37. C	*p. 568*
2. C	*p. 546*	20. D	*p. 555*	38. D	*p. 568*
3. C	*p. 547*	21. B	*p. 556*	39. A	*p. 568*
4. D	*p. 549*	22. D	*p. 556*	40. D	*p. 568*
5. A	*p. 549*	23. A	*p. 557*	41. D	*p. 569*
6. C	*p. 549*	24. C	*p. 558*	42. C	*p. 569*
7. A	*p. 550*	25. B	*p. 558*	43. B	*p. 573*
8. C	*p. 550*	26. C	*p. 559*	44. A	*p. 573*
9. C	*p. 550*	27. A	*p. 559*	45. A	*p. 574*
10. C	*p. 550*	28. B	*p. 559*	46. B	*p. 574*
11. C	*p. 550*	29. C	*p. 561*	47. C	*p. 575*
12. C	*p. 550*	30. D	*p. 565*	48. A	*p. 574*
13. B	*p. 551*	31. D	*p. 566*	49. D	*p. 574*
14. C	*p. 552*	32. D	*p. 566*	50. D	*p. 574*
15. A	*p. 553*	33. A	*p. 566*	51. C	*p. 575*
16. D	*p. 553*	34. B	*p. 567*	52. C	*p. 575*
17. C	*p. 554*	35. D	*p. 567*	53. D	*p. 575*
18. D	*p. 555*	36. B	*p. 567*		

Chapter 21: Answer Key

CASE STUDY

1. Acute respiratory failure is defined as a state of inadequate gas exchange resulting from the inability of the respiratory system to absorb oxygen and/or excrete carbon dioxide. Acute respiratory failure develops so quickly that the body's compensatory mechanisms do not have time to work. It is generally accepted that acute respiratory failure exists when the arterial blood gas shows an oxygenation level below 60 mmHg, a carbon dioxide level greater than 50 mmHg, and a pH of less than 7.30 on room air.

2. Management of asthma patients should focus on reversing bronchoconstriction and airway inflammation and edema. This will increase ventilation, oxygenation, and the elimination of carbon dioxide. First-line medications include oxygen, beta-agonists, and anticholinergics. The latter two are effective at reversing bronchoconstriction in the early stages of asthma. Corticosteroids are effective in reversing airway inflammation and edema. Magnesium administered intravenously helps relax bronchial smooth muscle tissue. Patients who are unresponsive to pharmacological agents but are not in imminent danger of losing their respiratory drive can benefit from noninvasive positive-pressure ventilation

(NPPV). NPPV helps keep the alveoli open, diminishes alveolar fluid accumulation, and assists in keeping smaller bronchioles open. This allows for more effective removal of carbon dioxide and decreases the work of breathing. Patients who are in imminent danger of respiratory arrest should be intubated without delay.

Management of the patient with an exacerbation of COPD focuses on improving oxygenation and carbon dioxide elimination, reversing bronchospasm, and treating the underlying cause of the exacerbation. Patients should receive high-flow, high-concentration oxygen using the appropriate device. Beta-agonists and anticholinergics are considered first-line treatments. If the patient's clinical condition suggests that infection has caused the exacerbation, antibiotics are administered. Indications for noninvasive positive-pressure ventilation and intubation are the same as those for asthma patients. Hyperventilation should be avoided.

Acute respiratory distress syndrome is not a primary disease, but a complication that occurs when a disease or traumatic insult produces a severe and progressive systemic response. It is characterized by impaired oxygenation, progressive hypoxemia, decreased lung compliance, and bilateral infiltrates. The goal for the critical care paramedic managing a patient with ARDS is to maintain oxygenation to an SpO_2 greater than 90 percent. If the patient is mechanically ventilated, the FiO_2 should ideally be kept to 50 percent or less. The tidal volumes should be adjusted to keep the peak inspiratory pressure to 35 cm H_2O, or less, to prevent hyperinflation and barotrauma to uninjured areas of the lungs. PEEP is a tool used to enable lower tidal volumes, rather than reduce alveolar edema as in asthma or COPD.

Patients with pneumonia mainly require oxygenation and ventilatory support. Severe cases of pneumonia may require the patient to be intubated because of respiratory compromise. Early antibiotic therapy has proven effective in reducing mortality and morbidity in this population.

CONTENT REVIEW

MULTIPLE CHOICE

1. A	p. 580	17. B	p. 588	33. B	p. 591
2. C	p. 581	18. A	p. 588	34. A	p. 591
3. B	p. 581	19. D	p. 588	35. D	p. 592
4. D	p. 582	20. C	p. 588	36. C	p. 592
5. C	p. 582	21. D	p. 588	37. B	p. 592
6. A	p. 585	22. B	p. 589	38. D	p. 592
7. D	p. 585	23. D	p. 589	39. A	p. 592
8. C	p. 585	24. C	p. 589	40. D	p. 592
9. A	p. 585	25. A	p. 589	41. B	p. 593
10. B	p. 586	26. B	p. 589	42. C	p. 593
11. D	p. 586	27. B	p. 590	43. D	p. 593
12. C	p. 586	28. A	p. 590	44. A	p. 594
13. A	p. 586	29. D	p. 590	45. B	p. 594
14. D	p. 586	30. C	p. 590	46. A	p. 594
15. C	p. 586	31. B	p. 591	47. C	p. 594
16. C	p. 588	32. A	p. 591	48. C	p. 594

49. B	p. 595	74. A	p. 605	99. C	p. 610
50. A	p. 595	75. B	p. 597	100. D	p. 610
51. C	p. 595	76. B	p. 605	101. D	p. 611
52. B	p. 595	77. C	p. 606	102. C	p. 611
53. D	p. 596	78. D	p. 606	103. C	p. 612
54. C	p. 596	79. B	p. 607	104. B	p. 612
55. D	p. 596	80. A	p. 607	105. D	p. 612
56. B	p. 596	81. B	p. 607	106. A	p. 612
57. C	p. 597	82. C	p. 607	107. D	p. 612
58. C	p. 598	83. B	p. 607	108. C	p. 613
59. A	p. 598	84. C	p. 607	109. B	p. 613
60. A	p. 598	85. A	p. 608	110. A	p. 613
61. B	p. 598	86. C	p. 608	111. B	p. 613
62. C	p. 598	87. B	p. 608	112. D	p. 613
63. A	p. 598	88. B	p. 608	113. C	p. 614
64. D	p. 598	89. D	p. 608	114. B	p. 614
65. A	p. 600	90. A	p. 608	115. D	p. 615
66. A	p. 600	91. C	p. 608	116. C	p. 615
67. B	p. 603	92. C	p. 608	117. A	p. 615
68. C	p. 603	93. D	p. 609	118. D	p. 615
69. A	p. 601	94. C	p. 609	119. D	p. 616
70. D	p. 603	95. D	p. 609	120. C	p. 616
71. D	p. 605	96. A	p. 610	121. B	p. 616
72. B	p. 605	97. B	p. 610	122. D	p. 616
73. B	p. 605	98. D	p. 610		

Chapter 22: Answer Key

CASE STUDY

1. Acute coronary syndrome (ACS) includes a spectrum of coronary artery disease processes ranging from myocardial ischemia to myocardial infarction. ACS is caused by a progressive narrowing of the lumen of the coronary arteries, causing an imbalance in oxygen supply and demand. ACS includes stable angina, unstable angina, and acute myocardial infarction.

2. Tests used to support the diagnosis of acute coronary syndrome include the electrocardiogram and serum cardiac enzyme markers. Although the ECG can be nondiagnostic, positive findings on ECG are often the catalyst for the initiation of fibrinolytic therapy or percutaneous coronary interventions. ECG can also be useful for screening for a pulmonary embolus or pericarditis. Serial testing of cardiac enzymes, such as CK-MB and troponin, is useful in diagnosing patients with acute myocardial infarction.

3. There are a number of pharmacological agents that may be used in the treatment of acute coronary syndrome. Supplemental oxygen should be administered through an appropriate device in order to increase the oxygen supply available to the myocardium.

   Nitrates are used to relax the smooth muscle of the coronary arteries. This improves coronary blood flow, increasing oxygen supply available to the myocardium. Nitrates reduce preload and afterload, which decreases myocardial oxygen demand. These drugs should be administered cautiously in patients with suspected right ventricular infarct.

   Analgesics are often administered in the treatment of acute coronary syndromes. One analgesic commonly used is morphine. Morphine reduces preload and afterload, which decreases cardiac contractility and lowers myocardial oxygen demand. Oxygen demand is also lowered because of a decrease in sympathetic discharge in response to pain.

Aspirin is the most common antiplatelet drug administered in acute coronary syndromes. Aspirin inhibits platelet aggregation at the site of the ruptured coronary artery plaque. Anticoagulants, such as heparin, inhibit further clot formation.

Beta blockers decrease heart rate and contractility, thereby reducing myocardial oxygen demand. Calcium channel blockers reduce myocardial oxygen demand by decreasing myocardial contractility. They also increase myocardial oxygen supply by improving coronary blood flow through the relaxation of smooth muscle.

Fibrinolytics are used to improve myocardial oxygen supply by lysing coronary thrombi.

CONTENT REVIEW

MULTIPLE CHOICE

1.	A	p. 623	27.	B	p. 633	53.	D	p. 646
2.	C	p. 624	28.	D	p. 633	54.	D	p. 647
3.	B	p. 624	29.	B	p. 633	55.	A	p. 647
4.	A	p. 626	30.	C	p. 634	56.	C	p. 650
5.	D	p. 624	31.	C	p. 634	57.	B	p. 650
6.	C	p. 627	32.	A	p. 635	58.	D	p. 651
7.	A	p. 627	33.	D	p. 635	59.	C	p. 651
8.	A	p. 628	34.	C	p. 635	60.	A	p. 652
9.	B	p. 627	35.	D	p. 636	61.	D	p. 652
10.	C	p. 627	36.	B	p. 637	62.	B	p. 652
11.	D	p. 627	37.	D	p. 638	63.	C	p. 652
12.	A	p. 628	38.	A	p. 638	64.	B	p. 654
13.	C	p. 628	39.	A	p. 638	65.	D	p. 655
14.	C	p. 629	40.	D	p. 638	66.	C	p. 655
15.	B	p. 629	41.	C	p. 639	67.	A	p. 655
16.	A	p. 629	42.	B	p. 639	68.	A	p. 655
17.	D	p. 629	43.	C	p. 640	69.	D	p. 657
18.	C	p. 630	44.	A	p. 640	70.	B	p. 657
19.	C	p. 630	45.	A	p. 641	71.	B	p. 658
20.	B	p. 631	46.	D	p. 641	72.	C	p. 664
21.	D	p. 631	47.	C	p. 642	73.	A	p. 664
22.	D	p. 631	48.	B	p. 642	74.	C	p. 664
23.	C	p. 632	49.	C	p. 643	75.	B	p. 672
24.	A	p. 632	50.	A	p. 644	76.	D	p. 672
25.	B	p. 632	51.	D	p. 645			
26.	C	p. 632	52.	A	p. 645			

Chapter 23: Answer Key

CASE STUDY

1. Proper management of airway, breathing, and circulation are important factors in preventing secondary injury in the neurologic patient. The neurons of the central nervous system are very sensitive and require adequate amounts of oxygen and glucose to function properly. If the supply of these materials is interrupted through hypoxia or hypoperfusion, or both, the tissues have very little reserve. Proper management of airway and breathing will help ensure the availability of adequate amounts of oxygen for the body's use. Efficacy of brain perfusion is measured by cerebral perfusion pressure (CPP). CPP is calculated by subtracting intracranial pressure (ICP) from the mean arterial pressure (MAP). As the ICP rises, the CPP will fall, assuming a constant blood pressure. If the central perfusion pressure falls below approximately 60 mmHg in adults, the brain loses its ability to autoregulate cerebral blood flow. The result is cerebral ischemia. As this worsens, the injured brain tissue becomes edematous. If cerebral edema is allowed to progress unchecked, it will ultimately cause herniation.

CONTENT REVIEW

MULTIPLE CHOICE

1.	C	p. 679	27.	A	p. 688	53.	A	p. 702
2.	A	p. 679	28.	C	p. 688	54.	C	p. 702
3.	C	p. 680	29.	D	p. 688	55.	D	p. 702
4.	C	p. 680	30.	D	p. 689	56.	B	p. 702
5.	B	p. 680	31.	B	p. 690	57.	D	p. 703
6.	B	p. 680	32.	D	p. 691	58.	D	p. 703
7.	D	p. 681	33.	C	p. 691	59.	C	p. 703
8.	A	p. 681	34.	D	p. 691	60.	A	p. 704
9.	C	p. 681	35.	A	p. 694	61.	C	p. 703
10.	C	p. 681	36.	C	p. 695	62.	B	p. 705
11.	B	p. 682	37.	B	p. 695	63.	D	p. 705
12.	D	p. 682	38.	C	p. 695	64.	B	p. 705
13.	A	p. 682	39.	B	p. 696	65.	C	p. 705
14.	C	p. 684	40.	B	p. 697	66.	B	p. 706
15.	B	p. 685	41.	B	p. 697	67.	C	p. 706
16.	A	p. 685	42.	A	p. 697	68.	A	p. 706
17.	D	p. 685	43.	A	p. 696	69.	D	p. 707
18.	B	p. 685	44.	B	p. 698	70.	D	p. 706
19.	C	p. 686	45.	B	p. 699	71.	B	p. 707
20.	A	p. 686	46.	D	p. 699	72.	C	p. 709
21.	D	p. 686	47.	B	p. 699	73.	A	p. 712
22.	B	p. 687	48.	C	p. 700	74.	C	p. 708
23.	B	p. 687	49.	A	p. 700	75.	D	p. 712
24.	D	p. 687	50.	C	p. 700	76.	B	p. 713
25.	C	p. 687	51.	D	p. 701	77.	C	p. 713
26.	B	p. 687	52.	B	p. 702	78.	A	p. 715

Chapter 24: Answer Key

CASE STUDY

1. Diagnostic studies used to determine gastrointestinal disease vary according to the disease process suspected. If GI bleeding is evident or suspected, endoscopy or colonoscopy, scintigraphy, and angiography can be used to assist in locating the source of the bleeding. Laboratory blood testing can have somewhat limited value in the early stages of a GI bleed since it may take several hours for changes in values, such as hemoglobin and hematocrit, to be evident. CT, MRI, ultrasound and X-rays can be helpful in diagnosing pancreatitis. Although levels of digestive enzymes in the blood are often tested in suspected pancreatitis, they are not, by themselves, diagnostic. A diagnosis is usually made after combining test results with imaging studies, reviewing the patient's history and the clinical presentation. Liver failure is diagnosed based primarily on clinical presentation and laboratory testing of liver function tests.

2. The critical care paramedic may encounter a variety of tubes or catheters used in the management of gastrointestinal disease. These may

include drainage tubes, feeding tubes, peritoneal dialysis catheters, and ostomy collection bags. It is of utmost importance that the critical care paramedic knows where the tube is placed, and what its purpose is, prior to transport. Proper placement of the tubes should be confirmed and the paramedic should be familiar with the type and amount of drainage that can be expected. Any collection devices should be emptied of their contents prior to transport, if at all possible.

CONTENT REVIEW

MULTIPLE CHOICE

1.	B	p. 720	21.	D	p. 730	41.	A	p. 735
2.	A	p. 721	22.	C	p. 730	42.	C	p. 736
3.	D	p. 721	23.	B	p. 730	43.	D	p. 736
4.	C	p. 722	24.	C	p. 731	44.	B	p. 736
5.	C	p. 722	25.	D	p. 731	45.	A	p. 736
6.	A	p. 722	26.	A	p. 731	46.	D	p. 736
7.	B	p. 722	27.	C	p. 731	47.	C	p. 737
8.	D	p. 722	28.	D	p. 731	48.	A	p. 737
9.	C	p. 722	29.	B	p. 732	49.	D	p. 737
10.	A	p. 722	30.	A	p. 733	50.	B	p. 737
11.	B	p. 722	31.	A	p. 733	51.	C	p. 738
12.	D	p. 722	32.	C	p. 733	52.	A	p. 738
13.	C	p. 726	33.	A	p. 734	53.	D	p. 738
14.	C	p. 727	34.	B	p. 734	54.	D	p. 739
15.	D	p. 728	35.	C	p. 734	55.	D	p. 739
16.	A	p. 728	36.	D	p. 734	56.	A	p. 739
17.	A	p. 729	37.	B	p. 735	57.	D	p. 739
18.	C	p. 729	38.	B	p. 735	58.	B	p. 739
19.	B	p. 730	39.	D	p. 735	59.	C	p. 739
20.	A	p. 730	40.	C	p. 735			

Chapter 25: Answer Key

CASE STUDIES

CASE STUDY #1

Peritoneal dialysis is one of the available renal replacement therapies used in the treatment of chronic renal failure. A catheter is surgically inserted into the patient's peritoneal cavity, allowing the infusion of dialyzing solution. The dialyzing solution dwells in the peritoneal cavity for a period of time, allowing the removal of toxins and excess water across the peritoneum's semipermeable membrane. The solution is then drained from the peritoneum. If peritoneal dialysis is not performed as scheduled, life-threatening physiological changes can occur. A major complication of peritoneal dialysis is peritonitis caused by contamination of the dialysis catheter. In peritoneal dialysis patients, the first sign of peritonitis may be the removal of cloudy fluid from the peritoneum during exchanges of dialyzing fluids. Care for this type of patient will be mostly supportive, with attention given to airway, respiratory, and circulatory status.

CASE STUDY #2

The patient in this case is diagnosed with diabetic ketoacidosis (DKA) secondary to a viral infection. The classic signs of DKA are hyperglycemia and acidosis. Acidosis occurs when the metabolism of fat causes a buildup of free fatty acids that reduce extracellular bicarbonate levels. These patients are often severely

dehydrated secondary to hyperglycemia-induced diuresis. Serum lab abnormalities may include increased potassium, BUN and creatinine, and hyperosmolality. DKA patients may present with Kussmaul-type respirations and may or may not have a discernable fruity breath odor caused by ketone bodies. The critical care paramedic should be primarily concerned with restoring the circulating volume of the patient with normal saline. Several liters may need to be given before the patient's volume status returns to normal. Regular insulin is given to address the patient's hyperglycemic state. Ordinarily, a loading dose is given, followed by a continuous infusion, and blood glucose levels are checked frequently to monitor progress. Administration of insulin will drive serum potassium back into the cells, leaving the patient at risk for hypokalemia. The critical care paramedic should frequently reassess the patient's vital signs and monitor for heart rhythm disturbances.

CASE STUDY #3

The patient in this case has a respiratory acidosis most likely caused by an exacerbation of COPD due to underlying pneumonia. The acidosis is caused by an excess buildup of carbon dioxide in the blood, and the ABG suggests an insidious onset since the kidneys have attempted to compensate. Treatment should focus on improving oxygenation and eliminating excess CO_2. This patient would benefit from high-flow, high-concentration oxygen and aerosolized beta-agonist and anticholinergic drugs. If the patient does not respond rapidly to these interventions and has no signs of imminent respiratory failure, noninvasive positive-pressure ventilation may be attempted. Any patient who shows signs of fatigue, altered mental status, or who is in danger of respiratory arrest should be intubated without delay.

CONTENT REVIEW

MULTIPLE CHOICE

1.	C	p. 752	12.	C	p. 755	23.	D	p. 760
2.	D	p. 752	13.	D	p. 756	24.	B	p. 760
3.	D	p. 752	14.	B	p. 756	25.	A	p. 760
4.	B	p. 751	15.	D	p. 757	26.	C	p. 760
5.	D	p. 752	16.	D	p. 757	27.	C	p. 760
6.	A	p. 752	17.	C	p. 757	28.	D	p. 760
7.	B	p. 753	18.	A	p. 759	29.	D	p. 760
8.	C	p. 753	19.	B	p. 759	30.	B	p. 763
9.	D	p. 753	20.	A	p. 759	31.	A	p. 763
10.	B	p. 755	21.	D	p. 759	32.	B	p. 763
11.	A	p. 755	22.	B	p. 760	33.	C	p. 767

Chapter 26: Answer Key

CASE STUDY

1. It is incumbent upon the critical care paramedic to be knowledgeable about the principles of infection control and the recognition and treatment of those infectious diseases that they may encounter in their work. It is the professional obligation of all health care workers to prevent the spread of infectious and communicable diseases between patients, themselves, coworkers, family, and friends. A good knowledge of communicable diseases and their modes of transmission will ensure that the critical

©2007 Pearson Education, Inc.
Critical Care Paramedic

care paramedic knows how best to take precautions against the spread of the disease.

2. Standard precautions incorporate the major components from Universal Precautions and Body Substance Isolation Precautions. Standard precautions apply to blood, all body fluids, secretions and excretions (except sweat), nonintact skin, and mucous membranes. Standard precautions include hand washing, wearing gloves, gowns, and adequate eye protection, and employing safety measures when dealing with sharps. Adequate cleaning and disinfecting procedures should be in place. Patient care equipment and linen should be handled in such a way so as to prevent cross contamination.

Airborne precautions are followed when caring for a patient with a known or suspected infectious disease that is spread by airborne droplet nuclei. When transporting a patient on airborne precautions, the CDC recommends a minimum of 6 to 12 air exchanges per hour, venting to the outdoors, separate air circulation between cab and patient compartment, keeping the door or window shut between the two compartments, and airing out the vehicle after transport. N95 respirators should be worn if pulmonary tuberculosis is suspected. If the patient can tolerate a surgical mask, one should be worn when he is being transported through public areas.

Droplet precautions are used when caring for a patient with known or suspected infection with pathogens that are spread by droplets generated by sneezing, coughing, talking, or suctioning. Patients should be placed so that they avoid contact within three feet of other people. When working within three feet of a patient, the provider should wear a mask. As with airborne precautions, the patient should wear a surgical mask in public areas if it can be tolerated.

Contact precautions are used with patients who are infected or colonized with pathogens capable of being transmitted by direct or indirect contact with the patient. Gloves should be worn when in the patient's room and should be changed when they become grossly contaminated, or between procedures. Gowns should be used whenever direct contact with the patient is expected or when significant contact with potentially contaminated surfaces or objects may occur. All nondisposable patient care equipment must be thoroughly cleaned and disinfected prior to being placed back in service.

CONTENT REVIEW

MULTIPLE CHOICE

1. C	p. 774	12. B	p. 776	23. D	p. 778	
2. A	p. 774	13. D	p. 776	24. C	p. 792	
3. A	p. 774	14. B	p. 781	25. B	p. 793	
4. A	p. 775	15. C	p. 785	26. B	p. 793	
5. B	p. 775	16. D	p. 782	27. D	p. 793	
6. C	p. 775	17. B	p. 787	28. C	p. 794	
7. D	p. 775	18. A	p. 789	29. A	p. 794	
8. B	p. 776	19. C	p. 790	30. B	p. 794	
9. B	p. 775	20. B	p. 790	31. D	p. 794	
10. A	p. 776	21. A	p. 791	32. C	p. 794	
11. B	p. 776	22. C	p. 791	33. A	p. 795	

34. A	p. 795	49. B	p. 798	64. B	p. 802
35. C	p. 795	50. D	p. 798	65. C	p. 802
36. A	p. 785	51. D	p. 798	66. A	p. 802
37. D	p. 795	52. B	p. 801	67. D	p. 801
38. C	p. 795	53. A	p. 801	68. D	p. 800
39. D	p. 785	54. C	p. 801	69. C	p. 802
40. C	p. 796	55. A	p. 801	70. B	p. 803
41. A	p. 796	56. D	p. 801	71. A	p. 802
42. B	p. 796	57. C	p. 801	72. D	p. 803
43. B	p. 796	58. B	p. 801	73. D	p. 805
44. A	p. 797	59. C	p. 802	74. C	p. 804
45. D	p. 797	60. B	p. 802	75. D	p. 805
46. A	p. 796	61. A	p. 802	76. D	p. 805
47. D	p. 797	62. D	p. 802		
48. C	p. 798	63. C	p. 802		

Chapter 27: Answer Key

CASE STUDIES

CASE STUDY #1

The infant in question is in respiratory failure, most likely secondary to a respiratory tract infection. The infant is wheezing, and although the possibility of foreign body obstruction should always be considered in children exhibiting wheezing for the first time, the history of two days of upper respiratory infection symptoms and fever make this concern less likely. Viral respiratory tract infections are very common in infants, and although these infections usually cause relatively mild disease, it is certainly not unusual for these infections to lead to respiratory failure. In this particular case, because of the lack of the classic "seal bark" cough or upper airway stridor, the possibility of a croup-type syndrome is also less likely. Fever, the gradual onset of symptoms, and wheezing point toward bronchiolitis as the most likely working diagnosis for this child. Respiratory syncytial virus (RSV) is the predominant causative agent for bronchial infections in children. The most important treatment for this patient would be reversing hypoxia with high-flow, high-concentration oxygen. Positive pressure ventilation should be used as necessary to correct hypoxia or hypercarbia. Beta-agonists may be helpful in reversing bronchospasm but steroids appear not to be helpful in most clinical trials.

CASE STUDY #2

This infant is most likely suffering from epiglottitis. Epiglottitis generally presents with a rapid onset of a fever and is often accompanied by a sore throat. The child may refuse to eat due to the irritation of the throat and may eventually resort to drooling as swallowing his own saliva becomes too painful. Due to the inflammation and edema of the epiglottis and surrounding structures, airway obstruction is of concern and treatment should focus on preventing this and preparing for emergent management of potential complete obstruction. The critical care paramedic should ensure a calm environment and administer blow-by oxygen. If the child has adequate air exchange, the throat should not be examined. Most epiglottitis cases have been caused by the *Haemophilus influenzae* type B virus, which is now commonly vaccinated against in children in the United States. Epiglottitis is being seen more in young adults.

CASE STUDY #3

The infant in question is displaying evidence of hypoperfusion. Because of the fever and petechial rash, it is most likely secondary to an overwhelming bacterial infection such as meningitis. Treatment for distributive shock secondary to sepsis includes expeditious administration of an appropriate broad-spectrum antibiotic and improving end-organ perfusion. High-flow, high-concentration oxygen should be administered, and blood pressure should be maintained at adequate levels using crystalloid fluids and vasopressors, as necessary.

CONTENT REVIEW

MULTIPLE CHOICE

1.	B	p. 814	11. A	p. 824	21. A	p. 832
2.	A	p. 815	12. B	p. 827	22. C	p. 833
3.	C	p. 817	13. C	p. 825	23. B	p. 833
4.	A	p. 817	14. D	p. 825	24. B	p. 833
5.	D	p. 818	15. C	p. 827	25. D	p. 834
6.	D	p. 820	16. B	p. 828	26. C	p. 833
7.	B	p. 821	17. A	p. 829	27. A	p. 836
8.	C	p. 827	18. C	p. 829	28. A	p. 813
9.	A	p. 824	19. B	p. 830	29. B	p. 813
10.	D	p. 822	20. D	p. 832	30. B	p. 813

Chapter 28: Answer Key

CASE STUDY

1a. Preeclampsia/Eclampsia: Preeclampsia is a syndrome of hypertension in pregnancy that is said to exist when hypertension and proteinuria coexist in the third trimester of pregnancy. This potentially life-threatening syndrome occurs in 6 to 8 percent of all live births. Fetal risks associated with preeclampsia include uteroplacental hypoperfusion, placental infarction, abruptio placentae, inhibited fetal growth, decreased amniotic fluid, and fetal demise. Maternal risks associated with preeclampsia include renal failure, hepatic failure, DIC, seizures, strokes, and death. Eclampsia is broadly defined as seizure activity or coma unrelated to other cerebral conditions in an obstetrical patient. Eclampsia is usually, but not always, associated with preeclampsia. Preeclampsia can be either mild or severe. Severe preeclampsia is said to exist when any of the following clinical or laboratory exam findings are present: SBP > 160 mmHg or DBP > 110 mmHg two times at least 6 hours apart, proteinuria > 5 g in 24 hours, cerebral or visual symptoms, oliguria, pulmonary edema, right upper quadrant pain, elevated liver enzymes, low platelet count, and restricted fetal growth. HELLP is an acronym for Hemolysis, Elevated Liver function tests, and Low Platelets that describes a subcategory of severe preeclampsia. Airway, breathing, and circulation need to be continuously assessed and managed in the preeclamptic and eclamptic patient. High-flow, high-concentration oxygen should be administered, and large bore IV access should be established. Urinary output should be monitored and urine should be assessed for protein. The transport environment should be as quiet and as low lit as possible to help prevent seizure activity. If pulmonary edema is present, IV morphine 2–5 mg and IV furosemide

20–120 mg can be administered and, in severe cases of respiratory distress, CPAP or endotracheal intubation may be necessary. If severe hypertension is present treatment with antihypertensives such as magnesium sulfate, hydralazine and labetalol may be necessary. If eclamptic seizures are prolonged or recurrent, administration of 2–4 mg of magnesium sulfate IV or IM should be considered.

1b. Amniotic Fluid Embolism: Amniotic fluid embolism (AFE) is thought to be associated with circulatory uptake of amniotic fluid into maternal circulation which then travels to the lungs. AFE is a rare complication of delivery that is associated with mortality rates of between 80 and 90 percent. The pathophysiology of AFE shares many of the same features as anaphylactic and septic shock. Vasospasm occurs, causing pulmonary hypertension, pulmonary edema, and severe hypoxia. Disseminated intravascular coagulation (DIC) is common with this emergency and is thought to be a result of the activation of the fibrinolytic system by the amniotic fluid. A patient with AFE has an acute onset of respiratory distress usually followed by pulmonary edema, shock out of proportion to actual blood loss, fever, chills, and diaphoresis. These signs and symptoms occur during or shortly after delivery. Management consists of ensuring oxygenation, supporting inadequate breathing, and providing circulatory support. The use of inotropic medication, fluid therapy, and blood transfusions are commonly used therapies. Additionally, bronchodilators, low dose heparin and steroids may be administered.

CONTENT REVIEW

MULTIPLE CHOICE

1.	C	p. 843	31. D	p. 852	61. C	p. 859
2.	D	p. 843	32. C	p. 852	62. C	p. 859
3.	B	p. 843	33. A	p. 852	63. B	p. 859
4.	C	p. 843	34. B	p. 853	64. A	p. 860
5.	A	p. 843	35. A	p. 853	65. C	p. 860
6.	B	p. 843	36. C	p. 853	66. D	p. 860
7.	A	p. 843	37. B	p. 853	67. B	p. 860
8.	B	p. 843	38. D	p. 853	68. D	p. 861
9.	A	p. 844	39. A	p. 853	69. C	p. 862
10.	C	p. 843	40. D	p. 853	70. A	p. 862
11.	C	p. 844	41. A	p. 853	71. D	p. 862
12.	A	p. 844	42. D	p. 854	72. B	p. 862
13.	D	p. 845	43. B	p. 854	73. C	p. 863
14.	D	p. 848	44. C	p. 854	74. B	p. 863
15.	B	p. 848	45. A	p. 854	75. A	p. 863
16.	C	p. 848	46. D	p. 854	76. D	p. 863
17.	C	p. 848	47. B	p. 854	77. C	p. 863
18.	A	p. 848	48. C	p. 854	78. D	p. 865
19.	C	p. 848	49. A	p. 854	79. B	p. 865
20.	B	p. 849	50. D	p. 854	80. A	p. 867
21.	A	p. 849	51. B	p. 855	81. C	p. 867
22.	B	p. 849	52. D	p. 855	82. C	p. 867
23.	D	p. 849	53. C	p. 856	83. B	p. 868
24.	B	p. 850	54. D	p. 857	84. D	p. 868
25.	D	p. 850	55. C	p. 857	85. C	p. 868
26.	C	p. 850	56. D	p. 858	86. A	p. 868
27.	C	p. 850	57. A	p. 859	87. B	p. 869
28.	D	p. 852	58. B	p. 859	88. C	p. 869
29.	A	p. 852	59. D	p. 859	89. D	p. 870
30.	D	p. 852	60. A	p. 859	90. C	p. 870

Chapter 29: Answer Key

CASE STUDY

1. Neonatal patients should have their airway, breathing, and circulation assessed, just like all other patients. It is important for the critical care paramedic to be knowledgeable about the differences in anatomy and physiology of infants as compared to adults. Some of these differences include: larger tongue and epiglottis, pliable trachea and bones, diminished pulmonary reserve capacity, higher metabolic rate, and inability to increase cardiac contractile force, among others. In addition, it is vital that the newborn be kept warm at all times as newborns have limited ability to maintain core temperature and cannot effectively induce shivering to generate heat.

2. As soon as the infant's head is clear of the vagina, the infant's mouth and nose should be suctioned with a bulb syringe. If it appears that the infant has aspirated meconium, nasopharyngeal and endotracheal suctioning of the infant prior to delivery of the thoracic cavity may limit the extent of meconium aspiration into the lower airways. Meconium may cause airway obstruction or contribute to the inactivation of alveolar surfactant. The infant should be carefully monitored and resuscitated as necessary.

3. Neonates are at significant risk of hypoglycemia due to poor glucose stores, inability to stimulate the release of glucose stores from the liver and increased metabolism that uses up the available glucose. They should be monitored closely until normal blood glucose levels are achieved. It is difficult to assess a neonate's level of mentation, so the critical care paramedic must be alert for the signs of hypoglycemia, which include: twitching, seizure activity, limpness, eye-rolling, high-pitched cry, apnea, or irregular respirations.

CONTENT REVIEW

MULTIPLE CHOICE

1.	D	p. 875	15.	C	p. 881	29.	B	p. 888
2.	D	p. 875	16.	B	p. 881	30.	B	p. 887
3.	B	p. 892	17.	D	p. 881	31.	C	p. 890
4.	C	p. 876	18.	D	p. 882	32.	A	p. 890
5.	D	p. 876	19.	A	p. 882	33.	A	p. 890
6.	A	p. 878	20.	D	p. 882	34.	B	p. 890
7.	D	p. 878	21.	C	p. 882	35.	D	p. 891
8.	B	p. 878	22.	B	p. 883	36.	C	p. 892
9.	A	p. 879	23.	A	p. 884	37.	B	p. 893
10.	B	p. 879	24.	C	p. 884	38.	A	p. 876
11.	C	p. 879	25.	C	p. 884	39.	B	p. 891
12.	D	p. 879	26.	C	p. 884	40.	D	p. 888
13.	C	p. 879	27.	D	p. 887			
14.	A	p. 879	28.	A	p. 887			

Chapter 30: Answer Key

CASE STUDY

1. Drowning is defined as death from suffocation due to submersion in liquid within 24 hours of insult. Survival past the 24-hour point is categorized as near-drowning.

2. The principle insult in drowning is hypoxia. When immersed, the initial natural tendency is to hold your breath, even though panic and hysteria make this very difficult. At some point, the stimulus to breathe overrides the voluntary ability of the victim to hold his breath, and he will gasp for air. This sudden influx of liquid will cause either laryngospasm, causing "dry drowning," or inhalation of the liquid, which would cause a "wet drowning." Up to 15 percent of drownings are dry and the remaining 85 percent are wet. When salt water enters the lungs, surfactant can be washed away and collapse of the alveoli occurs. In a freshwater drowning, the water moves from the alveolar space into the vascular space because of osmotic pressure. Although these are obviously different mechanisms, the principle problem remains hypoxia and correcting it remains the best determinant of prognosis. A high index of suspicion should be maintained for spinal and head injuries in these patients due to the high incidence of diving accidents often associated with drowning. Drowning which occurs in cold water causes core body function to slow down and allows hypothermic states to develop. This process causes blood to be shunted to coronary and cerebral circulation.

3. Regardless of the mechanism of injury, special attention must be given to the management of the patient's airway. If the patient remains hypoxic despite administration of high-flow, high-concentration oxygen, then positive pressure ventilation using at least 5 cm H_2O of PEEP should be initiated. Some patients may do well on noninvasive positive pressure ventilation, but some patients will require traditional intubation and ventilation. Decompression of the stomach via NG or OG tube can be very helpful, as many drowning victims swallow a great deal of water and that can prevent the diaphragm from fully expanding. Inhaled beta-agonists may be helpful in reversing bronchospasm and any cold induced bronchorrhea. Removal of excess fluid in the intravascular space may be accomplished by the use of diuretics. Finally, victims of cold water drowning who do not present as obviously dead should be resuscitated and warmed until normothermic.

CONTENT REVIEW

MULTIPLE CHOICE

1.	B	p. 897	16.	C	p. 904	31.	D	p. 907
2.	D	p. 897	17.	A	p. 905	32.	A	p. 907
3.	A	p. 897	18.	B	p. 905	33.	C	p. 907
4.	C	p. 897	19.	A	p. 905	34.	A	p. 907
5.	C	p. 897	20.	C	p. 904	35.	B	p. 908
6.	B	p. 899	21.	D	p. 904	36.	B	p. 908
7.	A	p. 899	22.	A	p. 905	37.	C	p. 908
8.	C	p. 900	23.	B	p. 904	38.	A	p. 910
9.	D	p. 900	24.	C	p. 905	39.	C	p. 912
10.	A	p. 901	25.	D	p. 905	40.	A	p. 911
11.	B	p. 901	26.	D	p. 905	41.	A	p. 911
12.	C	p. 901	27.	B	p. 906	42.	D	p. 909
13.	D	p. 903	28.	B	p. 906	43.	B	p. 912
14.	B	p. 903	29.	D	p. 906	44.	A	p. 912
15.	C	p. 903	30.	C	p. 905	45.	A	p. 912

Chapter 31: Answer Key

CASE STUDY

1a. The signs and symptoms of pulmonary overexpansion injuries are usually apparent soon after surfacing. Dyspnea, altered consciousness, difficulty in coordination of movement, chest pain, bleeding from the mouth and nose, weakness, and fatigue are all clues that an overexpansion injury may exist. The management of pulmonary overexpansion injuries is best performed in a hyperbaric chamber. The possibility that decompression sickness may accompany ascent barotraumas is very real and hyperbaric therapy can reduce the size of any gas emboli present. Management en route to the chamber consists of ensuring oxygenation, supporting inadequate breathing, and providing circulatory support.

1b. The signs and symptoms of decompression sickness start mildly and worsen as small bubbles expand and combine to form larger bubbles. Pain in joints and muscles are present in most patients and are usually apparent within 24 to 48 hours after surfacing. Additional signs and symptoms of severe decompression sickness include sensory impairment, headache, vertigo, loss of muscle coordination or paralysis, seizures, and coma. A severe manifestation known as "chokes" is seen in some worst-case scenarios, resulting in complaints of chest pain, dyspnea, and moderate to severe pulmonary edema. The definitive treatment for decompression sickness is recompression in a hyperbaric chamber so that the nitrogen in the body can safely exit over time. Management en route to the chamber consists of ensuring oxygenation, supporting inadequate breathing, and providing circulatory support. Diazepam or midazolam should be given to treat seizures or severe cramping.

CONTENT REVIEW

MULTIPLE CHOICE

1. B	p. 918	11. A	p. 923	21. D	p. 928
2. A	p. 918	12. B	p. 923	22. B	p. 929
3. C	p. 918	13. C	p. 924	23. B	p. 930
4. C	p. 919	14. D	p. 924	24. A	p. 931
5. A	p. 919	15. C	p. 925	25. B	p. 931
6. D	p. 919	16. B	p. 925	26. C	p. 930
7. D	p. 920	17. D	p. 926	27. A	p. 931
8. B	p. 920	18. A	p. 925	28. D	p. 932
9. B	p. 921	19. A	p. 925	29. D	p. 932
10. D	p. 923	20. C	p. 927		

Chapter 32: Answer Key

CASE STUDY

1. The role of a U.S. Poison Control Center (PCC) is to assist with the triage and management of patients with (potentially) toxic exposures. Critical care paramedics should take full advantage of the knowledge and resources available through consultation of a poison control center. They can be reached by phone at 800-222-1222.

2. Selective serotonin reuptake inhibitors (SSRI) work by interfering with the normal reuptake of serotonin in the brain. SSRI medications increase the availability of serotonin or other neurotransmitters (i.e., dopamine or norepinephrine) in the central nervous system. Mild overdoses lead to nausea, lethargy, tremors, and mild to moderate hypotension typically associated with reflex tachycardia. Massive overdoses can present with significant hypotension, severe agitation, tremor, or seizures. Respiratory distress (from hypoventilation or aspiration) and coma are possible. The coingestion of several different proserotonergic medications can lead to serotonin syndrome. SSRIs, MAO-Is, lithium, amphetamines, dextromethorphan, meperidine, and many other drugs all lead to increased serotonin levels. Patients with serotonin syndrome can present with altered mental status (delirium, agitation, seizures), autonomic instability (fever, tachycardia, hypertension, or hypotension), and neuromuscular derangements (myoclonus and rigidity). Patients with true serotonin syndrome often require hemodynamic monitoring, IV hydration, active control of hyperthermia, and benzodiazepines for rigidity. Paralysis and intubation may be necessary to achieve adequate oxygenation and ventilation in the compromised patient.

CONTENT REVIEW

MULTIPLE CHOICE

1. C	p. 937	24. B	p. 941	46. C	p. 948
2. D	p. 937	25. D	p. 942	47. B	p. 948
3. C	p. 938	26. C	p. 942,	48. B	p. 949
4. C	p. 938		943	49. D	p. 949
5. A	p. 938	27. D	p. 942	50. A	p. 949
6. B	p. 938	28. D	p. 939	51. C	p. 950
7. D	p. 939	29. C	p. 939	52. B	p. 950
8. B	p. 938	30. A	p. 942	53. D	p. 950
9. C	p. 939	31. C	p. 943	54. B	p. 950
10. D	p. 938	32. B	p. 945	55. C	p. 950
11. C	p. 938	33. D	p. 945	56. A	p. 950
12. A	p. 939	34. C	p. 945	57. D	p. 950
13. C	p. 940	35. B	p. 945	58. A	p. 951
14. A	p. 940	36. A	p. 946	59. B	p. 951
15. D	p. 940	37. D	p. 946	60. B	p. 952
16. B	p. 941	38. C	p. 946	61. C	p. 952
17. B	p. 941	39. D	p. 947	62. A	p. 953
18. A	p. 941	40. A	p. 947	63. D	p. 955
19. C	p. 941	41. B	p. 947	64. B	p. 955
20. A	p. 941	42. D	p. 947	65. C	p. 955
21. A	p. 939	43. D	p. 948	66. C	p. 955
22. C	p. 941	44. A	p. 948	67. D	p. 955
23. A	p. 941	45. A	p. 948	68. B	p. 955

Chapter 33: Answer Key

CASE STUDY

1. CBRNE agents are defined as chemical, biological, radiological, nuclear, and explosive agents or substances that possess the ability to cause illness or injury to exposed victims.

2. The first priority for the critical care paramedic is the safety of the crew and the patient. To ensure that the crew is not exposed to any hazardous substances, any casualty of a CBRNE or toxic industrial chemicals (TIC)/toxic industrial materials (TIM) incident must be thoroughly decontaminated and must not be a risk for off-gasing. Off-gasing is the emanation of vapor, usually from chemicals trapped in clothing or on the patient's body. With few exceptions, patients adequately decontaminated during initial care will not pose a threat to the critical care paramedic providing care for the patient during interfacility transport missions. In these rare instances, the critical care paramedic must wear appropriate chemical protective equipment and treat the patients as though they are still contaminated. Following care of these patients, it is critical to ensure that all personnel, equipment, supplies, and vehicles are free of contamination before being returned to service.

3. Incapacitating and irritant agents include the tear gases known formally as chlorobenzylidenemalononitrile (CS) and chloroacetophenone (CN), and common pepper spray, which is oleoresin capsicum (OC). These substances produce transient local pain and involuntary eye closure that can render the exposed patient temporarily incapable of normal activity. Law enforcement agencies commonly use these agents for riot control, barricade situations, and to control violent subjects. These agents cause immediate pain and burning sensation in exposed mucous membranes and skin. Clinical effects occur almost immediately following exposure, but seldom persist longer than a few minutes after exposure has ended. Although unlikely, bronchospasm is a concern following exposure to these types of agents. Acute exacerbation of pre-existing reactive airway disease may occur. In these cases, bronchoconstriction is usually transient when treated with bronchodilating agents.

CONTENT REVIEW

MULTIPLE CHOICE

1. C	*p. 962*	16. D	*p. 967*	31. D	*p. 974*
2. D	*p. 963*	17. D	*p. 970*	32. B	*p. 974*
3. B	*p. 963*	18. C	*p. 968*	33. B	*p. 977*
4. B	*p. 964*	19. A	*p. 968*	34. A	*p. 973*
5. D	*p. 965*	20. B	*p. 971*	35. C	*p. 976*
6. B	*p. 965*	21. B	*p. 968*	36. D	*p. 976*
7. C	*p. 964*	22. C	*p. 970*	37. D	*p. 976*
8. A	*p. 965*	23. D	*p. 969*	38. B	*p. 977*
9. B	*p. 968*	24. A	*p. 973*	39. D	*p. 972*
10. A	*p. 965*	25. C	*p. 973*	40. A	*p. 979*
11. C	*p. 965*	26. D	*p. 975*	41. B	*p. 979*
12. D	*p. 966*	27. B	*p. 973*	42. A	*p. 979*
13. B	*p. 969*	28. B	*p. 977*	43. A	*p. 980*
14. A	*p. 968*	29. B	*p. 973*	44. D	*p. 981*
15. B	*p. 967*	30. D	*p. 973*	45. C	*p. 983*

Chapter 34: Answer Key

CASE STUDY

1. Neurologic death, or brain death, is defined as the complete irreversible cessation of all brain and brain stem activity. The generally established criteria for brain death include: explained loss of consciousness, no motor response to painful stimuli, no brain stem reflexes, and apnea.

2. The organ donor is prepped and draped in normal surgical fashion according to established hospital procedure. A midline incision is made from just above the pubic bone to the sternal notch. The organs are exposed and examined for any obvious anatomical abnormalities. The surgical teams isolate the vasculature of each organ in preparation for removal from the body. The teams place cannulas into the great vessels to allow preservation solution to be flushed into the organs. When everything is ready, the aorta is cross-clamped, the chest and abdominal cavities are cooled rapidly using sterile ice, and cold preservation solutions are flushed through the vessels into the organs. The organs are further examined to ensure that the preservation solution flows well and that there are no vascular abnormalities. The organs are removed from the body and taken to a back table for further inspection and packaging. Once packaged, they are transported back to the transplant center for implantation into the recipient.

3. A variety of human tissue can be donated by anyone who has suffered a cardiac death and has a suitable medical and social history. This is unlike organ donation, which requires brain death and there are strict legislative requirements to determine brain death. Medical and social history requirements also differ between organ and tissue donors. Very few tissues are transplanted quickly and only under emergent situations. Organs have to be transplanted immediately and this is accomplished at a greater risk and expense. If waiting recipients do not receive the organ that they need, they will certainly die. Therefore, certain medical conditions are overlooked for organs, as long as the organ functions properly. Tissue donation does not overlook any disease. If there is a risk of transmission of communicable disease or a risk to the quality of the tissue, then the tissue is ruled unsuitable and is not recovered.

   Tissue donation involves all areas of the human body. Tissues that may be used for donation include: the dura mater, whole eyes or corneas, the mandible, skin grafts, the heart valves, bones and tendons and the greater saphenous and femoral veins.

CONTENT REVIEW

MULTIPLE CHOICE

1. A	*p. 990*	10. D	*p. 992*	19. C	*p. 995*
2. B	*p. 990*	11. A	*p. 992*	20. A	*p. 996*
3. D	*p. 990*	12. B	*p. 993*	21. A	*p. 997*
4. D	*p. 991*	13. B	*p. 994*	22. B	*p. 998*
5. C	*p. 991*	14. A	*p. 994*	23. D	*p. 998*
6. A	*p. 991*	15. D	*p. 994*	24. D	*p. 999*
7. D	*p. 991*	16. C	*p. 994*	25. C	*p. 994*
8. B	*p. 992*	17. C	*p. 994*		
9. C	*p. 992*	18. B	*p. 994*		

Chapter 35: Answer Key

CASE STUDY

1. Throughout the history of business, there has been continued evolution in the notion of what quality is, in both theory and practice. A fundamental tenet of quality is customer satisfaction. The purpose of business is to satisfy the customer. People have come to expect quality in every product or service. Health care, including EMS, is certainly no different. For your critical care service to maintain operational viability, the quality of service provided must be consistently sustained. All of the quality improvement initiatives, policies, and procedures should be meticulously documented to ensure a consistent application of the management practices.

2. A good QI program develops a process by which all aspects of clinical care and operational processes are evaluated and measured. These processes serve to provide key performance indicators (KPI) for your agency. Examples of retrospective analysis may include the critical care team patient care report and documentation, treatment evaluations, or hospital pickup times. Concurrent initiatives may be compiled by direct supervision of tasks or skills. Concurrent evaluations should also be included in the KPI report. These KPIs should also be very descriptive and tell the reader all of the details about measurement. The policy may include who is responsible for the measuring, why it is being measured, how to gather data, how to document the data, and who receives the report.

CONTENT REVIEW

MULTIPLE CHOICE

1. A	*p. 1004*	7. B	*p. 1007*	13. C	*p. 1011*
2. C	*p. 1004*	8. D	*p. 1008*	14. D	*p. 1012*
3. B	*p. 1006*	9. C	*p. 1008*	15. D	*p. 1013*
4. D	*p. 1006*	10. A	*p. 1009*	16. B	*p. 1016*
5. C	*p. 1006*	11. C	*p. 1010*		
6. A	*p. 1007*	12. B	*p. 1011*		

Chapter 36: Answer Key

CASE STUDY

1. Communication devices used before the critical care transport are mostly used by a communications specialist in the dispatch center and often include: telephones, radios, logging recorders, computer terminals, camera monitors, weather radar, mapping system, and fax machines. Communication devices used during and after the critical care transport may be used by and between: the pilot, air traffic, air traffic control, incident command, care providers, communication specialists, and receiving and sending hospitals.

2. The potential complications of illegible, incomplete, or inaccurate documentation have both medical and legal consequences. The medical consequences are naturally the most severe since care decisions may be made based on your submitted patient care report and if there are errors or omissions, the consequence can be poor patient care. In a court of law, what you document is many times what is debated, not what you actually did. Even though your patient care may have been exemplary on a particular transport, if the documentation does not reflect this, you may be found liable or negligent for the damages the plaintiff is claiming. Additionally, poor documentation practices will lead your program's administration, quality assurance committees, and billing departments to become more aware of your practices. These aforementioned intra-organizational departments rely heavily on the quality of the documentation provided by the critical care teams, and progressive correctional action may be taken against the critical care provider who continually fails to document appropriately.

CONTENT REVIEW

MULTIPLE CHOICE

1. D	*p. 1032*	10. D	*p. 1037*	19. B	*p. 1042*
2. A	*p. 1033*	11. A	*p. 1038*	20. D	*p. 1043*
3. D	*p. 1033*	12. C	*p. 1039*	21. C	*p. 1044*
4. B	*p. 1034*	13. B	*p. 1040*	22. D	*p. 1046*
5. D	*p. 1035*	14. C	*p. 1040*	23. A	*p. 1047*
6. C	*p. 1037*	15. D	*p. 1040*	24. C	*p. 1042*
7. B	*p. 1037*	16. B	*p. 1040*	25. B	*p. 1047*
8. A	*p. 1037*	17. D	*p. 1041*		
9. C	*p. 1037*	18. B	*p. 1042*		

Chapter 37: Answer Key

CASE STUDY

1. Some common hospital departments where the critical care paramedic may work alongside other health care providers include: the emergency department, critical care unit, cardiac catheterization and electrophysiology laboratory, diagnostic noninvasive cardiology laboratory, and interventional radiology suite.

2. The critical care paramedic skills that may be employed in the hospital setting include: patient assessment and reassessment, management of airway, ECG monitoring, patient movement and handling, charting and documentation tasks, medication administration, IV initiation, immobilization, equipment preparation (central lines, suturing, ECG, EEG, IABP, casting and splinting, and wound dressing), venous blood sampling, bedside cardiac enzyme testing, specialized monitoring (capnography, bedside BGL determination, and pulse oximetry), and aerosolized and nebulized bronchodilator therapy.

CONTENT REVIEW

MULTIPLE CHOICE

1. A	*p. 1053*	5. C	*p. 1055*	9. B	*p. 1061*
2. C	*p. 1053*	6. C	*p. 1056*	10. A	*p. 1053*
3. B	*p. 1053*	7. A	*p. 1057*		
4. D	*p. 1054*	8. D	*p. 1061*		

EMERGENCY DRUG CARDS

NITROPRUSSIDE SODIUM (Nitropress, Nipride)

Classification: Cardiovascular agent, antihypertensive agent, non-nitrate vasodilator
Actions: Relaxes venous and arterial smooth muscle, decreases preload, decreases afterload
Indications: Hypertensive emergency, hypertensive encephalopathy, cardiogenic shock
Contraindications: Hypotension, lactation, known hypersensitivity
Side effects: Hypotension, flushing, nausea/vomiting, thiocyanate poisoning (blurred vision, tinnitus, altered mental status, seizures)
Dose: 0.5–10 mcg/kg/min infusion
Special considerations: Monitor BP and cardiac rhythm closely, start low, titrate to effect. Caution in patients with renal and hepatic dysfunction. Administer in light-resistant container, metabolizes to thiocyanate. Infusions > 72 hrs increase risk of thiocyanate poisoning

NITROGLYCERIN IV (Tridil, Nitrostat IV)

Classification: Cardiovascular agent, vasodilator, nitrate
Actions: Smooth muscle relaxant of vascular and coronary smooth muscle, decreases systolic and diastolic BP, decreases cardiac workload, improves coronary artery perfusion
Indications: Ischemic chest pain, AMI, hypertension
Contraindications: Hypotension, known hypersensitivity
Side effects: Hypotension, headache, cardiac palpitations, reflexive tachycardia, flushing, methemoglobinemia
Dose: 5–50 mcg/min infusion
Special considerations: Monitor closely for development of hypotension

NESIRITIDE (Natrecor)

Classification: Cardiovascular agent, atrial natriuretic peptide hormone
Actions: Relaxes vascular smooth muscle, decreases preload, decreases afterload
Indications: CHF
Contraindications: Hypotension, valvular stenosis, restrictive or obstructive cardiomyopathies, cardiac tamponade
Side effects: Hypotension, cardiac dysrhythmia, angina, headache, palpitations
Dose: 2 mcg/kg IV push over 60 seconds, followed by a 0.01 mcg/kg/min maintenance infusion
Special considerations: Monitor BP and cardiac rhythm closely, caution in pregnant or lactating patients
Dedicated IV line: Do not administer in same IV line as other meds

NITROPRUSSIDE SODIUM

NITROGLYCERIN IV

NESIRITIDE

HYDRALAZINE HYDROCHLORIDE (Apresoline, Alazine)

Classification: Cardiovascular agent, non-nitrate vasodilator, antihypertensive agent

Actions: Direct arterial vasodilation via unknown mechanism results in decreased systolic and diastolic BP

Indications: Hypertensive emergency, first-line agent in pre-eclampsia, CHF, unexplained pulmonary hypertension

Contraindications: CAD, mitral valve disease, hypotension, AMI, known hypersensitivity, persistent tachycardia

Side effects: Hypotension, dizziness, headache, tachycardia, angina pectoris, nausea/vomiting, decreased hematocrit and hemoglobin

Dose: 5–40 mg IV push over 1–2 minutes

Special considerations: Monitor BP and cardiac rhythm closely, use caution when administering with beta blockers, hypotension may develop

NICARDIPINE HYDROCHLORIDE (Cardene, Cardene IV)

Classification: Cardiovascular agent, calcium channel blocker, antihypertensive agent

Actions: Decreases myocardial contractility, vascular smooth muscle dilation, decreased systemic vascular resistance

Indications: Hypertensive emergency, angina pectoris

Contraindications: Known hypersensitivity, lactation, advanced aortic stenosis

Side effects: Hypotension, palpitations, tachycardia, CNS disturbances

Dose: *Adult:* 5 mg/hr, can increase by 2.5 mg/hr q 15 minutes if needed. Max dose 15 mg/hour.
Pediatric: 1–3 mcg/kg/min for children 9 days–10 years old

Special considerations: Can be used alone or with beta blockers in treatment of stable angina. Can be used alone or with other antihypertensive agents for treatment of hypertension. Monitor patients closely, especially patients receiving multiple vasoactive medications. Use with caution in CHF, hepatic dysfunction, pregnancy

FENOLDOPAM MESYLATE (Corlopam)

Classification: Cardiovascular agent, non-nitrate vasodilator, antihypertensive agent, dopamine agonist

Actions: Dopamine receptor agonist, decreases peripheral vascular resistance. Decreases systolic and diastolic BP, increases renal blood flow

Indications: Severe hypertension

Contraindications: Known hypersensitivity, not for use with beta blockers

Side effects: Headache, nervousness, vertigo, hypotension, tachycardia, T-wave inversion, flushing, palpitations, dysrhythmias, AMI, heart failure, and increased creatinine, BUN, and glucose levels

Dose: 0.025–0.3 mcg/kg/min infusion, may be increased by 0.05–0.1 mcg/kg/min q 15 minutes

Special considerations: Use with caution in patients with asthma, hepatic cirrhosis, portal hypertension, and ariceal bleeding. Monitor BP and cardiac rhythm closely

HYDRALAZINE HYDROCHLORIDE

NICARDIPINE HYDROCHLORIDE

FENOLDOPAM MESYLATE

CLONIDINE HYDROCHLORIDE (Catapres, Dixaril)

Classification: Cardiovascular agent, CNS agent, analgesic
Actions: CNS alpha-adrenergic receptor stimulator, results in inhibition of sympathetic vasomotor centers and decreased nerve impulses. Reduces systolic and diastolic BP, produces bradycardia, and inhibits renin release from kidneys
Indications: Hypertension, especially useful if no IV access. Ethanol and opiate withdrawal syndrome
Contraindications: Hypotension, altered mental status, known hypersensitivity
Side effects: Hypotension, bradycardia/tachycardia, angioedema, weakness, somnolence
Dose: *Adult:* 0.1–0.2 mg oral/sublingual. *Pediatric:* 5–10 mcg/kg per day, divided over 8–12 hours
Special considerations: Monitor BP, airway, and cardiac rhythm closely

ENALAPRIL (Vasotec IV)

Classification: Cardiovascular agent, ACE inhibitor, antihypertensive agent
Actions: Inhibits the conversion of angiotensin I to angiotensin II, resulting in vasodilation and decreased preload and afterload
Indications: Mild to moderate hypertension, CHF, AMI
Contraindications: Hypotension, cardiogenic shock, known hypersensitivity
Side effects: Hypotension, tachycardia, palpitations, angioedema, nausea/vomiting, renal dysfunction, hyperkalemia
Dose: *Adult:* 1.25 mg slow IV push over 5 minutes, repeat q 6 hours. *Pediatric:* 5–10 mcg/kg IV q 8 hours
Special considerations: Caution in patients with renal dysfunction, renal artery stenosis, or who receive dialysis. Monitor BP and cardiac rhythm closely. Monitor lab values for hyperkalemia

ESMOLOL HYDROCHLORIDE (Brevibloc)

Classification: Parasympathomimetic, sympatholytic
Actions: Blocks beta-adrenergic receptors, inhibiting the effects of circulating catecholamines, resulting in negative dromotropic, chronotropic, and inotropic effects
Indications: Hypertensive emergency, SVT, PSVT, AMI
Contraindications: Cardiac failure, hypotension, AV heart block greater than a first degree, sinus bradycardia, moderate to severe CHF
Side effects: Hypotension, bradycardia, development of heart block, bronchospasm, headache, dizziness, confusion, nausea/vomiting
Dose: 500 mcg/kg over 1 minute, followed by a maintenance infusion of 50 mcg/kg/min. Can be increased q 5–10 minutes to a max of 300 mcg/kg/min
Special considerations: Use cautiously in patients with asthma, emphysema, CHF, or renal dysfunction. Monitor vital signs and cardiac rhythm closely, discontinue infusion immediately if heart block, bradycardia, or hypotension develops

CLONIDINE HYDROCHLORIDE

ENALAPRIL

ESMOLOL HYDROCHLORIDE

LABETALOL HYDROCHLORIDE (Normodyne, Trandate)

Classification: Parasympathomimetic, nonselective beta-adrenergic agonist, antihypertensive agent
Actions: Slows SA node discharge and AV node conduction. Decreased ventricular inotropy. Diminished peripheral vascular resistance. Longer half-life, duration of action compared to Esmolol
Indications: Hypertensive emergencies, especially those with increased ICP such as CVA, intracranial hemorrhage, traumatic brain injury
Contraindications: Bronchial asthma, bradycardia, hypotension, heart block, heart failure
Side effects: Bradycardia, hypotension, cardiac dysrhythmia, dizziness, fatigue, nausea/ vomiting, CHF
Dose: 20 mg IV push slowly over 2 minutes, can repeat 40–80 mg IV push q 10 minutes until desired effect to a max dose of 300 mg. Maintenance infusion 2 mg/min, titrate to effect
Special considerations: Monitor BP, cardiac rhythm closely, use with caution in COPD

DOPAMINE HYDROCHLORIDE (Intropin, Dopastat)

Classification: Sympathomimetic, α- and β-adrenergic agonist
Actions: Positive inotropic and chronotropic effects, peripheral vasoconstriction
Indications: Hypoperfusion secondary to AMI, CHF, sepsis, neurologically induced vasodilation, renal failure
Contraindications: Hypovolemia, pheochromocytoma, uncontrolled tachycardia, ventricular irritability, hypertension
Side effects: Tachycardia, hypertension, ventricular irritability, angina, anxiety, decreased peripheral perfusion, extravasation, tissue necrosis
Dose: *Adult:* titrate to effect. *Renal dose:* 2–5 mcg/kg/min. *Cardiac dose:* 5–15 mcg/kg/min. *Vasopressor dose:* > 15 mcg/kg/min. *Pediatric:* Start at 5 mcg/kg/min, titrate to effect
Special considerations: Be alert for cardiac compromise. Do not administer as IV bolus. Ensure IV patency, be alert for extravasation

DOBUTAMINE HYDROCHLORIDE (Dobutrex)

Classification: Sympathomimetic, β-adrenergic agonist, catecholamine
Actions: Positive inotropic and chronotropic effects
Indications: CHF, decompensating cardiomyopathy
Contraindications: Preexisting hypertension, tachycardia, acute coronary syndrome with ventricular irritability, idiopathic hypertropic subaortic stenosis, known history of hypersensitivity to sympathomimetic amines
Side effects: Tachycardia, hypertension, cardiac dysrhythmia, anginal pain, anxiety, decreased peripheral perfusion, extravasation, tissue necrosis, and nausea and vomiting
Dose: 2–20 mcg/kg/min, titrated to desired hemodynamic response
Special considerations: Do not administer as IV bolus, ensure IV patency and be alert for extravasation

LABETALOL HYDROCHLORIDE

DOPAMINE HYDROCHLORIDE

DOBUTAMINE HYDROCHLORIDE

PHENYLEPHRINE HYDROCHLORIDE (Neo-Synephrine)

Classification: Sympathomimetic, mydriatic, decongestant
Actions: Venous and arterial vasoconstriction results in increases in preload and elevated systolic and diastolic pressures
Indications: Vascular shock, BP maintenance during anesthesia
Contraindications: CAD, hypertension, ventricular tachycardia
Side effects: Tachycardia, hypertension, ventricular irritability, angina, anxiety, extravasation, tissue necrosis
Dose: 0.1–0.18 mg/min until the blood pressure stabilizes, followed by a 0.04–0.06 mg/min maintenance infusion
Special considerations: Use cautiously in patients with hyperthyroidism, diabetes mellitus, myocardial disease, cerebral arteriosclerosis, bradycardia

NOREPINEPHRINE BITARTRATE (Levarterenol, Levophed, Noradrenaline)

Classification: Sympathomimetic, alpha- and beta-adrenergic agonist
Actions: Alpha-adrenergic stimulation results in arterial and venous vasoconstriction
Indications: Septic shock, hypotension associated with sympathectomy, spinal cord injury, and poliomyelitis
Contraindications: Hypertension, shock secondary to hypovolemia
Side effects: Decreased renal perfusion, tachycardia, hypertension, cardiac dysrhythmia, decreased peripheral perfusion, extravasation, tissue necrosis
Dose: 0.5–1 mcg/min, titrate up to 30 mcg/min as needed to desired hemodynamic effect; typical therapeutic dose range 8–12 mcg/min
Special considerations: Monitor BP and cardiac rhythm, ensure IV patency.
Use caution in patients with hyperthyroidism, heart disease

EPINEPHRINE HYDROCHLORIDE (Adrenaline Chloride)

Classification: Sympathomimetic, alpha- and beta-adrenergic agonist, bronchodilator
Actions: Alpha- and beta-adrenergic stimulation results in increased chronotropy, inotropy, and dromotropy, peripheral vasoconstriction, and bronchodilation
Indications: Cardiac arrest, shock, bronchoconstriction
Contraindications: No contraindications in cardiac arrest. In the non-cardiac arrest, contraindications include hypertension, tachycardia, acute coronary syndrome, narrow angle glaucoma, and advanced age
Side effects: Tachycardia, hypertension, palpitations, cardiac dysrhythmias, tissue necrosis with infiltration, transient elevations in blood glucose levels
Dose: *Adult:*
       Anaphylaxis: 0.1–0.5 mg SQ/IM or IV
       Arrest rhythms: 1 mg IVP as needed q 3–5 minutes
       Refractory bradycardia: 2–10 mcg/min infusion
       Refractory hypotension: 1–4 mcg/min infusion, titrate to desired effect
    Pediatric:
       Anaphylaxis: 0.01 mcg/kg SQ/IM or IV
       Arrest rhythms: 0.01 mg/kg initial dose, 0.1 mg/kg subsequent doses IV push
       q 3–5 minutes followed by a 0.1–1 mcg/min infusion
Special considerations: Monitor BP and cardiac rhythm, protect from light

PHENYLEPHRINE HYDROCHLORIDE

NOREPINEPHRINE BITARTRATE

EPINEPHRINE HYDROCHLORIDE

VASOPRESSIN INJECTION (Pitressin)

Classification: Hormone, antidiuretic
Actions: ADH properties promote vascular smooth muscle constriction resulting in elevated systemic vascular resistance
Indications: Diabetes insipidus, polyuria secondary to ADH insufficiency, cardiac arrest, vasodilatory shock
Contraindications: Known hypersensitivity, chronic nephritis, advanced arteriosclerosis, ischemic heart disease. No contraindications in cardiac arrest
Side effects: Bronchoconstriction, pallor, nausea, abdominal cramping, angina, hypertension, dysrhythmia, respiratory congestion
Dose: *Non-arrest:* 10 units IV push. *Cardiac arrest:* 40 units IV push
Special considerations: Use with caution in CAD, pregnancy, epilepsy, asthma, heart failure

LIDOCAINE HYDROCHLORIDE (Xylocaine, Dilocaine)

Classification: Antiarrhythmic class IB, cardiovascular agent, CNS agent, local anesthetic
Actions: Suppresses ectopic ventricular foci, raises ventricular fibrillation threshold. Blunts ICP in RSI, though its efficacy is questioned. Local anesthetic properties
Indications: Ventricular ectopy and dysrhythmia
Contraindications: Known hypersensitivity, Stokes-Adams syndrome, ventricular ectopy in the presence of bradycardia
Side effects: Anxiety, seizures, hypotension, bradycardia, cardiac dysrhythmia, nausea/vomiting, drowsiness, paresthesia
Dose: *Adult:* 1–1.5 mg/kg IV over 3 minutes, repeat q 5–15 minutes to a max dose of 3 mg/kg followed by a maintenance infusion of 1–4 mg/min. *Pediatric:* 0.5–1 mg/kg followed by a maintenance infusion of 20–50 mcg/kg/min
Special considerations: Use with caution in renal, hepatic failure. Lidocaine toxicity

PROCAINAMIDE HYDROCHLORIDE (Pronestyl, Procan)

Classification: Cardiovascular agent, antiarrhythmic class IA
Actions: Suppresses conduction velocity through conduction system (atria, AV node, Purkinje system), prolongs atrial refractory period, negative inotropic and chronotropic effects
Indications: Ventricular dysrhythmias
Contraindications: Known drug allergy, myasthenia gravis, blood dyscrasias, AV conduction blocks, Torsades de Pointes, asymptomatic premature ventricular contraction, digitalis toxicity, hypotension
Side effects: Hypotension, conduction defects
Dose: 20 mg/min loading infusion until max dose of 17 mg/kg is reached, cessation of ectopy, hypotension develops, QRS or QT lengthens. Maintenance infusion 1–4 mg/min, titrated to effect
Special considerations: Monitor blood pressure and cardiac rhythm closely

VASOPRESSIN INJECTION

LIDOCAINE HYDROCHLORIDE

PROCAINAMIDE HYDROCHLORIDE

AMIODARONE HYDROCHLORIDE (Cordarone, Pacerone)

Classification: Cardiovascular agent, antiarrhythmic class III
Actions: Blocks sodium and potassium channels, increasing action potential and refractory period duration. Vascular smooth muscle relaxation results in decreased PVR and afterload
Indications: Ventricular dysrhythmia, atrial dysrhythmia refractory to other treatments
Contraindications: Known hypersensitivity to the drug, sinus bradycardia, second- or third-degree heart block, cardiogenic shock, and severe CHF
Side effects: Hypotension, bradycardia, AV blocks, ventricular dysrhythmia, pulmonary toxicity, anorexia, nausea/vomiting
Dose: *Adult:* For perfusing ventricular dysrhythmias administer 150 mg bolus IV over 10 minutes (15 mg/min) followed by a maintenance infusion of 1 mg/min over first 6 hours then 0.5 mg/min over the next 18 hours. For nonperfusing ventricular dysrhythmias administer 150 mg IV bolus, may be repeated once at 300 mg after 5–15 minutes. *Pediatric:* 5 mg/kg IV/IO rapid IV bolus, max dose 15 mg/kg
Special considerations: Correct hypokalemia or hypomagnesemia prior to administration, protect from light

ATROPINE SULFATE (Atropine)

Classification: Sympathomimetic, parasympatholytic, antimuscarinic agent
Actions: Blocks acetylcholine receptors, resulting in tachycardia and smooth muscle dilation. Used to reduce oral secretions prior to RSI
Indications: Increased parasympathetic tone, RSI
Contraindications: Known hypersensitivity to belladonna alkaloids
Side effects: Palpitations, tachycardia, dry mouth, dilated pupils, anxiety
Dose: *Adult cardiac:* 0.5 to 1 mg IVP q 3–5 minutes, max dose of 0.04 mg/kg. Adult organophosphate poisoning: 2–3 mg IVP, repeat as needed. *Pediatric:* 0.01–0.03 mg/kg IVP
Special considerations: Monitor blood pressure and cardiac rhythm closely, additive effect with other anticholinergic agents

ADENOSINE (Adenocard, Adenoscan)

Classification: Cardiovascular agent, antiarrhythmic class IA
Actions: Blocks K^+ channels in conduction system, slowing conduction through AV node and reentry pathways
Indications: SVT
Contraindications: AV block, sick sinus syndrome
Side effects: Heart block, VT/VF, flushing, palpitations, anxiety
Dose: 6 mg rapid IVP followed by 10–20 cc normal saline flush, may be repeated twice at 12 mg rapid IVP. Max dose 30 mg
Special considerations: Monitor heart rate and cardiac rhythm closely, warn patient of side effects including dizziness and LOC, effects potentiated with use of carbamazepine, dypyridamol, theophylline lessens effects

AMIODARONE HYDROCHLORIDE

ATROPINE SULFATE

ADENOSINE

MAGNESIUM SULFATE (Epsom Salt)

Classification: Gastrointestinal agent, laxative, electrolyte replacement, anticonvulsant
Actions: Decreases motor endplate sensitivity to acetylcholine and decreases excitability of motor nerve terminals resulting in smooth muscle relaxation
Indications: VT, preterm labor, bronchospasm
Contraindications: Heart block, renal disease, toxemia of pregnancy if delivery imminent
Side effects: Hypotension, tachycardia, maternal and neonatal respiratory depression, flushing, CNS depression, diaphoresis
Dose: *Adult:* 1–2 gm diluted in 100–250 mL D$_5$W, administered over 10–20 minutes
  Pediatric: 25–50 mg/kg IV or IM
Special considerations: Administer slowly. Monitor heart rate and cardiac rhythm closely, have calcium gluceptate or calcium gluconate available as antidote if OD occurs

DILTIAZEM (Cardizem, Cardizem Lyo-Ject, Cardizem IV)

Classification: Cardiovascular agent, calcium channel blocker, antihypertensive agent
Actions: Blocks calcium channels, slows velocity through SA and AV node, decreases myocardial contractility, and decreases peripheral vascular resistance
Indications: A-fib/A-flutter, SVT
Contraindications: Hypotension, bradycardia, AV block, known hypersensitivity to drug
Side effects: Hypotension, bradycardia, heart block, CHF
Dose: 0.25 mg/kg IV over 2 minutes, repeat 0.35 mg/kg IVP over 2 minutes followed by a maintenance infusion of 5–15 mg/min
Special considerations: Do not administer with IV beta blocker. Monitor vital signs, cardiac rhythm, and blood pressure. Not recommended for infusion over 24 hours duration

PROPRANOLOL HYDROCHLORIDE (Inderal, Apo-Propranolol)

Classification: Sympatholytic, beta-adrenergic antagonist, antihypertensive agent, antiarrhythmic class II
Actions: Blocks beta-2 adrenergic receptors. Stabilizes myocardial membrane and suppresses ectopic foci
Indications: Ventricular dysrhythmia, SVT, prolonged QT syndrome
Contraindications: Asthma, COPD, bradycardia, hypotension, acute CHF
Side effects: Hypotension, bradycardia, AV heart blocks, bronchospasm, decreased myocardial contractility, CHF
Dose: *Adult:* 1–3 mg slow IVP, repeat in 2 minutes if no response, then administer q 4 hours as needed. *Pediatric:* 0.01 mg/kg slow IVP, repeat if necessary to a max dose of 1 mg
Special considerations: Administer no faster than 1 mg/min, potentiation of side effects, use with caution in patients with lung disease

MAGNESIUM SULFATE

DILTIAZEM

PROPRANOLOL HYDROCHLORIDE

ACETYLSALICYLIC ACID (Aspirin)

Classification: CNS agent, analgesic, salicylate, antipyretic
Actions: Inhibits platelet aggregation by decreasing synthesis of blood coagulation factors VII, IX, and X. May also inhibit the action of vitamin K
Indications: Risk of MI, CAD, angina/MI
Contraindications: Allergy to salicylates, bleeding disorders, severe anemia, recent surgery, history of GI bleed
Side effects: Hypersensitivity reactions, anaphylaxis, bleeding, GI upset, thrombocytopenia, nausea/vomiting
Dose: 81–325 mg daily
Special considerations: Rule out allergy prior to administration

MILRINONE LACTATE (Primacor)

Classification: Cardiovascular agent, inotropic agent, vasodilator
Actions: Inhibits peak III cyclic AMP isoenzyme in cardiac and vascular muscle, resulting in an elevation of cyclic AMP and release of calcium. Positive inotropic effect and vasodilation follow
Indications: CHF
Contraindications: Known hypersensitivity, hypotension, aortic/pulmonic valve obstruction
Side effects: Dysrhythmias, hypotension, chest pain, cardiac ischemia, thrombocytopenia
Dose: 50 mcg/kg slow IVP over 10 minutes, followed by a maintenance infusion 0.375–0.75 mcg/kg/min
Special considerations: Monitor vital signs, cardiac rhythm, and blood pressure. Precipitates if infused with furosemide

INAMRINONE LACTATE (Inocor)

Classification: Cardiovascular agent, inotropic agent, vasodilator
Actions: Inhibits peak III cyclic AMP isoenzyme in cardiac and vascular muscle resulting in positive inotropic effects and arterial vasodilation. Increases CO, decreases preload, SVR, and PCWP
Indications: CHF
Contraindications: Hypersensitivity, aortic/pulmonic valve obstruction
Side effects: Hypotension, thrombocytopenia, pain or stiffness at injection site
Dose: 0.75 mcg/kg slow IVP over 2–3 minutes followed by a maintenance infusion of 5–10 mcg/kg/min
Special considerations: Do not mix with furosemide or dextrose-containing solutions. Monitor vital signs, cardiac rhythm, and blood pressure

ACETYLSALICYLIC ACID

MILRINONE LACTATE

INAMRINONE LACTATE

METOPROLOL TARTRATE (Lopressor, Norometoprolol)

Classification: Beta-adrenergic antagonist (sympatholytic), antihypertensive agent, autonomic nervous system agent

Actions: β-1 specific blocking agent. Results in decreased inotropy, chronotropy, and dromotropy

Indications: AMI, hypertension, CHF

Contraindications: Avoid in patients with second- or third-degree AV blocks preexisting bradycardia, hypotension, left ventricular failure, hypersensitivity

Side effects: Hypotension, bradydysrhythmias, bronchospasm, hypoglycemia, dizziness

Dose: *Adult:* 5 mg slow IVP repeated q 5 minutes up to 3 times if needed followed by a maintenance dose of 25–100 mg PO daily

Special considerations: Use with caution in inferior MI, MI with SA/AV node involvement. Monitor vital signs and cardiac rhythm closely

HEPARIN SODIUM (Hepalean)

Classification: Blood former, anticoagulant

Actions: Blocks the conversion of prothrombin to thrombin and fibrinogen to fibrin

Indications: Prophylaxis and treatment of pulmonary embolism in patients with new onset of atrial fibrillation, diagnosis and treatment of acute and chronic consumptive coagulopathies (DIC), prevention of clotting in arterial and cardiac surgery, prophylaxis and treatment of peripheral arterial embolism

Contraindications: Known hypersensitivity, severe thrombocytopenia, active bleeding, bleeding disorders, recent surgery, blood dyscrasia, advanced liver and kidney disease, severe hypertension, suspected intracranial hemorrhage

Side effects: Hemorrhage, thrombocytopenia, chest pain, anaphylactoid reactions, bronchospasm

Dose: Loading dose of 5,000–7,500 units IVP followed by a maintenance infusion based upon partial thromboplastin time (PTT) levels

Special considerations: Monitor partial thromboplastin time (PTT) levels frequently, especially after rebolus or adjusting continuous infusion. Monitor for bleeding. Protamine sulfate used as an antagonist in heparin overdosing. Use guided by PTT levels

ENOXAPARIN (Lovenox)

Classification: Blood former, anticoagulant, low molecular weight heparin

Actions: Low molecular weight heparin with antithrombotic properties. No effect on PT. Does effect thrombin time and activated thromboplastin time

Indications: Antithrombotic agent following surgery, prophylaxis for deep vein thrombosis (DVT) postoperatively, acute coronary syndrome, pulmonary emboli

Contraindications: Drug hypersensitivity, active major bleeding, hemorrhage disorders, recent surgery, blood dyscrasias

Side effects: Mild or severe allergic reaction, hemorrhage, thrombocytopenia, ecchymosis, anemia

Dose: DVT prophylaxis: 30 mg SQ bid. ACS: 1 mg/kg SQ q 2 hours for 2–8 days

Special considerations: No antagonist available, monitor for bleeding, PTT prior to administration, use with caution in patients with HTN, GI disease

METOPROLOL TARTRATE

HEPARIN SODIUM

ENOXAPARIN

WARFARIN SODIUM (Coumadin Sodium, Panwarfin)

Classification: Blood former, anticoagulant, oral anticoagulant
Actions: Depresses hepatic synthesis of vitamin K-dependent coagulation factors
Indications: Prophylaxis and treatment of DVT and pulmonary embolism, treatment of atrial fibrillation with embolization, coronary occlusion, TIA, prophalyxis in patients with prosthetic cardiac valves
Contraindications: Known hypersensitivity, hemorrhagic tendencies, vitamin C or K deficiency, hemophilia, coagulation factor deficiencies, blood dyscrasias, active bleeding, open wounds, extreme diastolic hypertension, cerebral vascular disease, pericarditis with acute MI, severe hepatic or renal disease
Side effects: Bleeding, abdominal pain and cramping, diarrhea, fatigue, nausea, fever, fluid retention, lethargy, liver damage
Dose: 50 mg IVP over 2 minutes
Special considerations: Consult drug compatibility chart as numerous medications react with warfarin. Use with caution in patients with alcoholism, lactation, debilitation, carcinoma, CHF, collagen diseases, hepatic and renal insufficiency, pancreatic disorders, vitamin K deficiency, hypothyroidism, hyperlipidemia, hypercholesterolemia, hereditary resistance to warfarin therapy

---

EPTIFIBATIDE (Integrilin)

Classification: Cardiovascular agent, antithrombotic agent, antiplatelet antibody, glycoprotein IIB/IIIA inhibitor
Actions: Selectively blocks platelet GPIIb/IIIa receptors, inhibiting platelet aggregation
Indications: ACS, need for coronary intervention (PCTA, stenting)
Contraindications: Active pathologic bleeding within 30 days, history of bleeding abnormalities, history of AV malformation, intracranial bleeding, brain tumor, history of recent trauma, uncontrolled hypertension with systolic BP > 200 mmHg, known hypersensitivity
Side effects: Bleeding, anemia, thrombocytopenia
Dose: 180 mcg/kg IV bolus upon diagnosis followed by a maintenance infusion of 2 mcg/kg/min for 72–96 hours
Special considerations: Monitor for bleeding, use with caution in patients with renal insufficiency or failure and those receiving oral anticoagulants or NSAID medications

---

ABCIXIMAB (ReoPro)

Classification: Blood former, anticoagulant, antithrombotic agent, antiplatelet agent, glycoprotein IIb/IIIa inhibitor
Actions: Selectively blocks platelet GPIIb/IIIa receptors, inhibiting platelet aggregation
Indications: ACS, need for coronary intervention (PCTA, stenting)
Contraindications: Active pathologic bleeding within 30 days, history of bleeding abnormalities, history of AV malformation, intracranial bleeding, brain tumor, history of recent trauma
Side effects: Bleeding, including life-threatening hemorrhage, bradycardia, AV blocks, atrial fibrillation, may precipitate hypotension and hematemesis
Dose: 0.25 mg/kg IV administered 10–60 minutes prior to the start of the intervention followed by a maintenance infusion of 10 mg/min for 12 hours after intervention
Special considerations: Monitor for bleeding, use cautiously in patients weighing < 75 kg, older adults, history of GI disease, and PCTA procedures lasting > 70 minutes. Do not agitate/shake vial

WARFARIN SODIUM

EPTIFIBATIDE

ABCIXIMAB

TIROFIBAN HYDROCHLORIDE (Aggrastat)

Classification: Blood former, anticoagulant, antiplatelet agent, glycoprotein IIb/IIIa inhibitor
Actions: Selectively blocks platelet GPIIb/IIIa receptors, inhibiting platelet aggregation
Indications: ACS, need for coronary intervention (PCTA, stenting)
Contraindications: Active pathologic bleeding within 30 days, history of bleeding abnormalities, history of AV malformation, intracranial bleeding, brain tumor, history of recent trauma
Side effects: Bleeding, vasovagal reaction, vertigo, bradycardia, anemia, thrombocytopenia
Dose: 0.4 mcg/kg/min IV for 30 minutes followed by a maintenance infusion of 0.1 mcg/kg/min
Special considerations: Monitor for bleeding, use cautiously with patients with platelet count < 150,000 mm^3

CLOPIDOGREL BISULFATE (Plavix)

Classification: Blood former, anticoagulant, antiplatelet agent
Actions: Inhibits the binding of adenosine diphosphate to its platelet receptor, preventing activation of GPIIb/IIIa complex and platelet aggregation
Indications: AMI, coronary intervention (PCTA, angioplasty), risk of CVA
Contraindications: Hypersensitivity, active pathological bleeding, lactating mothers
Side effects: Life-threatening bleeding, hypertension, syncope, palpitations
Dose: Recent MI: 75 mg PO daily. ACS: 300 mg PO followed by 75 mg daily
Special considerations: Monitor for bleeding, avoid unnecessary invasive procedures. Use with caution in patients receiving other drugs that may induce GI hemorrhage. Moderate concern in patients with hepatic impairment

TENECTEPLASE RECOMBINANT (TNKase)

Classification: Blood former, anticoagulant, thrombolytic enzyme
Actions: Activates plasminogen, converted to plasmin, breaks down fibrin mesh that binds clot, clot dissolves
Indications: AMI
Contraindications: Active internal bleeding, history of CVA, CNS surgery within past 2 months, neoplasm, AV malformations, severe uncontrolled hypertension
Relative contraindications: Recent major surgery, obstetrical delivery, organ biopsy, cerebrovascular disease, recent gastrointestinal or genitourinary bleeding, recent trauma, hypertension with a systolic BP $\geq$ 180 mmHg and/or diastolic BP $\geq$ 110 mmHg, high likelihood of left heart thrombus (ex: mitral stenosis with atrial fibrillation), acute pericarditis, subacute bacterial endocarditis, hemostatic defects, severe hepatic or renal disease, pregnancy, hemorrhagic ophthalmic conditions
Side effects: Bleeding, reperfusion dysrhythmias, cholesterol embolization
Dose: Administered IVP over 5 seconds

    < 60 kg = 30 mg
    60–70 kg = 35 mg
    70–80 kg = 40 mg
    80–90 kg = 45 mg
    > 90 kg = 50 mg

Special considerations: Monitor vital signs and cardiac rhythm, perform baseline neurologic assessment and reassess every 15 minutes. Monitor closely for evidence of internal bleeding. Provide direct pressure to any venipuncture sites for minimum 5 minutes if bleeding occurs. Do not administer any other medication through TNKase line. Should be used in combination with heparin sodium therapy

TIROFIBAN HYDROCHLORIDE

CLOPIDOGREL BISULFATE

TENECTEPLASE RECOMBINANT

RETEPLASE RECOMBINANT (Retavase, rt-PA)

Classification: Blood former, anticoagulant, thrombolytic enzyme
Actions: Activates plasminogen, converts endogenous plasminogan to plasmin, plasmin breaks down fibrin mesh that binds clot, clot dissolves
Indications: AMI
Contraindications: Active internal bleeding, history of CVA, CNS surgery within past 2 months, neoplasm, AV malformations, severe uncontrolled hypertension
Side effects: Bleeding, reperfusion dysrhythmias, anemia
Dose: 10 units IV over 2 minutes, can repeat after 30 minutes
Special considerations: Discontinue concomitant administration of heparin if bleeding develops, monitor bleeding sites

ALTEPLASE RECOMBINANT (Activase, t-PA, Actilyse)

Classification: Blood former, anticoagulant, thrombolytic enzyme
Actions: Activates plasminogen, converted to plasmin, breaks down fibrin mesh that binds clot, clot dissolves
Indications: AMI, acute ischemic stroke, acute pulmonary embolism
Contraindications: Active internal bleeding, history of CVA, CNS hemorrhage within past 2 months, recent trauma, AV malformation, bleeding disorders, uncontrolled hypertension
Side effects: Bleeding, reperfusion dysrhythmias, anemia
Dose: Acute MI
For weight > 67 kg:
15 mg IV over 2 minutes
50 mg IV over next 30 minutes
35 mg IV over next 60 minutes
For weight < 67 kg:
15 mg IVP over 2 minutes
0.75 mg IVP over the next 30 minutes
0.5 mg IVP over the next 60 minutes
Ischemic Stroke
0.9 mg/kg IV, with 10 percent of dose given as bolus over 1 minute
Maximum dose = 90 mg
Pulmonary Embolism:
100 mg IV over 2 hours
Special considerations: Monitor vital signs and cardiac rhythm, perform baseline neurologic assessment, and reassess every 15 minutes. Monitor closely for evidence of internal bleeding. Provide direct pressure to any venipuncture sites for minimum 5 minutes if bleeding occurs. Do not administer any other medication through TNKase line. Should be used in combination with heparin sodium therapy

PHENYTOIN SODIUM (Dilantin)

Classification: CNS agent, anticonvulsant, hydantoin
Actions: Thought to act on motor cortex, stabilizes seizure threshold, antidysrhythmic properties, also has antidysrhythmic properties beneficial for ventricular dsyrhythmias with QT prolongation
Indications: Grand mal, complex seizure activity
Contraindications: Allergy to phenytoin, hypoglycemic seizures, bradycardia, heart blocks, sick sinus syndrome
Side effects: Ataxia, slurred speech, confusion, CNS depression, nystagmus, hypotension with rapid administration, gingival hyperplasia with prolonged use, tissue necrosis with extravasation
Dose: *Adult:* 10–15 mg/kg slow IVP over 30 minutes, or single 1,000 mg loading dose followed with a maintenance dose 4–8 mg/kg slow IVP. *Digitalis toxicity:* 3–5 mg/kg slow IVP. *Pediatric:* 15–20 mg/kg slow IVP
Special considerations: Not compatible with dextrose containing IV solutions, do not administer faster than 50 mg/min, use with caution in patients with hepatic or renal disease

RETEPLASE RECOMBINANT

ALTEPLASE RECOMBINANT

PHENYTOIN SODIUM

PHENOBARBITAL SODIUM (Luminal, Barbital, Solfoton)

Classication: CNS agent, anticonvulsant, sedative-hypnotic, barbiturate
Actions: Inhibits nerve impulse transmission in the cerebral cortex via the ascending reticular activating system resulting in CNS depression and hypnotic effects. Controls the spread of seizures by raising the threshold for motor cortex stimuli
Indications: Grand mal and complex partial seizures, eclampsia, need for sedation
Contraindications: Allergy to barbiturates; significant hepatic, respiratory, or renal disease; significant hypotension
Side effects: Sedation, bradycardia, hypotension, respiratory depression, nystagmus, confusion, ataxia, somnolence
Dose: *Adult:* 100–250 mg IV over 5 minutes. *Pediatric:* 10–20 mg/kg IV over 5 minutes
Special considerations: Monitor for respiratory depression, use with caution in elderly, renal failure

---

FOSPHENYTOIN SODIUM (Cerebyx)

Classification: CNS agent, anticonvulsant, hydantoin
Actions: Prodrug that converts to phenytoin after administration. Thought to act on motor cortex, stabilizes seizure threshold, antidysrhythmic properties, also has antidysrhythmic properties beneficial for ventricular dsyrhythmias with QT prolongation
Indications: Grand mal, complex seizure activity
Contraindications: Allergy to phenytoin or hydantoin products, hypoglycemic seizures, bradycardia, heart blocks, sick sinus syndrome
Side effects: Ataxia, slurred speech, confusion, CNS depression, nystagmus, hypotension with rapid administration, gingival hyperplasia with prolonged use, tissue necrosis with extravasation
Dose: 15–20 mg PE/kg IV (PE = phenytoin equivalents) followed by a maintenance dose of 4–6 mg PE/kg slow IVP
Special considerations: Use with caution on patients with impaired hepatic, renal, or pulmonary function. Do not administer faster than 100–150 mg PE/min. Keep refrigerated prior to administration

---

MANNITOL (Osmitrol)

Classification: Electrolyte/water balance agents, osmotic diuretic
Actions: Hyperosmolar agent. Draws interstitial fluid into the intravascular space, increasing GFR, and decreases reabsorption of sodium, thus promoting water loss
Indications: Increased ICP
Contraindications: Hypotension, dehydration, acute pulmonary edema, anuria, known allergy
Side effects: Hypotension, dehydration, acidosis, electrolyte imbalances
Dose: 1.5–2 gm/kg IVP over 30–60 minutes
Special considerations: Use cautiously in patients with blood loss, hypotension, or dehydration. Monitor urinary output closely, be alert for transient hypertension, and use with caution in patients with poor left ventricular function or renal disease

PHENOBARBITAL SODIUM

FOSPHENYTOIN SODIUM

MANNITOL

METHYLPREDNISOLONE (Solu-Medrol, Medrol)

Classification: Hormone and synthetic substitute, corticosteroid, glucocorticoid, antiinflammatory
Actions: Antiinflammatory agent with immunosuppressive properties
Indications: Chronic and acute inflammation, swelling, bronchospasm, spinal cord injury
Contraindications: Suspected fungal infections, known hypersensitivity
Side effects: Edema, hypokalemia, hypotension, hypertension, hyperglycemia, CHF, delayed wound healing
Dose: *Spinal cord injury:* 30 mg/kg IV over 10–20 minutes, followed with a maintenance infusion 5.4 mg/kg/hr for next 23 hours. *Bronchospasm:* 40–125 mg IV over 2 minutes
Special considerations: Use with caution in patients with Cushing's syndrome, GI ulcerations, diabetes, or psychotic tendencies. Monitor for hyperglycemia in the non-diabetic patient

DEXAMETHASONE (Decadron, Hexadryl, Dexasone)

Classification: Hormone and synthetic substitute, corticosteroid, glucocorticoid
Actions: Potent antiinflammatory properties, crosses blood-brain barrier, giving it a role in managing increased ICP
Indications: Adrenal insufficiency, inflammatory conditions, allergic states, collagen diseases, hematologic disorders, Addisonian shock, neoplasm, rheumatic disorders, inflammatory GI diseases
Contraindications: Known allergy to the drug, systemic fungal infections, tuberculosis, varicella
Side effects: Edema, hypokalemia, hypotension, hypertension, hyperglycemia, CHF, delayed wound healing
Dose: *Adult:* 1–2 mg/kg followed by a maintenance infusion 1–1.5 mg/kg tapered dose over 4–6 hours. *Pediatric:* 0.5–1 mg/kg
Special considerations: Risk of CHF. Use cautiously in patients with hepatic and renal disease, GI ulceration, diabetes, seizure disorders, psychiatric disorders

NIMODIPINE (Nimotop)

Classification: Cardiovascular agent, calcium channel blocker
Actions: Calcium channel blocker, promotes smooth muscle relaxation. Preferentially binds to cerebral arteries, resulting in cerebral vasodilation
Indications: Vasospasm associated with SAH
Contraindications: Lactation
Side effects: Hypotension, tachycardia, ECG abnormalities, GI bleeding, peripheral edema
Dose: 60 mg PO or NG every 4 hours administered within 96 hours of subarachnoid hemorrhage, continued for 21 consecutive days
Special considerations: Caution when administered with other calcium channel blockers

METHYLPREDNISOLONE

DEXAMETHASONE

NIMODIPINE

ALBUTEROL (Proventil, Ventolin)

Classification: Sympathomimetic, beta-adrenergic agonist, bronchodilator
Actions: Beta-2 agonist with slight degree of beta-1 and alpha properties. Result in bronchodilation. Promotes insulin release, making it useful in treatment of hyperkalemia
Indications: Bronchospasm, hyperkalemia
Contraindications: Tachycardia, cardiac dysrhythmia, hypertension
Side effects: Tachycardia, hypertension, cardiac dysrhythmia, anxiety, palpitations, nausea/vomiting, dilated pupils
Dose: *Adult:* 2.5 mg in 3–5 mL of saline nebulized. *Pediatric:* 1.25 mg in 3–5 mL saline nebulized
Special considerations: Requires adequate tidal volume to distribute medication to distal airways

IPRATROPIUM BROMIDE (Atrovent)

Classification: Sympathomimetic, anticholinergic, bronchodilator
Actions: Blocks acetylcholine receptors on bronchial smooth muscle, resulting in a decrease of intracellular cyclic-GAMP and bronchodilation
Indications: Bronchoconstriction
Contraindications: Hypersensitivity. Not to be used as first-line agent for bronchoconstriction
Side effects: Tachycardia, dry mouth, palpitations, nervousness, headache
Dose: *Adult:* 500 mcg nebulized. *Pediatric:* 125–250 mcg nebulized
Special considerations: Often administered concurrently with albuterol

LEVALBUTEROL HYDROCHLORIDE (Xopenex)

Classification: Sympathomimetic, beta-adrenergic agonist, bronchodilator
Actions: Chemically related to albuterol with a higher specificity for beta-2 receptors and longer duration of action. Encourages bronchodilation, facilitates mucus drainage, and increases vital capacity
Indications: Bronchospasm
Contraindications: Hypersensitivity to levalbuterol or albuterol, age < 6 years, pregnancy
Side effects: Nervousness, palpitations, dry mouth, headache, tachycardia
Dose: *Adult:* 0.63–1.25 mg via nebulizer q 6–8 hours. *Pediatric:* 0.31–0.63 mg via nebulizer q 6–8 hours
Special considerations: Use with caution in patients with CVD, CAD, dysrhythmias, convulsive disorders, hyperthyroidism, and diabetes. Adequate tidal volume necessary to distribute medication to distal airways

ALBUTEROL

IPRATROPIUM BROMIDE

LEVALBUTEROL HYDROCHLORIDE

TERBUTALINE (Brethaire, Brethine, Bricanyl)

Classification: Sympathomimetic, beta-adrenergic agonist, bronchodilator
Actions: Beta-2 adrenergic receptor stimulant, results in bronchodilation, relaxation of peripheral vasculature, uterine muscle relaxation
Indications: Bronchospasm, preterm labor
Contraindications: Known hypersensitivity, severe hypertension, CAD, lactation, concurrent digitalis toxicity
Side effects: Tachycardia, hypertension, nervousness, palpitations, nausea/vomiting
Dose: *Adult:* 0.25 mg SQ, repeat q 15 minutes to a max dose 0.5 mg in 4 hours
  Pediatric: 0.005–0.01 mg/kg SQ repeat if necessary q 15–20 min to a max dose 0.4 mg
Special considerations: Monitor vital signs and cardiac monitor

HYDROCORTISONE SODIUM (A-Hydrocort, Solu-Cortef)

Classification: Skin and mucous membrane agent, antiinflammatory, hormone and synthetic substitute, corticosteroid, glucocorticoid, mineral corticoid
Actions: Short-acting synthetic steroid with immunosuppressant and antiinflammatory properties
Indications: Chronic restrictive airway disease
Contraindications: Idiopathic thrombocytopenic purpura, psychosis, Cushing's syndrome, acute hepatic dysfunction, age < 2 years
Side effects: Hypertension, hyperglycemia, flushing, tachycardia, anaphylactoid reactions, weight gain, mental disturbance, thrombocytopenia, muscle wasting
Dose: *Adult:* 100 mg IV q 6 hours. *Pediatric:* 1–2 mg/kg IV
Special considerations: Use with caution in patients with diabetes, hepatitis, convulsive disorders, hypothyroidism, gastritis, CHF, hypertension, renal insufficiency

SUCCINYLCHOLINE CHLORIDE (Anectine, Quelicin, Sucostrin)

Classification: Sympathomimetic, skeletal muscle relaxant: depolarizing
Actions: Blocks cholinergic receptors on motor endplate, produces depolarization and fasciculations. Subsequent nerve impulse transmission inhibited. Rapid onset, short acting
Indications: RSI
Contraindications: Personal or familial history of malignant hyperthermia, skeletal muscle myopathies. Use with caution in pediatric patients, patients with burns, and patients at risk for hyperkalemia
Side effects: Respiratory paralysis, malignant hyperthermia, muscular fasciculations, rhabdomyolysis. Increased intracranial, intragastric, and intraoccular pressure
Dose: *Adult:* 1–1.5 mg/kg IV. *Pediatric:* 1–2 mg/kg IV
Special considerations: Be prepared for endotracheal intubation immediately after administration of drug; if intubation unsuccessful, ventilatory assistance required. Eye care to prevent desiccation or abrasions. Shelf life of 30 days after removal from refrigeration

TERBUTALINE

HYDROCORTISONE SODIUM

SUCCINYLCHOLINE CHLORIDE

VECURONIUM (Norcuron)

Classification: Sympathomimetic, skeletal muscle relaxant: nondepolarizing
Actions: Blocks cholinergic receptors on motor endplate. Does not result in muscle depolarization, so fasciculations occur. Subsequent nerve impulse transmission inhibited
Indications: RSI, long-term paralysis after RSI
Contraindications: Known hypersensitivity
Side effects: Respiratory paralysis, malignant hyperthermia, rhabdomyolysis. Increased intracranial, intragastric, and intraoccular pressure. No fasciculations
Dose: *Defasciculating dose:* 0.1 mg/kg IV. *Adult paralyzing dose:* 0.08–0.10 mg/kg IV repeat q 1–2 hours. *Pediatric paralyzing dose:* 0.1 mg/kg IV repeat q 1–2 hours
Special considerations: Consider use of sedative or analgesic to decrease cardiovascular side effects. Be prepared for endotracheal intubation immediately after administration of drug. If intubation unsuccessful, ventilatory assistance required. Eye care to prevent desiccation, abrasions

PANCURONIUM BROMIDE (Pavulon)

Classification: Sympathomimetic, skeletal muscle relaxant: nondepolarizing
Actions: Blocks cholinergic receptors on motor endplate, does not result in muscle depolarization so no fasciculations occur. Subsequent nerve impulse transmission inhibited. Compared to other NMBAs, produces little histamine release resulting in less bronchospasm and hypotension
Indications: RSI, long-term paralysis after RSI
Contraindications: Known hypersensitivity
Side effects: Respiratory paralysis, malignant hyperthermia, rhabdomyolysis. Increased intracranial, intragastric, and intraocular pressure. No fasciculations. Tachycardia and ventricular ectopy
Dose: *Adult:* 0.04–0.10 mg/kg IV. *Pediatric:* 0.04–0.1 mg/kg IV
Special considerations: Consider use of sedative or analgesic to decrease cardiovascular side effects. Be prepared for endotracheal intubation immediately after administration of drug. If intubation unsuccessful, ventilatory assistance required. Eye care to prevent desiccation, abrasions

ROCURONIUM BROMIDE (Zemuron)

Classification: Sympathomimetic, skeletal muscle relaxant: nondepolarizing
Actions: Blocks cholinergic receptors on motor endplate, does not result in muscle depolarization, no fasciculations observed. Subsequent nerve impulse transmission inhibited
Indications: RSI, long-term paralysis after RSI
Contraindications: Known hypersensitivity
Side effects: Respiratory paralysis, malignant hyperthermia, rhabdomyolysis. Increased intracranial, intragastric, and intraoccular pressure. No fasciculations
Dose: *Adult:* RSI 0.6 mg/kg IV. Maintenance paralyzation 0.1–0.2 mg/kg IV q 1–2 hours or continuous infusion 0.01–0.012 mg/kg/min IV. *Pediatric (> 2 years):* 0.6 mg/kg IV
Special considerations: Consider use of sedative or analgesic to decrease cardiovascular side effects. Be prepared for endotracheal intubation immediately after administration of drug. If intubation unsuccessful, ventilatory assistance required. Eye care to prevent desiccation, abrasions

VECURONIUM

PANCURONIUM BROMIDE

ROCURONIUM BROMIDE

CISATRACURIUM BESYLATE (Nimbex)

Classification: Sympathomimetic, skeletal muscle relaxant: nondepolarizing
Actions: Blocks cholinergic receptors on motor endplate, does not result in muscle depolarization, no fasciculations observed. Subsequent nerve impulse transmission inhibited. Intermediate onset and duration compared to other NMBAs
Indications: RSI, long-term paralysis after RSI
Contraindications: Known hypersensitivity
Side effects: Respiratory paralysis, malignant hyperthermia, rhabdomyolysis. Increased intracranial, intragastric, and intraocular pressure. No fasciculations. Bradycardia, hypotension, flushing, bronchospasm
Dose: *Adult:* 0.15 mg/kg to 0.20 mg/kg IV followed by a maintenance infusion 1–3 mcg/kg/min to maintain paralysis. *Pediatric:* 0.1 mg/kg followed by 1–2 mcg/kg/min infusion to maintain paralysis
Special considerations: Use with caution in patients with electrolyte abnormalities, burns, neuromuscular disease, advanced age, decreased renal function, pregnancy

©2007 Pearson Education, Inc.

HYDROMORPHONE HYDROCHLORIDE (Dilaudid, Dilaudid-HP)

Classification: CNS agent, narcotic agonist
Actions: Semisynthetic derivative structurally similar to morphine, occupies opiate receptors. Compared to morphine, it has 8–10 times more potent analgesic effect, a more rapid onset, a shorter duration of action, a less hypnotic action, and a lower tendency to produce nausea/vomiting
Indications: Pain
Contraindications: Known hypersensitivity to hydromorphone, intolerance to opiate agonists, lactation
Side effects: Respiratory depression, hypotension, bradycardia/reflex tachycardia, nausea/vomiting, constipation, euphoria, vertigo, sedation, drowsiness
Dose: *Adult:* 1–4 mg IV, repeat as needed. *Pediatric:* 0.015 mg/kg, repeat as needed
Special considerations: Naloxone as antidote for OD

©2007 Pearson Education, Inc.

MORPHINE SULFATE (Duramorph, MS Contin)

Classification: CNS agent, narcotic agonist
Actions: Naturally occurring derivative of opium poppy. Binds with opiate receptors, produces mild vasodilation resulting in decreased preload, afterload, and myocardial oxygen demand
Indications: Pain, CHF
Contraindications: Allergy to opiates, decreased level of consciousness, hypotension, increased intracranial pressure, respiratory depression, convulsive disorder, ingested poisoning
Side effects: Respiratory depression, hypotension, localized allergic reaction with intravenous administration, nausea/vomiting, constipation, addiction with long-term use
Dose: *Adult:* 2–10 mg IV over 1–2 minutes, repeat as needed. *Pediatric:* 0.05–0.1 mg/kg IV, repeat as needed to max dose 15 mg
Special considerations: Be prepared to assist with ventilations or tracheal intubation if respiratory depression occurs. Action potentiated when used in combination with sedatives, hypnotics, or barbiturates. Naloxone as antidote for OD

©2007 Pearson Education, Inc.

CISATRACURIUM BESYLATE

HYDROMORPHONE HYDROCHLORIDE

MORPHINE SULFATE

MEPERIDINE HYDROCHLORIDE (Demerol)

Classification: CNS agent, narcotic agonist, analgesic
Actions: Synthetic opiate, acts as opiate receptor, analgesic effects mirror those of morphine at all dose ranges
Indications: Pain
Contraindications: Known hypersensitivity, seizure disorder
Side effects: Similar to morphine
Dose: *Adult:* 25–100 mg IV over 1–2 minutes, repeat as needed. *Pediatric:* 0.5–1.0 mg IV over 1–2 minutes, repeat as needed
Special considerations: Naloxone as antidote for OD

FENTANYL CITRATE (Sublimaze, Duragesic)

Classification: CNS agent, narcotic agonist, analgesic
Actions: Opioid analgesic, acts at opiate receptors, 10X more potent than morphine, shorter duration of action
Indications: Pain, RSI, sedation
Contraindications: Similar to morphine, patient receiving MAOI within previous 14 days, myasthenia gravis, active labor and delivery
Side effects: Similar to morphine, vertigo, delirium, euphoria, bradycardia, hypotension
Dose: *Adult:* 25–200 mcg IV over 1–2 minutes. *Pediatric:* 1–2 mcg/kg IV over 1–2 minutes
Special considerations: Use with caution in patients with head injury, advanced age, COPD, bradydysrhythmia, severe pulmonary, renal, or hepatic disease

KETOROLAC TROMETHAMINE (Toradol, Acular)

Classification: CNS agent, NSAID, analgesic, antipyretic
Actions: Peripherally acting analgesic, inhibits prostaglandin synthesis
Indications: Moderate to severe pain
Contraindications: Active labor/delivery, evidence of NSAID reaction, nasal polyps, angioedema, bronchospasm, renal failure, bleeding risk, active peptic ulcer disease, concomitant use of other NSAIDs
Side effects: Drowsiness, vertigo, headache, GI distress, nausea/vomiting
Dose: *Adult:* 30 mg IV, repeat q 6 hours to max dose 120 mg. Consider lesser dose of 15 mg IV if age > 65 years, weight > 50 kg, renal failure/impairment. *Pediatric:* 0.5 mg/kg IV to max dose 15 mg
Special considerations: May increase lithium and methotrexate levels and toxicity

MEPERIDINE HYDROCHLORIDE

FENTANYL CITRATE

KETOROLAC TROMETHAMINE

NALBUPHINE HYDROCHLORIDE (Nubain)

Classification: CNS agent, analgesic, narcotic agonist-antagonist
Actions: Synthetic opioid, actions at opiate receptor similar to morphine
Indications: Moderate to severe pain. Need to slow labor
Contraindications: Avoid long-term use in pregnancy to avoid fetal dependence
Side effects: Respiratory depression, hypotension, localized allergic reaction with intravenous administration, nausea/vomiting, constipation, addiction with long-term use
Dose: *Adult:* 5–10 mg IV as needed. *Pediatric:* 0.1–0.15 mg/kg IV as needed
Special considerations: Be prepared to assist with ventilations or tracheal intubation if respiratory depression occurs. Action potentiated when used in combination with sedatives, hypnotics, or barbiturates. Naloxone as antidote for OD

MIDAZOLAM HYDROCHLORIDE (Versed)

Classification: CNS agent, benzodiazepine anticonvulsant, sedative-hypnotic
Actions: Acts at GABA receptors, increases receptor affinity to GABA resulting in sedation, skeletal muscle relaxation, and sleep, at high doses
Indications: Anxiety, need for sedation, RSI, combativeness
Contraindications: Hypotension, decreased level of consciousness, hypoperfusion, alcohol intoxication, narrow angle glaucoma
Side effects: Hypotension, tachy/bradycardia, respiratory depression, altered level of consciousness
Dose: *Adult:* 1–2.5 mg IV over 1–2 minutes. *Pediatric:* 0.05–0.2 mg/kg IV over 2–3 minutes
Special considerations: Flumazenil 0.2–1 mg IV for benzodiazepine OD. Effects potentiated with combination analgesic/sedative/hypnotic therapy. Be alert for respiratory depression

DIAZEPAM (Valium)

Classification: CNS agent, benzodiazepine anticonvulsant, anxiolytic
Actions: Benzodiazepine derivative. Acts at GABA receptors, increases receptor affinity to GABA resulting in sedation, skeletal muscle relaxation, and sleep, at high doses
Indications: Anxiety, need for sedation, RSI, combativeness, seizures
Contraindications: Hypersensitivity, respiratory or cardiovascular depression
Side effects: CNS, cardiovascular, respiratory depression
Dose: *Adult:* 2–10 mg slow IVP, repeat as needed. *Pediatric:* 0.5–2 mg slow IVP, repeat as needed
Special considerations: Diastat available for rectal administration, flumazenil as antidote for OD

NALBUPHINE HYDROCHLORIDE

MIDAZOLAM HYDROCHLORIDE

DIAZEPAM

LORAZEPAM (Ativan)

Classification: CNS agent, benzodiazepine, sedative-hypnotic, anxiolytic
Actions: Acts at GABA receptors, increases receptor affinity to GABA resulting in sedation, skeletal muscle relaxation, and sleep, at high doses. Most potent of benzodiazepines
Indications: Anxiety, need for sedation, RSI, combativeness
Contraindications: Hypersensitivity, respiratory or cardiovascular depression
Side effects: Respiratory and cardiovascular depression, altered level of consciousness
Dose: *Adult:* 0.5–2 mg slow IVP repeat as needed. *Pediatric:* 0.03–0.05 mg/kg slow IVP to max dose 4 mg
Special considerations: Similar to midazolam, flumazenil as antidote

---

PROPOFOL (Diprivan)

Classification: CNS agent, general anesthesia, sedative-hypnotic
Actions: Exact mechanism of action unknown, thought to slow limbic system impulses. Rapid onset/half-life
Indications: Need for sedation, painful procedures, endotracheal intubation, mechanical ventilation
Contraindications: Known hypersensitivity, allergy to eggs
Side effects: Hypotension, decreased level of consciousness, respiratory depression, bradycardia, tachycardia, pain at injection site, acalculous cholecystitis with prolonged use
Dose: *Adult:* 2–2.5 mg/kg IVP over 1 minute followed by a maintenance infusion 6–12 mg/kg/hr. *Pediatric (> 3 years):* 2.5–3.5 mg/kg IV over 1 minute followed by a maintenance 7.5–18 mg/kg/hr.
Special considerations: Consider use of analgesic with propofol administration. Discontinue infusion for assessment

---

ETOMIDATE (Amidate)

Classification: CNS agent, general anesthesia
Actions: Exact mechanism of action unknown, thought to slow limbic system impulses. Rapid onset/half-life
Indications: RSI, need for anesthesia
Contraindications: Known allergy, pregnancy, adrenocortical function suppression
Side effects: Respiratory depression, bronchospasm, bruxism, vascular irritation, muscle rigidity
Dose: 0.1–0.3 mg/kg IV over 1 minute
Special considerations: No analgesic effects, side effects exacerbated with rapid administration

LORAZEPAM

PROPOFOL

ETOMIDATE

NALOXONE HYDROCHLORIDE (Narcan)

Classification: CNS agent, narcotic antagonist
Actions: Analog of oxymorphone. Blocks opiate receptors without opiate effects
Indications: Opioid OD
Contraindications: Known hypersensitivity
Side effects: Hypertension, tachycardia, ventricular dysrhythmias, abrupt withdrawal symptoms in long-term narcotic users and abusers
Dose: *Adult:* 0.4–2 mg IVP, IM, SQ q 2–3 minutes to max dose 10 mg. *Pediatric:* 0.01 mg/kg IV, IM, SQ q 2–3 minutes to max dose 10 mg
Special considerations: Be prepared for rapid withdrawal symptoms including agitation, rhythm disturbance, pulmonary edema, cardiovascular collapse

FLUMAZENIL (Mazicon, Romazicon)

Classification: CNS agent, benzodiazepine antagonist
Actions: Blocks GABA receptors in brain
Indications: Benzodiazepine OD
Contraindications: Known hypersensitivity, seizure history
Side effects: Hot flashes, pain at injection site, agitation, breakthrough seizures, elevated CNS response, anxiety
Dose: *Adult:* 0.2 mg IV q 1 minute as needed to max dose 1 mg. *Pediatric:* 0.01 mg/kg IV to max dose 0.2 mg
Special considerations: Phenobarbitol for seizure control after Flumazenil use

CEFAZOLIN SODIUM (Ancef, Kefzol, Zolicef)

Classification: Antiinfective, antibiotic, cephalosporin, first-generation
Actions: Cephalosporin-type bactericidal with action against both gram-positive and gram-negative bacteria
Indications: Skin or soft-tissue injury
Contraindications: Known hypersensitivity
Side effects: Nausea/vomiting, diarrhea, Stevens-Johnson syndrome
Dose: *Adult:* 1 gm/50 mL IV over 15–30 minutes q 8 hours. *Pediatric:* 25 mg/kg IV administered in 3 doses over 15–30 minutes q 8 hours
Special considerations: Monitor for allergic reaction. Use cautiously with patients with penicillin allergy

NALOXONE HYDROCHLORIDE

FLUMAZENIL

CEFAZOLIN SODIUM

CEFTRIAXONE SODIUM (Rocephin)

Classification: Antiinfective, antibiotic, cephalosporin, first-generation
Actions: Broad-spectrum cephalosporin-type bactericidal with action against gram-positive, gram-negative, aerobic and anaerobic organisms. Crosses blood-brain barrier
Indications: Otitis media, septicemia, meningitis, postoperative infection, preoperative prophylaxis
Contraindications: Allergy to cephalosporin group of antibiotics
Side effects: Nausea/vomiting, diarrhea, leucopenia, pain at injection site
Dose: *Adult:* 1–2 gm/100 mL IV daily. *Pediatric:* 50–75 mg/kg IV daily
Special considerations: Monitor for allergic reaction, use cautiously with patients with penicillin allergy

IMIPENEM-CILASTATIN SODIUM (Primaxin)

Classification: Antiinfective, beta-lactam antibiotic
Actions: Broad-spectrum carbopenem-type antibiotic with action against gram-positive, gram-negative, aerobic and anaerobic organisms
Indications: Need for broad-spectrum protection
Contraindications: Allergy to imipenem and its additives, especially lidocaine
Side effects: Nausea/vomiting, diarrhea, leucopenia, pain at injection site
Dose: *Adult:* 250–500 mg/100 mL over 1 hour q 6–8 hours. *Pediatric:* 10–15 mg/kg q 6 hours
Special considerations: Monitor for allergic reaction. Use cautiously in patients with impaired renal function

VANCOMYCIN HYDROCHLORIDE (Vancocin)

Classification: Antiinfective, antibiotic
Actions: Antibiotic agent with action against gram-positive, gram-negative, aerobic and anaerobic organisms, including methicillin-resistant staphylococcus aureus (MRSA)
Indications: Need for broad-spectrum antibiotic protection
Contraindications: Known hypersensitivity
Side effects: Nephrotoxicity: pseudomembranous colitis, ototoxicity, neutropenia, drug fever, pain at injection site
Dose: *Adult:* 0.5 g–1 g IV over 1 hour q 12 hours. *Pediatric:* 10 mg/kg IV over 1 hour q 6 hours
Special considerations: Monitor for allergic reaction. Monitor IV site for irritation, infiltration

CEFTRIAXONE SODIUM

IMIPENEM-CILASTATIN SODIUM

VANCOMYCIN HYDROCHLORIDE

GENTAMICIN SULFATE (Garamycin)

Classification: Antiinfective, aminoglycoside
Actions: Aminoglycoside-type antibiotic with action against infections in the central nervous, respiratory, and gastrointestinal systems
Indications: Individual system or systemic bacturemia
Contraindications: Known hypersensitivity to aminoglycosides
Side effects: Nephrotoxicity, neurotoxicity, confusion, urticaria, drug fever, nausea/vomiting, joint pain
Dose: *Adult:* 1.5–2 mg/kg IV over 1–1.5 hours. *Pediatric:* 6–7.5 mg/kg/day total IV in divided doses q 8 hours
Special considerations: Monitor for allergic reaction. Monitor IV site for irritation or infiltration

---

CLINDAMYCIN HYDROCHLORIDE (Cleocin, Dalacin)

Classification: Antiinfective, antibiotic
Actions: Bactericidal agent with action against anaerobic bacteria such as enterococcus, staphylococcus, and streptococcus
Indications: Severe infection, septicemia
Contraindications: Allergy to clindamycin or lincomycin
Side effects: Colitis, diarrhea, metallic taste, rash
Dose: *Adult:* 300–900 mg/IV over 1 hour. *Pediatric:* 20–40 mg/kg/day IV over 1 hour
Special considerations: Monitor for allergic reactions. Discontinue infusion if GI symptoms occur

---

AMPICILLIN/SULBACTAM SODIUM (Unasyn)

Classification: Antiinfective, antibiotic, aminopenicillin
Actions: Penicillin-class antibiotic with action against many gram-positive, gram-negative, and anaerobic organisms. Sulbactam component aids in treatment of resistant strains
Indications: Respiratory, urinary tract, and postoperative infections
Contraindications: Allergy to Unasyn and penicillin group agents
Side effects: Diarrhea, abdominal distension, flatulence, rash, facial swelling, candidiasis, fatigue
Dose: *Adult:* 1.5–3 gram (ampicillin equivalent)/100 mL IV over 30 minutes q 6 hours.
   Pediatric: > 40 kg receives full adult dosage in 50–100 mL IV over 30 minutes
   Children < 40 kg receive 300 mg/kg/day in 50–100 mL IV over 30 minutes
Special considerations: Monitor for allergic reactions

GENTAMICIN SULFATE

CLINDAMYCIN HYDROCHLORIDE

AMPICILLIN/SULBACTAM SODIUM

FLUCONAZOLE (Diflucan)

Classification: Antiinfective, antibiotic, antifungal
Actions: Inhibits fungal cytochrome P-450 sterol C-14 alpha-demethylation, preventing fungal growth
Indications: Candidemia and disseminated candidiasis, fungal pneumonia, cryptococcal meningitis
Contraindications: Allergy to fluconazole, or azole class of antifungals
Side effects: Nausea, headache, skin rash, diarrhea, liver insult
Dose: *Adult:* 200–400 mg/100 mL IV over 1 hour, maintenance dose 100–200 mg/100 mL IV over 1 hour daily. *Pediatric:* 6–12 mg/kg/50 mL IV over 1 hour, maintenance dose 3–6 mg/kg/50 mL IV over 1 hour daily
Special considerations: Monitor for allergic reaction. Use cautiously in patients with renal impairment

FUROSEMIDE (Lasix)

Classification: Loop diuretic, electrolyte and water balance agents
Actions: Blocks sodium reabsorption in renal tubules resulting in diuresis
Indications: CHF, fluid volume overload, mild impairment of renal function
Contraindications: Known hypersensitivity, anuria, hypotension, dehydration
Side effects: Cramping, diarrhea, nausea/vomiting, tinnitus, vertigo, headache, leucopenia, anemia, urticaria, rash, hypokalemia, dehydration
Dose: 1 mg/kg IV over 1–2 minutes
Special considerations: Monitor serum electrolytes

BUMETANIDE (Bumex)

Classification: Loop diuretic, electrolyte and water balance agents
Actions: Blocks sodium reabsorption in renal tubules resulting in diuresis 40x greater than furosemide. Shorter half-life than furosemide
Indications: CHF, fluid volume overload, mild impairment of renal function
Contraindications: Known hypersensitivity, anuria, hypotension, dehydration
Side effects: Cramping, diarrhea, nausea/vomiting, tinnitus, vertigo, headache, leucopenia, anemia, urticaria, rash, hypokalemia, dehydration
Dose: *Adult:* 0.5–2 mg IV over 1–2 minutes, repeat 4–5 hour to max dose 10 mg/day
Pediatric: 0.015–0.1 mg/kg every 6–24 hours, max dose 10 mg/day
Special considerations: Monitor serum electrolytes

FLUCONAZOLE

FUROSEMIDE

BUMETANIDE

RANITIDINE HYDROCHLORIDE (Zantac)

Classification: Gastrointestinal agent, H_2-receptor antagonist
Actions: Potent H_2-receptor antagonist, inhibits basal gastric acid secretion
Indications: Ulcers, ulcer prophylaxis, GI bleeding
Contraindications: Allergy to ranitidine or its additives
Side effects: Cardiac dysrhythmia, nausea/vomiting, rash, reversible mental confusion in the elderly, constipation
Dose: *Adult:* 50 mg/50 mL IVP over 15–30 minutes every 6–8 hours. *Pediatric:* 2–4 mg/kg/day in divided doses
Special considerations: Use cautiously in the elderly and the critically ill, mental status changes. Use cautiously in patients with hepatic and renal impairment

CIMETIDINE (Tagamet)

Classification: Gastrointestinal agent, H_2-receptor antagonist
Actions: Potent H_2-receptor antagonist with some H_1 effects. Inhibits basal gastric acid secretion, and indirectly reduces pepsin secretion
Indications: Ulcers, ulcer prophylaxis, GI bleeding
Contraindications: Allergy to cimetidine or its additives
Side effects: Cardiac dysrhythmia, nausea/vomiting, rash, drowsiness and reversible mental confusion in the elderly, impotence
Dose: *Adult:* 300 mg/50 mL over 15–30 minutes q 6–8 hours. *Pediatric:* 20–40 mg/kg/day PO in divided doses
Special considerations: Use cautiously in the elderly and the critically ill. Monitor for mental status changes. Use cautiously in patients with renal impairment

FAMOTIDINE (Pepcid)

Classification: Gastrointestinal agent, H_2-receptor antagonist
Actions: Potent H_2-receptor antagonist, inhibits basal gastric acid secretion
Indications: Ulcers, ulcer prophylaxis, GI bleeding
Contraindications: Allergy to famotidine or its additives
Side effects: Cardiac dysrhythmia, nausea/vomiting, rash, reversible mental confusion in the elderly, increased BUN and serum creatinine
Dose: *Adult:* 10–20 mg/10 mL IV over at least 2 minutes every 12 hours. *Pediatric:* 0.5 mg/kg every 8–12 hours, max dose 40 mg/day
Special considerations: Use cautiously in the elderly and critically ill. Monitor for mental status changes. Use cautiously in patients with renal impairment

RANITIDINE HYDROCHLORIDE

CIMETIDINE

FAMOTIDINE

PROMETHAZINE HYDROCHLORIDE (Phenergan, Histantil, Phenazine, Phencen)

Classification: Gastrointestinal agent, antiemetic, antivertigo agent, phenothiazine
Actions: Phenothiazine derivative with antipsychotic, H_1 receptor, and vomiting center blocking properties. At low doses, relatively free of extrapyramidal effects
Indications: Nausea/vomiting, medication administration, disease pathology
Contraindications: Allergy to promethazine, stenosing peptic ulcer, comatose state, bladder neck obstruction, narrow angle glaucoma
Side effects: Extrapyramidal symptoms with high doses or rapid intravenous administration, torticollis, oculogyric crisis, tongue protrusion, convulsive seizures, altered mental status, CNS depression, respiratory depression, cardiovascular depression, urticaria, leucopenia, dry mouth
Dose: *Adult:* 12.5–25 mg slow IVP q 4–6 hours or 25–50 mg IM. *Pediatric:* 0.25–0.5 mg/kg slow IVP q 4–6 hours or 12.5–25 mg IM
Special considerations: Treat extrapyramidal side effects with diphenhydramine 12.5–25 mg IV as needed

PROCHLORPERAZINE (Compazine)

Classification: Psychotherapeutic agent, phenothiazine, gastrointestinal agent, antiemetic
Actions: Exerts antiemetic effect via depressant action on the chemoreceptor trigger zone for vomiting in CNS
Indications: Nausea/vomiting, psychotic disorders, anxiety
Contraindications: Comatose state, CNS depression
Side effects: Extrapyramidal symptoms with high doses or rapid intravenous administration, torticollis, oculogyric crisis, tongue protrusion, convulsive seizures, altered mental status, CNS depression, respiratory depression, cardiovascular depression, urticaria, leucopenia, dry mouth
Dose: 2.5–10 mg slow IVP over 1–2 minutes, repeat q 6–8 hours as needed to max dose 40 mg/day
Special considerations: Treat extrapyramidal side effects with diphenhydramine 12.5–25 mg IV as needed

ONDANSETRON HYDROCHLORIDE (Zofran)

Classification: Gastrointestinal agent, antiemetic, serotonin 5-HT3-receptor antagonist
Actions: Not fully understood. Selective 5-HT3-receptor antagonist acts peripherally on vagal nerve terminals and centrally in the chemoreceptor trigger zone
Indications: Nausea/vomiting, medication administration
Contraindications: Allergy to ondansetron or its additives
Side effects: Hypotension, tachycardia, constipation, elevated liver enzymes, CNS depression
Dose: *Adult:* 4 mg IV over 2–5 minutes q 4–6 hours. *Pediatric (≥ 2 years):* 0.1 mg/kg slow IVP q 4–6 hours
Special considerations: Use cautiously in elderly and patients with renal impairment

PROMETHAZINE HYDROCHLORIDE

PROCHLORPERAZINE

ONDANSETRON HYDROCHLORIDE

DROTRECOGIN ALFA (Xigris)

Classification: Immunomodulator, recombinant human activated protein C
Actions: Recombinant form of exogenous activated protein C. Antiinflammatory mediator exerts an antithrombotic effect by inhibiting factors Va and VIIIa
Indications: Severe sepsis
Contraindications: Active internal bleeding, hemorrhagic stroke within past 3 months, intracranial/ intraspinal surgery within 2 months, trauma with an increased risk of life-threatening bleeding, presence of an epidural catheter
Side effects: Bleeding
Dose: 24 mcg/kg/hr infusion for 96 hours
Special considerations: Discontinue immediately if hemorrhage is witnessed or suspected

DROTRECOGIN ALFA